Synopsis of PATHOLOGY

Synopsis of
PATHOLOGY

W. A. D. Anderson
M.A., M.D., F.A.C.P., F.C.A.P.

Professor of Pathology, University of Miami School of
Medicine, Coral Gables, Florida; Director of
Pathology Laboratories, Jackson Memorial Hospital,
Miami, Florida

Thomas M. Scotti
A.B., M.D.

Professor of Pathology, University of Miami School of
Medicine, Coral Gables, Florida; Attending Pathologist,
Jackson Memorial Hospital, Miami, Florida

With 408 illustrations and 3 color plates

Seventh edition

The C. V. Mosby Company

Saint Louis   1968

To our wives
and children

Pathology is that branch of natural science which treats of the causes and nature of disease, together with the anatomical and functional changes incident thereto; the practice of human pathology is that specialty in the practice of medicine which may contribute to the diagnosis, treatment, observation and understanding of the progress of disease or medical condition in the human subject by means of information obtained by morphologic, microscopic, chemical, microbiologic, serologic or any other type of laboratory examination made on the patient or on any material obtained from the human body.

—approved definition of the College of American Pathologists

Preface

The approach and fusion of many basic science and clinical aspects of medicine make it increasingly difficult to define the limits of subjects to be included in a short presentation of pathology. The dynamic advances of medical science, based on new knowledge and concepts in the diverse fields of cytology, cytochemistry, microbiology, genetics, and immunopathology, as well as on clinical observation and practice, require attention in our consideration of the nature and mechanism of disease processes.

The task of presenting pathology in a concise but comprehensive form seems no less important as the difficulty increases. In fulfilling this task, we have kept in view the original purpose of a compact and condensed volume, one that is neither an elementary manual nor a large complete textbook or reference work. As such the book has been, and we hope will continue to be, useful to students in courses of general and systemic pathology, to clinicians who must maintain familiarity with the foundation sciences of medical practice, and to others in medical and paramedical fields who need knowledge of disease processes.

All chapters have been revised to improve them or to add new knowledge. In some instances they have been completely rewritten. A new chapter has been included that deals with ultrastructural and cytochemical features of normal and injured cells, cytogenetics, and inheritance patterns. The rapid advances in the various medical sciences serve as the basis of many of the changes throughout the text. To accomplish the welding of the new and exciting with the older but no less fundamental facts of morphology and function, without overemphasis or neglect, has been our challenging objective.

We are grateful to many people who have assisted with this revision by suggestions or more direct assistance. Generations of medical students have helped to mold this book by their eager and usually constructive criticism. Several colleagues have rendered valuable assistance by critically reading various portions. Our thanks also to our invaluable patient secretaries and particularly to Miss Edna Mae Everitt, who was assisted by Mrs. Louise Rhodes and Mrs. Virginia Martinez.

W. A. D. Anderson
Thomas M. Scotti

Contents

Color plates

Chapter 1

The cell and its behavior

The basic concepts concerning cells are the following: (1) Cells are the fundamental morphologic and functional units of the body. (2) All tissues are composed of cells and products of cells. (3) All cells are derived from preexisting cells, i.e., *omnis cellula e cellula* (aphorism of Rudolph Virchow, 1859). Developments in cell biology have advanced at a rapid rate in recent years, largely because of the progress that has been made in instrumental analysis (including electron microscopy and x-ray diffraction techniques) and the integration of cytology with other fields of biologic research (e.g., genetics, physiology, and biochemistry). As a result, new fields of study have come into being: *submicroscopic morphology* (ultrastructure), *molecular biology, cytogenetics, cell physiology,* and *cytochemistry.*

STRUCTURE AND FUNCTION OF CELLS

Cells vary in size and shape, but they have a number of characteristics in common. Each cell consists of a mass of *cytoplasm* and a *nucleus.* Surrounding the cell is a very thin *plasma membrane,* composed chiefly of lipids and protein, through which the exchange of materials takes place between the cell and its environment. The limiting membrane may be simple and smooth, or it may be a complex structure adapted to special functions of cells. For example, the numerous minute folds (microvilli) in the plasma membrane of epithelial cells in the intestine, renal tubules, and bile canaliculi increase the effective absorptive or secretory surface. Permeability of the cell membrane, one of its major functions, includes not only the process of diffusion or "passive transport" (in relation to water and certain solutes) but also the mechanism of "active transport" (as in the exchange of ions), which involves energy originating in the cell's own metabolism. Some substances are brought into the cell by *pinocytosis* (Gr. *pinein,* to drink). In this process the plasma membrane encircles fluid droplets in the environment

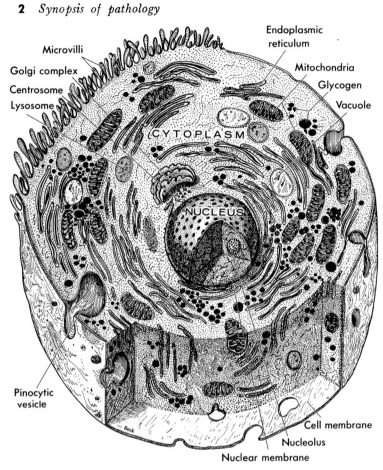

Microvilli

Golgi complex

Centrosome

Lysosome

Endoplasmic
reticulum

Mitochondria

Glycogen

Vacuole

CYTOPLASM

NUCLEUS

Pinocytic
vesicle

Cell membrane

Nucleolus

Nuclear membrane

Fig. 1-1. Diagram of a typical cell, based on electron microscopic appearances. (From Anthony, C. P.: Textbook of anatomy and physiology, ed. 7., St. Louis, 1967, The C. V. Mosby Co.).

(e.g., solutions of protein, glucose, hormones); it then invaginates into the cell and becomes pinched off, so that the fluids can be incorporated into the cytoplasm. For the induction of pinocytosis, certain substances other than water must be present in the environment, namely, certain amino acids, proteins, and salts. Carbohydrates and nucleic acid do not induce the process. Pinocytosis is somewhat like *phagocytosis* (Gr. *phagein,* to eat), a process whereby solid particles are ingested by a cell.

Outside the plasma membrane of some animal cells there is a cementlike substance, or *extraneous coat,* probably a sloughed-off by-product of the cell surface that is not essential for the integrity of the cell but apparently does play a significant role. The extraneous coat may have immunologic or filtration properties or may help in the maintenance of the microenvironment of the cell.

The plasma membrane connects with a membranous cytoplasmic network of tubules and vesicles, the *endoplasmic reticulum,* that courses throughout the cytoplasm to the nuclear membrane. Some of the cytoplasmic membranes are rough or granular *(ergastoplasm)* because of the attachment of dense granules to their outer surface. These granules, known as *ribosomes,* are present also in the cytoplasmic matrix outside the membrane system. They are composed of protein and ribonucleic acid (RNA) and serve as the centers for synthesis of proteins (including enzymes, the accelerators of chemical reactions within the cell). The ribosomes are responsible for the basophilic properties of cytoplasm. The rest of the endoplasmic reticulum is of the smooth-surfaced variety without a granular component.

The *Golgi complex,* or *body,* is generally considered to be a part of the agranular endoplasmic reticulum, although some investigators regard it as a separate membranous structure. The Golgi complex is apparently involved in the secretory activities of a cell, probably serving as a site where the products of secretion elaborated elsewhere in the cell are concentrated into granules or droplets prior to their liberation from the cell. The Golgi complex, in developing spermatids, participates in the formation of the *acrosome.*

Lysosomes are intracytoplasmic dense particles or vesicles, each surrounded by a single membrane, which contain hydrolytic enzymes and have a high content of acid phosphatase. There is a close relationship between the lysosomes and the Golgi complex. It is believed that the hydrolytic enzymes of the lysosomes influence phagocytosis and pinocytosis; it is also believed that they assist in the digestion of parts of the cell's own cytoplasm during starvation or in digestion of the cell after its death (autolysis). It is possible that cells may release lysosomal enzymes to produce lytic effects upon surrounding structures, as in the removal of bone by osteoclasts.

Mitochondria are granular, rodlike, or filamentous cytoplasmic organelles. Each mitochondrion is limited by a double (outer and

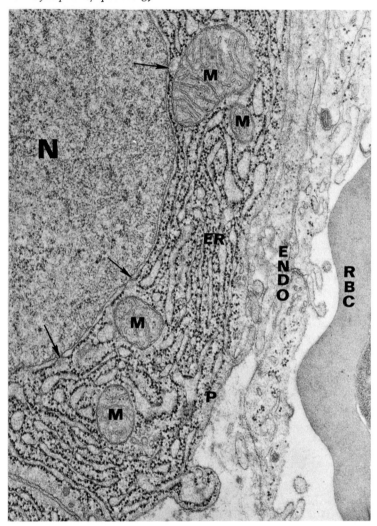

Fig. 1-2. Electron micrograph of the pancreatic acinar cell showing nucleus, cytoplasmic organelles, and adjacent capillary. The nucleus (**N**) is surrounded by a double-layered nuclear membrane with pores (arrows); the endoplasmic reticulum (**ER**) is of the rough type (with attachment of ribosomes); the mitochondria (**M**) vary in size and show characteristic internal membranes (cristae); next to the edge of the cell (**P**) are the capillary endothelium (**ENDO**) and a red blood cell (**RBC**) in the capillary lumen. (×52,500.) (Courtesy Dr. Douglas R. Anderson.)

inner) membrane. The inner membrane forms a series of complex infoldings (crests or cristae), which project into the mitochondrial cavity and are responsible for the characteristic striated appearance of the organelles. The mitochondria are the main "power plants" of the cell that supply the energy for its metabolic functions, the generation of energy being provided by the various intramitochondrial enzyme systems. The mitochondria are one of the major sources of adenosine triphosphate (ATP) in the cell. The mitochondrial membrane seems to be selectively permeable, so that the mitochondria swell or shrink as a result of chemical or osmotic changes in the cytoplasmic medium.

The *centrosome,* within which are two small granules called the *centrioles,* usually occupies the geometric center of the cell near the nucleus and is in close relationship to the Golgi complex. During cell division, two pairs of centrioles and surrounding astral rays appear; the pairs separate and become situated at the poles of the mitotic spindle. After mitosis each daughter cell receives two centrioles.

The *cytoplasmic matrix,* in which are embedded the various organelles, just mentioned, is a clear homogeneous substance with colloidal properties, such as those related to sol-gel transformations, viscosity changes, ameboid movements, spindle formation, and cell cleavage. In certain specialized cells the cytoplasmic matrix is the site of differentiation of fibrillar structures (e.g., keratin fibers, myofibrils, neurotubules). Much of the cytoplasmic matrix consists of water that contains electrolytes, soluble proteins and enzymes, lipids, carbohydrates, and soluble (transfer) RNA. Visible particles in the cytoplasm, other than the organelles, are called *inclusions* and comprise such structures as secretion granules, stored substances (lipids, glycogen), and various pigments.

The *nucleus* is the most conspicuous structure in a cell. It is present in all cells, although in the late stages of development of the human erythrocyte the nucleus disappears. The size and shape of the nucleus varies in different cells; generally, it is spherical or ovoid, but it may be indented or lobulated. Usually a single nucleus is present, but a few cells are binucleated (e.g., some plasma cells) or multinucleated (e.g., osteoclasts). The position of the nucleus in the cell is variable, being centrally or eccentrically located. As a rule, its position is constant for a given type of cell.

The nucleus serves as the control and regulating center of

most of the cell's activities and plays a fundamental role in cell division and heredity. The nucleus of a living cell is not clearly visible microscopically unless phase contrast microscopy is used, by which technique only the nuclear membrane and one or two nucleoli are observed in the interphase (nondividing) stage. The details of nuclear structure are best seen in fixed cells by means of routine staining procedures, by histochemical techniques, and especially by electron microscopy. The basic constituents are a *nuclear membrane,* filaments and granules of *chromatin* (considered to be the interphase form of chromosomes), one or more *nucleoli,* and the *nucleoplasm,* or *nuclear sap.* The latter, like the cytoplasm, is of a colloidal nature, being composed of water, electrolytes, protein (including enzymes), lipids, and carbohydrates. The most important chemical constituent in the nucleus is nucleic acid, of which there are two types: deoxyribonucleic acid (DNA) and ribonucleic acid (RNA). DNA is the more abundant, being present mainly in the chromatin. RNA is concentrated mostly in the nucleolus in the form of loosely bound, ribosome-like granules and also is found in small amounts in the chromatin. DNA, the essential component of genetic material, controls or directs protein synthesis within a cell, while RNA is concerned with the actual synthesis of protein.

In a high percentage of cells in females, but rarely in cells of males, a prominent mass of chromatin is found next to the nuclear membrane in interphase nuclei. This structure, known as the *sex chromatin* or *Barr body,* is present in persons with two or more X chromosomes; in fact, more than one Barr body may be present (the number of bodies is usually one less than the number of X chromosomes). By electron microscopy the *nuclear membrane* is seen to consist of two porous layers with a clear space between them. There appears to be a direct connection between the outer layer of the membrane and the endoplasmic reticulum. It is possible, therefore, that certain substances formed in the nucleus pass into the cytoplasm by means of this communication.

CELLULAR INJURY

The newer techniques of investigating cells (especially electron microscopy, ultracentrifugation, and cytochemistry) have increased our knowledge of the changes in the various cellular degenerations and infiltrations and in cell death. The details of these retrograde changes will be described in a later chapter.

Alterations in the specific components or organelles of a cell may be readily seen in the early stages of the development of these pathologic processes. It is generally believed that damage begins in and around the mitochondria. Structural, cytochemical, and biochemical alterations have been demonstrated in cells injured by various agents. Among the early changes that have been described are the following: shrunken, dense mitochondria; vesicular distention of the ergastoplasm; depletion of RNA granules with loss of cell basophilia; decrease in cytoplasmic glycogen; and a reduction or loss of enzymes such as adenosine triphosphatase (ATP-ase) and succino-dehydrogenase. These changes are followed by a swelling of the mitochondria with clearness of their matrix, the formation of large vesicles from the swollen endoplasmic reticulum, and the formation of lipid droplets in the vesicles and in the cytoplasmic matrix. As a result of the damage to the mitochondria and the subsequent interruption of the energy mechanisms within them, certain functional derangements may occur in the cell, including alterations in the "active transport" mechanism and cell membrane permeability (with changes in water and electrolyte content) and disturbances in the metabolism of carbohydrate, fat, and protein. Thus may be explained, at least in part, such pathologic processes as *cloudy swelling, hydropic degeneration, hyaline degeneration,* and *fatty metamorphosis.*

When cells in a living body are exposed to noxious agents, the damage may be serious enough to result in death of the cells. After cell death certain intracellular and extracellular enzymes cause nuclear and cytoplasmic changes that are visible in the light microscope. These structural alterations, which represent the histologic criteria of the process known as *necrosis,* are evident mainly in the nucleus (i.e., pyknosis, karyorrhexis, and karyolysis); but cytoplasmic changes such as coagulation of proteins, cytolysis, and contraction of cells may also be seen. In a normal piece of tissue that has been killed instantly by immersion in a fixative, the cell structure may remain apparently unaltered because of the sudden cessation of all enzymatic activity. Necrosis, which is a form of acute death of cells, is commonly differentiated from the process *necrobiosis.* The latter refers to the slow gradual death of cells that occurs as part of the constant turnover of cells in certain tissues (e.g., skin) after the cells have passed through a period of "senescence."

In contrast to the degenerative cellular changes, from which the cells may recover, the structural alterations in dead cells are irreversible. Although recognition of necrotic cells in the light microscope is based chiefly upon the prominent nuclear changes, submicroscopic morphologic alterations may be demonstrated in cytoplasmic organelles (particularly mitochondria and ergastoplasm), even before modifications in the nucleus become evident. Actually, the ultrastructural changes in dead cells are essentially an accentuation and progression of the early manifestations of cell injury described previously and include the following: severe swelling of the mitochondria with disappearance or disruption of the cristae and formation of dense particles or osmiophilic masses in the matrix; vesiculation, distortion, and fragmentation of mitochondrial membranes; breakdown of endoplasmic reticulum; clumping of nuclear chromatin; disruption and dissolution of the nucleolus; formation of intranuclear and intracytoplasmic blebs and vacuoles; focal cytoplasmic degradation, with fragments of cytoplasmic organelles in lysosomes (autophagic vacuoles); irregularity of nuclear and cytoplasmic membranes; and rupture and contraction of the cell.

THE CELL IN HEREDITY

Nuclear DNA is responsible for transmission of hereditary characteristics. The genetic information that is transmitted from generation to generation is coded in the DNA of the *genes,* the hereditary units of the chromosomes. The sequence of purine and pyrimidine bases in the DNA molecule forms the genetic code. Prior to cell division, DNA is able to replicate itself accurately so as to ensure the integrity of the genetic information during its transmission to future cells or generations. The DNA, through its genetic code, determines the biochemical processes of the cell by its control of protein synthesis. It dictates the specific sequence in which amino acids are incorporated into the polypeptides that combine to form structural proteins and enzymes. This information is transcribed to "messenger" RNA (formed in the nucleus upon a template or cast of DNA) and is carried by the RNA to the site of protein synthesis in the cytoplasm, the ribosomes.

The usually stable genetic and structural organization of chromosomes may be altered spontaneously, without apparent cause, or may be affected by injurious agents (e.g., ionizing radiation, chemicals, infections), thus leading to two types of chromosomal changes: (1) a change at the molecular level in the genetic material, occurring at definite points in the chromosome and usually involving individual gene loci without detectable microscopic alterations of the chromosomes (so-called *point mutation,* or *gene mutation*); and (2) *chromosomal aberrations,* recognizable microscopically and consisting of abnormalities of number or structure. The study of the microscopic appearance of chromosomes and their behavior during cell division is referred to as *cytogenetics.* The genetic makeup of an individual is called the *genotype,* and the expression of the genetic constitution (the physical, physiologic, and biochemical traits) is called the *phenotype.*

In point mutation there is a loss or change of function of a gene, caused by a defect in the DNA, which may lead to formation of an abnormal enzyme or other type of protein or may be responsible for lack of production of certain enzymes. Ex-

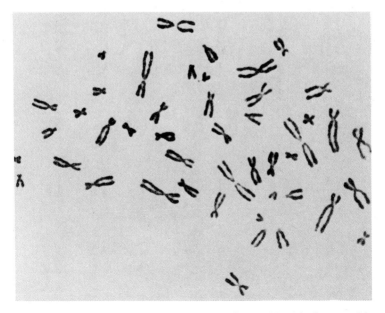

Fig. 1-3. Metaphase of a cultured, normal, female blood leukocyte with a diploid number of chromosomes (2n = 46). (From Sandberg, A. A.: CA 15:2-13, Jan.-Feb., 1965.)

amples of diseases characterized by such biochemical genetic disturbances are (1) the *hemoglobinopathies* (e.g., sickle cell disease), in which abnormal hemoglobins are produced by mutations in the genes controlling the formation of the globin portion of the hemoglobin molecule; and (2) *inborn errors of metabolism*, in which deficiency of a specific enzyme is evident (e.g., alcaptonuria, phenylketonuria, glycogen-storage diseases, galactosemia, cystinuria, homocystinuria, Wilson's hepatolenticular degeneration, and many others).

Chromosomal aberrations are characterized by alterations in number or in structure of chromosomes. It is to be remembered that normally each sex cell, or gamete, contributes 23 chromosomes to the fertilized ovum—22 autosomes and a Y or an X sex chromosome; the sperm contributes either a Y or an X

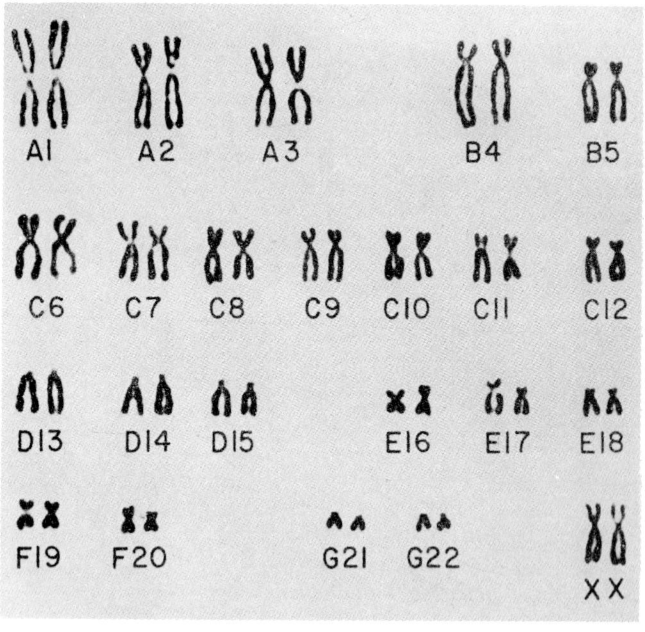

Fig. 1-4. Karyotype of metaphase shown in Fig. 1-3. The B5 chromosomes are somewhat shorter, relative to the B4 chromosomes, than usual. (From Sandberg, A. A.: CA 15:2-13, Jan.-Feb., 1965.)

chromosome and the ovum, only an X chromosome. Each cell of a normal person, except for the gametes, contains 46 chromosomes—22 pairs of homologous autosomes and a pair of sex chromosomes (XX in females, XY in males). Chromosomes are usually studied in cells that are grown in tissue cultures, either leukocytes obtained from the blood or cells derived from a small specimen of living tissue. The dividing cells are treated with colchicine, which halts them at the metaphase; then a hypotonic salt solution is added to cause swelling of the nuclei and separation of the chromatids while the centromeres are left intact. After the cells are fixed, placed on slides, stained, and examined microscopically, a photograph is made and enlarged in order to obtain more detail. Each chromosome is cut out of the picture, arranged in pairs, and classified into seven groups (A through G) on the basis of size of chromosomes and position of the centromere, and each pair of autosomal chromosomes is numbered in the order of decreasing size. The X chromosome (resembling those of the C6-12 group, especially chromosome 6) and the Y chromosome (similar to the G21-22 chromosomes) are not numbered. This systematic arrangement of the photographs of the chromosomes is referred to as the *karyotype*. (The word *idiogram* is sometimes used synonymously, but strictly this term is applied to a diagrammatic representation of a karyotype.) By means of a more recent technique, using a special computer, the time needed to process the chromosomes has been reduced considerably. The computer is programmed to count the number of chromosomes, measure their length, and recognize other morphologic features in an unenlarged photograph of chromosomes that have not been rearranged. Sandberg and co-workers have used successfully a "direct" fixation method of studying freshly aspirated bone marrow, which does not require culturing of cells or treatment with colchicine.

An abnormal number of chromosomes may result from *nondisjunction* in meiosis—a failure of the usual separation of two chromosomes of a pair, so that one daughter cell receives both and the other daughter cell receives neither chromosome of the pair. A gamete with an extra chromosome (24 chromosomes) fertilizing a normal gamete (23 chromosomes) results in a trisomic zygote. Such an abnormality is seen in *mongolism* (Down's syndrome), in which there is a *trisomy* of one of the autosomal chromosomes, number 21, with the result that there is a total of 47 chromosomes in that individual. Other congenital abnor-

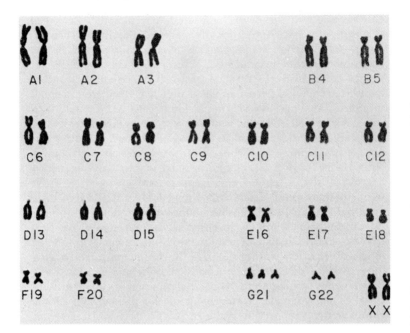

Fig. 1-5. Karyotype from a female patient with mongolism (Down's syndrome). Note the trisomy (extra chromosome) in Group G21. (From Sandberg, A. A.: CA **15**:2-13, Jan.-Feb., 1965.)

malities with trisomy of autosomal chromosomes have been described, e.g., trisomy of chromosome 18. When only one chromosome is present instead of the usual pair, the abnormality is referred to as a *monosomy*. In the monosomic state known as Turner's syndrome, only one sex chromosome exists, an X chromosome. Monosomes with only a Y chromosome are not known to occur.

In *Klinefelter's syndrome* (seminiferous tubule dysgenesis) there is a phenotypic male with small testes, frequently gynecomastia, and sometimes mental retardation. The cells usually have a Barr body (sex chromatin) in the nucleus and 47 chromosomes, including 22 pairs of autosomes and two X and one Y sex chromosomes. Some have 48 or 49 chromosomes with a sex chromosome composition of XXXY, XXYY, XXXXY, or XXXYY. Even *mosaicism* has been identified, i.e., the presence of cells in the same individual that differ in their chromosomal constitution, a defect that may arise during mitosis after fertilization, perhaps as a result of nondisjunction or complete loss of a chromosome in the early stages of growth of the zygote. For example, some cells may contain XY chromosomes, while others contain XXY chromosomes (expressed as XY/XXY); another mosaic type may be XY/XXXY.

A patient with *Turner's syndrome* (ovarian dysgenesis) is usually a phenotypic female with amenorrhea, hypoplastic ovaries or absence of ovarian tissue, which is replaced by fibrous tissue, and other physical abnormalities. The chromosomal number is usually 45, one less than normal, with 22 pairs of autosomes and a single X sex chromosome, expressed as XO. The nuclei of the cells are usually negative for Barr bodies (sex chromatin). Mosaicism also may be noted, e.g., XO/XY, XO/XX, XO/XXX, or XO/XYY.

Certain hereditary diseases are characterized by structural aberrations of the chromosomes: *deletion,* which is a loss of a portion of a chromosome; *duplication,* which is the presence of an extra piece of a chromosome; *inversion,* which is the fragmentation of a chromosome, followed by a rejoining of the fragments in such a way that they are inverted or reversed with respect to the rest of the chromosome; *translocation,* which is the transfer of a portion of one chromosome to a nonhomologous chromosome; and *isochromosomes,* which are abnormal chromosomes resulting from division of the centromere perpendicularly to the long axis of a chromosome, rather than parallel to it. Although mongolism is usually associated with an aberration in the number of chromosomes, as noted earlier (e.g., trisomy of chromosome 21), a few of the patients with this disease have translocation of an extra chromosome 21 onto another chromosome, e.g., number 15. The Philadelphia chromosome (Ph[1]) is an anomaly observed in the leukocytes of patients with chronic granulocytic leukemia. This is an abbreviated 21 autosome with its long arms substantially shortened, an example of deletion. In the forms of acute leukemia, aneuploidy (an abnormal number of chromosomes) has been demonstrated in bone marrow cells, particularly when prepared by the "direct" fixation technique. Chromosomal abnormalities, such as breakage with translocation or deletions, including an anomaly similar to the Philadelphia chromosome of leukemia, have recently been observed in patients who have been using LSD-25.

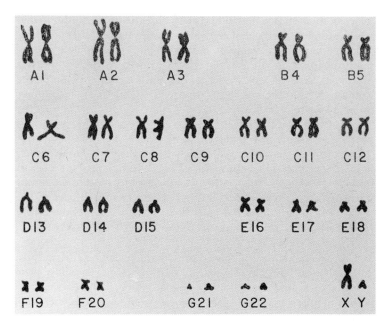

Fig. 1-6. Karyotype from a patient with chronic myelocytic leukemia. Note abbreviated G21 chromosome with long arms substantially shortened, the Philadelphia (Ph¹) chromosome. (From Sandberg A. A.: CA 15:2-13, Jan.-Feb., 1965.)

INHERITANCE PATTERNS

Inherited disorders resulting from mutant genes are known as *autosomal* or *sex-linked,* depending upon whether the affected genes are in the autosomes or in the sex chromosomes. A *dominant* disease is one that is clinically manifest in an individual who has only one mutant gene (a *heterozygous* state). A person with two abnormal dominant genes (a homozygous state) would be phenotypically similar to the heterozygote. However, since diseases related to dominant genes are so uncommon, it is extremely unlikely in practice to encounter such a homozygous individual, because the latter can result only from mating of two affected persons. A *recessive* disease is one that is apparent only in a *homozygous* subject; it is not evident in a heterozygote, but the latter is a carrier of the condition.

The patterns of hereditary transmission are classified according to the classic mendelian categories. A variety of patterns of inheritance have been observed, some simple, others complex. Those that are readily recognized are the simple patterns produced by rare genes at a single locus that include *autosomal dominant, autosomal recessive, sex-linked dominant,* and *sex-linked recessive.* In almost all of the sex-linked disorders the mutant gene is on the X chromosome, and this is the entity referred to when the term *sex-linked* is used without qualification. Well-substantiated examples of Y-linked traits are rare, occurring only in males.

Although the concepts of dominance and recessiveness are being presented here according to the simple hereditary patterns, it should be emphasized that some genes are neither strictly dominant nor strictly recessive. In one form of hereditary transmission, a harmful gene occurring alone in an individual (heterozygote) may produce a mild effect, but when there are two of the genes in the same person (homozygote), a greater degree of the abnormality may appear. This is referred to as *intermediate inheritance.* As an example, patients who are heterozygotes for an abnormal hemoglobin may have abnormal red cells but are asymptomatic (sickle cell trait), whereas those who are homozygous develop severe effects, including hemolytic anemia (e.g., sickle cell anemia). Other concepts such as *incomplete dominance, codominance, penetrance,* and *expressivity* are not considered in this chapter.

In the autosomal forms of inheritance, dominant or recessive, males and females tend to be equally affected. When dominant, the disorder is transmitted directly from affected person to affected person, appearing in every generation, as a rule, without skips or breaks in continuity. About half of the children of an affected parent will be affected. An autosomal recessive disease characteristically appears in siblings whose parents, offspring, and other relatives are usually phenotypically normal. The parents of an affected child are generally both heterozygous carriers. Typically, one out of four children of two heterozygous parents is affected (homozygous). An increase in the occurrence of the recessive condition occurs in consanguineous marriages because of the greater proportion of carriers marrying other carriers.

In sex-linked dominant states (when mating is between an affected and a normal person) the affected male transmits the disorder to all daughters, not to sons; the affected female who is heterozygous transmits it to half the offspring, male or female, and a homozygous female transmits it to all her children. In sex-linked recessive disorders the abnormality is expressed by all males who possess the mutant gene on the X chromosome, since it is not paired with a normal gene on the genetically inert Y chromosome. Males are neither heterozygous nor homozygous with reference to the X-linked gene, but are known as *hemizygous*. Females must be homozygous for expression of the trait. A heterozygous female appears normal but is a carrier of the mutant gene. An affected father (mating with a normal mother) does not transmit the disease directly to his sons; and the disease appears only in males after mating of a carrier female and a normal male. It is rare to see serious sex-linked recessive disorders (e.g., hemophilia) in females because mating of an affected male and a carrier female, which would be necessary, is an uncommon occurrence.

Examples of diseases inherited according to these four patterns are (1) *autosomal dominant:* Marfan's syndrome, Huntington's chorea, osteogenesis imperfecta, Milroy's disease, von Recklinghausen's neurofibromatosis, and familial intestinal polyposis; (2) *autosomal recessive:* galactosemia, phenylketonuria, alkaptonuria, fibrocystic disease of the pancreas, Wilson's disease, and Tay-Sachs disease (amaurotic family idiocy); (3) *sex-linked recessive:* hemophilia A; pseudohypertrophic muscular dystrophy (Duchenne type), congenital agammaglobulinemia, and glucose-6-phosphate dehydrogenase deficiency (e.g., favism); and (4) *sex-linked dominant:* vitamin D–resistant (hypophosphatemic) rickets.

Chromosomal aberrations generally do not show the familial tendencies as seen in the truly inherited disorders related to mutant genes. In many of the chromosomal anomalies, transmission to the next generation is not possible because of their tendency to produce severe abnormalities and sterility. There is some evidence that about one fifth of spontaneous abortions may be caused by chromosomal aberrations. In several family studies, one chromosomal disorder, mongolism, was observed to have been transmitted through subsequent generations, thus designated familial mongolism.

In addition to the diseases that are the direct result of mutant genes or chromosomal aberrations, there are certain disorders, such as hypertension, atherosclerosis, and some of the congenital malformations, that probably result from the interaction of genetic and environmental factors. It is difficult to assess the exact role that heredity plays in these diseases, but it is usually regarded as a predisposing factor. It is to be noted that the term *congenital,* meaning born with, is not synonymous with the term *hereditary.* A congenital disease may or may not be hereditary. Also, while many hereditary diseases are congenital, in the sense that manifestations are present at birth, in some of them the clinical features do not appear until later in life. A *familial disease* is one that tends to run in families or affects two or more siblings in a particular family, and it may be either genetic in origin or caused by environmental factors.

In certain hereditary disorders, clinical manifestation of the genetic defect may not be apparent unless some environmental influence supervenes. For example, persons with a deficiency in the activity of the enzyme glucose-6-phosphate dehydrogenase (G-6-PD) in the erythrocytes may show no ill effects and the affected red blood cells may not be associated with any decrease in life-span, unless the patient is exposed to certain chemical or other toxic agents. Drugs such as the antimalarial compound primaquine result in increased destruction of the genetically defective red cells, causing hemolytic anemia *(primaquine sensitivity).* Some patients who develop hemolytic anemia as a result of sensitivity to the fava bean or its pollen *(favism)* are known to have G-6-PD deficiency of the erythrocytes.

Chapter 2

Retrograde disturbances

Among the fundamental results of injury to tissues are the *retrograde cellular changes,* i.e., atrophy, degeneration, and necrosis (cell death). A wide variety of injurious agents, including bacterial and chemical poisons, trauma, radiant energy, heat, ischemia, and nutritional disturbances, cause such effects. Retrograde cellular changes may or may not be accompanied by an inflammatory reaction, depending on the degree of damage to the cells, and the rate at which cells die and set free toxic decomposition products. Closely related to the retrograde cellular changes are *infiltrations or depositions,* i.e., the abnormal accumulation of substances in tissues (within or between cells), e.g., adiposity (adipose tissue infiltration) and deposition of amyloid, urates, calcium, or pigments. The degenerative changes, as well as the infiltrations or depositions, are often looked upon as disturbances of metabolism of various substances, e.g., protein, fat, carbohydrate, mineral, or pigment.

ATROPHY

Atrophy is an acquired decrease in size of organs, or cells, which were once of normal proportions. This is to be distinguished from certain congenital abnormalities: *agenesia,* which denotes complete absence of an organ or tissue; *aplasia,* which indicates almost complete failure of development; and *hypoplasia,* which is a failure of full development.

Atrophy of an organ or tissue may be caused by a reduction in size or in number of component cells, or in both. When atrophy affects cells, the organ or tissue is usually, but not necessarily, reduced in size. Frequently the atrophied cells are replaced by connective tissue or fat, which helps to maintain the size of the organ. In certain atrophic parenchymal cells an accumulation of a granular yellowish brown pigment (lipofuscin) occurs, as in the heart, which causes a brown appearance of the organ grossly (brown atrophy). Function is disturbed by atrophy if the reserve capacity of the organ is encroached upon.

The general cause of atrophy is inadequate nutrition of the cells, which in turn results from a variety of causes. The disturbed cellular nutrition leads to a negative balance between the metabolic processes, anabolism and catabolism, resulting in a progressive breakdown of cellular constituents and decrease in cell mass. If the causative agent is removed, restoration of equilibrium between these processes with recovery of the cell may occur. Persistence of the disturbed equilibrium causes slow death of cells, thus accounting for the reduction in number of cells. In certain organs a normal, or *physiologic, atrophy* occurs at certain periods of life, as in the thymus at puberty and in the breast and uterus after the menopause.

Whether the atrophy that occurs in many organs and tissues in advanced age *(senile atrophy)* is physiologic or pathologic is a debatable point. During this period, endocrine changes bring about the atrophy of some tissues, e.g., the breasts. Lymphoid tissues, elastic tissues (as in the skin and blood vessels), bones (osteoporosis), and the nervous system all participate prominently. The possibility that ischemia resulting from arteriosclerosis contributes to atrophy in some of the tissues must be considered. *Pathologic atrophy* may be either general or local.

General atrophy. A major cause of general atrophy, involving widespread tissues and organs of the body, is starvation or inanition. The atrophy of starvation results from the using up of stored carbohydrate, fat, and eventually protein. It may be caused by lesions of the digestive tract, such as an obstructing tumor of the esophagus, or by loss of appetite without organic cause (anorexia nervosa), as well as by lack of essential foodstuffs. The central nervous system, bones, and muscles that are in active use participate less in the atrophy than do other tissues of the body. The basis for the generalized wasting (cachexia) of advanced cancer is not always certain, but in some instances it is a nutritive disturbance related to an inadequate food intake. Senile atrophy is a form of general atrophy, which, to a certain extent, may be physiologic; but the atrophy of some of the tissues or organs may, at least in part, be caused by pathologic influences, e.g., circulatory insufficiency brought about by arteriosclerosis.

Local atrophy. Local atrophy may be caused by disuse of a part, by ischemia, by pressure, by loss of endocrine stimulation, or by unknown causes.

Disuse atrophy. Forced inactivity of muscle soon results in decrease in size, the atrophy being particularly great when there is loss of motor nerve supply. It is not certain whether the interruption of the nerve supply leads to an absence of a "trophic" (nutritional) influence. Glandular organs forced to inactivity by occlusion of their ducts soon show atrophy of their functional cells. In the case of the pancreas, occlusion of the duct results in atrophy of the acinar tissue, while the endocrine islet tissue, the secretion of which goes directly into the bloodstream, remains relatively unaffected.

Ischemic atrophy. A slow, progressive narrowing of the arteries (as in atherosclerosis), in the absence of an adequate collateral circulation, may result in atrophy of an organ or tissue. A similar effect may be produced by pressure upon a vessel by an extrinsic tumor or other mass.

Pressure atrophy. Pressure atrophy is commonly the result of prolonged or continuous pressure upon a local area or group of cells. Pressure apparently affects cells by interfering with blood flow and tissue fluid circulation, thus preventing proper nutriment from reaching and being absorbed by the cells. Pressure exerted by a growing tumor causes such atrophy of the adjacent nontumor tissue. Amyloid deposited within tissue spaces brings about atrophy of the adjacent cells. The constant pulsating pressure of an aneurysm causes atrophy of any tissue, even bone, on which it impinges. Obstruction of a ureter with distention of the pelvis of the kidney (hydronephrosis) eventually leads to severe atrophy of renal tissue.

Endocrine atrophy. Endocrine atrophy occurs in organs that depend for their functional activity on endocrine stimulation, and it results whenever such stimulation decreases or ceases. Cessation of pituitary activity results in atrophic changes in the thyroid, adrenals, ovaries, and other organs that are influenced by pituitary hormones (Simmonds' disease, p. 668). Long-term administration of adrenal steroids may suppress the release of adrenocorticotropic hormone (ACTH) from the pituitary gland and lead to adrenal cortical atrophy. Prolonged hyperfunction of an endocrine gland (e.g., thyroid, islets of pancreas) may be followed by atrophy of the gland *(exhaustion atrophy)*.

Idiopathic atrophy. Idiopathic atrophy is a rare type of atrophy in which the cause has not yet been identified. Some investigators have attributed it to an unknown toxic influence, thus it is sometimes called "toxic atrophy." Some cases of Addison's disease (p. 706) have as their basis an idiopathic bilateral atrophy of the adrenal cortices; however, it has not been proved that this disease is not the result of adrenal cortical necrosis. The presence of circulating antibodies against adrenal tissue in some patients with Addison's disease has suggested the possible role of autoimmunity.

DEGENERATIONS AND CERTAIN INFILTRATIONS

A form of cellular injury is *degeneration,* characterized by a disturbance of intracellular metabolism, a swelling of the cell, and an accumulation in the cytoplasm of substances that normally are invisible, absent, or present only in small amounts. The degeneration is named—according to the nature of the abnormally accumulated material—albuminous (cloudy swelling), hydropic, fatty, hyaline, etc. These degenerative changes vary in severity and usually are reversible. However, severe degenerations may proceed to death of the cells.

Cloudy swelling (albuminous or parenchymatous degeneration). Most acute infections and toxic conditions are accompanied by some degree of cloudy swelling. It is the mildest and most common type of degeneration and is easily reversible. It is best seen in the liver and kidneys and sometimes in the heart. The name is descriptive of the gross appearance. The affected organ is swollen, so that the capsule is tense and the cut surface bulges. The tissue appears more opaque (cloudy) than normal, pale, and soft. Microscopically the affected cells are swollen and have a granular cytoplasm, the granules being of a protein or albuminous nature and caused, at least in part, by changes in the mitochondria. The ultrastructural and cytochemical alterations have already been described in Chapter 1 (see Cellular injury). The swelling of the cell mainly results from an increased water content of the cytoplasm, although increase in the water content of the organ as a whole may not be demonstrable. It has been postulated that the energy function of the damaged mitochondria is disturbed, leading to a diminished output of ATP. The decrease in ATP impairs cellular membrane permeability and the "active transport" mechanism of the cell, which normally maintain a low concentration of intracellular sodium. The result is an increase in sodium ion within the cell, followed by an increased water content. Generally the nucleus is unaffected in cloudy swelling, but in one investigation a decrease in DNA of the nucleus was detected. The RNA of the cell, as noted previously, may also be diminished after injury

Table 2-1. *Commonly used tissue stains*

Use	Stain	Comment
Routine histologic study	Hematoxylin and eosin	A good routine method; nuclei stain blue; cytoplasm, pink
Connective tissue (particularly collagen)	Azocarmine	Collagen and reticulum stain dark blue; valuable for study of renal glomerular basement membrane
	Mallory's aniline blue	Collagen stains blue
	Masson's trichrome	Collagen stains blue or green (See below for muscle)
	van Gieson's	Collagen stains red (See below for muscle)
Reticulum	Ammoniacal silver impregnation	Reticulum fibers stain black
	Periodic acid–Schiff (PAS)	Reticulum fibers stain rose to purple red; staining of collagen varies from pale to deep pink; valuable for demonstrating most basement membranes
Elastic tissue	Verhoeff's	Elastic fibers stain black
Muscle	Masson's trichrome	Muscle fibers stain red
	van Gieson's	Muscle fibers stain yellow
	Phosphotungstic acid hematoxylin	Striations in striated muscle fibers appear dark blue
Fibrin	Weigert's modified Gram stain	Fibrin stains violet
Amyloid	Congo red	Amyloid stains orange-red (ordinary light microscopy); green birefringence on polarization microscopy
	Methyl or crystal violet	Amyloid stains purple-red (metachromatic reaction)
	Thioflavine-T	Yellow fluorescence of amyloid in ultraviolet light
	Iodine	Amyloid stains mahogany brown
	Silver	Amyloid stains dark brown to black; used on frozen sections
Glycogen	Best's carmine	Glycogen stains red; fixation in alcohol-formalin or Carnoy's solution is recommended

Table 2-1. *Commonly used tissue stains*—cont'd

Use	Stain	Comment
Glycogen— cont'd	Periodic acid–Schiff before and after digestion with saliva or diastase	Glycogen stains purple-red with PAS; digestion removes glycogen, resulting in negative reaction with PAS
Mucin	Mayer's mucicarmine Also methods listed under Acid mucopolysaccharides	Mucin stains red (See below)
Acid mucopolysaccharides	Periodic acid–Schiff Toluidine blue or thionine Alcian blue	A purple-red reaction is positive Acid mucopolysaccharides stain metachromatically (purple-red) Acid mucopolysaccharides stain blue-green
Fat	Scharlach R (scarlet red) and Sudan III Osmic acid	Neutral fat and lipids stain orange to red; used on frozen sections; stains mineral oil Fat stains black; does not stain mineral oil
Bacteria	Giemsa stain Gram's stain for paraffin sections; Brown and Brenn stain; MacCallum-Goodpasture stain; and Glynn's method	Bacteria stain blue Gram-positive bacteria stain blue or blue-black, and gram-negative bacteria stain red with these methods
Acid-fast bacteria (tubercle bacilli, lepra bacilli, and others)	Ziehl-Neelsen stain Fite-Faraco oil fuchsin method	Acid-fast bacilli stain red Acid-fast bacilli stain red; valuable for demonstrating lepra bacilli
Spirochetes	Levaditi's method Warthin-Starry method	Spirochetes appear black; entire tissue block is stained before paraffin embedding Spirochetes appear black; paraffin sections are stained
Fungi	Periodic acid–Schiff	Mycelial fungi and yeasts stain purple-red

Continued on next page.

Table 2-1. *Commonly used tissue stains*—cont'd

Use	Stain	Comment
Fungi—cont'd	Gridley fungus stain	Hyphae are deep purple; conidia, rose to purple; yeast capsules, deep purple
	Methods for mucin in addition to periodic acid–Schiff (See above)	To demonstrate *Cryptococcus neoformans (Torula histolytica)* which produces abundant mucin
	Methenamine silver	Cell walls of fungi stain black
	Acridine orange fluorescent stain	Fungi stain red, yellow, yellow-green, or green when examined with blue light
Actinomyces	Mallory's Gram method	Mycelia stain blue; peripheral clubs stain red
Nocardia	Gram's stain	Organisms are gram-positive
	Ziehl-Neelsen stain	Some species of *Nocardia* are acid fast
Amebae	Iron hematoxylin stain	Nuclei stain black; cytoplasm, gray
Other tissue parasites	Azure-eosin methods	Generally, rickettsiae are blue; *Leishmania* and leishmanial forms of trypanosomes appear with deep blue kinetoplasts and lighter blue trophonuclei; toxoplasmata appear with blue-stained chromatin; and plasmodia with deep blue chromatin and lighter blue cytoplasm
Inclusion bodies	Schleifstein's method	For Negri bodies which stain magenta red
	Lendrum's phloxine-tartrazine method	Inclusion bodies stain red; recommended for oxyphilic inclusions, other than Negri bodies
Free iron	Perls' ferrocyanide reaction (Prussian-blue method)	Hemosiderin stains blue
Calcium	von Kóssa's silver method	Calcium appears black
Urates	de Galantha stain	Urates appear black
Argentaffin granules	Masson-Fontana silver method	Argentaffin granules (e.g., in carcinoids) stain black

Table 2-1. *Commonly used tissue stains*—cont'd

Use	Stain	Comment
Melanin	Masson-Fontana silver method	Melanin stains dark brown to black
	Dopa reaction (incubation in di-hydroxyphenyl-alanine solution)	Frozen sections required; melanoblasts stain black (dopa-positive); melanin maintains natural dark brown color
Nervous tissue	Bodian silver method	Nerve fibers and neurofibrils stain blue-black
	Weil-Weigert (Lillie's variant)	Myelin stains blue-black
	Cajal's gold-sublimate method	Must be fixed in formalin ammonium bromide; frozen sections required; proto-plasmic astrocytes appear black
	Mallory's phospho-tungstic acid–hematoxylin	Neuroglial fibrils stain blue
	Thionine	Nissl substance of nerve cells stains dark blue

to the cell. The parenchymal cells of the liver and convoluted tubular cells of the kidney show the change most severely. Fresh tissue is essential for recognition, as postmortem autolytic changes are confusing.

Hydropic degeneration. In cloudy swelling there is some imbibition of water into the cell, but in hydropic degeneration this is of greater degree. Hydropic degeneration is a more severe form of cellular injury than cloudy swelling, but it too is reversible. The cytoplasm is greatly swollen, pale, clear, and watery in appearance. When larger vacuoles appear, the term "vacuolar degeneration" is often used. The latter is a characteristic lesion affecting the renal tubular epithelium in potassium deficiency (p. 383).

Fatty metamorphosis. Fatty metamorphosis, or fatty change, is an abnormal accumulation of lipid *in parenchymal cells* of a tissue or organ where normally lipid is not demonstrable histologically. This process is to be differentiated from interstitial fatty infiltration, or adiposity, a condition characterized by the abnormal accumulation of adipose tissue in the stroma of parenchymatous organs (i.e., *between* parenchymal cells). Fatty metamorphosis is a disturbance of fat metabolism, but often the involved cells also exhibit an alteration of the intracellular proteins in the form of cloudy swelling or hydropic degeneration. Fatty change, although a more serious disturbance than the latter degenerative lesions, is generally reversible, but when severe, it may result in death of cells (necrosis). Functional impairment of affected organs sometimes occurs when the process is extensive. In preparations of ordinary paraffin sections the intracellular lipid is dissolved out, so that it appears as small or large vacuoles in the cytoplasm. Special staining procedures, including use of frozen sections, are available for demonstration of the lipid (Table 2-1).

Fatty metamorphosis is seen most frequently in parenchymatous organs, particularly liver, kidneys, and heart. The gross appearance of the affected organ depends upon the amount of fatty change. Little or no alteration is observed when there is only a slight degree of involvement. With a more severe degree of change the liver is enlarged, yellow, and decreased in consistency; the margins are rounded; the cut surface is greasy and bulges; and the lobular markings are obscured when the change is diffuse, but may be accentuated if the lipid is limited to a particular zone of the hepatic lobules (e.g., centrolobular regions). Microscopically, the vacuoles in the cytoplasm of the hepatic cells may be tiny and numerous or may be large, sometimes replacing the cell and pushing aside the nucleus. In some areas there may be rupture of the membranes of adjacent cells with confluence of large vacuoles, producing so-called "lipid cysts." It is said that these lipid cysts may rupture into sinusoids and release the lipid into the venous circulation as fat emboli.

The fatty kidney may be normal in size or slightly enlarged, and the cut surfaces are pale grayish brown or yellowish brown and soft or friable. Microscopically, small vacuoles are found mainly in the epithelial cells of the convoluted tubules, particularly the proximal.

In the heart, fatty change affects the myocardium and may be patchy or diffuse. In patchy involvement, such as occurs in severe anemias, the change is best seen in the subendocardial region of the ventricles as irregular yellow streaks or lines alternating with lines of unaffected muscle, producing the so-called "tigroid," or "tabby cat," or "thrush breast" appearance. In diffuse fatty change, usually caused by severe infections or

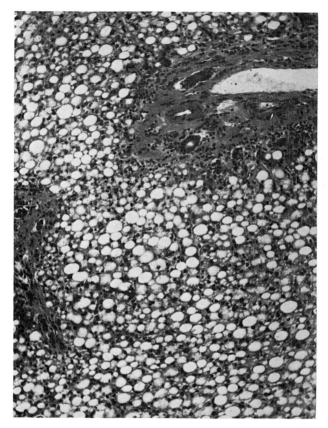

Fig. 2-1. Extreme fatty change of the liver.

toxic states, the entire myocardium is pale yellow or yellowish brown, soft, and flabby when the condition is severe; but lesser degrees are detected only upon histologic examination. Microscopically, a fine vacuolization is observed within the sarcoplasm of myocardial fibers in ordinary paraffin sections. The minute droplets are often less distinct than the small or large vacuoles usually seen in liver or renal tubular cells.

Fatty metamorphosis in the kidney, heart, and liver may be caused by a variety of noxious agents, such as toxins of infectious diseases, phosphorus, carbon tetrachloride, chloroform, and also by anoxia resulting from circulatory insufficiency or severe

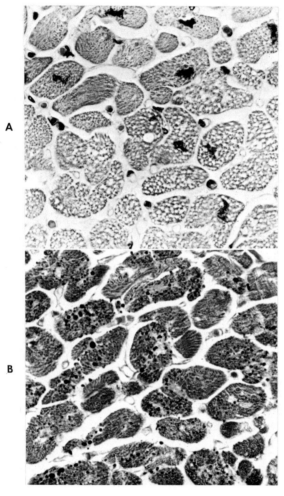

Fig. 2-2. A, Fatty degeneration of myocardium. Rather uniform, fine vacuolization in myocardial fibers. **B,** Fatty degeneration of myocardium in phosphorus poisoning. Black droplets in myocardial fibers are globules of fat (osmic acid stain). Note occasional fat globules in interstitial tissue, which appear to have been expelled from fibers. (From Scotti, T. M.: Heart. In Anderson, W. A. D., editor: Pathology, ed. 5, St. Louis, 1966, The C. V. Mosby Co.)

anemias. The change occurring in the injured cells is caused by impaired intracellular metabolism and is commonly referred to as "fatty degeneration." Some of the lipid may be derived from phospholipids of intracellular membrane systems undergoing degradation, which may be the ultrastructural manifestation of what previously was called "fat phanerosis," or "unmasking" of preexistent lipids. Much of the lipid, however, may accumulate because of the inability of the injured cell to eliminate it, which could result from the impairment of energy-producing enzyme reactions caused by degradation of mitochondria and endoplasmic reticulum.

An inadequate diet, as in starvation or chronic alcoholism, results in a deficiency of lipotropic substances (e.g., choline and methionine), which normally aid in removal of fat from cells. Such a deficiency produces an abnormal accumulation of intracellular lipid, particularly in the liver, perhaps by causing damage to the mitochondria and endoplasmic reticulum and thus interfering with the utilization and elimination of lipid. In chronic alcoholism the possibility that ethanol itself produces an injurious effect upon parenchymal cells must be considered. Excessive mobilization of fat resulting from overfeeding may cause a fatty liver, since more lipid is brought to the cells than can be metabolized; in this instance a relative deficiency of lipotropic substances may be responsible. This form of fatty metamorphosis was formerly called "parenchymal fatty infiltration." A deficiency of intracellular carbohydrate, such as occurs in diabetes mellitus or starvation, is another cause of fatty change in the liver. Apparently, decreased liver glycogen leads to an increased oxidation of fat in hepatic cells, with a resultant increase of mobilization of lipid from the fat depots.

Adiposity (interstitial fat infiltration). In adiposity, which is commonly associated with generalized obesity, there is an abnormal or excessive accumulation of adipose tissue (adult fat cells) between parenchymal cells of an organ. The increase in adult fat cells is believed to result from the transformation of interstitial connective tissue cells after the deposition of lipid within them. The heart and pancreas are the two organs principally affected. In the heart the adipose tissue appears between myocardial fibers and frequently is continuous with the overlying epicardial fat, which usually is increased in amount. Atrophy of muscle fibers may occur. Only rarely will myocardial adiposity produce clinical manifestations. In the pancreas there is an

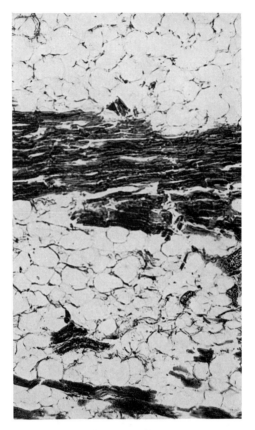

Fig. 2-3. Fatty infiltration of heart. Adipose tissue between myocardial fibers. (From Anderson, W. A. D., editor: Pathology, ed. 5, St. Louis, 1966, The C. V. Mosby Co.)

accumulation of adipose tissue in the interlobular septa that may affect also the interacinar stroma within the lobules. Usually, fatty infiltration of the pancreas produces no functional disturbance of the acinar tissue or islets. Areas of necrosis or atrophy in an organ or tissue may be replaced by adipose tissue (so-called "fatty replacement").

Hyaline degeneration and extracellular hyalins. The term *hyaline* is a descriptive adjective used to qualify any translucent, homogeneous, structureless material that stains with eosin. There

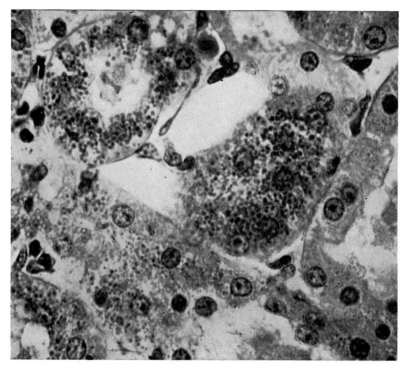

Fig. 2-4. Hyaline droplet degeneration of epithelial cells lining renal tubules. (From Anderson, W. A. D., editor: Pathology, ed. 5, St. Louis, 1966, The C. V. Mosby Co.)

is a variety of intracellular or extracellular hyaline substances *(or hyalins)*, which are mainly of a protein nature. To speak of a substance as a hyalin does not disclose its specific chemical nature nor its localization. Certain types of hyalin, such as amyloid, have distinctive characteristics or staining reactions and hence are separable from the general group.

After injury to certain cells a hyaline change of varying degree may take place in the cytoplasm, which is termed *hyaline degeneration*. This represents a disturbance of protein metabolism within the cell and is a more serious change than cloudy swelling or hydropic degeneration. Examples of this intracellular change are as follows: (1) *hyaline droplet degeneration of renal tubular epithelium*, particularly in proximal convoluted tubules, which is characterized by numerous, closely grouped, minute, hyaline droplets within the cytoplasm, representing either a coagulation of the intracellular protein or protein that has passed through injured and abnormally permeable glomeruli and has been reabsorbed into tubular cells (perhaps by pinocytosis); (2) *Mallory bodies,* which are hyaline masses within degenerating liver cells in active nutritional ("alcoholic") cirrhosis; (3) *Councilman bodies,* which are hyaline masses in liver cells in yellow fever; (4) *acidophilic bodies,* which are hyaline rounded masses in liver cells in viral hepatitis; (5) *Crooke's hyaline change* in basophils of pituitary gland in Cushing's disease; (6) *Russell-Fuchs bodies,* which are rounded hyaline masses that contain gamma globulin formed apparently in response to antigenic stimuli, thus probably not a true degenerative process; and (7) *Zenker's (waxy) degeneration,* which is a hyaline change in voluntary muscle originally described by Zenker in cases of typhoid fever but also seen in other severe infections. The alteration is not caused by the localization of the infection in the muscle but rather by the toxins or excess accumulation of lactic acid. The lesion is best seen in the rectus abdominis and diaphragmatic muscles. The involved muscle is very pale and friable, so that rupture of the fibers and small hemorrhages are frequent. Microscopically, the affected fibers are swollen, they lose their striations, and they have a hyaline appearance. When advanced, the lesion progresses to necrosis.

Extracellular hyaline substances include connective tissue hyalin, fibrinoid, vascular hyalin, and amyloid. The last-named type of hyalin will be discussed in the next section. *Hyaline change in connective tissue* is common, occurring in old scars, in thickened serosae (e.g., pleura) after chronic inflammation, in a thickened capsule of the spleen, in the intima of arteries (atherosclerosis), in the stroma of tumors (e.g., leiomyomas), and in other sites. The change actually is a physical alteration of the collagen fibers, which become fused to form a homogeneous, acellular area, but the collagen retains its usual staining quality. This change is sometimes referred to as "hyaline degeneration" of connective tissue, but it is better called "hyalinization."

Fibrinoid represents altered collagen which appears homogeneous and stains deeply eosinophilic so that it resembles fibrin. Fibrinoid change (often called "fibrinoid degeneration" or "fibrinoid necrosis") is a characteristic lesion in many of the generalized collagen diseases associated with hypersensitivity

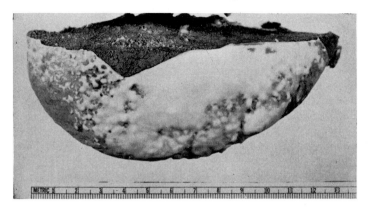

Fig. 2-5. Hyalinization of the splenic capsule.

(e.g., polyarteritis nodosa, rheumatic fever, systemic lupus erythematosus, etc.); it is also present in the arteriolar walls in malignant hypertension. Studies have shown that fibrinoid consists of a mixture of substances including fragments of collagen, acid mucopolysaccharide, fibrin, and in certain situations also gamma globulin.

Vascular hyalin occurs in the walls of arterioles in the hyaline form of arteriolosclerosis. Despite several thorough electron microscopic studies of vascular hyalin, the origin of this substance is still not settled. Some investigators believe that the hyaline deposits are derived from plasma proteins filtering through the endothelium and are deposited predominantly within intimal spaces, while the larger deposits infiltrate the adjacent elastic tissue and smooth muscle of the media. Others claim that the hyalin is essentially an excessive elaboration of endothelial and smooth muscle cell basement membrane material, which is followed by atrophy and disappearance of smooth muscle.

Last it should be mentioned that certain substances of a different nature may have a hyaline appearance, e.g., protein casts in the lumen of renal tubules, colloid in thyroid acini, clumped masses of fibrin, inspissated secretions in glandular ducts, and thrombi in small blood vessels as in thrombotic thrombocytopenic purpura.

Amyloid deposition (amyloidosis). Amyloid is a hyaline material characterized by deposition intercellularly, rather than in cells, and by specific staining reactions with iodine, methyl violet, Congo red, silver, and thioflavine-T (Table 2-1). By electron microscopy, amyloid is seen to be made up primarily of fine fibrils, which are different from collagen or elastin. The exact chemical composition is unknown, but protein fractions and a sulfate-bearing polysaccharide have been identified, and it is considered by some investigators to be a glycoprotein in which a mucopolysaccharide is attached to a globulin. It has been demonstrated in certain studies that mucopolysaccharide is not a significant part of the amyloid fibers themselves but that it represents the ground substance in which amyloid is deposited. There is some question also as to whether gamma globulin is a part of the amyloid fibril or whether it is nonspecifically present in the amyloid deposits. Amyloid is probably not a single chemical substance but a series of closely related protein compounds. The disappearance of Congo red from the blood one hour after intravenous injection is a useful clinical test for amyloidosis. Other diagnostic tests include biopsy of rectal mucosa and needle biopsy of organs, e.g., liver or kidney.

Exact causative and pathogenetic factors in amyloidosis are still unknown, but some disturbance of protein metabolism is involved. Experimentally it has been produced in animals by various stimuli, such as repeated injections of bacterial toxins and sodium caseinate, or by vitamin C deficiency. Horses hyperimmunized for production of diphtheria antitoxin may develop amyloidosis. In man some of the conditions in which amyloid is found are characterized by hyperglobulinemia. One of the theories indicates that amyloid is the result of an antigen-antibody reaction and represents the tissue localization of a circulating abnormal protein complex. Another hypothesis considers a soluble precursor of amyloid to be a glycoprotein (the carbohydrate portion of which is sulfated), formed from proliferating plasma cells, mainly in the red pulp of the spleen. The glycoprotein circulating in the blood and a sulfated mucopolysaccharide formed by endothelial cells combine to produce the complex, amyloid. A third theory, which is supported by recent electron microscopic and autoradiographic evidence, emphasizes the role of the reticuloendothelial system in the production of amyloid locally. It is believed that the reticuloendothelial cells are activated by a wide variety of immunological or other stimuli to produce amyloid fibrils and that possibly a local decrease in pH about these metabolically active cells accelerates the local precipitation of amyloid.

Amyloidosis may be classified as (1) secondary (usually secondary to chronic infections or other chronic inflammations); (2) primary or idiopathic, which may be (a) systemic or (b) localized; (3) associated with multiple myeloma; and (4) hereditary forms. The hyaline material found in the islets of the pancreas in diabetic and nondiabetic persons is probably a form of amyloidosis also.

The commonest form is *secondary amyloidosis* associated with chronic tissue-destructive infections (e.g., tuberculosis, leprosy, syphilis), with other chronic inflammations (e.g., rheumatoid arthritis, regional enteritis, chronic ulcerative colitis), and sometimes with certain malignant neoplasms (e.g., Hodgkin's disease). The organs most frequently involved in the secondary form are the spleen, kidneys, liver, and adrenals. Blood vessel walls tend to be affected first and most prominently in these organs. The earliest amyloid deposits are characteristically subendothelial, along reticulin fibers ("perireticulin amyloidosis") in contrast to the deposition in primary or similar forms of amyloidosis, in which deposits are along collagen fibers ("pericollagen amyloidosis").

The amyloid *spleen* is enlarged, firm, and of rubbery or elastic consistency. On the cut surface the amyloid areas have a characteristic, pale translucent appearance. The involvement may be focal or diffuse. In the *focal form* (sago spleen) the deposition is in arteriolar walls and extends into surrounding lymph follicles. The involved foci are prominently pale and translucent against the red background of the remainder of the spleen. In the *diffuse form* (lardaceous spleen) there is widespread deposition between the fibrous reticulum of the spleen, the follicles tending to be spared.

Considerable amyloid deposition in the *liver* causes it to be enlarged, firm, and unusually translucent. Deposition tends to occur first in the midzonal region of the liver lobule, appearing in the space between the sinus endothelium and the liver cells. In the liver, as elsewhere, the deposition of amyloid tends to cause pressure atrophy of the parenchymatous cells.

Amyloid disease of the *kidney* is occasionally severe enough to disturb renal function and give a picture of renal disease. With glomerular involvement the nephrotic syndrome may occur. Amyloid is deposited chiefly in glomeruli and blood vessel walls.

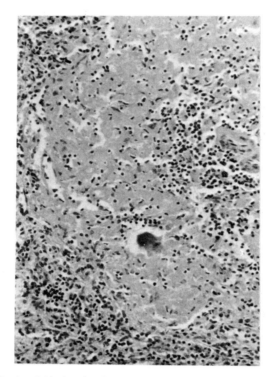

Fig. 2-6. Amyloidosis of spleen. (From Anderson, W. A. D., editor: Pathology, ed. 5, St. Louis, 1966, The C. V. Mosby Co.)

In the glomeruli the amyloid is deposited between the basement membrane and the endothelial lining of the capillaries. The capillaries are narrowed and finally obliterated so that the glomerulus becomes functionless and secondary changes develop in the tubules. Amyloid may also be deposited beneath the basement membrane of some of the tubules.

Primary systemic amyloidosis also occurs but is rare. It is not associated with known diseases. Mesenchymal rather than parenchymatous tissues tend to be involved. Amyloid may be deposited in irregular masses or in the form of "rings" in fatty tissue. A *primary localized amyloidosis* forming tumorlike nodules has been described in many areas, including the respiratory tract, tongue, pharynx, thyroid, etc. Primary amyloidosis restricted to the heart has been reported in elderly patients. The amyloid in the primary systemic or localized form tends to stain atypically. *Multiple myelomas* may be complicated by amyloidosis that is similar to primary systemic amyloidosis in its tissue distribution and variable staining reaction. Several *hereditary forms of amyloidosis* have been described. One of these is associated with familial Mediterranean fever, an autosomal recessive disorder in which renal involvement is the most prominent lesion. Other organs are affected as in the usual secondary form, except that deposits of amyloid in the liver are not striking. Another is the neuropathic type, transmitted by an autosomal dominant gene, with amyloid deposition as in the classic primary systemic form but with prominent involvement of the peripheral nerves and sympathetic ganglia. An autosomal, probably dominant, hereditary amyloidosis with myocardiopathy and progressive cardiac insufficiency has also been reported.

Mucinous degeneration. Mucin is a clear, structureless material, which stains lightly with basic dyes (hematoxylin). In certain epithelial tumors and in some catarrhal inflammations of mucous membranes, an excess is secreted by the epithelial cells. A somewhat similar (mucoid or myxomatous) material may be formed by connective tissue (normally in the umbilical cord) and is found in the subcutaneous tissue in thyroid deficiency (myxedema) and in the connective tissue tumors called myxomas. Actually the designation "mucinous degeneration," which is commonly used for these epithelial and connective tissue disturbances, does not seem to be appropriate. The alteration appears to be one of overproduction of mucin, although secondary adverse effects may be produced in cells surrounded by the abundant material. What is probably a true regressive cellular change is so-called *basophilic (mucinous) degeneration* of myocardial fibers, characterized by the appearance of a blue intrasarcoplasmic substance, which has the staining quality of mucoprotein or acid mucopolysaccharide. The cause of this lesion is not certain, but it may be a form of ischemia. A similar change has been described in voluntary skeletal muscle in myxedema.

Disturbances of purine metabolism. Uric acid, derived mainly from nucleoproteins of food and body tissues, is important under pathologic conditions in the formation of uric acid calculi and so-called "uric acid infarcts" of the kidneys and in gout. *Gout,* a genetic disturbance of purine metabolism, is characterized by

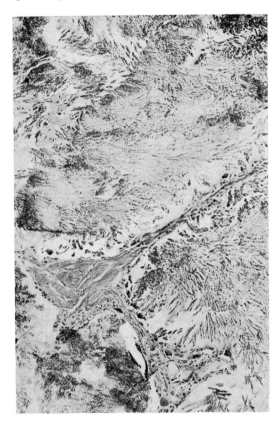

Fig. 2-7. Tophus of gout. Massive crystalline deposits, about which there are some multinucleated giant cells. (From Anderson, W. A. D., editor: Pathology, ed. 5, St. Louis, 1966, The C. V. Mosby Co.)

deposition of crystalline urates in cartilaginous tissues and ligaments about joints, in synovial membranes and tendon sheaths, in cartilages of the ears, in eyelids, in subcutaneous tissues about joints, in heart valves, and in interstitial tissues and tubules of the medullae of the kidneys. The deposits form small masses (tophi), which may be visible or palpable clinically (Fig. 2-7). Microscopically, tophi consist of masses of needlelike crystals or amorphous granules of urates surrounded by a foreign body reaction (lymphocytes, plasma cells, macrophages, giant cells, and fibrous tissue). Most cases of gout occur in men.

In many newborn infants, and occasionally in adults, urate deposits in the pyramids of the kidneys form yellowish gray streaks of crystalline material. The uric acid and urates are within the lumina of collecting tubules and normally are excreted without damage to the kidney. These so-called *uric acid infarcts* elicit no inflammatory reaction. A hyperuricemic syndrome occurs in children, first described by Lesch and Nyhan, and is characterized by self-destruction behavior (chewing one's own lips and fingers) and associated with mental retardation, cerebral palsy, and athetosis.

Disturbances of glycogen distribution. Glucose is not identifiable histologically in tissues, but glycogen can be demonstrated by Best's carmine stain after fixation in alcohol or Carnoy's fluid or by periodic acid–Schiff (PAS) stain (Table 2-1). The normal liver of a well-nourished individual contains abundant glycogen in the cytoplasm of the hepatic cells. In ordinary sections this gives the hepatic cells a foamy or finely reticulated appearance. Postmortem tissues may show a little of this appearance, but may show a greater change if only a short time has elapsed between food intake and death. Glycogen is normally quite abundant in various other tissues such as skin, muscle, heart, and parathyroid glands. Histochemical methods have indicated that potassium and glycogen are closely related in the heart and liver and that the potassium appears to invest the glycogen droplets intimately. Excess glycogen within cells is usually regarded as a form of "infiltration," but some consider it a "degeneration." Glycogen may be increased in areas of inflammatory reaction around dead tissues.

Diabetes mellitus that is inadequately controlled by insulin shows depletion of the normal store of glycogen in the liver and skin. In the presence of glycosuria, excess glycogen content may be demonstrable in renal tubules, particularly in the cells lining the lower proximal convoluted tubules and Henle's loops. The glycogen content of hepatic cell nuclei is often increased in diabetes (p. 533).

One form of glycogen-storage disease (von Gierke's disease), a rare inborn defect of glycogen metabolism, is characterized by abnormal amounts of glycogen in certain organs of infants, particularly the liver and kidneys. It is associated with an enzyme defect of glucose-6-phosphatase. A cardiac form (which has been called Pompe's disease) has been seen that is associated with a deficiency of a lysosomal enzyme, α-1,4-glucosidase. It is part

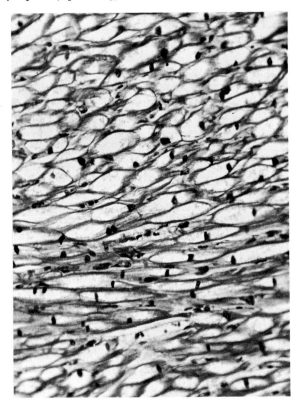

Fig. 2-8. Glycogen-storage disease of myocardium. In formalin-fixed, hematoxylin and eosin–stained histologic preparations, the muscle fibers appear as clear spaces surrounded by a thin rim of sarcoplasm.

of a generalized glycogenosis in which the major manifestation is in the heart. The sarcoplasm of the myocardial fibers is replaced by glycogen, so that the fibers appear as hollow cylinders surrounded by a thin rim of sarcoplasm. The heart is enlarged. Pompe's disease is usually fatal before 8 months of age (p. 487). A localized form of glycogen disease in the heart, forming tumorlike nodules, also occurs.

NECROSIS

The most serious effect of injury is death, which may be of the body as a whole (somatic death) or of localized areas of tissue or certain cells. Cell or tissue death within the living body is termed *necrosis* and is recognizable by the changes that the dead tissues and cells undergo after their death. As mentioned previously (p. 7), the earliest change in necrotic cells seen by light microscopy appears to be in the nucleus. Most investigators, however, have identified ultrastructural alterations in the cytoplasmic membranes and particulate systems and disturbances in their functions before any nuclear changes, although in certain experimental models of cell injury, clumping of nuclear chromatin has been observed almost as early as some of the cytoplasmic alterations. Whether or not the release of enzyme from the lysosomes is responsible for initiating the cellular changes leading to cell death is not settled; but it is generally accepted that these, as well as extracellular enzymes, act upon the cells after their death to produce the morphologic effects that are characteristic of necrosis.

Necrosis may be caused by almost any type of severe injury. Macroscopic areas of dead tissue tend to be opaque; i.e., the normal translucency of most living tissues is lost, and a whitish or yellowish color is assumed. However, gross appearances of necrotic tissue may differ, varying with the type of tissue affected and the causative agent, so that several types are described.

Microscopic recognition of necrosis is aided by nuclear changes in necrotic cells. The nucleus may shrink and stain more intensely basophilic (pyknosis), or it may fragment (karyorrhexis). More commonly the nucleus simply loses its ability to stain differentially with basic dyes (karyolysis), so that it fades and eventually is indistinguishable. Necrotic tissue tends to stain diffusely with red acid dyes such as eosin, with lack of any blue or hematoxylin-staining material. Any calcium that precipitates in the necrotic material stains with hematoxylin, thus appearing as bluish masses.

Coagulation necrosis. Coagulation necrosis is commonly produced by the cutting off of blood supply, i.e., in infarction, and is characterized by a protoplasmic coagulative process. In such necrosis general architectural features may be preserved for a considerable period, although cellular detail is lost.

Caseous necrosis. Caseous necrosis is so called because of a cheesy macroscopic appearance. It is particularly characteristic of the necrotic tissue resulting from tuberculous infection. Microscopically, the architectural outline of the necrotic tissue is completely lost.

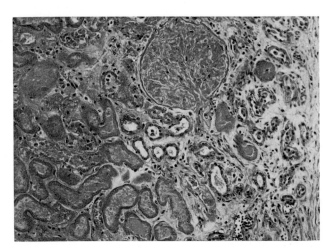

Fig. 2-9. Coagulation necrosis as seen at the margin of an infarct of the kidney. The outlines of a glomerulus and tubules are evident although individual cells and their nuclei are not discernible in the necrotic area.

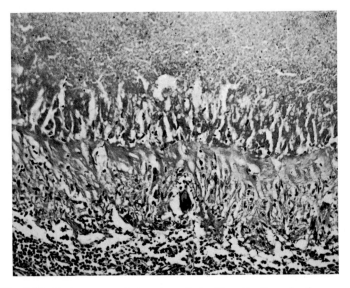

Fig. 2-10. Caseous necrosis in tuberculosis. Necrotic tissue in the upper part of the figure lacks both structural outlines and discernible individual cells and their nuclei.

Gummatous necrosis. Gummatous necrosis results from syphilis and resembles both caseous and coagulation necrosis microscopically, but in the gross form it has a more rubbery consistency.

Liquefactive necrosis. In liquefactive necrosis the dead area softens and eventually liquefies. It is especially characteristic of necrosis in the central nervous system. It may follow other types of necrosis in other tissues, and the term may be applied to the liquefaction of pus in abscesses.

Fat necrosis. Fat necrosis is most commonly the result of pancreatic disease, which allows release of enzymes that act upon fat. The traditional concept is that lipase, and possibly other enzymes from the pancreas, permeate the fat causing hydrolysis of the neutral fat, and the free fatty acids that are split off in this process combine with calcium and other cations in the tissue fluid. An alternative theory is that the fat-cell membrane is damaged by pancreatic enzymes (amylase, lecithin, or both), then lipase, and possibly other enzymes are freed from the cytoplasm and cell membrane complexes that cause self-digestion of the cell fat. The fat of the pancreas, omentum, or other intra-abdominal tissues shows whitish opaque nodules of very characteristic appearance. A zone of congestion and leukocytes surrounds the necrotic area. Eventually calcium tends to be deposited in these areas, and a foreign body reaction occurs around them. In rare instances of acute pancreatitis, foci of fat necrosis may occur outside the abdominal cavity (e.g., subcutaneous tissue). Fat necrosis may also occur in the breast and other subcutaneous areas, from trauma, toxic agents, circulatory disturbances, and injection. There is necrosis of the fat cells, with release of neutral fat into tissues and its subsequent change into fatty acids or soaps. An inflammatory reaction occurs, often of foreign body type with formation of giant cells, and a tumor-like mass may result.

Gangrene. In the strict sense the term *gangrene* refers to necrotic tissue in which there is putrefaction resulting from invasion by saprophytic bacteria (e.g., moist gangrene). By usage, however, the term is also applied to massive areas of necrosis, even without invasion by saprophytes (e.g., dry gangrene). *Dry gangrene* (or mummification) is a term usually applied to ischemic necrosis of a portion of an extremity, i.e., an infarction of the extremity. The tissue becomes dried out, greenish yellow, and finally dark brown or black. Inflammatory

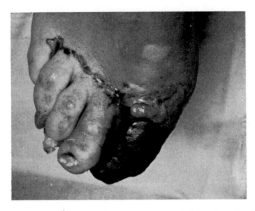

Fig. 2-11. Diabetic gangrene of the great toe. White female, 53 years of age. (From Gore, I.: Blood and lymphatic vessels. In Anderson, W. A. D., editor: Pathology, ed. 5, St. Louis, 1966, The C. V. Mosby Co.)

reaction in the adjacent living tissue causes a sharp line of demarcation separating healthy and dead tissues. In *moist gangrene,* which may be found in almost any part of the body, saprophytic organisms invade the dead tissue through wounds or from the respiratory or intestinal tract, causing putrefactive changes. *Gas gangrene* occurs when the invading saprophytes are of the gas-forming group (e.g., the Welch bacillus).

Senile gangrene is a necrosis in an extremity resulting from interference with blood supply by arteriosclerosis. It is often a dry type but may be moist and putrefactive. *Diabetic gangrene* is similar and also caused by arteriosclerosis, but it tends to occur at an earlier age. Gangrenous extremities resulting from interference with blood supply may also be caused by Raynaud's disease (vascular spasm), ergot poisoning (vascular spasm), and thromboangiitis obliterans (endarteritis).

POSTMORTEM CHANGES

Somatic death, or death of the body as a whole, is followed by some early changes with which some familiarity is necessary.

Rigor mortis. Rigor mortis is a stiffening of muscles resulting from a chemical change in which there is precipitation of protein. It begins first in involuntary muscles, affects voluntary muscles in about four to ten hours, and passes off in three or four days. Since time of appearance and degree of rigor mortis are affected by a number of conditions, it is unreliable as an indicator of the exact time of death.

Livor mortis. Livor mortis is the reddish discoloration of dependent portions of the body resulting from the gravitational sinking of blood. Internal organs, such as the lungs, as well as the skin are affected. Hemolysis of red cells occurs with varying rapidity after death, and hemoglobin may lightly stain the aortic lining or serous surfaces. Hemoglobin staining may be hastened in death from infections, particularly if caused by hemolytic organisms.

Postmortem clots. Postmortem clots are described in a subsequent section (p. 100) and compared with antemortem clots, or thrombi (q.v.).

Autolysis. Autolysis is the self-digestion or breakdown of tissues caused by ferments released in the body after death. In some tissues, such as the mucosa of the stomach or gallbladder, autolytic changes are rapid, and good microscopic preparations of such tissues may be difficult to obtain post mortem. In general, the highly differentiated tissues (e.g., the ganglion cells in the nervous system and glandular epithelium) undergo more rapid autolysis than do supporting or connective tissue structures. Early autolysis results in loss of cellular detail in staining and may cause some confusion in differentiation from such degenerative processes as cloudy swelling. In autolysis there is no inflammatory cell response, in contrast to that which may be seen in relation to necrotic tissue.

Putrefaction. Putrefaction in the dead body follows entrance of saprophytes, usually from the intestinal tract. It results in production of gases and a greenish discoloration of tissues. Gas-producing saprophytes may cause a foamy or spongy appearance of organs, particularly the liver.

CALCIFICATION

Calcium salts are normally deposited only in bone and teeth, but pathologic calcification is frequent in soft tissues and as concretions (calculi) in excretory or secretory passages. The calcium deposits contain calcium phosphate, calcium carbonate, and variable amounts of other salts, the composition being similar to that in normal bone. Frequent sites of pathologic calcification are blood vessel walls and kidneys; but some tissues contain calcium deposits with such regularity that it may be a normal event (e.g., pineal gland in adults). Pathologic calcification is commonly classified as *dystrophic* or *metastatic*.

Dystrophic calcification. Dystrophic calcification is the deposition in dead or degenerating tissue. This is the most frequent type of pathologic calcification, occurring in areas of tuberculous necrosis, in blood vessels in arteriosclerosis, in areas of fatty degeneration and necrosis, in degenerating thyroid tissue, in degenerating tumors, etc. A retained ectopic fetus may become calcified (lithopedion). Dystrophic calcification is not dependent upon an increase in the calcium content of the blood but appears to be influenced by a local relative alkalinity of the damaged tissue.

Metastatic calcification. Metastatic calcification is a precipitation of calcium salts resulting from a disturbance in calcium and phosphorus metabolism and is often associated with an excess of calcium in the circulating blood. It occurs particularly as a result of hyperparathyroidism (p. 695) but also is seen in hypervitaminosis D (pp. 253 and 395) and in some conditions associated with destructive bone lesions, particularly tumors. The calcification tends to occur mainly in the kidneys, lungs, gastric mucosa, and media of blood vessels. In addition any degenerating or necrotic tissue tends to become infiltrated by the excess calcium circulating in the blood.

Calcinosis. Calcinosis is a disorder of unknown cause characterized by calcification, particularly in or under the skin. Circumscribed and generalized forms occur, the latter often having calcium deposits in tendons, fasciae, muscles, and nerves. Progressive systemic sclerosis (scleroderma) may have an associated calcinosis.

Pathologic ossification. In extraosseous sites pathologic ossification is characterized by the formation of bone structures, such as lamellae, lacunae, and sometimes marrow and is accompanied by calcification. Such heteroplastic bone formation occurs in a variety of tissues and is frequent in an injured eye with chronic inflammation. *Myositis ossificans* is a pathologic calcification and ossification that may occur in a localized form after trauma to a muscle, or it may progress to involve also tendons, fasciae, and ligaments.

PIGMENTATION

In a number of conditions colored materials are deposited in the skin or internal tissues. Although considered here together, they have nothing in common except the pigment deposition. There are two classes of pigmentation: (1) *endogenous,* in which the colored substance is produced within the body, and (2) *exogenous,* in which the pigment is introduced into the body by way of the intestinal tract, skin, or lungs.

Endogenous pigmentation

There are three types of pigments produced within the body: *melanins, those related to hemoglobin, and lipochromes.*

Melanin. Melanin, an insoluble polymer of high molecular weight, forms the normal coloring matter of the skin and the uveal tract and retina of the eye. It is produced in the skin by melanoblasts (melanocytes) situated in the basal layers of the epidermis. These specialized cells may be distinguished, even though they contain no pigment at the time, by the dopa reaction (p. 819). The precursor is tyrosine, which by a series of oxidations under the influence of the enzyme tyrosinase forms melanin. Pigment-carrying cells are present in the subepithelial tissues. The amount of melanin in the skin is increased by exposure to sunlight. Skin pigmentation is increased in Addison's disease (p. 706), and pigmented spots are common in association with multiple neurofibromatosis. Patchy areas lacking pigment also occur, and there may be a congenital absence of melanin pigment (albinism) resulting from a genetically transmitted lack of tyrosinase.

Partial albinism is a rare congenital defect with permanent absence of melanin pigment in various areas of the body (e.g., white forelock and spotting of the skin, a simple dominant condition; or albinism of the eye alone, a sex-linked recessive disorder). The also rare total albinism, involving skin, eyes, and hair, is transmitted as a simple recessive. Vitiligo is an acquired depigmentation of areas of the skin, in which the size and distribution of the lesions may alter.

Benign pigmented nevi and malignant melanomas are tumors composed of melanoblasts. The amount of pigment found in such tumors shows extreme variation. Melanomas commonly arise from the skin or eye.

A melanocyte-stimulating hormone is produced by the pituitary gland. This hormone appears to be mainly responsible for the increased melanin pigmentation of the skin in Addison's disease and in pregnancy. Hydrocortisone from the adrenal cortex inhibits the release of the melanocyte-stimulating hormone, and adrenal medullary hormones appear to interfere with the action of the melanocyte-stimulating hormone on the melanocytes. Pigmentation may follow the administration of estrogens or of corticotropin but not of cortisone.

Ochronosis is a rare type of pigmentation by a melanin, in which cartilage is affected. Discoloration of the cartilage of the ear and nose may be visible through the skin. Ocular and renal tubular pigmentation also may be present. Most cases result from an inborn error of metabolism evidenced by alkaptonuria.

Ochronosis appears to be a genetic defect of phenylalanine and tyrosine intermediary metabolism, resulting in abnormal accumulation of homogentisic acid, which tends to localize selectively in cartilage. Oxidation of homogentisic acid in the presence of alkali produces the dark urine (alkaptonuria), which is the main evidence of the disease in early life. Ocular pigmentation, with brownish blue spots on the sclera or on margins of the cornea, is a common finding. In later years osteoarthritis of severe degree may develop and is the main clinical disturbance. The spine, knees, shoulders, and hips are most frequently affected.

Melanosis coli is a black discoloration of the mucosa of the large intestine, occurring in chronically constipated persons. The pigment resembles but is not a true melanin (p. 647).

Hemoglobin-related pigments. Hemoglobin, the pigment of red blood cells, is a combination of a pigment complex, *heme,* plus a protein, *globin*. The heme fraction consists of iron and protoporphyrin III. Several types of pigments are related to hemoglobin: hemosiderin, bilirubin (hematoidin), hematin, and the porphyrins.

Hemosiderin. Hemosiderin appears as golden brown, varying-sized, refractive crystals and granules of pigment, formed locally when hemoglobin breaks down in tissues (e.g., as the result of hemorrhage) or systemically when there is excessive destruction of erythrocytes in the circulation. Hemosiderin is formed within phagocytic cells of the reticuloendothelial system, and the time for its production may be as short as one day. Hemosiderin has no exact chemical composition but contains loosely bound iron, which gives a Prussian blue reaction (a blue color with potassium ferrocyanide and hydrochloric acid). The iron is present mainly in the ferric form.

The normal continuous breakdown of red blood cells in the reticuloendothelial system results in some hemosiderin deposition in the liver and spleen. Pathologic excess of hemosiderin deposit (hemosiderosis) occurs in these organs and elsewhere whenever there is excessive breakdown of blood. Such occurs systemically in hemolytic anemias (e.g., pernicious anemia, sickle cell anemia), or after numerous blood transfusions, and locally in areas of hemorrhage or in passive congestion of an organ, where stagnation in capillaries results in increased blood destruction. In the spleen, hemosiderin pigment is found in phagocytic cells of the pulp and sinuses. In the liver the pigment is found both in the phagocytic Kupffer cells of the sinusoids and in the liver cells. In the kidney, tubular lining cells, as well as interstitial tissue and endothelial cells, may contain pigment. In the lung, hemosiderin pigment is often abundant in large mononuclear phagocytic cells in alveoli when there is chronic congestion. These pigmented alveolar macrophages are often called "heart failure cells" because of their association with circulatory failure. Cardiac failure is the most common cause of pulmonary hemosiderosis, but idiopathic forms also occur, usually in association with repeated pulmonary hemorrhages. A related syndrome

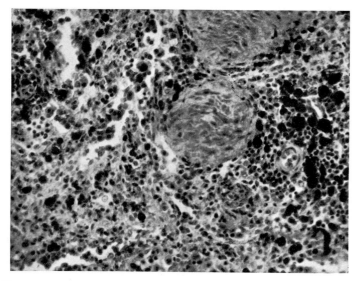

Fig. 2-12. Hemosiderin pigment in the spleen.

(Goodpasture's disease) is characterized by pulmonary hemorrhage and glomerulonephritis.

Primary, or *idiopathic, hemochromatosis* is a rare disturbance of iron-pigment metabolism, occurring almost exclusively in males of middle life and beyond (80% between 35 and 60 years of age). It is sometimes familial. It is usually characterized clinically by cirrhosis of the liver, diabetes mellitus, and skin pigmentation ("bronzed diabetes"), but the diabetes or the skin pigmentation is occasionally absent. Splenomegaly often accompanies the hepatic cirrhosis, and ascites may be present in late stages. Endocrine disturbances are sometimes present, and cardiac complications may occur late in the disease. Primary carcinoma of the liver is a terminal complication in about 7% of cases.

Hemochromatosis appears to be caused by an excess absorption of iron, with gradual accumulation over the years of storage forms of iron in the tissues. Excess iron occurs particularly in the liver, pancreas, heart, skin, and endocrine glands. Iron is ordinarily absorbed from the diet through the duodenal mucosa in amounts of about 1.5 mg. per day. According to some investigators an excess absorption is prevented normally by a protective mechanism ("mucosal block"), which becomes deranged in idiopathic hemochromatosis. Further, it is believed that the abnormality of absorption is based upon a genetic metabolic disturbance. Another view, discounting the idea of a genetic mucosal block defect, is that iron overloading is the result of excessive intake of iron and that idiopathic hemochromatosis is a variant of portal cirrhosis. There is evidence that in hemochromatosis there is an increased tissue avidity for iron. In hemochromatosis the increased absorption of iron may be roughly six times normal amounts. The serum iron level is high, and the total amount of iron in the body is increased from a normal of 4 to 5 grams to 25 to 50 grams. The liver contains the most iron, with increased amounts also in the pancreas, thyroid, pituitary, salivary glands, and myocardium. There is little increase of iron in the spleen and bone marrow, the excess iron being predominantly in epithelial or parenchymatous cells rather than in the reticuloendothelial system. The excess iron may be mobilized from the body by repeated phlebotomy. The degree of injury from the excess of stored iron is uncertain, and it is not known whether the fibrosis of the liver and pancreas is caused by the iron or simply occurs concurrently.

The liver is enlarged and shows a portal type of cirrhosis with irregular hepatic nodules separated by thick fibrous bands. Hemosiderin is demonstrable predominantly in liver cells (not always distributed uniformly throughout) but is also present in the connective tissue, Kupffer cells, and epithelial cells of bile ducts. The pancreas is enlarged, hard, and pigmented, with variable degrees of fibrosis. Pigmentation in the skin is often caused by an increase of melanin, but in about 50% of the cases there is also demonstrable hemosiderin in the skin. The heart almost always has an increased iron content with hemosiderin in muscle fibers. An excess of a yellowish fatty pigment, lipofuscin (hemofuscin), may be present in the heart, in walls of blood vessels and connective tissues of the involved organs, and in the smooth muscle of the intestinal tract.

Transfusional siderosis ("exogenous hemochromatosis") is an excessive iron storage in tissues as a result of multiple transfusions, usually given for the treatment of refractory anemia. It occurs in young adults of both sexes. The excess iron is deposited first and predominantly in the spleen and reticuloendothelial system. The skin, liver, and pancreas all may show siderosis, but great degrees of fibrosis of the liver and pancreas are not usually present. Apparently siderosis must be present in these organs for prolonged periods before advanced fibrosis develops. The heart is not pigmented, and lipofuscin is not increased.

Siderosis of the liver is relatively frequent and severe in the Bantu race in South Africa. It may be associated with hepatic portal fibrosis or with fully developed hepatic cirrhosis. The evidence suggests that the siderosis is related to Bantu dietary habits and iron intake.

Bilirubin and hematoidin. Bile pigment is formed from the breakdown of hemoglobin by reticuloendothelial cells, particularly in the spleen, liver, and bone marrow. Excessive bilirubin in the circulation causes the yellowish pigmentation known as jaundice, or icterus (p. 512).

A benign hepatic disease, chronic idiopathic jaundice, has been described by Dubin and Johnson, and by Sprinz and Nelson (see also p. 488). The disease appears to be an inborn metabolic error, in which the jaundice is caused by excess direct-reacting bilirubin in serum. The liver is heavily pigmented, particularly about central zones of the lobules, by a brown pigment in parenchymal cells. The pigment bears a resemblance to a lipofuscin. Except for the pigmentation, there are no consistent changes in the liver. The abundant pigment may cause a black or greenish black discoloration of the liver grossly, and one term that has been proposed for the condition is "black-liver jaundice" ("mavrohepatic icterus").

Hematoidin is a pigment closely related to or identical with bilirubin and formed in tissues from hemoglobin. Like that of hemosiderin, its formation is intracellular, but several days are required to produce hematoidin. It is formed mainly in tissues wherein a good oxygen supply is lacking. Hence it is often found where there is breakdown of blood in dead or dying tissues, as in infarcts, and usually appears extracellularly. Hematoidin may be seen as amorphous yellow granules or sheaves of crystals, which are frequently burr shaped. It does not give the Prussian blue reaction for free iron, since it is iron free but it does give the Gmelin reaction for bile.

Hematin and malarial pigment. Hematin, which may be formed by the action of acids or alkalies on hemoglobin, is not a normal breakdown product of hemoglobin or a precursor of hemosiderin and bile pigments. However, there is a possibility of its formation in some cases of intravascular hemolysis or hemoglobinemia. In such cases it rapidly combines with blood proteins to form methemalbumin. In the tissues, hematin appears as minute, rather uniform-sized rhomboid, dark brown pigment granules. Sometimes it is mistaken for hemosiderin, but its iron is firmly bound so that it fails to give a Prussian blue reaction as does hemosiderin.

In massive hemoglobinurias such as may result from transfusion reactions, casts of hematin pigment may be formed in renal tubules by the action of an acid urine and are a contributing factor in the resulting renal failure.

Malarial pigment is a closely related (hematin) compound formed by action of the malarial parasite on the hemoglobin in the red blood cell. Massive deposits of this brown pigment, which fails to stain for iron, are formed in reticuloendothelial cells of the spleen and liver (p. 220). In malignant pernicious malaria the pigment is especially seen in red blood cells within capillaries and other small vessels of many organs, particularly the brain. Formalin pigment, a hematin, is formed in tissues containing much blood when they are exposed to prolonged fixation in formalin, especially if it is acidified.

Porphyrins. Porphyrins are pigments that are normally found in minute amounts in the urine. In a rare inborn metabolic disturbance, congenital (erythropoietic) porphyria, large amounts of porphyrins are found in the urine, which is colored Burgundy red. Individuals having this disease are abnormally sensitive to light. This erythropoietic porphyria appears in infancy or childhood, transmitted as a mendelian recessive characteristic. It appears to be caused by an abnormal (increased) porphyrin formation in the bone marrow. Splenomegaly is commonly present. Hepatic porphyria, apparently an autosomal dominant disorder, occurs in adults, with high concentrations of porphyrins and porphyrin precursors in the liver. It may occur in an intermittent acute or a chronic cutaneous form. Acquired porphyrinuria occurs as a result of various conditions (e.g., lead poisoning and other chemical intoxications, hemolytic anemia, pernicious anemia, liver diseases, and carcinoma).

Lipochrome pigments. Lipoid pigments are found in small amounts in various places in the body. Some of these are probably related to carotene, a vegetable pigment ingested with food. The yellowish pigment of the corpus luteum is a lipochrome. Certain lipochromes are said to be the result of wear and tear of tissues. Brown atrophy of the heart is a senile condition in which lipochrome pigments are visible at the nuclear poles of heart muscle fibers. The heart has a brownish discoloration and is small as a result of atrophy of the muscle fibers.

Exogenous pigmentation

Colored materials may gain entrance to the body by inspiration, ingestion, and inoculation into the skin. Pigmentation of the lung by inspired substances such as carbon forms an important group of pulmonary conditions known as the pneumoconioses (p. 478).

Silver poisoning (argyria). Silver poisoning may cause a permanent pigmentation of the skin. Excessive administration of a silver compound over a long period of time results in deposition of pigment in the upper layers of the corium, immediately under the epithelium, and around sweat and sebaceous glands. The skin acquires an unpleasant, permanent, ashen gray hue. In severe cases pigment is present in the kidney and liver as well. The pigment, an insoluble albuminate of silver, appears to be deposited between the connective tissue cells of the skin and in the basement membranes in the liver and kidneys.

Lead poisoning (plumbism). Lead poisoning may cause pigmentation of oral mucosa. A line of deep blue pigmentation develops at the junction of teeth and gums because of the formation of lead sulfide.

Carotenemia. Carotenemia is a pale yellowish discoloration of the skin resulting from excessive ingestion of plant pigments, such as the carotene found in carrots. No deleterious effects are known.

Tattoos. Tattoos are pigments introduced into the skin by a needle or other sharp instrument for decorative purposes. The pigment may be seen as small granules held in the corium by macrophages. Infections, such as serum hepatitis or syphilis, may be introduced at the time of tattooing by unclean habits of the operator.

Chapter 3

Inflammation and repair

INFLAMMATION

Inflammation is the local reactive change in tissues following injury or irritation. Wright defines inflammation as "the process by means of which cells and exudate accumulate in irritated tissues and tend to protect them from further injury." It is a progressive reaction in living tissues, accompanied or followed by the process of repair or healing. The agents causing the injury and hence leading to inflammation may be of bacteriologic, physical, chemical, or traumatic nature. The irritant apparently induces direct injury of cells, their resulting altered metabolism liberating materials which initiate the inflammatory process. Inflammation is the most common and fundamental pathologic reaction and in general is protective, tending to localize or dispose of the injurious agent and to set the stage for repairs. In the local area there are vascular effects, disturbances of fluid exchange, and emigration of the white blood cells (leukocytes) from the blood into the tissues. The accumulation of fluid and cells is referred to as an exudate. The cells of the local area show some effect of the injury, which may vary from mild degenerative changes to massive death and destruction. These alterative changes in tissue are essential in the initiation of the vascular, exudative, and reparative changes which follow.

Vascular reactions in acute inflammation

After a local acute injury there sometimes occurs a momentary or transitory contraction of vessels, and hence local anemia. This evanescent constriction is rapidly replaced by hyperemia of the part, resulting from dilatation of arterioles, capillaries, and venules. The increased rate of flow also is transitory and gives way to a slowing of the current in the dilated vessels, which progresses to capillary and venular stagnation and stasis. The local changes in the blood flow are important in that they affect the passage of fluid and leukocytes through the vessel walls and thus bring about the formation of an exudate. The increased passage of fluid through the vessel walls is caused by elevation

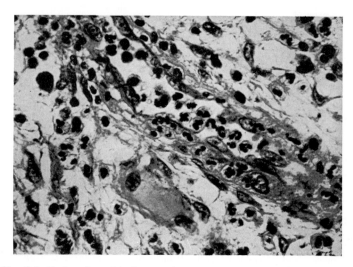

Fig. 3-1. Emigration of leukocytes in a nasal polyp. Vessel in the center contains a number of granulocytes; others are seen in the wall of the vessel, apparently in the process of emigrating. (×640.) (From Anderson, W. A. D., and McCutcheon, M.: Inflammation. In Anderson, W. A. D., editor: Pathology, ed. 5, St. Louis, 1966, The C. V. Mosby Co.)

of capillary pressure and increased vascular permeability. The traditional concept is that the increased vascular permeability associated with inflammation occurs in the capillaries. However, evidence from recent investigations, mainly by electron microscopy, suggest that venules (20 to 30μ in diameter) contribute substantially to the fluid of the exudate; indeed, these studies show that the venules may be the most permeable segment of the microcirculation. Further, it has been demonstrated that increased permeability, under the influence of vasoactive substances, may be caused not only by the intensification of the physiologic mechanism of fluid exudation but also by the appearance of intercellular gaps in the endothelium through which even the larger molecules of the plasma (e.g., protein) could pass. According to Menkin there is a permeability factor, *leukotaxine,* a nitrogenous substance liberated by injured tissue, which affects the permeability of the vascular endothelium and also causes the migration of polymorphonuclear leukocytes into the injured area. Other observers agree that proteolytic enzymes acting on damaged tissues and blood substrate release a polypeptide of low molecular weight that acts to increase vascular permeability in the locally injured area. Among the polypeptides considered to be mediators of the inflammatory process, in addition to leukotaxine, are *bradykinin* and *kallidin*. Certain serum proteins (globulins) may increase endothelial permeability. Spector suggests that damaged cells release substances that cause liberation of 5-hydroxytryptamine and histamine and then activate the permeability-globulin precursor. Local vasodilatation and active hyperemia are important in supplying leukocytes to the area and in formation of an exudate. The slowing of the blood flow in small vessels allows the leukocytes to line up along the vessel walls (*margination* of leukocytes) instead of being carried in the axial stream. The leukocytes pass through the vessel wall and tissue spaces by ameboid motion.

Histamine and certain of the other chemical substances that produce increased vascular permeability are also considered to be involved in the development of vascular dilatation, although neurogenic influences, such as local axon reflexes, may play a less important role in this vascular response. The slowing of the blood current results from increased viscosity of the blood and possibly from swelling and irregularity of the endothelial lining of the vessels.

Exudation. The accumulation of an exudate of fluid and cells in the area of injury is dependent on the vascular effects. The fluid (serous) part of the exudate is largely plasma from the blood and, when abundant, may be referred to as inflammatory edema. The fluid coagulates with the precipitation of an abundant network of fibrin. The inflamed area tends to be walled off, and the injurious agent is localized by the fibrinous material and by thrombotic occlusion of draining lymphatics. When immunity is present, localization of bacterial irritants is aided also by agglutinins, the invading organisms adhering to each other and to the tissues. The early fixation of a bacterial irritant in the area allows time in which leukocytes can assemble for phagocytosis. Neutrophilic leukocytes migrate through the vessel walls by ameboid motion, apparently by dissecting into and passing through the cellular junctions of inflamed endothelium. This is aided in some cases by attraction to the site of injury by a chemical stimulus, a process referred to as *chemotaxis*. Leukotaxine may contain a factor concerned in this process. Bacteria and products of injured tissue act as chemotaxic agents, intensifying the emigration of neutrophilic leukocytes from blood vessels and directing them toward the injurious agent, leading them to the actual contact with the foreign particle which makes phagocytosis possible. Adenine compounds released by the breakdown of nucleoproteins in injured tissue appear to promote chemotaxis and also to stimulate leukocyte formation in the bone marrow. Viruses apparently do not attract leukocytes. The inflammatory cell response is probably evoked by products of cells damaged by viruses, rather than by the viruses themselves.

The mechanism of the directional movement has been thought to depend on changes in surface tension, but McCutcheon has presented reasons for considering it to be caused by a directional orientation of colloidal changes within the cell. Chemotaxis is a directional reaction superimposed on ameboid motion. The rate of motion probably is not influenced. Toxic degenerative changes of leukocytes may interfere with chemotaxis and with rate of motion. Negative chemotaxis is a repelling of leukocytes by certain substances (e.g., silicic acid). Monocytes are slower in chemotactic motion, and lymphocytes have little or no chemotactic activity. Positive chemotaxis is of great value in placing leukocytes in position to phagocytize bacteria and to form a wall about bacteria to prevent their spread.

Menkin has demonstrated an injury factor (necrosin) in inflammatory exudates of animals, associated with the euglobulin fraction, which when injected induces tissue damage and initiates the inflammatory process. The significance of this material in inflammation is not yet fully known. Menkin has suggested also that local changes in hydrogen ion concentration affect the leukocytes and influence the type of cell found in the exudate. The initial response in acute inflammation is an exudate in which neutrophilic leukocytes predominate. The subsequent development of a local acidosis injures these cells, and at a pH of about 6.9 the monocytes (macrophages) tend to survive and predominate. Others have found that there may be little correlation between the pH and the type of cell in the exudate. In infections with pyogenic organisms, bacterial toxins and enzymes are probably largely responsible for the dissolution of tissues and destruction of leukocytes, which result in a purulent exudate and abscess formation. Proteoltyic enzymes released from dead neutrophils lyse dead tissue, cells, and fibrin, contributing much to the formation of pus; in fact, it is by this

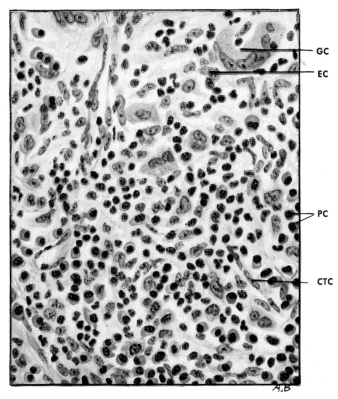

Plate 1. Chronic inflammatory cells. Study in cell structure to show plasma cells **(PC)**, connective tissue cells **(CTC)**, giant cells **(GC)**, and epithelioid cells **(EC)**. (From McCarthy, L.: Histopathology of skin diseases, St. Louis, 1931, The C. V. Mosby Co.)

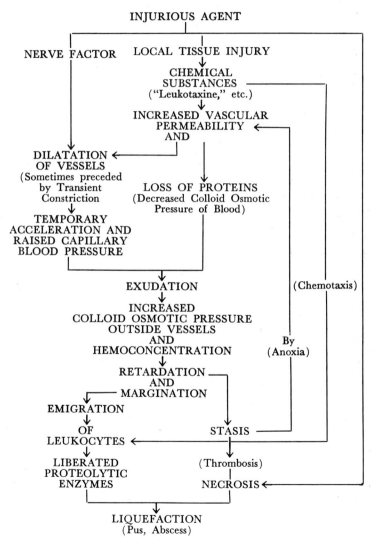

Fig. 3-2. Mechanism of inflammation.

means that suppuration occurs in nonbacterial lesions (e.g., after turpentine injection).

The action of fibrinous exudate and agglutinins in localization of a bacterial irritant may be opposed by "spreading factors." The effect of these substances, which are believed to include an enzyme (hyaluronidase), is to reduce the viscosity of body fluids and thus to promote a free permeation of tissues. Spreading factors are produced by certain invasive bacteria, such as *Clostridium welchii* and the pneumococcus. They are also found in testicular tissue, some snake venoms, and in malignant tumors. Coagulation and fibrin formation are important changes in the fluid of inflammatory edema that tend to localize infection. Reduction of lymph flow by lymphatic thrombosis may also assist in limiting some infections.

The fluid of an exudate usually has a specific gravity of 1.020 or higher, due mainly to an abundant content of serum proteins. Ordinary edema fluid (a transudate) has a distinctly lower specific gravity. Antibodies of the blood are brought into the tissues with the exudate.

In inflammatory processes there is frequently an increase in the number of circulating leukocytes (leukocytosis). This is stimulated by distintegration of leukocytes in tissues, apparently due to some globulin-like factor produced in the area which acts on the bone marrow. The proportion of immature forms of neutrophilic leukocytes in the peripheral blood is increased. Leukocytosis is another factor which aids in quickly bringing great numbers of phagocytic cells to the area of injury. In certain infections, such as typhoid fever, influenza, and most viral diseases, leukocytosis is absent, or there may be actual decrease of circulating leukocytes (leukopenia). In bacterial diseases ordinarily accompanied by leukocytosis, leukopenia is an unfavorable sign suggesting overwhelming infection. Fever is also an accompaniment of many inflammations, due to toxic products from bacteria or protein disintegration.

Corticoids, such as hydrocortisone, appear to inhibit the development of an inflammatory reaction but without impeding necrosis as a result of the injurious agent.

Cells of inflammation. Cells in an inflammatory exudate may include various types of leukocytes, red blood cells, macrophages, and giant cells.

Neutrophils. Neutrophilic leukocytes are the important cells of most acute inflammations. They migrate through the vessel walls and proceed by their ameboid activity to the site of injury, influenced by chemotaxis. Their function is phagocytosis of bacteria and tissue fragments, under the stimulus of opsonins and other tropins. They disintegrate and release substances that stimulate leukocytosis and proteolytic ferments (leukoproteases), which liquefy the injured cells. Enzymes demonstrated in neutrophils include nucleases, nucleotidases, trypsin, etc. The leukocytes tend to increase progressively until the irritant is overcome, provided the bone marrow is capable of increased production. Leukocytes are recognized by their segmented or lobulated nucleus. Faintly stained fine granules are present in their cytoplasm.

Lymphocytes. The lymphocytes are not present in significant numbers in acute inflammatory reactions except in lymph nodes and in the nervous system. However, they are numerous and important in many subacute and chronic inflammations. The lymphocytes are rounded cells, each with a relatively large dark nucleus and very scanty cytoplasm. It has been demonstrated that lymphoblasts, when studied in tissue culture, have a characteristic type of locomotion and shape which enables their differentiation from other cells which often are morphologically similar (e.g., myeloblasts, monocytes). Lymphocytes are rarely phagocytic, but it has been maintained by Maximow and others that lymphocytes may be transformed into large mononuclear cells (macrophages) which have an active phagocytic function. The exact role of the lymphocyte in antibody formation has been debated for years, although some recent evidence suggests that the cells are concerned with synthesis of antibody. There is no question that lymphocytes react to foreign antigens in certain immune responses, and thus are regarded as immunocompetent cells. For example, the cells accumulate in lesions of the delayed hypersensitivity type and at the site of rejection of cell or tissue transplants. It has been suggested that the thymus is the source of these immunologically competent cells or that it secretes a substance which permits development of lymphocytes. Adrenal cortical activity appears to exert some control over lymphocytes and antibody production. Administration of cortisone causes lysis of the cells. The lymphocyte is rich in adenosinase, which may be active in the destruction of toxic products of protein metabolism. It has also been suggested that the lymphocyte has a function in protein synthesis, acting as a carrier of reserve nucleoprotein.

Plasma cells. Plasma cells may be present in small numbers in acute and subacute inflammations but are particularly characteristic of chronic inflammation. Plasma cells are slightly larger than lymphocytes and have a basophilic cytoplasm which contains ribonucleic acid, and an eccentric nucleus in which the chromatin is collected in small masses around the periphery to give it a cartwheel or clock-face appearance. They are rarely seen in the circulating blood. The evidence suggests that they are derived from stem reticular cells which become differentiated. Little is known of their function, but much evidence suggests that plasma cells are concerned in production of antibody and other globulins. Immature plasma cells appear to be the main producers of antibody, which is found where reticulum cells are stimulated by antigen to develop into plasma cells. The plasma cell elaborates protein substances which accumulate in the ergastoplasm and under certain conditions may become condensed into acidophilic intracellular hyaline bodies (Russell bodies). Experimentally these bodies may be produced by antigenic stimulus, and antibody may be a component of such bodies. Plasma cell hyperplasia occurs during immunization. Antibodies are demonstrable in plasma cells by fluorescent microscopy and radioautography. Gamma globulins and specific antibodies have been demonstrated in tissue extracts composed largely of plasma cells. In cases of agammaglobulinemia there is a lack of plasma cells, and plasmacytomas may be accompanied by hyperglobulinemia.

Eosinophils. Eosinophils have large reddish granules in their cytoplasm, and lobulation of the nucleus is less marked than in the neutrophilic polymorphonuclear leukocytes. Little is known of their function. Some evidence has suggested that they are a source of blood histamine. Although capable of phagocytosis, this does not seem to be a common activity. They are numerous in allergic inflammations of the nose, sinuses, and bronchi (asthma). They also appear as a reaction to certain parasites, especially worms, and may be present in increased numbers in the blood. Subacute and chronic inflammations in the uterus, fallopian tubes, and intestinal tract (especially the appendix) often show numerous eosinophils.

Circulating eosinophils decrease in number under conditions of stress due to increased pituitary-adrenal cortical activity. When there is normal pituitary and adrenal cortical activity, epinephrine injection produces a decrease of circulating eosinophils. A decrease of this kind following the administration of adrenocorticotropic hormone of the pituitary (ACTH) is an indication of adrenal cortical response to the stimulating hormone.

Basophils. Basophils are present normally in small numbers in the blood (0.5%). Their cytoplasm contains granules with a strong affinity for basic dyes and may alter the color of such dyes (metachromasia). The metachromasia appears to be due to heparin content. The basophil also contains histamine, and nearly all the histamine in the bloodstream is carried by the basophil. The heparin content may be significant in blood coagulation and in fat transport and clearing in the bloodstream. Because of its histamine content, the basophil has a role in allergy, and particularly in the histamine shock of anaphylaxis. Mast cells, which also contain basophilic, metachromatic cytoplasmic granules, are found in connective tissues and sometimes appear particularly numerous in perivascular connective tissues. They have many similarities to the basophils of the blood. Mast cells have been shown to contain histamine, heparin, and 5-hydroxytryptamine. Their exact functional significance in relation to these substances is still undergoing clarification. It has been suggested that a function of mast cells is to store and release mucopolysaccharides for connective tissues. Mast cells may be present in increased numbers in some chronic or healing inflammations. The skin lesions of urticaria pigmentosa are characterized by large numbers of mast cells.

Macrophages. These large phagocytic cells are described under a variety of names, being termed monocytes, histiocytes, large mononuclear cells, polyblasts, endothelial cells, clasmatocytes, etc. They may be derived from monocytes, and perhaps also from lymphocytes, which have wandered from the bloodstream into the tissues. The majority of the macrophages, however, arise locally from the cells of the reticuloendothelial system, both those lining certain vascular spaces (sinusoids of liver, spleen, lymph nodes, and bone marrow) and those which are intimately mingled with fibroblasts in nearly all tissues. They also comprise the septal cells of the lung. The corresponding cells in the nervous system are the microglial cells.

Macrophages are large rounded or oval cells, with an oval or indented nucleus and abundant relatively dense cytoplasm devoid of specific granules. They are highly important in both acute and chronic inflammatory reactions. In acute inflammations they appear later than the polymorphonuclear leukocytes but may persist after the latter have broken down. They are actively mobile, slower in chemotactic movement than neutrophilic leukocytes, but highly phagocytic, ingesting bacteria, foreign material, and degenerating leukocytes, red cells, and tissue cells. Macrophages contain nucleases, proteinases, and carbohydrases and are rich in lipases. Thus they act as scavengers and prepare the way for repair. They are the predominant and characteristic cells in certain inflammatory processes, as in typhoid fever, and in tuberculosis, in which they are transformed into "epithelioid" cells by the waxy material of the capsule of the tubercle bacillus. Acquired resistance to bacterial infections depends in part on the presence of numerous macrophages in the tissues. Antibody production has been considered a function of mononuclear phagocytes, but this is still somewhat debatable. Macrophages in fixed tissues form bilirubin from hemoglobin.

Erythrocytes. Red blood cells appear in the exudate by passage through the excessively permeable vessel walls in the area of inflammation (diapedesis). In other cases there are small hemorrhages due to rupture of injured vessel walls, so that red cells are more abundant in the exudate. An exudate of hemorrhagic character is present in reactions to certain organisms, such as those of anthrax.

Giant cells. Multinucleated cells of giant size are generally present when there are materials which resist absorption, e.g., foreign bodies and bone, and are a particular feature of certain inflammatory processes, as in tuberculosis, and foreign body reactions. They appear to be formed by fusion of monocytes around some insoluble material, although nuclear division without cytoplasmic division probably occurs also. The Langhans giant cell of tuberculosis usually has peripheral nuclei, and foreign body giant cells have diffuse or central nuclei, but probably they are essentially the same. Other types of giant cells, not concerned with inflammation, are osteoclasts, megakaryocytes, tumor giant cells, and syncytial giant cells found in repair of muscle, nerves, and epithelium.

Phagocytosis. Phagocytosis is the process of ingestion of foreign material or particulate matter. Its importance in the inflammatory reaction and as a defense of the body was first stressed by Metchnikoff. The neutrophilic leukocytes and the large mononuclear cells or macrophages are the important phagocytic cells, although a number of other cells exhibit lesser

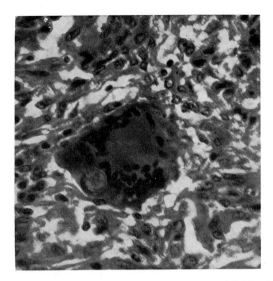

Fig. 3-3. Phagocytosis of the pathogenic fungus *Coccidioides immitis* by a giant cell in the human lung. Double-contoured organism is seen in the midst of nuclei. (×420.) (From Anderson, W. A. D., and Mc-Cutcheon, M.: Inflammation. In Anderson, W. A. D., editor: Pathology, ed. 5, St. Louis, 1966, The C. V. Mosby Co.)

degrees of phagocytic power. Macrophages occur as monocytes in the blood, as wandering cells in all organs, and as cells lining the sinusoids of the liver, spleen, and lymph nodes. The phagocytes are motile and in the case of the neutrophils are chemically attracted to the material to be ingested (chemotaxis). The actual mechanism of ingestion probably depends on surface tension changes. The phagocytosis of bacteria is influenced by the nature of their surfaces and is aided by substances present in tissue fluids, such as opsonins, tropins, and agglutinins. The more highly virulent bacteria tend to resist phagocytosis.

After being engulfed, bacteria, tissue and cell fragments, foreign particles, etc. tend to be digested by cellular enzymes. Not all bacteria are killed by phagocytosis. Some continue to live and even multiply within the phagocytes. This is true of the organisms of histoplasmosis, kala-azar, and leprosy. Tubercle bacilli also have considerable resistance to intracellular digestion.

Signs of acute inflammation

The classic clinical signs of an acute inflammation on the surface of the body, where it can be seen and felt, are swelling, heat, redness, pain, and disturbance of function. The swelling is due to the edema, exudation, and congestion in the area. The inflamed area feels hot in comparison with surrounding areas because the dilated vessels bring a large amount of warm blood to the area. The heat is only that of the interior of the body. The redness results from the vascular dilatation and congestion. Pain is due to the swelling and tension on tissues caused by the exudate, with pressure on nerves. The accumulation of chemical substances or of hydrogen ions in the area may contribute to the pain by their action on the nerve endings. The cells and tissues involved by inflammation have their normal function disturbed.

Types of inflammation

Classification of inflammation may be according to (1) duration and severity, as acute, subacute, and chronic; (2) the predominant nature of exudate, as serous, fibrinous, hemorrhagic, purulent, and catarrhal; and (3) the causative agent, as tuberculous, syphilitic, staphylococcic, foreign body reaction, allergic, etc. These classifications can often be combined. The ending "itis" is added to the name of an organ or tissue to indicate an inflammatory process, e.g., appendicitis—inflammation of the appendix; hepatitis—inflammation of the liver; dermatitis, inflammation of the skin. The various constituents of exudates often occur in combination, so that the reaction may be termed serofibrinous, fibrinopurulent, seromucinous, mucopurulent, etc. The inflammatory reactions induced by specific pathogenic organisms are described in Chapters 5 to 9, inclusive.

In some inflammatory processes proliferation (i.e., multiplication of cells) or necrosis may be more prominent than exudation. Proliferation is not great in most acute inflammations caused by bacteria, except in typhoid fever, in which there is early multiplication of mononuclear cells, but many viral infections stimulate proliferation in their early stages. In subacute inflammations proliferation is usually evident, and in chronic inflammations connective tissue proliferation is often predominant.

Necrosis may be a very prominent part of the inflammatory picture in certain infections, e.g., gas gangrene.

Acute inflammation. The acute inflammations are those which have a rapid course, the lesions clinically exhibiting the classic signs of heat, redness, swelling, and pain, or they are associated with severe or sharp constitutional reactions. Pathologically the prominent features are vascular changes and exudation of fluid and neutrophils, but there is insufficient time for development of connective tissue or accumulation of lymphocytes and plasma cells. An acute inflammation may subside or proceed to subacute or chronic phases.

Subacute inflammation. Subacute inflammation is considered a transitional phase between acute and chronic stages. The exudative changes of acute inflammation are still present, while the proliferative changes characteristic of a chronic process have begun. The use of this term probably has little value except for those cases which cannot clearly be classed as either acute or chronic.

Chronic inflammation. Chronic inflammation is a process in which exudative changes are prolonged, and proliferation (especially of connective tissues) forms a prominent feature. It may be simply a late stage of a more acute process, or the inflammation may be essentially chronic (productive) from the beginning. The latter is likely to be the case with organisms of low virulence whose pathogenicity tends to be nearly balanced by the resistance of the body. The predominant cells in chronic inflammation are lymphocytes, plasma cells, and macrophages, although a few polymorphonuclear leukocytes may be present. The proliferative activity, leading to the production of abundant scar tissue, may in itself be distinctly harmful. This is the case in chronic nephritis, in which the progressive glomerular scarring eventually results in functional failure of the kidneys.

Serous inflammation. Serous exudates, in which there is outpouring of abundant fluid in the inflammatory reaction, occur particularly in acute inflammations of serous cavities. The fluid contains a larger amount of protein and tends to have a higher specific gravity than a transudate. However, the specific gravity of fluids in serous cavities is not always an accurate guide to their nature. If fibrin precipitates from the fluid and appears on the inflamed surfaces, the exudate is termed serofibrinous. Reactions in other areas, such as some early acute inflammations of the skin, also may have an exudate of a predominantly serous nature.

Fibrinous inflammation. An abundance of fibrin in an exudate is frequently seen in inflammations of serous surfaces, such as the pericardium and peritoneum. It is also seen in the reaction to diphtheria bacilli, in which the fibrin entangles cells and necrotic material to form a false membrane on the surface. Fibrin formation decreases permeability of tissues and contributes to localization in acute inflammatory processes.

Hemorrhagic inflammation. Exudates containing so large a proportion of red blood cells as to have a grossly bloody appearance are usually due to highly virulent organisms which damage small blood vessels. The reactions in severe cases of smallpox, anthrax, and meningococcal and hemolytic streptococcal infections are often hemorrhagic.

Purulent (suppurative) inflammation. Purulent inflammations are those in which there is production of pus, which is a creamy, semifluid opaque substance containing mainly liquefied necrotic material and many neutrophilic leukocytes (pus cells), both intact and disintegrated. A suppurative reaction results from a number of injurious agents, mainly bacterial, but also from some chemicals such as turpentine and Aleuronat. Bacteria that commonly result in abundant pus production (pyogenic organisms) include staphylococci, gonococci, pyocyaneus bacilli, etc. Suppurative inflammation may be (1) on a surface, (2) localized in the tissues (abscess), or (3) diffusely spreading through tissue spaces (phlegmon or cellulitis).

An *abscess* is a localized area of pus accumulation within a tissue. It is found in an acute inflammation in which there is circumscribed destruction of tissue and a collection of many neutrophils, which undergo disintegration. Thus a cavity is formed that contains the pus. Abscesses are fluctuant swellings because of their semifluid consistency. Healing is facilitated by drainage and removal of the purulent material; otherwise a relatively slow process of absorption is necessary. Abscesses may become walled off by fibrous tissue, or they may spread and extend and the bacteria gain entrance into the bloodstream (pyemia) and form new (metastatic) abscesses in distant tissues. Boils or furuncles are small abscesses of the skin. A carbuncle is a more extensive or spreading abscess of the skin which tends to discharge at several points.

Most, but not all, acute inflammations in which neutrophils predominate in the exudate are purulent, i.e., produce pus. A common example in which pus production does not usually occur

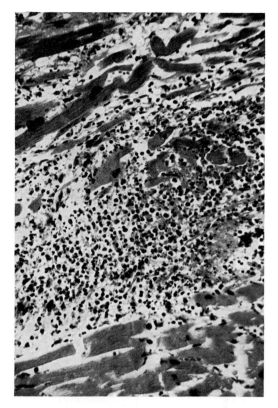

Fig. 3-4. Small abscess of the myocardium. Local collection of pus cells has replaced muscle fibers, undissolved fragments of which are seen near the edge of the lesion. (×370.) (From Anderson, W. A. D., and Mc-Cutcheon, M.: Inflammation. In Anderson, W. A. D., editor: Pathology, ed. 5, St. Louis, 1966, The C. V. Mosby Co.)

is pneumococcal (lobar) pneumonia (p. 450), although leukocytes are abundant in the alveolar exudate.

Phlegmonous inflammation. Phlegmonous inflammation (cellulitis) is characterized by a diffuse spread through tissue spaces. It causes the involved area to be tense, hard, and rigid. Very highly virulent strains of streptococci and other organisms may produce an acute diffuse spreading inflammation without any actual liquefaction and pus production. Actually, the term *cellulitis* may be used for this nonsuppurative, diffuse, spreading

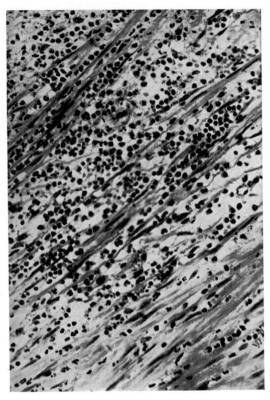

Fig. 3-5. Phlegmon of the appendix. Fibers of muscularis are separated by exudate in which many polymorphonuclear leukocytes are recognizable. Lesion is not circumscribed. (×270.) (From Anderson, W. A. D., and McCutcheon, M.: Inflammation. In Anderson, W. A. D., editor: Pathology, ed. 5, St. Louis, 1966, The C. V. Mosby Co.)

inflammation as well as for a suppurative one; the latter is more strictly referred to as a *phlegmon*.

Catarrhal inflammation. Catarrhal inflammation is a superficial and usually mild inflammation of mucous surfaces, in which mucinous material forms a prominent part of the exudate. It is commonly seen in inflammations of the upper respiratory tract and of the large intestine.

Pseudomembranous inflammation. Inflammations on mucous

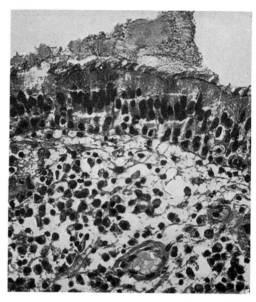

Fig. 3-6. Catarrhal inflammation in a nasal polyp. Tissue is edematous and infiltrated with leukocytes. Observe the mucous secretion beyond the ciliated epithelial cells at the top of the photograph. (×350.) (From Anderson, W. A. D., and McCutcheon, M.: Inflammation. In Anderson, W. A. D., editor: Pathology, ed. 5, St. Louis, 1966, The C. V. Mosby Co.)

surfaces caused by a powerful necrotizing agent, such as diphtheria toxin or certain irritant gases, are characterized by formation of a false membrane. The surface pseudomembrane is composed of necrotic epithelium, coagulated plasma, and fibrin (p. 119).

Ulcer. Ulcer is a loss of continuity or substance from a surface, skin, or mucous membrane, with inflammation of adjacent tissue. Necrotic tissue discharged from the surface, leaving the ulcer, is termed a slough.

Allergic inflammation. In allergy or hypersensitivity there is an alteration or heightening of tissue reactivity (hyperergy) to an antigen. The *Arthus phenomenon* is a marked local allergic inflammation and necrosis which results when an antigen is injected into the skin of an animal previously sensitized to the same antigenic protein. Altered sensitivity or allergy is probably an important factor in many diseases of both bacterial and other origins.

Disorders produced by hypersensitivity may be divided into two categories. In the first are the primary diseases of hypersensitivity, caused by agents which are not intrinsically harmful, including the hypersensitive reactions to pollens, dusts, foodstuffs, drugs and various industrial chemicals. The effects include the general group of anaphylactic reactions and the conditions of bronchial asthma and hay fever. The most commonly recognized allergic conditions affect the mucosa of the respiratory tract and nasal sinuses, the skin, and the mucosa of the gastrointestinal tract.

A nonprotein substance can induce specific sensitivity if its chemical constitution is such that it attaches to a normal protein of the body, producing thus a new "foreign" protein which stimulates production of specific antibodies. Such seems to be the mechanism by which sulfonamides and other drugs may produce hypersensitivity reactions.

It appears established that polyarteritis nodosa (p. 304) may be produced as a hypersensitivity reaction to certain antigens and that it has resulted from sensitivity to various drugs. Other lesions that can result from hypersensitivity include pneumonitis, myocarditis, focal necrosis of lymph nodes and spleen, focal collagen degeneration, tuberculoid granulomas in the viscera, purpura, agranulocytosis, hemolytic anemia, enteritis, arthritis, and glomerulonephritis.

In the allergic inflammations of the respiratory tract, such as asthma, one sees hyperplasia and hypersecretory activity of the mucous glands and goblet cells. The tissue is edematous, and eosinophils form a large and prominent proportion of the inflammatory cells. The basement membrane underlying mucosal epithelium becomes thickened and hyalinized. In more transient pneumonitis from hypersensitivity there is damage to alveolar capillaries, with exudation of fluid, hyaline alveolar membranes, focal exudation of leukocytes, and, in the more severe reactions, capillary thrombosis or rupture with hemorrhage into alveoli. Similar pulmonary lesions are sometimes seen in polyarteritis nodosa, rheumatic fever, and disseminated lupus erythematosus.

Myocarditis resulting from hypersensitivity is characterized by focal inflammatory infiltration, in which mononuclear cells may predominate but are accompanied by eosinophils and neutrophils. Some myocardial fibers may become necrotic in areas of intense inflammation. Such myocarditis may be seen in anaphylactic serum sickness, in allergic reactions to drugs such as penicillin, and in severe asthma.

Much experimental and clinical evidence indicates that glomerulonephritis (p. 363) is a lesion produced as a result of a hypersensitivity reaction. In human glomerulonephritis this is often related to a streptococcal infection, such as scarlet fever or tonsillitis, the evidence of glomerulonephritis appearing after a latent period long enough to permit development of antibody and hypersensitivity. Less frequently, acute nephritis has been noted to occur when a food to which the person had become sensitized was ingested. In experimental nephritis, comparable glomerular lesions can be produced by antigens possessing no primary toxicity; they appear only after a latent period sufficient to allow the development of hypersensitivity.

Suggestive but not conclusive is the evidence that hypersensitivity is important in a group of diseases characterized by widespread focal degeneration of collagen fibers and by endothelial and vascular injury. These conditions, which include rheumatic fever, rheumatoid arthritis, and disseminated lupus erythematosus, like polyarteritis nodosa, may have features of a type that hypersensitivity reactions are known to produce, such as fever, arthritis, purpura, cutaneous eruptions, pneumonitis, myocarditis, sterile pericarditis or pleuritis, necrosis and inflammation of arteries, and focal collagen degeneration called "fibrinoid degeneration." Fluorescent antibody techniques show that in these lesions there is a concentration of globulin, presumably antibody globulin, and little albumin.

Fibrinoid degeneration is characterized by the appearance of an eosinophilic, homogeneous, refractile substance with some of the staining properties of fibrin. At least in part or in some instances fibrinoid material does appear to be fibrin, i.e., derived from fibrinogen. There may be more than one kind of fibrinoid material, and some appears to be associated with precipitation of the acid mucopolysaccharide of the ground substance of connective tissue.

In the second category of diseases of hypersensitivity are conditions in which the causative agents (microorganisms, viruses, parasites) are themselves injurious, but in which the disease process may be intensified or modified by the development of hypersensitivity. Characteristic of tuberculous infection, this is known as the tuberculin type of hypersensitivity. The tissue reaction which results is important in chronic infections and may intensify the tissue damage and destruction. The intensified tissue reaction does not appear to be essential for the development of acquired immunity.

On the basis of experimental work, hypersensitivity has been divided into two types: (1) *immediate,* in which the reaction rapidly develops following administration of the antigen; and (2) *delayed,* in which the response occurs after twenty-four to forty-eight hours. A more fundamental difference between the two is that immediate hypersensitivity is associated with specific circulating antibodies, while in delayed hypersensitivity the reaction is mediated by antibody fixed to cells and is not dependent upon the usual serum antibodies. Examples of the immediate reaction are the Arthus phenomenon, anaphylactic shock, serum sickness, and certain other sensitivities to drugs, foods, or dusts. The classic example of delayed reaction is the tuberculin-type hypersensitivity. The tissue reactions that occur in certain infectious diseases, the rejection of homologous transplants, and autoimmune diseases show characteristics of delayed hypersensitivity.

Autoimmunity refers to an abnormal immunologic state in an individual that may result in damage to his own cells or tissues. Normally there is a mechanism in the body that prevents it from forming antibodies against its own antigens; but when this mechanism breaks down, certain "autoantibodies" form that react with the patient's own tissues. Among the theories that have been proposed to explain this abnormal state are the following: (1) normally, tissues and proteins (such as the ocular lens, myelin, thyroglobulin, spermatozoa) do not come in contact with antibody-forming cells, but as a result of injury or disease, they may be released into the bloodstream or infiltrated by antibody-forming cells, so that antibodies against the tissue antigens may be formed; (2) mutation of a gene occurs that controls antibody production in immunocompetent cells, altering their immunologic tolerance, so that a "forbidden" pattern of antibody occurs—namely, formation of antibody against tissue that was previously tolerated; (3) tissue antigen is altered by injury or disease or as a result of a somatic mutation, so that the body recognizes it as "foreign"; and (4) a foreign antigen (e.g., bacteria) in the body may stimulate antibodies against certain tissue antigens as well as against itself ("cross-reactive" antibodies).

Examples of autoimmune diseases are Hashimoto's disease of the thyroid gland, acquired hemolytic anemia, "allergic" encephalomyelitis, some forms of aspermatogenesis, and uveitis. Rheumatic fever, diffuse glomerulonephritis, rheumatoid arthritis, and certain of the other collagen diseases may be the result of autoimmunity.

Granulomatous inflammation. A number of infectious agents produce a chronic inflammation with predominant participation by reticuloendothelial cells and characterized by development of focal nodules composed predominantly of mononuclear types of cells and frequently proliferation of fibrous tissue. Multinucleated giant cells are often present. Such lesions are common in tuberculosis, leprosy, syphilis, various mycotic and protozoal infections, and in foreign body reactions.

Foreign body reaction. Foreign materials which are too large to be ingested by phagocytes become surrounded by macrophages, which fuse to form large multinucleated giant cells. Chronic inflammatory cells and fibroblastic proliferation appear in the surrounding tissue. The foreign material may gradually dissolve or, if indigestible, remain surrounded by giant cells and

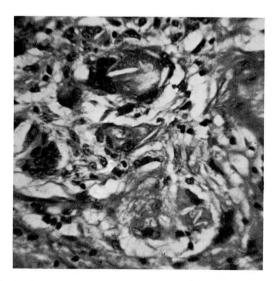

Fig. 3-7. Foreign body reaction with crystalline material in giant cells.

connective tissue. A foreign body reaction is seen around surgical sutures, cholesterol crystals, waxy materials, ingrowing hairs (e.g., in a pilonidal sinus), talcum powder from a surgeon's gloves in wounds, etc.

REPAIR OR HEALING

Repair or healing of an injured tissue (e.g., an area of inflammation or a wound) may be brought about by one or more of three processes: (1) *Resolution* (or restoration of the involved part to a normal state) may occur when the injury is slight and there is degeneration of parenchymal cells without necrosis, as in certain inflammations. After subsidence of the inflammatory response and recovery of the degenerated cells, the area is restored to normal. (2) *Healing by granulation tissue or scar formation* may take place if resolution is delayed or if the injury is severe enough to produce destruction of tissue. (3) There may be replacement of destroyed or lost cells by proliferating cells of similar type from adjacent living cells *(regeneration)*.

Repair by scar formation

A connective tissue reaction is a fundamental part of the response of the body to injury when tissue destruction occurs. Whether this reparative process is considered as part of inflammation or as a separate process is immaterial. Proliferative and reparative activity tends to follow the vascular and exudative phenomena of inflammation and often proceeds coincidentally. The final healed state is achieved by development of a connective tissue scar and by regeneration of cells. The degree of each and the balance between scarring and regeneration depend primarily on the nature and extent of the destroyed tissue.

The connective tissue cells which react to injury are the fibrocytes and the histiocytes (macrophages). The functions of the latter have already been noted. The changes of repair begin as a proliferation of young connective tissue cells (fibroblasts) and multiplication of small blood vessels by mitotic division of connective tissue and endothelial cells, respectively. The elongated fibroblasts and buds of endothelial cells grow into and permeate the exudate, producing a highly vascularized, reddish granular mass termed *granulation tissue*. The granulation tissue replaces the exudate and fills any gaps in the tissue.

This loose and highly vascularized young connective tissue is very resistant to infection. The replacement of necrotic material, exudate, or a thrombus by granulation tissue is referred to as *organization.*

A large abscess cavity or a tuberculous cavity from which the contents have been discharged may not be filled by granulation tissue; rather, a fibrous wall may form around it. If, however, the cavity can be collapsed so that the walls are in contact, healing may be completed.

In the healing of a surface wound or ulcer there is proliferation of epithelial cells at the edge, the cells gradually growing from the periphery to cover over the surface gap. When the area to be covered is too large, the epithelial cells may be unable to complete the covering process. If any skin appendages (e.g., hair follicles) persist in the depths of a wound, they may contribute proliferating epithelium to help cover the defect. Skin grafting may be used to supply other foci of epithelial cells from which extension can occur.

When organization is complete and the defect has been filled by granulation tissue, the capillaries decrease in size and number and largely disappear. The connective tissue shrinks, becomes condensed, develops more collagenous fibers, and acquires the appearance of adult connective tissue. The scar (cicatrix) thus produced is transformed slowly from a soft, red area to a pale or white, shrunken, firm fibrous tissue. Shrinkage or contracture may produce deformities of internal organs or disability if the scar is situated over a joint.

Adhesions of serous surfaces, as between visceral and parietal layers of peritoneum, pleura, or pericardium, frequently result from the organization of fibrinous exudates on apposing surfaces. In the pericardium the effect may be to obliterate the sac and throw an added functional burden on the heart. Adhesions as a result of arthritis may limit the movement of a joint.

The healing of a clean uninfected incised wound, in which there is little destruction of tissue and where the edges of the wound are held in apposition, occurs with a minimum of granulation and scar tissue and is referred to as "primary union," or "healing by first intention." The migrating and proliferating epithelium from the wound margins advances beneath the fibrin clot and eventually covers the defect. In the earlier stages of healing, according to recent work, the epithelium extends down into the wound along the sides of the incision, but as healing in

Fig. 3-8

Fig. 3-9

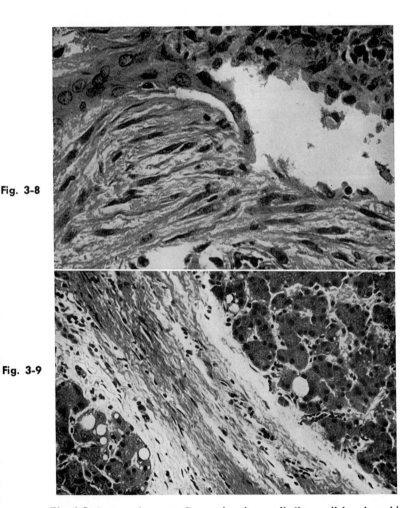

Fig. 3-8. Scar, early stage. Connective tissue cells lie parallel and are bipolar, provided with processes, and separated by extracellular collagen fibers. (×370.) (From Anderson, W. A. D., and McCutcheon, M.: Inflammation. In Anderson, W. A. D., editor: Pathology, ed. 5, St. Louis, 1966, The C. V. Mosby Co.)

Fig. 3-9. Scar, late stage, in cirrhotic liver. Scar composed largely of collagen fibers with scanty elongated nuclei of connective tissue cells. (×180.) (From Anderson, W. A. D., and McCutcheon, M.: Inflammation. In Anderson, W. A. D., editor: Pathology, ed. 5, St. Louis, 1966, The C. V. Mosby Co.)

the dermis occurs, the epithelial ingrowths regress and the surface epithelium completes its regeneration. Tensile strength, which is the factor that combats dehiscence of a surgical wound, increases progressively from the fourth to the fourteenth or fifteenth day of the healing process and is related to collagen formation. If there is much loss of tissue or if there is infection, the healing process is more delayed ("secondary union"), and greater scarring results. In this circumstance the infection must be overcome and the tissue defect be filled in by growth of granulation tissue. The granulation tissue must be built up slowly from the bottom and sides of the wound, and epithelium grows over the granulation tissue. In extensive, full-thickness wounds, it appears that a bed of granulation tissue is necessary before the defect undergoes epithelialization.

The nature and efficiency of the healing process may be influenced by various factors. The state of nutrition is of importance. Vitamin C is essential for proper collagen formation, and in severe deficiency of this vitamin, wounds fail to heal properly and are easily disrupted. Proper healing of bone is promoted by a sufficiency of vitamins C and D. An adequate protein diet also may be important, as some experiments have indicated that wound healing is delayed when plasma proteins are sufficiently reduced. Local factors that delay healing of a wound include excessive trauma of tissue during operation, poor blood supply to area, hematoma (collection of blood) in and about the wound, and infection. Foreign substances vary widely in the type of tissue response that they elicit. Certain metal alloys used to hold fractured bone fragments in position elicit only little tissue response and do not delay healing. Similarly, certain suture materials, such as silk, cotton, and some synthetic fibers, produce relatively little inflammatory response in tissues as compared with other materials, such as catgut. Sulfonamides applied to wounds cause some reaction in tissues but apparently not sufficient to retard healing seriously. Experimentally, administration of cortisone or ACTH appears to depress formation of granulation tissue and delay wound healing.

Regeneration

Regeneration is the replacement of lost or destroyed tissue by newly formed similar tissue, which is accomplished by proliferation of the adjacent living specialized cells. Physiologic regeneration is the reproduction of tissue lost by the normal wear of life, e.g., of surface epithelium, red blood cells, etc. Regeneration also acts to replace tissues destroyed by disease. Capacity for regeneration decreases as age increases and also is affected by the state of nutrition of the individual. The most important factor, however, is the type of tissue destroyed. The more highly specialized the tissue, the less is the capacity for regeneration. Thus, connective tissue regenerates most readily, whereas ganglion cells of the central nervous system have no ability to regenerate. The power of various tissues to regenerate may be outlined as follows:

Blood-forming tissues—regenerate readily

Bone—regenerates readily from periosteum or endosteum, with preliminary formation of uncalcified osteoid tissue

Cartilage—regenerates to some extent from perichondrium

Connective tissue—regenerates very readily

Glandular epithelium—individual cells regenerate, but specialized structures are not so readily formed; e.g., in the kidney, tubular epithelial cells regenerate easily, but whole tubular or glomerular structures are not replaced after their destruction

Liver—shows marked capacity for regeneration, provided its blood supply and connective tissue framework are intact

Myocardium—achieves practically no regeneration, except possibly in infancy

Neuroglial tissue—regenerates quite readily

Neurons of the central nervous system—have no power of regeneration

Peripheral nerve fibers—regenerate easily if the injured ends are in apposition

Striated voluntary muscle—has a limited capacity for replacement after a destruction of limited size

Surface epithelium—has marked capacity for regeneration, but in the skin associated structures such as hair follicles and sweat glands do not regenerate if completely destroyed

When tissues without the ability to regenerate are destroyed, repair is by connective tissue, or, in the central nervous system, by neuroglial cells. Even in tissues with good regenerative ability, such as the liver, the repair of extensive destruction is largely by connective tissue.

TRANSPLANTATION

Transplantation (or grafting) is not only a procedure for studying the reaction of a host to foreign cells or tissues, but also a useful procedure employed in the surgical repair or replacement of diseased tissues or organs.

Transplants (grafts) and the usual response to them by a

normal recipient (host) are as follows. An *autograft* is a tissue of one site engrafted to another site in the same individual. Such a graft is usually accepted and survives, causing a minimum of inflammatory reaction. A *homograft* is a tissue of one individual transplanted to another of the same species. A homograft between two genetically identical members of a species (e.g., monozygous twins or members of inbred strains) is an *isograft* (*isogeneic,* or *syngeneic* graft) that is accepted by the host; one between two genetically different members of the same species is an *allograft* (*allogeneic* graft). The latter excites an inflammatory reaction in the host's tissue, characterized by proliferation of cells (especially lymphocytes and fibroblasts). The graft undergoes necrosis and is rejected. This immunologic mechanism is referred to as the *homograft reaction.* A transplant between members of different species is a *heterograft (xenograft),* which induces more intense reaction and is more rapidly rejected than an allogeneic graft. It should be noted that isografts, which actually behave biologically like autografts, are separated from the group of homografts by some authors who consider only the allogeneic grafts as true homografts.

The immune response to a graft may be suppressed by several means, including whole body irradiation, the administration of certain drugs and steroid hormones, or a combination of irradiation and treatment with drugs or steroids. An unfortunate complication of such therapy is an increased susceptibility of the individual to infectious diseases. A serious consequence of homotransplantation that has been demonstrated in experimental animals and is theoretically possible in humans is the *graft-versus-host reaction;* i.e., a graft that contains immunologically competent cells may produce antibodies that can react against the antigens of the host's tissues.

Chapter 4

Disturbances of body water, electrolytes, and circulation of blood

For the maintenance of health there must be a proper distribution and normal balance of fluids and their electrolytes throughout the body, namely, in the intravascular, interstitial-lymph, and intracellular compartments. For the continuance of a state of equilibrium it is necessary that there be a normal circulation of blood and lymph and a constant, dynamic exchange of fluids and electrolytes among the body compartments through their intervening permeable membranes. When disturbances arise, they are either (1) abnormalities of body water (including electrolytes) and/or disturbances in the volume of circulating blood (i.e., edema, dehydration, electrolyte deficits and excesses, hyperemia, hemorrhage, and shock); or (2) disorders interfering with the circulation of blood (e.g., thrombosis and embolism) and their consequences (i.e., ischemia and infarction).

EDEMA

Edema is an excess of fluid within tissue spaces and/or serous cavities, either localized or generalized. An excessive accumulation of fluid in the pleural, pericardial, and peritoneal cavities is known as *hydrothorax, hydropericardium,* and *hydroperitoneum (ascites)* respectively. *Anasarca (dropsy)* is a generalized edema that is evident particularly in the subcutaneous tissues and in the body cavities. Subcutaneous edema causes swelling of the part, and the overlying tissue is usually tense. When severe, it "pits on pressure"; i.e., digital pressure displaces fluid from the tissue and leaves a dent, which slowly fills in as fluid flows back into the area after release of pressure *(pitting edema)*. Generally, an edematous organ is heavier and larger than normal, it may be boggy, and the capsule or covering serous surface may be stretched and glistening. The cut surface exudes fluid, which in the case of the lung may be frothy, since it is contained in alveoli where it is mixed with air. Microscopically, the fluid may be very pale and barely stained, or it appears as an acidophilic material, the density of which varies in direct proportion to the amount of protein it contains.

Factors that govern the interchange between intravascular fluid (blood plasma) and interstitial fluid and that serve to maintain normal volumes in these compartments are: (1) hydrostatic pressure of the blood, tending to force fluid through capillary walls; (2) colloid osmotic pressure of plasma proteins, which tends to hold fluid in the vessels and to draw it from tissues into the blood; (3) permeability of vascular endothelium; (4) extravascular tissue factors (hydrostatic pressure and osmotic pressure), which normally are so low they do not counteract the action of the same type of forces in the vessels; (5) normal concentration of sodium in intravascular and interstitial fluids; and (6) free flow of lymph in the lymphatic vessels, which normally serve as a route for return of some of the extravascular fluid and its protein to the blood. Disturbances in any of these factors may lead to edema. Although edema may result from any one of the following mechanisms, frequently several factors are operative at the same time in a particular disorder.

Increased hydrostatic pressure in capillaries. Normally the hydrostatic pressure in the arterial end of capillaries is such that the reverse force exerted by plasma proteins is overcome and fluid flows into intercellular spaces; whereas in the venous end of capillaries the hydrostatic pressure is low and the fluid that has not been carried away by lymphatics is drawn from tissue spaces into the blood. This balance of hydrostatic pressure is upset by passive or venous congestion. The generalized venous congestion of heart failure is the most common cause. Hence, cardiac failure is commonly associated with widespread edema *(cardiac edema)*. However, in cardiac failure, sodium retention also influences the development of edema. Localized venous congestion may also cause edema, e.g., edema of the lower extremities resulting from thrombosis of the iliac veins or from pressure on these veins by a tumor or a pregnant uterus, or ascites associated with portal congestion in cirrhosis of the liver. It is to be noted that additional factors are operative in the development of ascites in hepatic cirrhosis, e.g., hypoproteinemia, renal retention of sodium and water, and increased production of lymph in the liver because of intrahepatic passive congestion. Also, edema may occur elsewhere in the body because of the low plasma proteins and sodium and water retention.

Decreased plasma colloid osmotic pressure. The osmotic pressure of any body fluid is dependent upon the concentration of its active chemical constituents, including the electrolytes. The largest part of the total osmotic pressure of the plasma is caused by the crystalloids, but since they readily diffuse through the vascular membrane, they are not effective in the interchange of the fluids. The nondiffusible colloids, particularly the proteins, which are more abundant in the blood plasma than in the interstitial tissue, make up a relatively small part of the total osmotic pressure of the blood, but they represent the effective part *(colloid osmotic pressure)* that promotes the exchange of water between the intravascular and interstitial compartments.

Edema is caused by a lowering of the colloid osmotic pressure of blood, which results when there is a decrease in plasma proteins (hypoproteinemia), particularly in the albumin fraction, since the osmotic attraction of plasma depends largely upon the albumin content. Edema tends to appear when the plasma albumin is reduced to a level below 2.5 grams per 100 ml. A common cause of hypoproteinemic edema is renal disease associated with prominent loss of protein in the urine, e.g., in the nephrotic syndrome *(renal, or nephrotic, edema)*. This type of edema may also be caused by the failure of sufficient formation of serum albumin, as in undernourishment from famine *(nutritional edema)* or in *hepatic disease* (e.g., cirrhosis). However, it has been shown that hypoproteinemia is not always present in starvation, so that perhaps other factors, such as sodium and water retention, may play a role. Also, in renal and liver diseases, sodium and water retention as well as other factors contribute to the edema.

Increased vascular permeability. Vascular endothelium acts as a semipermeable membrane in that normally water, crystalloids, and dissolved gases pass through it freely but only a very small amount of protein is permitted to pass through. Agents that are injurious to the endothelium increase its permeability to protein colloids. Diffusion of proteins, which occurs apparently through the walls of the venules as well as the capillaries, lowers the plasma osmotic pressure and increases the interstitial fluid osmotic pressure, both factors favoring the development of edema. Systemic edema resulting from increased endothelial permeability occurs in a variety of conditions, including *severe infections, anaphylactic reactions, poisonings* with drugs and chemicals, and *anoxia,* such as may occur in secondary shock. The generalized edema in *acute glomerulonephritis* may be caused by increased vascular permeability, although retention of sodium and water and hypoalbuminemia may be significant causative factors also. Local edema resulting from increased endothelial permeability is seen in the inflammatory reaction *(inflammatory edema)* and in *angioneurotic edema,* the latter being allergic or neurogenic in origin.

Tissue factors. Normally the tissue fluid colloid osmotic pressure is so small that it is insignificant in opposing the osmotic pressure of the plasma. However, in clinical states associated with increased vascular permeability or when there is lymphatic obstruction, the protein concentration of the interstitial fluid increases, which assists the production of edema. An *increased sodium concentration* of tissue fluid occurring in those states characterized by renal retention of this ion contributes to edema. The relatively low hydrostatic pressure of the interstitial fluid in certain areas of the body (e.g., in the subcutaneous tissues of the eyelids and external genitalia) enhances the edema caused by other factors.

Lymphatic obstruction. *Lymphedema* is the term applied to an increase of interstitial fluid resulting from interference with the flow of lymph from an area of the body. This may be caused by surgical removal of the axillary lymph nodes, as in radical mastectomy for cancer of the breast. Lymphatic obstruction may be caused by infiltrating cells of a malignant neoplasm, by extrinsic pressure of tumors, by inflammatory fibrosis, or by parasites (as in filariasis). An enlargement of the scrotum or an extremity resulting from lymphedema and associated fibrosis is often referred to as *elephantiasis.* Congenital lymphedema is caused by abnormal development of the lymphatic vessels, which causes defective lymph drainage (e.g., *Milroy's disease*).

Sodium and water retention. Retention of sodium occurs when its excretion in the urine is less than the intake. The excess sodium results in a retention of water. With progressive retention of sodium and water there is expansion of the extracellular fluid volume, both intravascularly and interstitially, with resultant edema. At first the retention of sodium produces an increased concentration of this ion in the extracellular fluids, so that *hypertonicity* exists. In response to this state, water is retained until normal concentration of sodium *(isotonicity)* is reached. As a rule, the amounts of sodium and water retained are proportionate, so that the serum in edematous patients contains a normal concentration of sodium *(normonatremic edema)*. In some patients a greater amount of water is retained, so that there is a low concentration of sodium *(hypotonicity)* in the plasma and interstitial fluid *(hyponatremic edema)*, despite an excess of total body sodium.

The retention of these substances occurs in a variety of edematous states, as in *congestive heart failure, hepatic cirrhosis,* the *nephrotic syndrome,* and possibly *acute glomerulonephritis.* This mechanism of edema production may be secondary in these conditions, although some writers believe that it is primary in cardiac failure, resulting from decreased cardiac output and renal blood flow (forward failure) or from an increase in circulating aldosterone. The retention of sodium may be caused by intrinsic renal mechanisms or extrarenal hormonal or neural influences, e.g., reduction in glomerular filtration, enhanced tubular reabsorption, and increased filtration factor in the kidneys; and increased secretion of aldosterone or decreased rate of inactivation of aldosterone by the liver. A factor causing or contributing to retention of water is increased secretion of antidiuretic hormone (ADH). The stimulus for aldosterone secretion may be a reduction in the volume of extracellular fluid, particularly the intravascular phase, sodium deprivation, positive potassium balance, or oversecretion of a trophic hormone (possibly angiotensin). Other hormones besides aldosterone that enhance renal tubular absorption of sodium are ACTH, testosterone, progesterone, and estrogen. Premenstrual edema may be related to the sodium-retaining properties of progesterone and estrogen.

DEHYDRATION

Dehydration is a disturbance of water balance in which body water is below the normal level; but there is also an accompanying abnormality of the electrolytes. Dehydration may be the result of water depletion or of sodium depletion, but usually both types of depletion exist in a given case, although one or the other may predominate.

Water depletion (primary dehydration). Pure *water depletion,* or *primary dehydration,* occurs as a result of restriction of intake of water, as in a patient who has a severe physical or mental illness and cannot or refuses to drink or in an unfortunate person in the desert or at sea without fresh water. The increased sodium concentration (hypertonicity) that occurs in the extracellular fluids draws water from the cells (intracellular dehydration), which results in thirst; it also stimulates the release of ADH, leading to oliguria. In addition to thirst and oliguria, decreased salivary flow, dryness of mouth, weakness, and subsequently mental disturbances are characteristic features. Death occurs in seven to ten days, as a rule, after complete water deprivation.

Sodium depletion (**secondary dehydration**). *Sodium depletion,* or *secondary dehydration,* is caused by loss of electrolyte-containing fluids from the body, which occurs commonly by means of vomiting, diarrhea, pancreatic and biliary fistulas, and continuous aspiration through intubation. It may also result from excessive perspiration when only water is taken as a replacement or from loss of sodium in the urine in certain conditions such as Addison's disease, diabetic acidosis, cerebral salt-wasting syndrome, and in some instances of chronic renal disease. Lack of sodium in the diet does not cause sodium depletion in a healthy subject, as a rule, because the kidney can conserve this ion effectively. As a result of sodium depletion, the extracellular fluid becomes hypotonic, inhibiting the release of ADH, so that the kidneys excrete water in an attempt to maintain normal extracellular sodium concentration. The result is a decrease in the volumes of the plasma and interstitial fluid, but because the extracellular fluids are hypotonic in relation to the intracellular fluid, water flows into the cells. Nausea, vomiting, cramps, lassitude, headache, and loss of weight are common symptoms. Alterations of serum potassium and chloride and a disturbance of acid-base balance may also appear. The lowered blood volume may result in decreased cardiac output, low blood pressure, a tendency to orthostatic fainting, and decreased glomerular filtration with subsequent nitrogen retention. When there is a great reduction in the volume of extracellular fluid, peripheral circulatory failure (shock) may develop.

ELECTROLYTE DISTURBANCES

The electrolytes play a significant role in the maintenance of osmotic pressures and of normal balance and distribution of the body fluids, and are also concerned with the preservation of acid-base balance and of normal neuromuscular irritability. In the extracellular fluids the electrolytes that are highest in concentration are sodium and chloride ions, next are bicarbonate ions, and in comparatively low concentration are potassium, magnesium, phosphate, and sulfate ions. The blood plasma and interstitial fluid have a similar chemical composition, except for the presence of a larger amount of protein in the former, which is responsible for adjustments of the concentration of diffusible ions in order to preserve the total cation-anion equivalence (Gibbs-Donnan equilibrium). The intracellular water, in contrast, has a high concentration of potassium and a low concentration of sodium and chloride. It contains more phosphate, sulfate, magnesium, and protein but less bicarbonate than the extracellular fluids.

A *decreased sodium concentration* in the plasma *(hyponatremia)* may be brought about by sodium depletion (depletional hyponatremia) or by retention of water over and above the retention of sodium (dilutional hyponatremia). Sodium depletion was discussed on p. 87. Dilutional hyponatremia occurs in such states as overhydration (water intoxication), congestive heart failure and cirrhosis of the liver with impaired water diuresis, and other entities thought to be caused by an excess secretion of ADH. Usually hyponatremia, especially when severe, results in various clinical manifestations. Instances of "asymptomatic hyponatremia" have been described in patients with the salt-wasting or salt-losing syndromes associated with cerebral or pulmonary disease (tuberculosis, bronchogenic carcinoma) or without evidence of other disease (idiopathic).

An *increased sodium concentration* in the blood *(hypernatremia)* occurs when there is either an output of water in excess of sodium or a severe restriction of water with dehydration (see water depletion, p. 86). It may occur in patients with cerebral lesions (encephalomalacia, hemorrhage, lacerations, malignant tumors, and meningitis), which probably interfere with production of ADH, causing an acute diabetes insipidus that is not compensated by adequate water intake. In primary aldosteronism, hypernatremia develops while potassium concentration is decreased. Acute salt poisoning has been reported in infants who were inadvertently given a formula containing salt instead of sugar. Central nervous system alterations may be produced by hypernatremia. There is a relationship between excess sodium and hypertension.

Hypopotassemia (hypokalemia) is caused by inadequate intake (as in starvation) or by excessive loss of potassium from the body (as in vomiting, diarrhea, diuresis, adrenal cortical hyperactivity, administration of adrenocortical hormones, and surgical trauma). In familial periodic paralysis there is hypokalemia without an increased excretion of potassium. It is probable that in this disease the potassium is shifted into the muscle cells. The effects of hypokalemia include foci of necrosis and leukocytic infiltration in the myocardium, electrocardiographic changes, fatty degeneration and necrosis of renal tubular epithelium, vacuolar nephropathy, and metabolic alkalosis.

Hyperpotassemia (hyperkalemia) does not occur as commonly as hypopotassemia. It may be seen in patients who receive excessive administrations of potassium parenterally or by mouth, in acute renal failure and in chronic renal disease with inability to excrete potassium, and in adrenal insufficiency with resultant retention of potassium. It may also result from a shift of cell potassium to the extracellular fluids as a result of injury to cells by noxious agents (e.g., anoxia in late stages of secondary shock) or in destruction of cells (e.g., extensive hemolysis of red blood cells). The effects of hyperkalemia include paresthesias, flaccid paralysis, listlessness, mental confusion, decline in blood pressure, and certain electrocardiographic changes.

A decreased concentration of chloride in the plasma *(hypochloremia)* occurs in vomiting, adrenal insufficiency, acute infections, and renal failure. *Hyperchloremia* may be seen in patients receiving parenteral administrations of hypertonic sodium chloride solutions and in those suffering from water depletion. Alterations in acid-base balance may result with changes in chloride concentration; hypochloremia is counterbalanced by increased bicarbonate concentration causing metabolic alkalosis; hyperchloremia is associated with decreased bicarbonate concentration and metabolic acidosis.

The concentration of magnesium of the plasma is decreased *(hypomagnesemia)* in chronic alcoholism, prolonged diuresis in congestive heart failure, rehydration therapy for dehydration in diabetic acidosis, and starvation. It causes muscular twitching, choreiform movements, convulsions, and coma. *Hypermagnesemia* is seen in severe dehydration, untreated diabetic acidosis, renal failure, or excess administration of magnesium. Clinical features include muscle relaxation, lethargy, coma, and respiratory failure.

HYPEREMIA (CONGESTION)

An increased volume of blood within dilated blood vessels in an organ or a part of the body is referred to as *hyperemia,* or *congestion.* It may be rapid in onset (*acute* congestion) or may occur gradually and be prolonged (*chronic* congestion).

Active hyperemia. Active hyperemia is the result of increased arterial blood to a part, is usually acute, and is characterized by dilatation of arterioles and capillaries. It occurs during functional activity of any tissue (e.g., exercised muscle) and as a result of emotion or heat (flushing of skin). It also occurs in the early stages of inflammation. Usually the only change in active hyperemia is a deep pink or red appearance of the affected tissue (*erythema*). In the case of acute inflammation the additional factor of endothelial damage causes edema.

Passive hyperemia. Passive hyperemia is brought about by diminished venous blood flow from an area and is characterized by dilatation of the veins and capillaries. It may be acute but

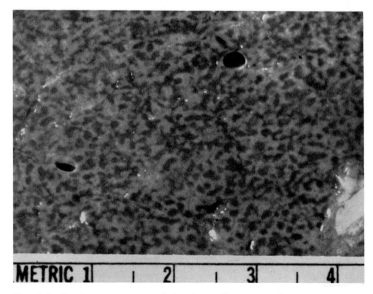

Fig. 4-1. Passive congestion of the liver. The cut surface of the organ shows a "nutmeg" appearance from the centrolobular zonal accumulation of blood.

often is prolonged, resulting in chronic passive congestion. *Hypostatic congestion* is a form of passive hyperemia that involves the dependent portion of an organ and is caused by gravitation of the blood in a relaxed vascular system. *Local venous congestion* is caused by interference with the venous outflow from an organ or a part of the body, as in venous thrombosis, extrinsic pressure on a vein by a tumor or other masses, and constriction by ligatures, tight bandages, scar tissue, hernia, volvulus, etc. The severity of the congestion depends upon the adequacy of the collateral circulation. *Systemic venous congestion* is observed in congestive heart failure, affects organs and tissues throughout the body, and is commonly associated with dyspnea, cyanosis, and edema.

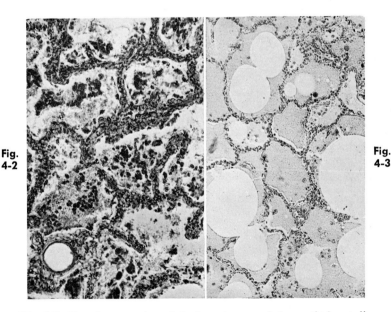

Fig. 4-2. Chronic congestion of the lung in case of rheumatic heart disease with mitral insufficiency. Alveolar walls are thickened. Alveolar spaces contain pigment-laden macrophages and precipitated protein. (From Millard, M.: Lung, pleura, and mediastinum. In Anderson, W. A. D., editor: Pathology, ed. 5, St. Louis, 1966, The C. V. Mosby Co.)

Fig. 4-3. Pulmonary edema. Vacuoles of entrapped air in some alveoli. (From Millard, M.: Lung, pleura, and mediastinum. In Anderson, W. A. D., editor: Pathology, ed. 5, St. Louis, 1966, The C. V. Mosby Co.)

In certain organs chronic passive congestion produces characteristic changes. The *liver* is enlarged and the cut surface has a mottled appearance, resembling the cut surface of a nutmeg *(nutmeg liver)*. The mottling is caused by redness of the central part of the liver lobules around the central veins, contrasted with grayish peripheral portions of the lobules. Because of the anoxia of continued congestion, the liver cells in the centrolobular zones undergo fatty metamorphosis and/or atrophy. In more severe congestion, necrosis of the cells occurs.

The congested *spleen* is enlarged and has a tense capsule and a dark red, firm cut surface. The sinuses are engorged with blood. In long-standing cases the trabeculae and walls of the sinusoids undergo fibrosis, and the malpighian corpuscles are atrophic. Iron deposits are likely to occur in passive congestion caused by portal hypertension. They occur in areas of hemorrhage and are followed by fibrosis (siderofibrotic nodules, or Gandy-Gamna nodules).

Chronic passive congestion of the *lung* results in edema and extravasation of red blood cells from the distended capillaries into alveolar spaces. The hemoglobin of the red cells breaks down, forming hemosiderin, which is ingested by macrophages. The hemosiderin-laden macrophages are sometimes referred to as "heart failure cells" because of their frequent association with congestive heart failure. In long-standing cases fibrosis of the edematous alveolar walls develops, and this together with the brownish pigmentation of hemosiderin produces a gross appearance of the lung called "brown induration" (p. 468).

HEMORRHAGE

Hemorrhage denotes escape of blood from the cardiovascular system, usually the result of *rupture* of a vessel or the heart. Extravasation of erythrocytes because of their passage through apparently unruptured capillary walls is known as *hemorrhage by diapedesis*.

Hemorrhage may be classified as (1) *capillary, venous, arterial,* or *cardiac* (depending on origin); (2) *external* or *internal* (in relation to the body); (3) *traumatic* (when incident to various wounds) or *spontaneous* (when it occurs in the absence of obvious trauma); and (4) according to type of lesion, e.g., *petechiae* (minute hemorrhagic spots, usually of capillary origin), *ecchymoses* (larger, blotchy areas of extravasated blood), *purpura* (characterized by spontaneous hemorrhages, varying in size from petechiae to ecchymoses throughout various tissues of the body), *hematoma* (localized collection of blood, forming tumorlike swelling in the tissue), *apoplexy* (copious effusion of blood in an organ, as in the brain).

Hemorrhages may be designated according to their location, e.g., *epistaxis* (bleeding from the nose); *hemoptysis* (expectoration of blood from hemorrhage in the lungs or elsewhere in the respiratory tract); *hematemesis* (vomiting of blood); *melena* (presence of dark, decomposed blood in the stools); *hemothorax, hemopericardium, hemoperitoneum* (hemorrhage in the pleural, pericardial, and peritoneal cavities, respectively); and *hematuria* (blood in the urine).

Local hemorrhages may be caused by trauma, as in abrasions, lacerations, contusions, fractures, and penetrating injuries; or it may occur in the absence of trauma (i.e., spontaneously) as a result of rupture of diseased vessels or the heart (e.g., atherosclerosis, cystic medial degeneration, inflammations, and congenital defects of arteries, which cause weakening of arterial walls, often with aneurysmal formation; erosions and ulcerations of the gastrointestinal tract, producing discontinuity of vascular walls; neoplastic invasion of vessels; and infarct of the myocardium). Hypertension (high blood pressure) may be a factor in the development of local hemorrhage, particularly if there is underlying disease of the arteries (e.g., in cerebral atherosclerosis).

Systemic hemorrhages are seen in a group of disorders characterized by a *hemorrhagic diathesis* (i.e., a hemorrhagic tendency), in which multiple tissues and organs are involved, often simultaneously. These disorders are caused by defects of the coagulation mechanism, by defects of the vascular walls, or by both, e.g., hemophilia, hypoprothrombinemia, hypofibrinogenemia, the various purpuras associated with platelet deficiencies, hereditary hemorrhagic telangiectasia, vitamin C deficiency, Schönlein-Henoch ("anaphylactoid") purpura, and purpuras associated with endothelial damage caused by anoxia, chemicals, snake venom, fulminating infections, etc.

The effects of hemorrhage may be local or systemic. The *local effects* may be of a mechanical nature and will depend on the size and the location of the hemorrhage, e.g., subdural hematoma with pressure on the brain; pericardial hemorrhage causing interference with filling of the cardiac chambers— *cardiac tamponade;* and hemorrhage in the larynx, causing swelling of tissues and narrowing of the lumen, resulting in asphyxiation. If the hemorrhage is slight, it may be completely resorbed, leaving little or no trace behind, or it may undergo fibrosis (organization). Discoloration may occur at the site because of breakdown of erythrocytes and formation of hemo-globin-derived pigments. *Systemic effects* of hemorrhage depend upon the rapidity of bleeding (acute or chronic) and the amount of blood loss. Acute hemorrhage may be massive enough to cause peripheral circulatory failure (shock) and death. A tran-sient anemia may result from acute blood loss, which may be followed by response of the bone marrow to produce erythro-cytes. Chronic blood loss leads to an iron-deficiency anemia of the hypochromic type. Certain compensatory mechanisms may be activated as a result of a sudden loss of a considerable amount of blood: (1) Lowered blood pressure affects the presso-receptors, altering impulses to the cardiac and vasomotor centers and resulting in increased cardiac rate, peripheral vasoconstric-tion, and increased secretion of catecholamines (the latter con-tributing to the vasoconstriction). (2) Lack of oxygen in the circulation (a) activates the chemoreceptors and (b) increases renal secretion of a vasoexcitor material (VEM) or renin (which is important in the formation of angiotensin), and both contrib-ute to peripheral vasoconstriction. (3) Under the influence of epi-nephrine the spleen contracts and discharges blood into the cir-culation. These mechanisms assist in the recovery of the blood pressure and divert the blood from the less vital to the vital organs (viz., heart and brain).

SHOCK

Shock is a circulatory disturbance characterized by a disparity between the effective circulating blood volume and the volume capacity of the vascular system. A transient form, so-called "pri-mary shock," results from a neurogenic vasodilatation with pooling of blood in the peripheral microcirculation, particularly in the splanchnic area, and diversion of blood from the brain, leading to prostration and unconsciousness. This condition occurs immediately after trauma or may result from pain due to various causes or from emotional reactions (e.g., fear, grief, and emotion associated with the sight of blood or a wound). The more serious, and sometimes fatal, disorder is true shock, often referred to as "secondary shock," which tends toward progressive circula-tory failure with resultant damage to the body tissues. This is the form usually meant when the term "shock" is used without qualification and the one that is to be discussed. Among the usual clinical manifestations are weakness, cold moist skin, collapse of superficial veins, shallow respirations, rapid weak pulse, low blood pressure, and oliguria.

The *causes* of shock include many forms of injury and disease, e.g., trauma, hemorrhage, burns, surgical operations, bacterial infections, drug toxicity, ionizing radiation, intestinal obstruction, perforated viscera, dehydration, and cardiac insufficiency (as in myocardial infarction). The types of shock are generally classified on the basis of the principal cause, e.g., traumatic shock, hemorrhagic shock, surgical shock, septic (or endotoxin) shock, cardiac shock, and so forth.

The basic hemodynamic mechanism of shock is summarized as follows: *reduction of effective circulating blood volume* → *decreased venous return to heart* → *decreased cardiac output* → *reduced blood flow* → *reduced delivery of oxygen to tissues (anoxia).* The one major feature in the pathogenesis of shock is the reduction of blood flow and resultant anoxic state of the tissues to the point where metabolic needs are no longer met. If the anoxic state is permitted to continue, it aggravates and perpetuates the circulatory deficiency. Each of the clinical states mentioned previously sets this hemodynamic mechanism into motion by means of one or more of the following *initiating factors:* (1) reduction of actual blood volume because of (a) local loss of blood and/or plasma at the site of a wound, burn, or operation, or (b) escape of fluid into the interstitial compartment as a result of generalized increased vascular permeability, or (c) loss of fluid as by dehydration; (2) increased capacity of the vascular system, as by vasodilatation, in the peripheral microcirculation with pooling of blood, in essence, a reduction of effective circulating blood volume; and (3) decreased cardiac output, as in myocardial infarction or cardiac tamponade. In the type of septic shock caused by powerful endotoxins of gram-negative organisms ("endotoxin shock"), the initiating events are not as well understood as in other forms of shock. On the basis of experimental work there is evidence that vasoconstriction in the microcirculation or thrombosis in these minute vessels may be the initiating factor by impeding the venous return to the heart. Certain hemodynamic studies in cases of clinical septic shock, however, suggest that in some patients peripheral vasodilatation may be the initiating factor, perhaps caused by circulating polypeptides (plasma kinins) activated by endotoxins, possibly through release of proteolytic enzymes from cells injured by the toxins. When shock is associated with actual loss of blood volume, it is termed *hypovolemic;* that which is not accompanied by actual loss of blood, as in vasodilatation with peripheral pooling of blood or in cardiac shock, is known as *normovolemic.*

Vasoconstriction of the peripheral small vessels (other than that which may be produced by the direct effect of endotoxins in "endotoxin shock") is the basic compensatory phenomenon in shock, resulting from neural and hormonal influences in response to diminished blood volume and anoxia. The participation of pressoreceptors, chemoreceptors, catecholamines, and humoral factors (e.g., renin, vasoexcitor material) from hypoxic kidneys is similar to that already discussed in relation to acute hemorrhage (q.v.). While peripheral vasoconstriction aids in maintaining systemic blood pressure, it may, if prolonged, accentuate the anoxic effects upon the tissues, particularly in the splanchnic region, already present as a result of the initial reduction in blood volume. The persistent vasoconstriction may lead to ischemic necrosis of certain organs (e.g., liver and intestines) and ultimately to paralysis of vascular muscle (vasodilatation) and decreased venous return to the heart. Thus a state of *irreversibility,* or decompensation, in shock ensues by the establishment of a "vicious circle."

A number of other mechanisms have been suggested as being responsible for irreversibility in shock as follows: (1) Ischemic myocardium causes decreased cardiac output, thus perpetuating the vicious circle. (2) Cerebral ischemia results in depression of the vasomotor center with consequent vasodilatation and pooling of the blood in the peripheral circulation, reducing the venous return to the heart and lessening the cardiac output. (3) As a result of the hypoxic state, a vasodilator material (VDM) is released from the liver, spleen, and skeletal muscle and, unable to be inactivated by the hypoxic liver, causes terminal vessels to be refractory to epinephrine, resulting in vasodilatation. (4) A product of bacterial activity (e.g., endotoxin) derived from the intestinal flora is absorbed in the circulation; and, since the antibacterial defense mechanism of the reticuloendothelial system of the liver and spleen is impaired by anoxia (especially as a result of persistent vasoconstriction), the resulting endotoxemia accentuates the vasoconstriction that was originally induced as a compensatory mechanism. The endotoxins elicit this effect by stimulating sympathetic activity. It is within the realm of speculation that endotoxins may produce the opposite effect in some patients, namely, microcirculatory vasodilatation, by means of its activation of vasoactive plasma kinins. (5) Hemorrhagic lesions in the intestines, caused by persistent vasoconstriction or by thrombosis in minute vessels, leads to loss of blood and serum into the intestinal lumen and a reduced circulating blood volume. This mechanism is much more characteristic of shock induced experimentally in dogs than of naturally occurring shock in man. (6) Decreased venous return may result from multiple intravascular thrombi. The tendency to thrombosis is the result of several possible factors, including stasis and sludging of blood, anaerobic metabolism with excess of lactic acid in the blood that neutralizes the normally present heparin, increased coagulability of the blood because of the release of a clot-promoting factor caused by the catecholamines in the circulation, and endothelial damage resulting from anoxia or noxious products released from damaged tissue. (7) The hypoxic state causes damage to capillaries and venules leading to vasodilatation and/or increased vascular permeability with escape of fluid to the interstitial spaces, both resulting in a decreased return of venous blood to the heart.

The *morphologic changes* in shock include capillovenous hyperemia; petechiae in serous cavities; edema, at least in certain organs such as the lungs; congested gastrointestinal mucosa, with petechiae and acute ulcers, especially in the stomach; degenerative changes in the kidneys, liver, heart, and adrenal glands; foci of necrosis in the lymph nodes, spleen, pancreas, and liver; and the characteristic lesion in the kidneys known as "hemoglobinuric nephrosis," or "lower nephron nephrosis" (p. 385). The blood is hypercoagulable in the early stages of shock but is later characterized by hypocoagulability and fibrinolysis.

THROMBOSIS

A *thrombus* is a mass formed from the constituents of the blood within the vessels or the heart during life; the process of its formation is known as *thrombosis*. The typical thrombus is initiated by clumping of the platelets and is further developed by coagulation of the blood (fibrin formation). A thrombus consisting entirely of erythrocytes or of platelets is not as common. Sometimes referred to as an "antemortem clot," a thrombus is to be differentiated from a clot that forms extravascularly in an area of hemorrhage or from that occurring within the vessels after death (postmortem clot).

Formation and structure of a thrombus. The initial event in thrombosis appears to be the adherence of platelets to the lining endothelium. A small mound of agglutinated platelets forms the *primary platelet thrombus.* Disintegration of some of the platelets causes liberation of a substance that is used in the generation of plasma thromboplastin, which initiates the clotting mechanism; thromboplastin converts prothrombin to thrombin, which in turn, reacts with fibrinogen to form fibrin. Whether or not tissue thromboplastin from an injured vessel wall contributes to the initial formation of a thrombus is uncertain. As the thrombus develops, the platelets project from the vessel wall in the form of lamellae, bent in the direction of blood flow, and these in turn branch out as secondary lamellae, giving rise to a coral-like mass. The bands of platelets, outlined by leukocytes and interlaid with fibrin, erythrocytes, and other leukocytes, are known as the *lines of Zahn,* which appear grossly as wavy, pale gray-white striae. The characteristic structure of the thrombus depends upon the velocity of blood flow. When the mass grows sufficiently large to obstruct the flow of blood, a homogeneous, dark red coagulum, lacking the lamellar arrangement of platelets, forms upon the coralline thrombus and is sometimes referred to as the "tail." The propagated part of the thrombus, occurring in a relatively stagnant column of blood proximally (toward the heart) in a vein, is at first unattached to the vessel wall. If it proceeds to the next tributary of the vein, a new platelet thrombus may form at the site of contact with flowing blood, followed by the events previously outlined.

Etiology. Three factors predispose to the formation of a thrombus: (1) changes in the vessel wall; (2) changes in blood flow (e.g., slowing, stasis, and eddying of the current); and (3) changes in the blood constituents. An alteration of the lining endothelium is perhaps the most important factor causing thrombosis. This is operative in a wide variety of conditions, e.g., atherosclerosis of the aorta or its branches; inflammation of the wall of arteries (as in polyarteritis nodosa, thromboangiitis obliterans), or of veins (thrombophlebitis), or of heart valves; physical or chemical injury of a vessel; and ischemic injury of the heart wall (as in myocardial infarction). The importance of changes in the blood flow is indicated by the frequency of thrombosis in the veins, where slowness and stasis are more likely to occur than in the arteries. Thrombi occur frequently in the veins of the lower extremities in bedridden patients, especially in those with heart disease, which is attended by slowing of the peripheral circulation, and in those in the post-operative period. Thrombosis is common in varicose veins, where stasis and eddying of the blood are present. Eddying of the bloodstream promotes thrombus formation in an aortic aneurysm. There is evidence that stasis of the blood produces alterations of the endothelium and that this may be the means by which stasis predisposes to thrombosis. Changes in the blood constituents favoring thrombosis include increase in number and adhesiveness of platelets (as in the postoperative and puerperal states, accidental trauma, cancer, and certain peripheral vascular diseases), increased viscosity of blood (as in polycythemia), release of thromboplastic-like substance (as in visceral carcinoma), and increase in fibrinogen and other clotting factors of the blood (as in pregnancy).

Types and fate of thrombi. A thrombus that completely obstructs the lumen of a vessel is referred to as *occlusive;* one that extends along a vessel from the primary occlusive part is a *propagating* thrombus. A nonocclusive thrombus adherent to the wall is known as *mural* or *parietal*. When the latter occurs in the heart, it may be *pedunculated* or may appear as a rounded mass, which may become dislodged and move about freely in the chamber (a ball thrombus). Thrombi occurring on the valves of the heart as a result of underlying damage (infectious or noninfectious) are known as *vegetations*.

Various changes occur in thrombi. There may be a *softening* in the center of a large sterile thrombus caused by proteolytic enzymes released from disintegrating leukocytes or in an infected (septic) thrombus that is invaded by pyogenic organisms; the latter may give rise to septic emboli and abscesses in distant organs. *Dissolution* and removal of a small thrombus may occur. *Healing* of a thrombus is accomplished by the process of organization, proceeding from the periphery toward the center. Some degree of circulation may be reestablished through an occlusive thrombus by contraction of the mass and by formation of newly formed vascular channels *(canalization)* within it. *Calcification* occurs in some organizing thrombi, especially in small veins *(phleboliths)*. There may be *detachment* of a whole thrombus or parts of it before it undergoes organization, forming emboli that are transported elsewhere.

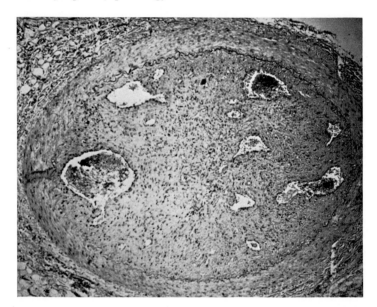

Fig. 4-4. Organized and recanalized arterial thrombus. The wavy dark line is the internal elastic lamina.

Effects of thrombi. The local effects of thrombosis result from the interference of the circulation in an organ or part of the body. The effects depend upon the size and type of a thrombus, the degree of vascular occlusion, the kind of vessel involved, the degree of collateral circulation, and the organ affected. Thrombotic occlusion of a vein may lead to stasis of blood, edema, and even necrosis in the area drained by the vessel. Occlusive arterial thrombi may cause localized ischemic necrosis *(infarct)* in an organ or *gangrene* of an extremity. If collateral circulation is adequate, little or no change may result from the vascular obstruction. A pedunculated or ball thrombus in the left atrium of the heart may suddenly occlude the mitral orifice and cause dyspnea, cyanosis, syncope, and even death. Detached masses of thrombi, set free in the circulation, result in *embolism* with its serious consequences (q.v.).

Postmortem intravascular clot. It is important to distinguish between a thrombus and an intravascular postmortem clot at autopsy. A thrombus tends to be dry, friable, and mottled gray-white and red; is adherent to the lining endothelium; exhibits lines of Zahn; and sometimes produces distention of the affected vessel. A postmortem clot is moist, elastic, homogeneous, and without lines of Zahn; is not adherent to the lining endothelium; forms a cast of the vessel and its branches or tributaries; and is deep red throughout ("currant-jelly" clot), when clotting takes place rapidly after death, or layered with a lower deep red part consisting of settled erythrocytes and an uppermost gray-yellow plasma layer ("chicken-fat clot"), when clotting occurs slowly.

EMBOLISM

Embolism is a partial or complete obstruction of some part of the vascular system by any mass carried there in the circulation; the transported material is an *embolus*.

Emboli are classified as *solid* (detached thrombi, fragments of tissue, clumps of tumor cells, etc.); *liquid* (fat globules); or *gaseous* (air). They may be *bland* or *septic*. They are also designated according to their location—*venous, arterial,* or *lymphatic.* A *paradoxical* embolus is one that arises in the venous circulation but enters the arterial side, or vice versa, usually through an arteriovenous communication such as a patent foramen ovale or some other septal defect in the heart. An embolus that travels against the flow of blood is a *retrograde* embolus.

The *effects* of emboli, as with thrombi, may be caused by the obstruction of the circulation in an organ or a part of the body, so that infarcts or gangrene may occur. Septic emboli may produce foci of inflammation, abscesses, and "mycotic" aneurysms at the sites of blockage. Dissemination of a malignant neoplasm occurs, locally or systemically, by means of tumor emboli in the bloodstream or in the lymphatics. Sudden death may result from emboli in the pulmonary or coronary arterial vessels.

Thromboembolism. The most frequent type of embolus is a detached thrombus or portion of one, which arises in the venous or arterial circulation. The arterial emboli arise usually from mural thrombi in the heart (left ventricle or atrium), from vegetations on the aortic or mitral valves, and occasionally from thrombi on atheromatous plaques or in aneurysms of the aorta. They produce occlusions most frequently in the spleen, kidneys, brain, and lower extremities, often with resultant infarcts in the organs and gangrene in the limbs. Septic emboli (as from vegetations of bacterial endocarditis) may cause abscesses or arteritis with formation of "mycotic" aneurysms. Coronary arterial embolism occurs in rare instances. *Venous* emboli originate most commonly from thrombi in veins of the lower extremities, less frequently from thrombi in the pelvic veins or in the right side of the heart, and rarely from thrombi in veins of the upper extremities. The most significant complication of venous embolism is the obstruction of the pulmonary arterial circulation. The effects of *pulmonary embolism* include sudden or delayed death, infarction, and hemorrhage. Death is usually related to a large embolus in one or both main pulmonary arteries, sometimes in the form of a "saddle embolus" overriding the bifurcation of the vessel; or it may be found in the right ventricle obstructing the outflow tract. Sudden death is attributed to one or several of the following mechanisms: asphyxia; acute cor pulmonale; diminished cardiac output with arterial hypotension, coronary insufficiency and myocardial failure, cerebral anoxemia, or generalized anoxemia with peripheral circulatory failure; vagopulmonic reflex causing widespread pulmonary and coronary vascular spasm; a reflex eventuating in peripheral circulatory failure; and a reflex producing cardiac standstill. Chronic cor pulmonale may result from widespread organized pulmonary emboli in the smaller vessels after recurrent thromboembolism.

Fat embolism. Fat *globules* enter the circulation from fat-bearing sites most commonly as a result of trauma to bones, particularly after fractures of the long bones. Fat embolism may also be caused by contusion or laceration of adipose tissue; and in the absence of trauma it may occur in association with extensive cutaneous burns, inflammation in fatty marrow or adipose tissue, fatty livers, and decompression sickness. Fat emboli may also arise from extrinsic fat or oil introduced into the body for therapeutic or other purposes. The minute emboli in the pulmonary circulation do not produce infarcts of the lungs but may cause congestion, edema, and focal hemorrhages. Respiratory symptoms may occur with extensive involvement. Systemic fat embolism results from the passage of the globules through the pulmonary capillaries and are disseminated to the brain, kidneys, heart, and other organs. Death may result from cerebral involvement. Microinfarcts and focal hemorrhages may be observed in the brain.

Amniotic fluid embolism. Amniotic fluid embolism may be a cause of severe or fatal shock coming on during or soon after labor. Although the incidence is low, it is an important cause of

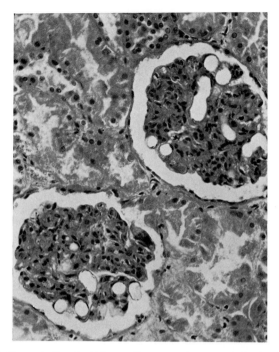

Fig. 4-5. Fat embolism in kidney. Clear, prominent vacuoles in glomerular capillaries are fat emboli (dissolved out in preparation of section). (From Scotti, T. M.: Disturbances of body water, electrolytes, and circulation of blood. In Anderson, W. A. D., editor: Pathology, ed. 5, St. Louis, 1966, The C. V. Mosby Co.)

obstetric death. The pulmonary vessels contain the components of amniotic fluid—epithelial squames, vernix caseosa, and sometimes mucus and lanugo hairs—admixed with leukocytes. Pulmonary edema may be present. It is not always clear how the amniotic fluid enters the circulation from the uterus, although in some instances it is probably accomplished through tears or surgical incisions in the myometrium or endocervix. Death may result from mechanical blockage of the pulmonary circulation, superimposed reflex vascular spasms, or "anaphylactoid" reaction. In some patients disseminated thrombosis and resultant afibrinogenemia (with a hemorrhagic tendency) may appear as a result of thromboplastin entering the circulation along with amniotic fluid.

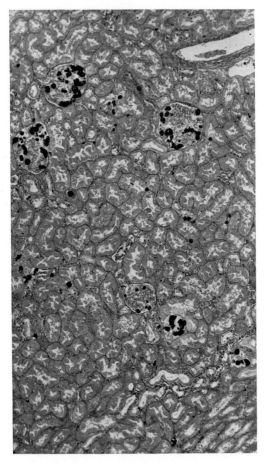

Fig. 4-6. Fat embolism in kidney. Glomerular capillaries and interstitial vessels contain fat globules (stained with osmic acid). (From Scotti, T. M.: Disturbances of body water, electrolytes, and circulation of blood. In Anderson, W. A. D., editor: Pathology, ed. 5, St. Louis, 1966, The C. V. Mosby Co.)

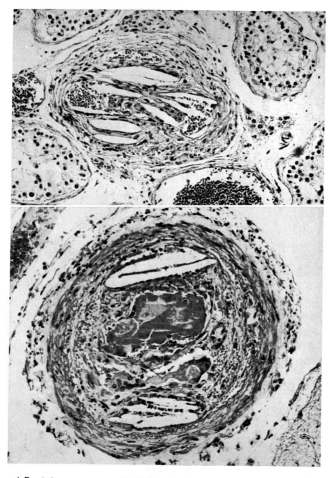

Fig. 4-7. Atheromatous emboli in arteries of the testicle (upper) and meninges (lower). The slitlike spaces are areas. from which lipid (cholesterol) crystals have been dissolved in preparation of the sections. (From Winter, W. J.: Arch. Path. **64:**137, 1957.)

Air embolism. *Venous air embolism* may occur as a complication of surgical operations, particularly of the chest and neck, during which air may be sucked into opened veins. Air may also be introduced into veins by various diagnostic or therapeutic procedures (e.g., during peritoneoscopy, induction of pneumoperitoneum). Venous embolism is also known to occur after the accidental injection of air, by means of a syringe, into endometrial veins during attempted abortion. Death may result from pulmonary embolism, and in such cases frothy ·blood is usually found in the right side of the heart at autopsy. *Arterial air embolism* may result from introduction of air into a pulmonary vein during thoracic operations or induction of pneumothorax. Since the air enters the systemic circulation, air bubbles may be found in the coronary or cerebral arteries. In such instances, smaller amounts may produce death than in the case of venous air embolism.

Decompression sickness. When divers or workers in caissons descend to levels of high pressure, the amount of gases held in solution in the blood and tissues increases. If the pressure is rapidly reduced during ascent to normal pressure, the gases (particularly nitrogen) come out of solution as bubbles in the blood and tissues, causing a variety of symptoms depending on their location (*caisson disease,* or *diver's palsy*). The same effect may be produced in aviators who ascend from normal atmos-

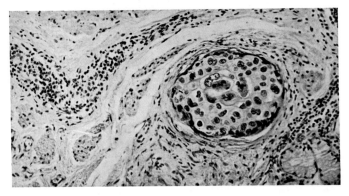

Fig. 4-8. Tumor embolism. Cells of a squamous carcinoma occupying the lumen of a blood vessel.

pheric pressure to low atmospheric pressures of high altitudes.

Other types of embolism. In *bone marrow embolism,* fragments of marrow (*adipose tissue* and marrow cells) enter the venous circulation after bone fractures or as a result of sternal puncture, closed chest cardiac massage, or bone marrow infarction (as in hemoglobin C and S disease). Sometimes fat embolism (liquid *globules* of fat) is associated with bone marrow embolism. *Atheromatous embolism* may result when fragments of eroded atheromatous plaques enter the arterial circulation. Emboli of other tissues may sometimes appear (e.g., *placental fragments, cerebral* or *hepatic tissues,* and *clumps of tumor cells*). *Bacteria, parasites,* and certain *foreign bodies* entering the circulation (e.g., needles, shrapnel, bullets, polyethylene catheters) are other forms of emboli.

ISCHEMIA

Ischemia refers to the diminution or the obliteration of the blood supply to a localized area of the body. As a result, the affected part is deprived of vital nutritional substances, particularly oxygen, while certain potentially injurious, metabolic products accumulate in the area. The term, ischemia, is generally used in reference to interference with arterial blood flow to a part; but it should be noted that venous obstruction may also cause local tissue damage because of stagnant anoxia and lack of removal of metabolites.

Causes of ischemia include thrombosis, embolism, arteriosclerosis, polyarteritis nodosa, thromboangiitis obliterans, vasospasm (as in Raynaud's disease, hypothermia, ergotism), outside pressure on a vessel by tumors or other masses, and constriction by a ligature or volvulus. The extent of damage depends upon (1) the rapidity of development of ischemia (gradual or sudden), (2) the degree of occlusion (partial or complete), (3) the vulnerability of the organ or tissue involved, and (4) the degree of sufficiency of the collateral circulation.

Among the changes associated with gradual incomplete ischemia are degenerations, atrophy, and fibrosis and/or adipose tissue replacement (gliosis in the central nervous system). The change associated with sudden, complete ischemia is usually necrosis (infarct or gangrene), but in the case of acute myocardial ischemia, sudden death may ensue. In instances in which the collateral circulation is good, an occlusion of a vessel may not be associated with visible effect.

INFARCTION

An *infarct* is a localized area of ischemic necrosis, resulting from some form of circulatory insufficiency. The process whereby this lesion is developed is known as *infarction*. Causes of infarcts are those noted in the previous section discussing ischemia, particularly thrombosis and embolism. Arterial obstructions produce infarcts more frequently than do venous obstructions.

Infarcts are most common in the spleen, kidneys, lungs, intestines, heart, and brain. Cardiac infarcts usually are the result of coronary arterial thrombosis rather than embolism and are an important cause of disability and death (p. 347). Intestinal infarcts involve a segment of the bowel, are associated with paralytic intestinal obstruction, and unless surgical relief is prompt, result in death from peritonitis or shock (p. 642).

In the lung, because of its abundant circulation, infarction follows pulmonary embolism only when there is already some interference with the circulation, such as chronic passive congestion. The liver likewise has an abundant circulation, and in this organ infarction is rare.

In the spleen, kidneys, and lungs, an infarct forms a slightly raised pyramidal mass of dead tissue, with its base at the periphery of the organ and its apex toward the point of arterial obstruction. In the myocardium the pattern of an infarct is more irregular. Shortly after the vascular obstruction the area becomes red and congested as a result of dilatation of the vessels and flowing of blood into the part from adjacent vessels. Hemorrhage occurs as a result of ischemic damage to vessel walls and is particularly severe in infarcts of the lungs and spleen. The area becomes swollen and edematous. In some cases the amount of redness, congestion, and hemorrhage is slight. Degenerative changes appear, and within forty-eight hours (sometimes as early as twelve to twenty-four hours) necrosis is evident, first affecting the parenchymatous tissue, but eventually the less sensitive supporting connective tissue is affected as well.

The tissue around certain infarcts responds to breakdown products of the necrotic tissue by an inflammatory reaction (hyperemia and infiltration of neutrophils, and if the area is covered by a serous layer, a fibrinous exudate may occur on the surface). The necrosis is of the coagulative type, except in the brain where it is liquefactive. The infarct is gradually decolorized, as erythrocytes are lysed and removed from the area, and forms a yellow-white opaque area (*pale* or *white* infarct).

Hematoidin and hemosiderin may be seen microscopically in some infarcts. However, in organs composed of soft, loose tissue (e.g., lungs and intestines), and especially in organs with a double blood supply (e.g., lungs), infarcts tend to remain hemorrhagic *(red infarcts)*. Healing of an infarct is accomplished by removal of dead tissue and replacement by fibrous tissue (organization), so that an older infarct shrinks beneath the surface of an organ and appears as a pale, depressed area.

Chapter 5

Bacterial infections

I nfectious diseases are caused by a variety of microorganisms, including bacteria. Pathogenic bacteria have the ability not only to establish and reproduce themselves within the host but also to elaborate certain metabolic products, including toxins, which participate in the development of the disease. The organisms are transmitted by direct contact with infected animals or human beings or by means of contaminated food, water, milk, or other substances that may harbor the infectious agents, i.e., fomites. A characteristic of these diseases is a period of incubation, i.e., an interval of time between the invasion of the body by the organisms and the appearance of clinical manifestations, which may vary from a few minutes or hours to weeks or months, or even longer. The microorganisms enter the body through various routes (portals of entry), i.e., skin and mucous membranes, respiratory tract, alimentary tract, and genitourinary tract.

The course of an infection depends upon (1) the organism, its nature, virulence, invasiveness, specificity, portal of entry into the body, and number (dose) and upon (2) the resistance to the organism and its growth and spread. The resistance is influenced not only by such factors as the age, nutrition, etc. of the person but also by the various immunologic (and allergic) mechanisms which alter the reaction to the infection. Spreading or localization of an infection depends not only on the invasiveness of the organisms and spreading factors which it may produce, but also on immunologic phenomena. The lymphoid and reticuloendothelial tissues are important in resistance to infections by production of antibodies and by phagocytic activity (p. 64). Fluorescent labeling of antibodies has demonstrated their presence in plasma cells and also has been a useful technique of demonstrating the localization of antibodies in various infections.

Individuals with hypogammaglobulinemia or agammaglobulinemia have lessened resistance to infections. Such persons, children or adults, have recurrent infections, diminished or absent circulating gamma globulin (although other blood proteins may be normal in amount), inability to form circulating antibodies in response to administered antigens or infecting organisms, and absence of heterologous blood-group isoagglutinins. Lymphoid tissue in nodes, the spleen, or elsewhere may show absence of germinal centers and of plasma cells.

The various *effects of infection,* local and systemic, are summarized in Fig. 5-1. The local effect is inflammation, which may be represented by one or more types (i.e., acute, chronic, nonspecific, purulent, necrotizing, ulcerative, granulomatous, etc.), depending on the organism. The term *nonspecific* is often used when the inflammatory reaction does not conform to any distinctive histologic pattern. Spread of an infection may be by contiguity (cellulitis or phlegmon); by lymphatics (lymphangitis, lymphadenitis); by other natural passages (bronchi, ureters); by bloodstream (bacteremia, septicemia, pyemia, toxemia); or by a combination of these means. A significant effect is the production of antibodies. The antibodies may be beneficial to the body in that they tend to destroy or immobilize the invading organisms or neutralize their toxins (immunity); or they may sensitize the tissues of the host, resulting in a hypersensitivity state. Hypersensitivity is important in certain infectious diseases because of its influence upon the character of the lesions and the progress of the disease. The intense tissue reactions, usually associated with this state, may be detrimental to the host and even severe enough to cause the death of the patient. An unsettled question is whether hypersensitivity reactions ever enhance immunity by serving as a defense mechanism against infection.

Bacteremia, the circulation of organisms in the bloodstream without clinical evidence of their presence, is probably frequent, is usually transient, and in most cases leads to no distant injury or new focus of infection. The term *septicemia* is applied when the bacteria and their toxins in the circulation are associated with clinical manifestations such as chills, fever, and petechial hemorrhages of skin. Pathologic changes associated with septicemia include (1) degenerative changes in parenchymatous organs; (2) foci of necrosis and reticuloendothelial hyperplasia in lymph nodes, spleen, liver, and bone marrow; (3) acute splenitis; (4) congestion and hemorrhages (e.g., in skin, serosae, and adrenal glands) and generalized edema; and (5) acute inflammation in various organs (e.g., bacterial endocarditis, meningitis).

The term *pyemia* is used for that type of septicemia (septico-

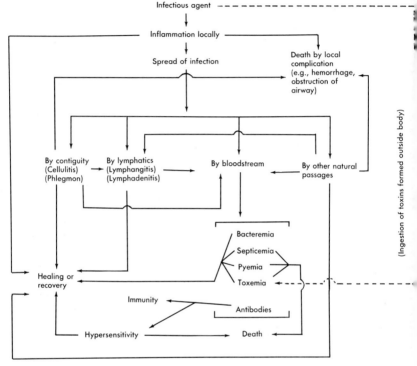

Fig. 5-1. Effects of infection.

pyemia) in which pyogenic organisms are spread by the blood and result in multiple abscesses in distant areas. *Sapremia* is the presence in the blood of injurious substances resulting from the growth of saprophytic bacteria in necrotic tissue. *Toxemia* is the effect on the tissues of circulating bacterial toxins, whether or not the bacterial organisms are also circulating in the blood. Toxemia is of prime importance as the effect of certain organisms, e.g., in diphtheria, tetanus, and botulism. However, unlike diphtheria and tetanus, in which the toxins are derived from organisms within tissues of the host, the toxins of botulism are formed outside the body and ingested, causing a pure toxemia without invasion of the host's tissues by the organisms. In severe infections with toxemia, shock may develop.

The various recent chemotherapeutic and antibiotic agents so effective in a wide range of infections apparently act by influencing or inhibiting growth of organisms rather than by augmentation of natural defense mechanisms.

STAPHYLOCOCCAL INFECTION

Staphylococci are pus-producing organisms of the genus *Micrococcus,* which grow in grapelike or irregular clusters and are gram-positive and aerobic, but facultatively anaerobic. The main pathogenic types are the golden *Staphylococcus aureus* and the white *Staphylococcus epidermidis.* In cultures a hemolysin is produced, which by laking of red cells produces a clear zone around colonies on blood agar plates. Staphylococci produce an exotoxin, which originally was believed to contain several fractions, referred to as leukocidin, hemolysin, acute killing fraction, skin-necrotizing fraction, and nephrotoxin. Staphylococcus toxin is very potent in producing local necrosis, apparently acting by localized direct injury of cells. Treatment of the toxin by formalin (producing toxoid) removes its injurious properties, though it is still active in stimulating antibody formation. Toxoid is of some value in immunization of individuals subject to staphylococcal infections. There has been an increase of these infections in recent years because of the appearance of strains of staphylococci that are resistant to antimicrobial agents.

Wherever a foothold is gained in the body, staphylococci tend to produce a localized abscess. The skin is most commonly affected, with the production of furuncles (boils) and carbuncles. Staphylococci are commonly present on healthy skin, and although most are saprophytic, some forms are pathogenic. Predisposing factors of lowered resistance or abrasions allow these to enter tissues and produce lesions.

Furuncle. Furuncles usually start about hair follicles, with production of a small localized but painful abscess. The abscess ruptures and discharges its pus on the surface, and healing follows. The inflammation may extend and burrow in the subepithelial tissues, and a number of discrete areas of necrosis form in the skin from which pus is discharged.

Carbuncle. The more extensive lesion, a carbuncle, is particularly dangerous on the upper lip or upper half of the face, where thrombophlebitic extension may lead to cavernous sinus and meningeal involvement.

Staphylococcal septicemia. *Staphylococcal septicemia* may occur by extension from any localized focus. This is an extremely dangerous condition with a mortality (without antibiotic therapy) of about 80%. It results in multiple pyemic abscesses in kidneys, heart, lungs, joints, etc. In some of these cases the original focus may be difficult to identify because it has healed or is hidden among the multiple lesions.

Suppurative nephritis. When caused by staphylococci, suppurative nephritis may appear as a focal disease resulting from pyemia ("pyemic kidney") or as a suppurative pyelonephritis.

Staphylococcal endocarditis. Staphylococcal endocarditis is one form of acute endocarditis (p. 338) and has large, soft vegetations.

Staphylococcal pneumonia. Staphylococcal pneumonia represents 5% or less of bacterial pneumonias. It may be a primary infection, but more often it occurs when resistance is depressed, as by epidemic influenza. It also occurs as a complication of pertussis, measles, mucoviscidosis, leukemia, and various chronic debilitating diseases. It is often rapidly fatal, with an alveolar exudate of hemorrhagic and edematous character, although abscess formation occurs if life continues for more than three or four days.

Osteomyelitis. Osteomyelitis is commonly a localized staphylococcal infection in bone (p. 837). The organisms reach the bone by the bloodstream from some primary, and often inconspicuous, focus. The localization in a certain site may be determined by some particular stress or injury to the bone.

Food poisoning. Food poisoning is sometimes caused by growth of staphylococci in spoiled food. The manifestations are the result of ingestion of enterotoxin elaborated by the organisms in the food and not by a true infection of the intestinal tract.

STREPTOCOCCAL INFECTION

Streptococci are gram-positive, spherical organisms that grow in chains. They are widely distributed and very common bacteria which are associated with a diversity of lesions, including tonsillitis, otitis media, cellulitis, appendicitis, wound infections, puerperal infections, bronchopneumonia, endocarditis, erysipelas, scarlet fever, and certain abscesses. Also associated with streptococcal infection are glomerulonephritis and rheumatic fever.

It is no longer held that specific strains of streptococci are responsible for scarlet fever and erysipelas. The hemolytic streptococci, although pyogenic, tend to produce a diffuse and spreading type of inflammation rather than the circumscribed abscesses so characteristic of staphylococci. In addition to their pyogenicity and invasiveness, the hemolytic streptococci may produce an erythrogenic or rash-producing exotoxin. Other demonstrable toxins include a fibrinolysin, which dissolves fibrin, a hemolysin, which acts on red cells, and a leukocidin, which kills leukocytes. These toxins are probably factors in the invasive power of the hemolytic streptococci.

The nonsuppurative inflammatory diseases, rheumatic fever and diffuse proliferative glomerulonephritis, are considered to be complications of infections caused by Group A, beta-hemolytic streptococci, not as infective lesions resulting from invasion by organisms but as poststreptococcal hypersensitivity diseases.

Wound infection. Invasion of streptococci through any wound of the skin, even a small cut or abrasion, may result in a dangerous infection. The organisms may spread rapidly in subcutaneous tissues, producing a cellulitis, with diffuse suppuration in later stages. Spread is often along lymphatics, with the formation of reddish streaks (lymphangitis). The lymphatic glands, when they are reached, also become swollen and tender (lymphadenitis). The more virulent infections reach the bloodstream and produce general septicemia. This may be associated with severe symptoms, chills, a high fever, and a rapidly developing hemolytic anemia. Focal pyogenic lesions are not as common with streptococcal septicemia as they are in the staphylococcal pyemia, although lungs, joints, or heart valves may be affected. Toxic degenerative changes (cloudy swelling and fatty degeneration) are severe in the heart, liver, and kidneys, and the spleen is enlarged, soft, and of purplish red color on the cut surface (acute splenic tumor).

Puerperal endometritis and myometritis are particularly dangerous forms of streptococcal wound infection. The raw surfaces of the postpartum uterus facilitate invasion, and rapid spread may occur by infection of lymphatics and blood vessels.

Erysipelas. Erysipelas, is a spreading streptococcal infection of the skin. The organisms enter through some minute wound or abrasion. Spread occurs by lymphatics, which are especially involved. The lesion appears as an elevated reddened area of skin with an irregular advancing margin. The inflammatory reaction in the corium is characterized by neutrophils, lymphocytes, and mononuclear wandering cells. Suppuration is unusual unless deeper parts of the skin and subcutaneous tissues are invaded.

Scarlet fever (scarlatina). Scarlet fever is caused by a strain of hemolytic streptococci in which production of an erythrogenic or rash-producing exotoxin is a prominent characteristic. The infection is usually a local one, with sore throat, accompanied by fever and a widespread skin rash. It is frequently complicated by glomerulonephritis or otitis media.

The organism produces a potent exotoxin, which by injection into the skin may be used to demonstrate susceptibility or immunity to the toxin (the Dick test). In susceptible persons a bright red swollen area develops in about twenty-four hours. If the serum from a scarlet fever convalescent is injected into the skin of a patient suffering from the disease, the rash is blanched in that area because of local neutralization of the toxin (Schultz-Charlton phenomenon).

An inflammatory lesion of the throat is constantly present. Occasionally invasion by the streptococci produces suppurative lesions, but most of the distant manifestations are due to toxin production. The skin rash shows marked vascular dilatation, and in late stages the lesion is infiltrated by leukocytes. A generalized lymphoid hyperplasia and some degree of acute splenic tumor are usually present. Cloudy swelling of the heart, liver, and kidneys accompanies the infection.

Acute glomerulonephritis is a complication which often develops during convalescence. It usually clears up completely but may give rise to a subacute or chronic glomerulonephritis and progress to a fatal ending. The result depends on the severity of the injury to glomeruli. The damage is believed to be caused not by the streptococci themselves but by their toxins, and the lesion may be a manifestation of an allergic reaction.

Streptococcal sore throat. The hemolytic streptococcus is a common cause of sore throat (nasopharyngitis), which sometimes occurs in epidemic form. Direct spread from one person to another is common, but milk-borne epidemics also have occurred. Possible complications include peritonsillar abscess, cellulitis (Ludwig's angina), otitis media, sinusitis, septicemia, rheumatic fever, and glomerulonephritis.

Streptococcal bronchopneumonia. The streptococcus is particularly important as a cause of bronchopneumonia complicating other infections, such as epidemic influenza (p. 166).

Streptococcal endocarditis. The hemolytic streptococcus is one of the organisms which may cause acute ulcerative valvular endocarditis. *Streptococcus viridans* is the common cause of the more prolonged subacute bacterial endocarditis (p. 336).

PNEUMOCOCCAL INFECTION

The principal disease caused by the pneumococcus is lobar pneumonia (p. 450). Less commonly, it is the etiologic agent in peritonitis (in children), endocarditis, and meningitis.

MENINGOCOCCAL INFECTION

The meningococci *(Neisseria intracellularis)* are gram-negative organisms which are pathogenic for man only and are the cause of epidemic cerebrospinal meningitis (spotted fever).

The organisms probably enter the body from the nasopharynx, where the local infection may be so mild that the patient is not aware of it. The bacteria invade the bloodstream and localize in meninges, skin, and sometimes joints, heart, and other tissues. Prior to localization of the organisms in the tissues, the bacteria in the blood may be unaccompanied by symptoms or signs (bacteremia); but in some cases, generalized clinical manifestations (e.g., fever, chills, malaise, etc.), without signs of local inflammation, may appear (septicemia). The meningeal infection produces a purulent exudate, and often there is also some involvement of brain tissue (p. 904). The septicemic stage presents skin involvement with reddish petechial lesions of the skin, which are caused by thrombotic involvement of the capillaries. Septicemia without meningeal involvement is not uncommon. Occasionally the septicemia is fulminant and overwhelming and may lead to rapid death with peripheral circulatory failure. In some of these cases there is hemorrhage into the adrenals, in addition to cutaneous hemorrhages (Waterhouse-Friderichsen syndrome, p. 706).

GONOCOCCAL INFECTION

The gonococcus, described by Neisser in 1879, is a gram-negative pyogenic organism, characteristically seen in diplococcal form within the cytoplasm of neutrophils. Gonorrhea is a disease of venereal nature, the primary acute infection involving the urethra in the male and the urethra, cervix, and Bartholin's glands in the female. In the acute stage the inflammation is characterized by congestion, swelling, and a profuse purulent exudate.

Although in many cases the condition rapidly subsides and may completely clear up, there is often spread or development of chronicity. In the male, spread occurs to the posterior urethra, with involvement of the prostate, seminal vesicles, and epididymis. Spread by the bloodstream may lead to joint involvement (arthritis). Healing may cause damage by fibrosis, which in a joint causes decreased mobility. Fibrosis in the epididymis may result in sterility, and in the urethra it produces stricture and interference with urination. In the female, spread from the cervix results in salpingitis following a transient and mild endometritis (p. 742). Peritonitis of the upper part of the abdomen (perihepatitis) is an occasional complication in young women. In healing it may lead to thin ("violin string") adhesions between the liver and abdominal wall. Proctitis, an uncommon lesion, is more prevalent in females than in males.

Gonococcal endocarditis may result from spread of the organism via the bloodstream. It is an acute destructive valvular involvement, with very large and friable vegetations. This is an infrequent complication of gonorrhea today.

Gonococcal nonvenereal infection in infancy particularly involves the conjunctiva and vagina. In newborn infants an acute conjunctivitis may arise from organisms acquired in passage through the birth canal. It produces severe injury of the cornea and blindness, but its occurrence is prevented in most cases by a routine prophylactic instillation of silver solution or penicillin into the infant's conjunctival sac.

Vulvovaginitis caused by the gonococcus occurs in female infants, whereas the more cornified adult vaginal mucosa resists the infection. It is usually due to contact with materials contaminated by gonorrheal pus. The infection is usually mild and complications are uncommon.

BACILLUS PYOCYANEUS INFECTION

Infections due to *Bacillus pyocyaneus (Pseudomonas aeruginosa)* are usually local and mild. Superficial skin wounds and the lower urinary tract are the most frequent sites. Otitis media or externa and infections of the nasal fossa may also occur. The lesions caused by *Pseudomonas* are characterized by the presence of a blue-green purulent exudate, and often by necrosis. More serious lesions include corneal ulcer, pneumonia, pyelonephritis, endocarditis, and meningitis. Necrotic, ulcerative skin lesions (ecthyma gangrenosum) may accompany *Pseudomonas* sepsis. Septicemia is a serious complication that may result in shock and death. *Pseudomonas* infections are particularly prevalent in debilitated patients and in those receiving prolonged antibiotic therapy, which suppresses other bacteria, allowing the resistant *Pseudomonas* organisms to flourish.

DIPHTHERIA

Diphtheria is a disease in which the organism forms a characteristic local lesion on the mucosa of the pharynx or upper respiratory passages. Widespread effects are produced by formation of a powerful exotoxin (toxemia) rather than by invasion or by spread of the organisms through the bloodstream. The function of the exotoxin is to inhibit the inflammatory reaction of the tissues, thus enabling the bacteria to become established. If the inflammatory response is inadequate, the bacteria proliferate rapidly, and the toxin produced soon overwhelms the defense mechanism. *Corynebacterium diphtheriae* may be identified in cultures by swabs obtained from involved mucosa and spread on Loeffler's medium. The diphtheria virulence test is a method of determining whether a strain of *C. diphtheriae* is capable of forming significant quantities of the exotoxin. Diphtheria is most common in children between 2 and 10 years of age, which is the period of greatest susceptibility. Immunity to diphtheria depends upon immunity to the toxin due to the possession of a requisite amount of antitoxin. In the Schick test to determine immunity, a minute amount of toxin is injected intracutaneously. If antitoxin (immunity) is present, no reaction occurs. A positive local reaction of congestion and inflammation, reaching a peak in about four days, indicates lack of immunity. Evanescent passive immunity is produced by injection of antitoxin contained in the serum from immunized horses. More lasting (active) immunity results from injection of modified toxin or toxoid.

The local lesion of diphtheria on the mucosa of the pharynx, larynx, trachea, or elsewhere is characterized by formation of a false membrane. This is composed of necrotic surface tissue welded together by fibrin and infiltrated by leukocytes. The term *diphtheritic membrane* frequently is used for such a pseudomembranous layer on a mucosal surface, whether it is caused by *C. diphtheriae*, or other bacteria, or by injurious chemicals such as strong acids, alkalies, or heavy metal salts. Marked

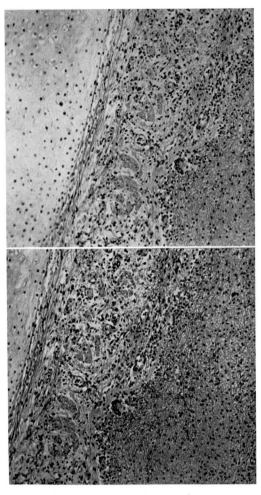

Fig. 5-2. Diphtheritic tracheitis. Note the tracheal cartilage on the left, the edema and inflammatory infiltration of the tracheal wall, and the diphtheritic membrane on the right, with its abundant fibrin and inflammatory cells.

cervical lymphadenitis with prominent enlargement of the nodes (bull neck) may occur in severe forms of diphtheria.

In the pharynx the diphtheritic membrane is closely adherent, but in the trachea and bronchi the membrane is more easily detached and often coughed up in large fragments. The chief danger of the membrane is obstruction of respiratory passages, and asphyxiation is one of the major causes of death in diphtheria. The mechanical obstruction due to the membrane is enhanced by local inflammatory swelling and edema and by laryngeal spasm. Occasionally the diphtheria organism attacks other mucous membranes, such as of the nose, conjunctiva, or vagina. Other primary sites of infection may be the umbilical cord (diphtheria neonatorum), the genital tract (e.g., in circumcision), and traumatic wounds or burns.

The more distant effects of diphtheria are also serious, and mortality is frequently due to circulatory failure. This is contributed to by relaxation of blood vessels from loss of vasomotor control as well as by toxic degenerative changes in the myocardium. Myocarditis has been reported in 70% of fatal cases of diphtheria. It may be a late manifestation after apparent improvement. The heart is enlarged, dilated, flabby, and pale. There is a primary toxic degeneration of myocardial fibers, which elicits an inflammatory response and culminates in scarring. Bronchopneumonia, due to streptococci or other organisms, is a common complication. Degenerative changes occur in the liver, adrenals, and kidneys. In some cases the kidneys show, in addition, an acute interstitial nephritis (p. 387). Nerve paralyses are common and are due to degenerative changes in nerve fibers. The muscles of the palate and of the eyes are most frequently paralyzed.

PERTUSSIS (WHOOPING COUGH)

Whooping cough, caused by *Haemophilus pertussis*, is an important infection of early childhood. The major changes are in the air passages and lungs. Tracheitis, bronchitis, and bronchiolitis with excessive production of thick mucus are the most prominent findings. Emphysema is usually present. Secondary bronchopneumonia is a common complication.

INTESTINAL INFECTIONS

The intestinal infections are considered in Chapter 20, typhoid fever on p. 622, paratyphoid fever on p. 624, bacillary dysentery on p. 625, and cholera on p. 626. Food poisoning caused by infection (botulism, staphylococcal, and *Salmonella* infection) is discussed on pp. 114 and 625.

TETANUS

In tetanus, as in diphtheria, there is production of a powerful exotoxin with distant and far-reaching effects, although growth of the bacteria remains localized, with little or no invasion. The organism, *Clostridium tetani,* is an anaerobic rod, gram-positive, and forming characteristic terminal spores. The spores are very resistant and are common in dust and soil which has been contaminated by excreta. Infection occurs particularly in deep penetrating wounds which are soiled by such dirt and in which growth is promoted by anaerobic conditions and by the presence of injured or dead tissues. The disease has also been known to result from infected burns, omphalitis (tetanus neonatorum), surgical procedures (contaminated sutures, dressings, plaster casts), and endometritis (puerperal sepsis or attempted abortions). The incubation period varies from three or four days up to several months. The more severe and serious cases have shorter incubation periods.

The tetanus toxin has a direct effect upon the central nervous system. Whether carried there by the bloodstream or by nerve fibers is a matter of debate. Hyperexcitability of the nervous system results and gives rise to muscular spasms and convulsions. The spasms often begin in the masseter muscles, and hence the term *lockjaw.* No specific anatomic changes are usually recognizable in the nervous system or elsewhere by ordinary methods of examination, although chromatolysis of cells of motor nuclei and perivascular demyelination have been described in patients living three days or more.

GAS GANGRENE

Gas gangrene is an infection by one or more pathogenic anaerobes of the saccharolytic group of the genus *Clostridium* (*Cl. welchii, Cl. septique, Cl. oedematiens*). These organisms, being anaerobic, thrive best in dead tissue and where oxygen tension is low. Hence this infection is particularly likely to complicate wounds in which there are destruction of tissues, absence of free drainage, and some interference with circulation. The condition develops in a few hours up to a few days after infection of the wound or dead tissue. A limb in which

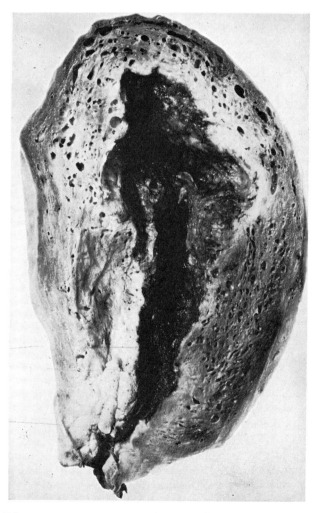

Fig. 5-3. Puerperal endometritis and myometritis. *(Clostridium welchii)*. Note the sponginess of the myometrium, caused by gas formation.

the circulation has been cut off may have very massive involvement. In other cases of wound infection there is an active, spreading involvement of muscle. Gas production makes the tissue crepitant, and bubbles of gas may appear when the tissue is pressed upon. Muscle particularly is involved, the dead muscle appearing brown and opaque. The necrosis appears to be a direct action on the muscle fiber of alpha toxin (lecithinase) in *Cl. welchii* infections. Other toxins and enzymes produced by the organisms enhance their effect, e.g., hyaluronidase, collagenase, leukocidin, deoxyribonuclease, fibrinolysin, and hemolytic toxins. Later the skin and other tissues become affected and appear yellowish, greenish, or black and putrefactive. The pigmentation is the result of breakdown of red blood cells in the lesion. Associated with the necrosis there are congestion and edema, a relatively sparse leukocytic infiltration, hemorrhages, and thromboses of minute vessels. In severe cases, systemic reactions include fever, tachycardia, nausea, vomiting, prostration, and shock. Anemia caused by hemolysis may develop rapidly. In terminal stages there may be wide dissemination of the organisms. However, in most cases where such widespread involvement of tissues is found at autopsy, the spread has been post mortem (see postmortem changes, p. 44). Various internal organs, such as the liver, are found to be spongy and full of gas.

Puerperal infection with *Cl. welchii* or related organisms occasionally occurs, the anaerobes gaining a foothold in the necrotic material inevitably left in the uterus following delivery of the child. The wall of the uterus becomes involved, and terminally there may be extensive spread throughout the body.

ANTHRAX

Anthrax is a septicemic bacterial infection due to a large square-ended, gram-positive, encapsulated bacillus, which readily forms highly resistant spores. The disease is enzootic in certain regions among sheep, cattle, and other herbivorous animals. Human infection is mainly among persons who handle the hides or hair of infected animals, and hence the disease is most common among tanners, butchers, brush and hair workers, and woolsorters. Infection is by way of the gastrointestinal tract in animals, but in man this is uncommon.

Anthrax in man is commonly an infection of the skin (malignant pustule) or of the lungs (woolsorters' disease). The essential features of anthrax lesions are acute congestion, hemorrhages, and effusions of bloodstained serous fluid.

Malignant pustule is the common form of anthrax in man. The organism enters through a small abrasion of the hand, face, or neck, and in five or six days a reddened vesicle appears. This vesicle contains hemorrhagic fluid and many organisms. The vesicle breaks down and forms a depressed blackened scab, surrounded by satellite pinkish vesicles and a broad zone of edema. The lesion is often relatively painless, apparently due to axonal degeneration of local nerve fibers of the skin. The microscopic features of the lesion are an acute hemorrhagic, inflammatory exudate with relatively few neutrophils and necrosis of tissue of the coagulative type. The local lymph nodes are swollen because of acute lymphadenitis. Spread does not occur to underlying muscle. Healing and recovery may occur, or in severe cases with bloodstream invasion there is septicemia, with rapid collapse and death.

In occasional cases the primary local lesion is in the nasal mucosa, from which perineural lymphatic spread to the brain may result in a peculiarly hemorrhagic *meningitis*.

Woolsorters' disease occurs among workers in woolsorting and brush making. The infection enters by the respiratory tract. A localized lesion forms in a bronchus, from which spread produces a hemorrhagic bronchopneumonia.

In fatal cases of anthrax the blood vessels are sometimes filled with the large bacilli, a finding often prominent on low-power examination.

PLAGUE

Plague is an acute, highly fatal, infectious disease caused by *Pasteurella pestis*. It is primarily a disease of rats and other rodents and is transmitted to man by fleas. Cases have occurred in western United States, where endemic foci of sylvatic plague exist among California ground squirrels. India and China are important endemic centers of plague.

The disease has been classified into bubonic, septicemic, and pneumonic forms, according to whether the lymphatic system, blood, or lungs are involved primarily.

In the bubonic form, following a fleabite or contact with infected material, spread occurs to lymph nodes, usually without development of a lesion at the site of entry, although a small lesion (vesicle, pustule, or ulcer) may appear. The involved lymph nodes (buboes) are necrotic and enlarged by intense congestion and hemorrhagic edema. Areas of suppuration may be associated with the acute necrotizing hemorrhagic inflammation. The tissues surrounding the lymph nodes are involved in the reaction. Septicemic spread may follow, with involvement of many tissues, including the lungs (secondary pneumonic plague). There is a pronounced destructive effect on blood vessels, and marked congestion of all organs and extensive hemorrhagic extravasations are usual. Primary pneumonic plague spreads from person to person by droplets of infected sputum. Bronchioles and alveoli are distended by a hemorrhagic exudate containing little fibrin and many organisms. Necrosis of pulmonary tissue is conspicuous in areas. Primary septicemic plague is probably acquired through mucous membranes of the mouth, throat, and conjunctiva. Localizing lesions are not clinically apparent.

TULAREMIA

Tularemia is an infectious disease caused by *Pasteurella tularensis*. It is characterized by necrosis, with subacute and chronic granulomatous lesions in lymph nodes, liver, spleen, and lungs. Wild rabbits form a reservoir of the disease, and most human cases result from the handling of infected rabbits. The condition also occurs in ground squirrels, wild rats, and mice. The organisms are transferred among animals by the wood tick. Although most human infections are caused by the handling of infected carcasses, transfer also may be by the bites of ticks and deer flies. Transmission by ingestion of contaminated food or water is possible.

The clinical types of the disease are (1) ulceroglandular, in which a primary lesion forms at the site of inoculation in the skin and is followed by enlargement of regional lymph nodes; (2) oculoglandular, wherein the primary involvement is in the conjunctiva and is followed by lymph node enlargement; (3) typhoid type, in which septicemic manifestations occur while the primary point of inoculation and the lymph node enlargement are not obvious; (3) intestinal form, caused by ingestion of organisms in contaminated food or water; and (5) primary pneumonic form caused by inhalation of material from cultures or contaminated particles. Septicemia may occur in any of the forms of the disease in addition to the typhoid type. Most cases are of the ulceroglandular type. Specific agglutinins, useful in diagnosis, develop during the second week of the infection. The

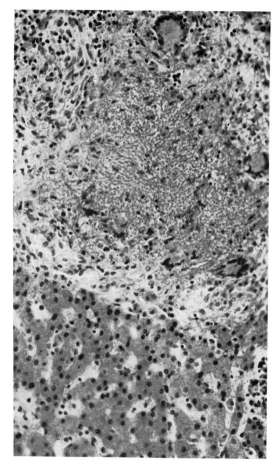

Fig. 5-4. Tularemia. Granulomatous reaction in liver very closely simulates tuberculosis. (From Hopps, H. C.: Bacterial diseases. In Anderson, W. A. D., editor: Pathology, ed. 5, St. Louis, 1966, The C. V. Mosby Co.)

disease has a mortality of about 4%. A nonfatal attack confers lasting immunity.

In tularemia there are two effects in human tissues: (1) a necrotizing effect caused by the organism, producing areas of suppuration or caseous necrosis, and (2) a tissue reaction in which monocytes and epithelioid cells predominate. These granulomatous lesions, with or without caseous centers, resemble those of tuberculosis. In early lesions the necrosis tends to predominate, while in old lesions the cellular reaction and fibrosis are more prominent.

The characteristic lesions of focal caseous necrosis and mononuclear cell reaction are found in the lymph nodes draining the primary lesions and also commonly in the spleen (70%), liver (55%), and lung (70%). The pulmonary involvement, which may be primary or more often secondary to one of the other forms of the disease, is a nodular or confluent pneumonia with mononuclear exudate and a tendency to caseous necrosis of exudate and alveolar walls (p. 462). In fatal cases the necrotizing factor in tularemic lesions is particularly prominent, whereas in specimens from the nonfatal cases the epithelioid cell reaction is more striking and there may be multinucleated giant cells of the Langhans type. The organisms are found in the lesions of lower animals but are scarce and usually not demonstrable in human lesions.

UNDULANT FEVER (BRUCELLOSIS)

Undulant fever has become recognized within recent years as a frequent and widespread infectious disease. The *Brucella* organisms causing the disease are of three strains: *Br. abortus,* the bovine strain from cattle; *Br. suis,* the porcine strain from swine; and *Br. melitensis,* the caprine strain from goats. The term *undulant fever* refers to the intermittent febrile periods, which are a common manifestation. The organisms enter the body through abrasions of the skin and mucous membranes after direct contact with tissues or body fluids of infected animals; less frequently they enter through ingestion of contaminated milk or milk products. Positive diagnosis depends largely on laboratory procedures. The mortality is low, and the lesions found post mortem have varied from slight reticuloendothelial hyperplasia to granulomatous lesions of spleen and lymph nodes resembling tuberculosis or sarcoidosis, since the granulomas are usually of the noncaseating type. However, in the more chronic forms of the disease, suppuration and caseation occasionally occur, particularly in *Br. suis* infections. Endocarditis, meningitis, and arthritis caused by *Br. abortus* have been reported.

MYCOPLASMA

Organisms of the genus *Mycoplasma,* or pleuropneumonia-like organisms (PPLO), are very small (125 to 250 mμ), pleomorphic bodies that have no rigid cell wall, such as bacteria do, but they are bounded by a plasma membrane. The PPLO are classified somewhere between the large viruses and the bacteria, but they are distinguished from the rickettsiae. Many instances of what was formerly called "primary atypical pneumonia" or "virus pneumonia" have been shown recently to be caused by *M. pneumoniae* (Eaton's agent). The organism is probably transmitted by infected respiratory secretions. An increase in titers of cold agglutinins in the serum is a feature of this disease. The more specific complement fixation, indirect hemagglutination, and fluorescent antibody tests are more useful diagnostic procedures. *M. hominis* type 1 has produced exudative pharyngitis in human volunteers under experimental conditions. Its relationship and that of other *Mycoplasma* organisms to naturally occurring pharyngitis is under investigation. Genitourinary tract infections, particularly urethritis and infections of the female genital system, and the Reiter's syndrome (arthritis, nongonococcal urethritis, and conjunctivitis) have been attributed by some investigators to PPLO.

Chapter 6

Tuberculosis

Tuberculosis is still a serious disease and a major cause of death in certain parts of the world; although in other areas, as in the United States, the mortality rate is steadily declining. In 1900 there were 200 deaths per 100,000 population in the United States; but in 1963 the death rate was only 4.9 per 100,000. The high mortality rate that was associated with infancy and early adult life years ago has been greatly reduced. Today most of the deaths occur in the elderly.

The prevalence of tuberculosis also has decreased over the past fifty years, but not at the same rate as the mortality. Despite the decline in the prevalence and mortality of the disease, particularly as a result of better socioeconomic conditions, earlier and more efficient diagnosis, and improvement in therapy, tuberculosis is still a significant health hazard in the United States. Over 50,000 new active cases are reported each year, and well over 300,000 active and inactive cases of tuberculosis are under medical supervision.

The causative organism, *Mycobacterium tuberculosis*, stimulates a specific granulomatous tissue reaction characterized by caseous necrosis, pale mononuclear "epithelioid" cells, and giant cells with multiple peripheral nuclei. Human and bovine strains of the organism are important. Most pulmonary tuberculosis is caused by the human type, but in countries where bovine tuberculosis is common, the bovine type is quite commonly found in intestinal, bone, and joint tuberculosis in children. Infection with the latter type is spread by milk from infected cows and has become rare in certain countries, such as the United States, because of pasteurization of milk and eradication of tuberculosis in cattle. Infection with the human strain takes place by means of inhalation directly into the lungs of organisms contained in droplets or dust. In most cases resistance is sufficient to overcome infection with a small dose of organisms. After this early infection there is an enhanced sensitivity or allergy to products of the organism, as manifested by a reaction to a tuberculin skin test. The lung is the organ most frequently affected, but the lymph nodes, intestine, kidney, brain, meninges, spleen, and liver are also commonly involved. Spread in the body occurs by direct extension, lymphatics, bloodstream, and natural passages such as bronchi.

TUBERCLE BACILLUS

The tubercle bacillus, discovered by Koch in 1882, belongs to the group of mycobacteria. This group of acid-fast bacilli also

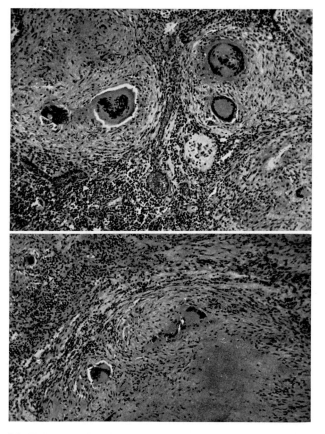

Fig. 6-1. Tuberculosis of the lymph node. Note the caseation, epithelioid cells, and characteristic multinucleated giant cells.

includes the bacillus of leprosy and certain anonymous or atypical mycobacteria. Human and bovine strains of the tubercle bacillus commonly infect man, but human infection with the avian strain is very rare. The human strain is virulent in man and the guinea pig, but rabbits and fowls are resistant. The bovine strain, in addition to infecting cattle, is virulent for the rabbit, guinea pig, and man. The human and bovine strains, while distinguishable by cultural methods, are best differentiated by studying their relative virulence for rabbits.

The tubercle bacillus is a slender rod with a somewhat beaded or granular appearance. It can be stained in smears or tissues by the Ziehl-Neelsen method, which consists of staining by hot basic fuchsin and decolorization by acid. The organisms, being acid fast, retain the dye and are colored red. When the organisms are scanty, a concentration method, using antiformin, may be useful. When the organisms are small in number, staining methods may fail, but inoculation of infected material into guinea pigs will reveal their presence, for this animal will develop characteristic tuberculous lesions within six weeks.

Tubercle bacilli do not have exotoxins or endotoxins to account for their effects; however, certain chemical fractions have been isolated from them that on injection cause reproduction of the cellular reactions of tuberculosis. These chemical fractions include lipids, polysaccharides, and proteins. One of the lipids, a phosphatide, is taken up by phagocytic mononuclear cells and converts them into epithelioid cells and derivative giant cells, the characteristic cells of tuberculous lesions. Certain waxes, higher hydroxy acids, are responsible for the acid fastness of the bacilli and on injection induce the formation of multinucleated giant cells. The polysaccharides have a chemotactic effect on neutrophils, causing an accumulation of these cells at the site of injection. The proteins induce a neutrophilic and macrophage response and stimulate the monocytes to form epithelioid cells and giant cells. Sensitization of the tissues is attributed to this protein fraction.

ROUTES OF INFECTION

The routes of infection of tuberculosis are as follows: (1) Direct infection of the lung by inhalation of organisms contained in droplets or dust particles is the most important method of infection in man. (2) Infection through the alimentary tract occurs in bovine bacillus infection by ingestion of contaminated milk. The organisms enter through the mucosa and the lymphoid tissues of the tonsils or pharynx to involve cervical lymph nodes or through the intestine to reach mesenteric lymph nodes. No lesion may be left at the point of entry. In the United States, primary infection by the alimentary tract is rare. (3) Infection through the skin is rare, but it may occur in surgeons and pathologists who handle infected tissues. It usually results in a local lesion rather than in generalized infection. (4) Congenital infection may occur when there are placental lesions, but this is rare and unimportant.

TISSUE REACTIONS

The typical lesion in tuberculosis is a chronic granulomatous inflammation with formation of localized nodules known as tubercles, which consist of aggregates of mononuclear (epithelioid) cells, giant cells, and a border of lymphocytes. Caseation necrosis is frequently present in the centers of the tubercles.

When tubercle bacilli are injected into tissues, there is a prompt outpouring of polymorphonuclear leukocytes. Very rapidly, however, the reaction becomes mononuclear. These phagocytic cells are derived from histiocytes and rapidly engulf the organisms and degenerated leukocytes. The fatty material thus engulfed becomes dispersed in fine particles throughout the cell, giving it a distinctive appearance with resemblance to an epithelial cell. These transformed macrophages are called epithelioid cells. They have large, oval, pale nuclei and abundant pale, eosin-staining cytoplasm and are bound together by irregular branching processes. Cell boundaries are often indistinct, and the appearance is that of a syncytium. Near the central part of the cluster of epithelioid cells there may be one or more giant cells. These are formed by fusion of epithelioid cells or possibly by amitotic division of nuclei without cellular division. The nuclei usually form a ring about the periphery or cluster at one or more poles of the giant cell (Langhans giant cell), but occasionally they are scattered uniformly throughout the cytoplasm, resembling a foreign body giant cell.

Caseous necrosis develops in the center of the tubercle at about the end of the second week after injection of the tubercle bacilli. The necrosis is probably the result of acquired hypersensitivity to the tuberculoproteins, which can develop in about ten to fourteen days after inoculation of the organisms in a previously uninfected animal. There is a possibility that avascularity of the tubercle contributes to the necrosis. No blood vessels are present within the tubercle itself. The necrotic material is granular and cheesy in its gross appearance, and usually no residual histologic evidence of tissue structure can be seen in it. Lymphocytes border the periphery of the epithelioid cluster, and as the lesion ages, fibrosis develops around the tubercle.

The several elements that compose the tubercle vary quantitatively. When dosage and virulence of the organisms are low and resistance is high, epithelioid cells are predominant, giant cells may be scarce, and there is little or no necrosis. This type of lesion is often termed a "hard tubercle." On the other hand, when the dosage and virulence are high in comparison with resistance, necrosis may predominate and epithelioid cells may be relatively scarce. These are termed "soft tubercles."

The smallest tubercles are of microscopic size, but their enlargement or fusion produces visible lesions. The smallest of these, about the size of a millet seed, are little grayish areas, 1 or 2 mm. in diameter, with or without a minute yellowish point of necrosis in their centers.

The aforementioned reactions are essentially productive, but in certain situations tuberculous inflammation may be exudative. On serous surfaces such as the peritoneum and in tuberculous pneumonia and tuberculous meningitis, there may be a serofibrinous exudate in addition to tubercle formation. Rare cases of nonreactive (acute caseating) tuberculosis occur and are characterized by necrosis and many organisms but minimal reaction in surrounding tissue. Cortisone administration may cause a similar failure of tissue response.

If the tubercle is very small, healing may result in its disappearance or replacement by a fibrous scar. A considerable amount of caseous material may not be absorbed but becomes calcified by the deposition of calcium salts. This tendency to calcification is comparable to calcium deposition in any devitalized tissues in the body (dystrophic calcification) and possibly depends on a localized increased alkalinity of the necrotic material. While calcified tuberculous lesions ordinarily are considered healed, it is sometimes possible to demonstrate living tubercle bacilli in them. Under certain circumstances, the necrotic material of tubercles can be disposed of by natural passages; e.g., a tubercle in the lung may rupture into a bronchus and the caseous mass be transferred by bronchial passages, leaving a cavity. As a result, progression of the disease may occur throughout the lung, or the infective material may be coughed up and inhaled into the opposite lung or be swallowed into the gastrointestinal tract.

Chemotherapeutic agents may have an effect on the progress of tuberculosis and also may produce a change in the tissue reactions and microscopic appearance. *Streptomycin* promotes healing of surface lesions and liquefaction of the content of tuberculous cavities. In such lesions the tubercle bacilli may be demonstrable by staining although they may not grow on culture media or produce disease on injection into susceptible animals. *Isoniazid* treatment may result in the presence of numerous multinucleated giant cells of foreign body type and of atypical appearance and location. The contents of cavities and caseous nodules tend to become liquefied with a marked polymorphonuclear leukocytic reaction.

RESISTANCE AND HYPERSENSITIVITY

As with any other infection, the development and course of tuberculosis are dependent upon the virulence, dosage, and portal of entry of the organisms; but also important are the variable factors in the host: (1) native and acquired resistance and (2) hypersensitivity. Differences in native resistance are both racial and individual. Negroes and American Indians are more susceptible than Caucasians, although certain environmental factors probably contribute to the decreased resistance. There is evidence that heredity or genetic factors play a role in individual resistance. Significant environmental factors that tend to decrease native resistance include malnutrition, physical and psychological stress, fatigue, and certain diseases, e.g., diabetes mellitus and alcoholism. There is a high incidence of tuberculosis in patients with silicosis, but the reason for this is not clear— whether it is caused by decreased pulmonary resistance brought about by the injurious effects of silica or to enhancement of growth and virulence of the organisms resulting from a synergism between the silica and tubercle bacilli. Other factors, such as overcrowding and slum conditions, are favorable for exposure to infection.

Age and sex appear to influence susceptibility. While infants, young adults, and the elderly are susceptible to the disease, children in the age group of 5 to 14 years are more resistant. Today it appears that tuberculosis in the United States is becoming a disease of older persons, particularly men. Resistance

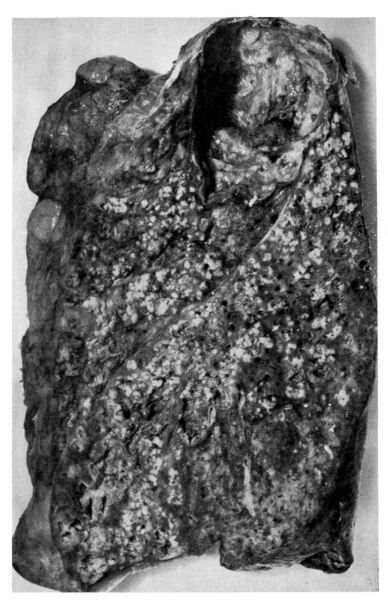

Fig. 6-2. Pulmonary tuberculosis. Note the large cavity at the apex and the spread throughout the rest of the lung.

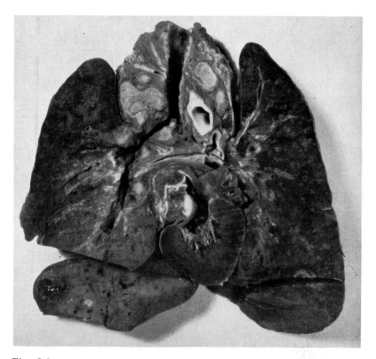

Fig. 6-3. Primary tuberculosis. Large caseous masses in the mediastinal lymph nodes.

in males and females is similar until puberty, but during the reproductive period the disease is more serious in females. From about 40 years of age on, mortality is greater in men and increases progressively with advancing age.

The problem of acquired resistance (immunity) and hypersensitivity is a complex one. A certain degree of immunity results from a previous infection, but it does not appear to be related to specific, circulating antibodies. Although antibodies have been demonstrated in the sera of tuberculous patients, these have not been found to be protective against the bacilli. This acquired immunity appears to be a cellular phenomenon, whereby macrophages proliferate and inhibit further growth of tubercle bacilli. Hypersensitivity to bacterial products also occurs as a result of infection with tubercle bacilli, and it is characterized by an accelerated and intense inflammatory reaction, with tissue destruction and caseous necrosis. Although hypersensitivity develops shortly after the first infection by tubercle bacilli, the reaction tends to be more severe in a host who has previously been infected. However, at the same time that this vehement tissue reaction is taking place, there is an apparent attempt to localize the infection, which is a feature of immunity. When the immunity factor is dominant, the proliferative (macrophagic and fibroblastic) response is prominent and there is a tendency toward healing of the lesions. The hypersensitivity reaction is especially severe in a host with low resistance who is infected by a large dose of virulent organisms. Although some investigators have suggested that acquired immunity and hypersensitivity in tuberculosis are different manifestations of the same mechanism, there is a strong opinion that the two processes are independent, at least partially.

MILIARY TUBERCULOSIS AND SINGLE ORGAN DISEASE

Miliary tuberculosis is the result of widespread dissemination of large numbers of tubercle bacilli by the bloodstream. When the dissemination is massive, myriads of tiny miliary tubercles develop in the lungs, spleen, liver, kidneys, meninges, and other organs. The tubercles are seen as grayish nodules, 1 or 2 mm. in diameter, fairly uniform in size, studding the outer and cut surfaces of affected organs. The patient exhibits fever and intense intoxication, and death usually results in a few weeks. Less massive discharge of bacilli into the circulation may give rise to subacute and chronic forms of miliary tuberculosis.

The spread of such large numbers of tubercle bacilli by the blood may be the result of tuberculous infection of a vessel wall from an adjacent lesion (as in the lung or mediastinal lymph node), followed by rupture of an intimal tuberculous lesion into the lumen. Occasionally a lesion of the thoracic duct similarly causes massive vascular spread. Miliary dissemination commonly may be from an extrapulmonary lesion into the draining lymphatic system, and in turn into the venous system.

Organisms spread in small numbers by the bloodstream may cause a few clinically silent tuberculous lesions, particularly in spleen, liver, or kidney. Many such lesions heal and are seen as rounded, grayish white fibrous or calcified nodules a few millimeters in diameter. Sometimes a few bacilli in the circulation may result in progressive disease in only a single tissue or organ, accounting for the extrapulmonary clinical form known as "single organ," "isolated organ," or "local metastatic" tuberculosis, as in bone, kidney, adrenal gland, fallopian tube, or epididymis. This type of disease may be clinically manifest while the the initial (e.g., pulmonary) lesion from which it arose is still active; or frequently it does not become apparent until years after the initial lesion has healed. Prior to the days of effective chemotherapy these localized, extrapulmonary lesions were treated principally by surgery and often were referred to as "surgical tuberculosis."

PULMONARY TUBERCULOSIS

Primary tuberculosis. The primary type of pulmonary tuberculosis is characterized by development of a small peripheral or subpleural tubercle (sometimes multiple), which may develop in any portion of any lobe. It is more frequent in the lower or middle part of the lung and is rarely at the apex.

This tuberculous lesion was minutely studied by Ghon and is frequently termed the *Ghon tubercle*. It develops to a size of 1 to 3 cm., and from it spread occurs by lymphatics to mediastinal lymph nodes, which become greatly enlarged and caseous. The combination of the peripheral lung lesion and enlargement of the tracheobronchial lymph nodes is characteristic, and the two lesions together are called the *primary* (or *Ghon*) *complex*. Progression by direct extension or by bronchial, lymphatic, or bloodstream dissemination may occur, but in most cases there is healing by resolution, fibrosis, or calcification. Frequently in adult lungs healed remnants of primary tuberculous infection may be found by careful search. In the few patients who develop progressive disease, direct extension of the pulmonary lesion and bronchial dissemination to other parts of the lung occur. Involvement of the bronchi, with subsequent rupture of lesions into the lumen, results either from the pulmonary lesion itself or from an adjacent caseous lymph node. Small and large areas of tuberculous bronchopneumonia are scattered throughout the lung. When a significant degree of immunity exists, the lesions are likely to be of a proliferative nature. In a poorly resistant patient, however, especially when a large number of bacilli have been disseminated and tissue hypersensitivity has developed, an extensive pneumonia with exudation and severe caseation necrosis may be produced ("caseous pneumonia").

Cavitation, which occasionally occurs in the progressive lesions, is not as striking a feature as it is in reinfection tuberculosis. Other possible complications of bronchial spread may result from coughing up of infected material and from initiation of lesions in the opposite lung, larynx, and intestines.

Lymphohematogenous spread may lead to generalized miliary tuberculosis or to localized, progressive disease in a single site (i.e., single, or isolated, organ tuberculosis).

Primary pulmonary tuberculosis has been referred to commonly as "childhood type." While it is true that this is the usual manifestation of the disease in children and infants, it may also appear in adolescents and adults not previously infected. Most cases of bovine tuberculous infection from milk occur in childhood, but as already mentioned, the bovine bacillus accounts for only a small proportion of tuberculosis cases. The infection occurs by way of the alimentary tract with involvement of cervical or mesenteric lymph nodes.

Reinfection tuberculosis. Reinfection tuberculosis is also re-

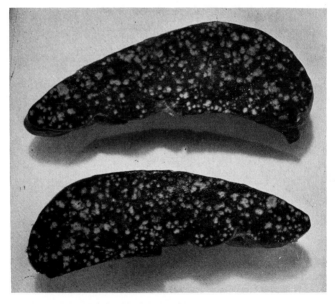

Fig. 6-4. Miliary tuberculosis of the spleen.

ferred to as "adult, "post-primary," or "secondary" type. This is the type most commonly seen in adults, although it may appear in adolescents. The patient has had a previous infection, which might have been detected by a positive tuberculin skin test but, otherwise, usually remained clinically unnoticed. The interval between the primary infection and reinfection tuberculosis is variable, often many years. A debated problem is

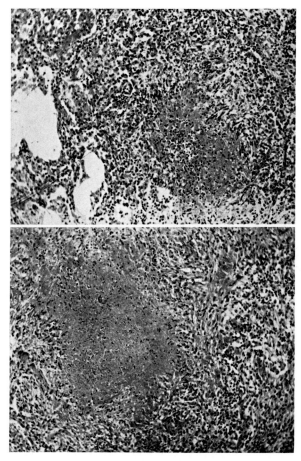

Fig. 6-5. Miliary tubercles in the lung. Note the focal areas of caseous necrosis, about which there is relatively little epithelioid cell formation.

whether reinfection tuberculosis represents a fresh infection from without or a lighting up or reinvasion from a partially healed earlier lesion in which tubercle bacilli have remained viable. There is no doubt that both types can and do occur, and it is generally considered that exogenous reinfection is the more frequent process in older adults, while endogenous reactivation is the more common mechanism in the younger patients.

In adult pulmonary tuberculosis there is a very constant localization of lesions in the upper part of the lung (apical region). The reason for this has never been adequately explained.

A localized pneumonic focus develops in the subapical portion of the lung consisting of exudative and proliferative features, usually with some caseation. If the infection is overcome, healing occurs with fibrosis, leaving a depressed fibrous scar at or near the apex. The scar is often blackened by coal dust pigment, and occasionally ossified. Such scars are very commonly found at autopsy. It is to be noted that other diseases may also produce apical scars, e.g., localized silicotic lesions and histoplasmosis. The regional lymph nodes are usually normal or involved only slightly in these healed cases.

If the lesion progresses, the tubercles coalesce to form a nodular, expanding mass with more extensive caseation necrosis. Healing and fibrosis about the margins result in a fibrocaseous lesion, which in some cases is well walled off and may be stationary. If healing is less complete, irregular extensions into the adjacent lung tissue occur. When a bronchial wall becomes involved in such extension, the caseous material is discharged and coughed up, leaving a cavity in the lung. Such cavities may be as large as 4 or 5 cm. and may have thickened, fibrocaseous walls and rough, irregular linings. Secondary infection by inhaled organisms is usual in these cavities. Severe hemorrhage may occur into a cavity, but hemorrhage is usually slight or entirely lacking as a result of the narrowing of the lumen of involved vessels by intimal thickening (endarteritis obliterans) and thrombosis. The thickened vessels are sometimes seen as firm cords traversing the cavity.

Spread to uninvolved portions of the lung from the active apical lesion may occur as a result of bronchial dissemination of the organisms. Isolated tuberculous nodules may appear, and in places the tubercles coalesce, replacing large areas of parenchyma. Some of the foci undergo caseation necrosis and are surrounded by fibrous tissue (fibrocaseous tuberculosis). Multiple cavities are likely to form in the involved areas. In addition to the role they play in cavitation, the bronchi may be involved by mucosal tuberculous lesions (endobronchial tuberculosis), strictures, and dilatation (bronchiectasis). Patches of pulmonary collapse are usually present. Fibrosis of the lung may be severe enough in some cases to produce pulmonary hypertension and cor pulmonale. With progressive disease of the lungs, the pleura is commonly affected (pleural effusions, fibrinous pleuritis, tuberculous empyema, or fibrosis with partial or complete obliteration of the pleural cavity). Foci of tuberculosis, with little or no caseation necrosis, may be present in the regional lymph nodes. Lesions in the opposite lung, the larynx, or the intestines may result from bronchial spread of the infection.

Hematogenous dissemination may lead to miliary tuberculosis in many organs, including the lungs, or to localized progressive disease in a single tissue or organ (isolated organ tuberculosis). [When a large number of bacilli are spread by way of the bronchi, in the presence of a high degree of hypersensitivity and relatively low immunity, a caseous tuberculous pneumonia develops and progresses rapidly to a fatal ending (galloping consumption).] With such an event the involved portions of the lung are gray white or yellow white, consolidated, and airless. Microscopically there is a massive caseation, the alveoli being filled with necrotic material. There is some protein-containing exudate, and few epithelioid or giant cells are formed.

Healing of tuberculous cavities of the lung is most commonly by inspissated caseous contents filling the lumen and becoming surrounded by contracted scar tissue. The bronchi entering the area become narrowed and finally have their lumina occluded. Rarely there may be healing by scar tissue with no caseous remnants remaining, or there may be "open healing," the cavity remaining open and in communication with bronchi, the fibrous wall tending to develop an epithelial lining. There is evidence that streptomycin therapy promotes regression and healing of tuberculous lesions, particularly those that are recent and predominantly exudative.

EXTRAPULMONARY TUBERCULOSIS

Tuberculous pericarditis. Tuberculous involvement in the pericardium is usually an extension from the lungs or mediastinal lymph nodes. It is characterized by extreme thickening

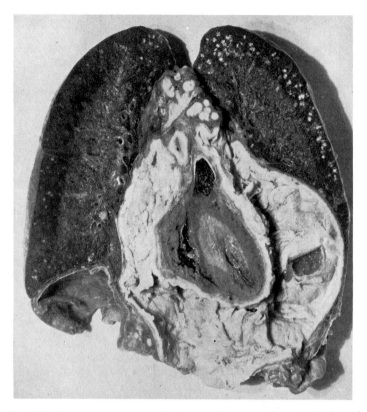

Fig. 6-6. Tuberculous pericarditis. Note the tremendous thickening of the pericardium, the caseation of the mediastinal lymph nodes, and the tubercles in the lungs.

of visceral and parietal layers because of the tuberculous lesions, frequently with much caseation necrosis, and because of organizing fibrinous exudate. (See p. 326.)

Intestinal tuberculosis. Intestinal tuberculosis is usually a complication of pulmonary tuberculosis resulting from swallowing infected sputum. It begins in lymphoid tissue of the ileum or cecum and results in ulcers whose long axes run transversely. (See Fig. 6-7, p. 145, and p. 631.)

Tuberculous peritonitis. Peritoneal tuberculosis may be localized around an infected mesenteric node, fallopian tube, or

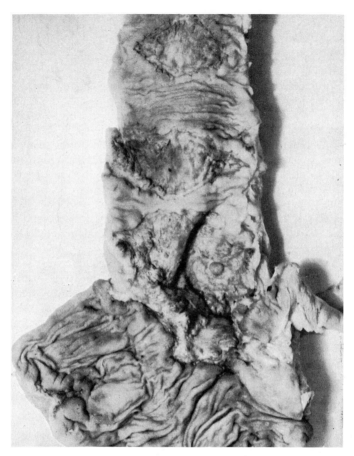

Fig. 6-7. Tuberculous enteritis, terminal ileum. Note the oval ulcers which tend to encircle the bowel.

other visceral lesion. A general form also occurs in which both visceral and parietal peritoneum become studded with tiny tubercles. There may be abundant peritoneal exudate (wet form) or a fibrinous exudate causing marked adhesions of viscera (dry or plastic form). (See p. 661.)

Tuberculosis of larynx. The larynx most often becomes infected by sputum from pulmonary lesions. Ulceration is usual, and there may be considerable destruction or fibrosis.

Tuberculosis of kidney. The kidney is usually involved in generalized miliary tuberculosis. Hematogenous spread of tubercle bacilli also causes isolated organ tuberculosis resulting in a chronic ulcerative type of tuberculous pyonephrosis. (See p. 393.)

Tuberculosis of ureter and bladder. Tuberculosis of the ureter and bladder is usually secondary to involvement of the kidney, and in the bladder it is most prominent around ureteral openings. Cystitis often gives the first evidence of renal infection.

Tuberculosis of male genitalia. Male genital organs are most often involved by hematogenous spread. The epididymis, seminal vesicles, and prostate are often infected, but involvement of the testis is less common and usually is secondary to the lesion in the epididymis. Another possible source of infection of the prostate is infected urine from a tuberculous kidney; and the prostate disease, in turn, may extend to the seminal vesicles and epididymis.

Tuberculosis of female genitalia. Of the female genitalia the fallopian tubes are most commonly involved, and from them the infection may spread to the endometrium or to the peritoneal cavity. (See p. 744.) Infection of the tubes is by way of the bloodstream.

Tuberculous meningitis. Except when occurring as part of a miliary tuberculosis, meningeal infection is usually a spread from a caseous focus in the brain substance or choroid plexus. An abundant translucent exudate covers basal portions of the brain. The exudate is less noticeable over the convexities of the brain. Minute tubercles may be seen along the course of blood vessels and are frequently obvious on the margins of the Sylvian fissure. In the nervous tissue itself localized, tumorlike tuberculous lesions (tuberculomas) may develop to considerable size. (See p. 906.)

Tuberculosis of bones and joints. Children are particularly susceptible to tuberculosis of the bones and joints, which is sometimes due to bovine infection. Spongy bone especially is attacked. Tuberculosis of the bodies of vertebrae (Pott's disease) may cause deformities such as kyphosis. (See p. 839.)

Tuberculosis of skin. There are several types of tuberculous skin lesions, of which *lupus vulgaris* is most common. *Tuberculides* are skin lesions which histologically resemble tuberculosis, but in which the organisms are rarely demonstrable.

ATYPICAL MYCOBACTERIOSIS

There has been a growing awareness in recent years of a group of mycobacteria that resemble *Mycobacterium tuberculosis,* but differ from it in several respects, and are known as the "atypical," "anonymous," or "unclassified" mycobacteria. Many of these organisms produce colonial pigmentation, and all of them are nonpathogenic for guinea pigs. They include Group I: photochromogens (*M. kansasii*—"yellow bacillus"); Group II: scotochromogens (*M. scrofulaceum*—"orange bacillus"); Group III: nonphotochromogens ("Battey bacillus"); and Group IV: rapid growers *(M. fortuitum).*

The disease caused in man by these organisms (atypical mycobacteriosis) may be localized or disseminated. The localized form is most common in the lungs, particularly in middle-aged persons, and in the cervical lymph nodes of children. Rarely the bones and joints may be affected. While any of the atypical mycobacteria may be identified with pulmonary disease, one of the photochromogens or the nonphotochromogens is usually the responsible agent. Most of the cases of cervical lymphadenopathy (in the United States) are caused by the scotochromogens. The mode of transmission of the infection is not known, and evidence of man-to-man transmission is lacking. The microscopic appearance of the local disease is similar to that of tuberculosis. Although there are certain differences, it is generally believed that it is impossible to make a positive differential histopathologic diagnosis between the two. The pulmonary disease simulates tuberculosis clinically and radiologically.

Disseminated atypical mycobacteriosis is rare and fatal, usually occurring in young children debilitated by other diseases or receiving steroid therapy. Lesions are most frequent in lymph nodes, the reticuloendothelial system, and bones, being characterized by varying degrees of noncaseous necrosis, hypertrophy and hyperplasia of the reticuloendothelial cells, and numerous acid-fast bacilli within and outside histiocytes. Granulomas and caseous necrosis are rarely seen.

M. balnei and *M. ulcerans,* which cause tuberculoid skin lesions, are also atypical mycobacteria but are generally considered separately from the previous four groups. *M. balnei* has been incriminated as a cause of swimming pool granuloma.

Chapter 7

Rickettsial and viral diseases

Rickettsial and viral diseases are considered together because they are closely related biologically. Both are caused by obligate intracellular parasites that multiply only when they are in living cells by utilizing the enzyme systems of these cells. Because of their complex growth requirements, they cannot be cultivated on lifeless media. They may be propagated in living animals, in tissue cultures, or in the cells of the membranes of the developing chick embryo. On the other hand, bacteria generally are able to live independently, so that they exist and multiply extracellularly within the tissues of a host, and they can be cultivated on cell-free media. There are a few bacteria with partial enzyme deficiencies that often grow within cells, but even these can be grown on special cell-free media (e.g., *Bartonella bacilliformis*).

Rickettsiae are considered to be intermediate between bacteria and viruses in regard to morphologic features and independent metabolic activity; but they are more closely related to bacteria, resembling them in several respects. They are visible by light microscopy (when appropriate stains are used), appearing as small, pleomorphic coccobacillary forms. Also, like bacteria, they are retained by the Berkefeld filter, reproduce by binary fission, contain both nucleic acids (RNA and DNA), possess certain metabolic enzymes, and are susceptible to antibiotics. However, although they possess a certain degree of independent metabolic activity, they are greatly dependent upon the intracellular enzymes of the host for much of their metabolism.

Viruses, on the other hand, are devoid of any enzymes for their own metabolic functions and are totally dependent upon the enzymes of the infected cells. A virus, in its simple form, consists of an outer coat of protein and an inner core of nucleic acid—either RNA or DNA, not both. The protein portion is antigenic and is responsible for most of the immunologic reactions induced by viruses. Because of their very small size, viruses can be seen only with the electron microscope, with the exception of some of the large viruses that are just barely visible with the light microscope (e.g., the intracytoplasmic "elementary bodies" of smallpox).

The causative agents of psittacosis, lymphogranuloma venereum, trachoma, and inclusion conjunctivitis, were formerly classified as viruses but are now grouped separately, between the rickettsiae and the viruses. These obligate intracellular parasites, sometimes called "pseudoviruses," bear a resemblance to the rickettsiae in size, staining characteristics, reproduction by binary fission, possession of both RNA and DNA, and susceptibility to antibiotics; but they have a more limited capacity for independent metabolic activity. It has been suggested that this psittacosis-lymphogranuloma-trachoma group of agents be named the *Bedsoniae* after Bedson, who made the first comprehensive study of the psittacosis agent. They are also referred to as *Chlamydiae*.

RICKETTSIAL DISEASES

The rickettsiae lead an intracellular existence in the tissues of many arthropods. These organisms usually do not injure their arthropod hosts and in several instances are transmitted from generation to generation by inclusion in the ova. Of the many

Table 7-1. *Rickettsial diseases of man*

	Etiologic agent	Vector	Distribution
Typhus fever			
Epidemic	*R. Prowazeki*	Lice	Europe, Africa, Asia, Central and South America
Endemic	*R. mooseri*	Rat flea	Worldwide
Spotted fever group			
Rocky Mountain spotted fever	*R. rickettsi*	Ticks	Worldwide
Boutonneuse fever	*R. conori*	Ticks	Mediterranean area
Rickettsialpox	*R. akari*	Mites	New York
Tsutsugamushi disease	*R. tsutsugamushi*	Mites	Western Pacific area
Q fever	*R. burneti*	Ticks?	Australia, United States
Trench fever	*R. quintana*	Lice	Europe

rickettsiae inhabiting arthropod tissues, the ones listed in Table 7-1 are known to be pathogenic for man. *Bartonella bacilliformis*, the cause of Carrión's disease, is not included with the rickettsiae but is closely related to them and will be discussed in this chapter for the sake of convenience.

Rickettsial diseases clinically are acute fevers, usually with characteristic skin eruptions and with variable mortality in different outbreaks. Clinically variant forms are seen, partly as a result of variation in virulence and partly because of strain modifications from prolonged residence in different arthropod and mammalian hosts. Immunologic studies have shown, however, that all rickettsial diseases known at present fall into one or another of the foregoing groups.

Typhus group. Epidemic or human typhus is numerically the most important of the rickettsial diseases. About 15,000,000 cases with over 3,000,000 deaths occurred during and shortly after World War I. In World War II devastating epidemics did not occur, a fact which probably may be attributed largely to improved delousing methods and prophylactic vaccination. The etiologic agent, *R. prowazeki* (Fig. 7-1), is carried from man to man by the infected louse, *Pediculus humanus*. The organisms, which multiply in the intestinal lining cells and are

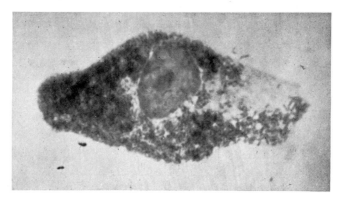

Fig. 7-1. Typhus rickettsiae. Photomicrograph showing a serosal cell almost completely filled with *Rickettsia prowazeki;* Giemsa-stained film preparation from the scrotal sac of an infected guinea pig. (Courtesy Dr. Henry Pinkerton.)

present in the feces of the louse, gain entrance to dermal capillaries through the puncture wound made by the louse in feeding.

Endemic or murine typhus, with a reservoir in wild rats, is transmitted to man by the bite of the rat flea. This type is clinically milder, and slight but definite immunologic differences between it and epidemic louse-borne typhus have been demonstrated. Presumably murine typhus may be transformed into epidemic typhus by repeated louse transfer, but this has not been proved.

The gross pathology of typhus is not impressive; no changes other than splenic enlargement and cloudy swelling of the organs are seen. Microscopically there is found a generalized proliferative reaction of the endothelium of small blood vessels, often leading to thrombosis and caused by the growth of rickettsiae in the cytoplasm of the endothelial cells. Localized perivascular collections of mononuclear cells (the so-called typhus nodules) are also characteristic. Demonstration of the organisms is difficult and requires perfect fixation and staining. Fixation in Regaud's fluid and staining by the Giemsa method are most satisfactory. Lesions are seen most strikingly in the skin, myocardium, and brain. In the myocardium, in addition to the vascular lesions, a diffuse infiltration of mononuclear cells between the muscle fibers is seen, with myocardial fiber degeneration in some instances. In the brain the characteristic focal lesions center around minute damaged capillaries. Petechial hemorrhages, perivascular cuffing, and glial nodes are also seen, so that the picture resembles that of the various types of viral encephalitis. Interstitial pneumonitis, characterized by the accumulation of mononuclear cells in the alveolar walls, often appears to be part of the picture of uncomplicated typhus.

Clinically typhus is characterized by headache, mild chills, and fever which reaches its height at the end of the first week and terminates by rapid lysis, in uncomplicated cases, on the fourteenth to sixteenth days. The characteristic rash appears between the fourth and eighth days. It consists of pink macules and papules 2 to 5 mm. in diameter, which later become hemorrhagic because of thrombosis of the skin capillaries. In the second week, delirium, stupor, or even coma may be seen as a result of the encephalitis. Gangrene of the skin from vascular occlusion is occasionally seen. Death may be due to the myocarditis, to the encephalitis, to secondary bronchopneumonia, or to generalized toxemia. There is evidence that a shocklike condition with peripheral circulatory failure, hemoconcentration, and low blood pressure also may be important in many fatal cases.

The natural mortality is 20 to 70% in epidemic typhus and 2 to 3% in murine typhus. It is practically nil in young children and very high in the aged. Antibiotics such as chloramphenicol and the tetracyclines have greatly improved the prognosis.

Spotted fever group. The spotted fever group, in addition to Rocky Mountain spotted fever of the United States and Brazilian spotted fever, includes fièvre boutonneuse of the Mediterranean countries, South African tick-bite fever, and rickettsialpox. The clinical picture of Rocky Mountain spotted fever is similar to that of typhus, but the rash appears earlier (on the second to fifth day), is more hemorrhagic, appears first on the extremities, and involves the palms and soles. Cases have occurred in all sections of the United States. It is endemic in the South Atlantic states, where the largest number of infections are reported. In fièvre boutonneuse a local lesion at the portal of entry and regional lymphadenitis are reported. All of these diseases except rickettsialpox are carried by ticks, and the rickettsiae are found in the cytoplasm and also in compact clusters in the nuclei of the cells of many tissues in ticks, including the salivary glands. Several varieties of ticks and several intermediate mammalian hosts are involved in the epidemiology of different varieties within this group. The mortality in Rocky Mountain spotted fever in different localities and from various strains ranges from 1% up to 95% (average, 20%) without chemotherapy.

Pathologically the changes in spotted fever (Fig. 7-2) are much like those in typhus. Differential microscopic diagnosis can be made only by an experienced observer. Rickettsiae are found in the smooth muscle cells of arterioles as well as in the endothelial cells, while in typhus the organisms are confined to the endothelium. The pathologic physiology and modes of death are those already described for typhus.

Rickettsialpox is carried from the house mouse to man by a mite. The etiologic agent, *R. akari,* localizes in the nuclei of infected yolk sac cells. The rash in this disease passes through a vesicular stage. Little is known of the systemic pathologic changes in man, since the disease has no mortality.

Tsutsugamushi group. The tsutsugamushi group of diseases occurs in Japan, China, Sumatra, Australia, and several other countries and islands along the western Pacific coast. This group

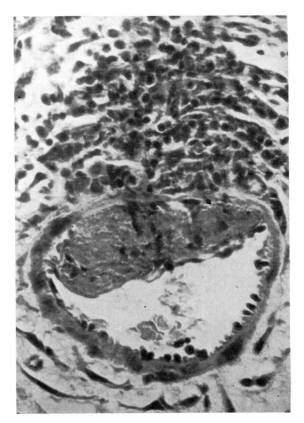

Fig. 7-2. Rocky Mountain spotted fever, showing the characteristic vascular pathology. A fibrin thrombus partially occludes the lumen of the vessel, and there is a focal perivascular collection of lymphocytes and macrophages. (Courtesy Dr. Henry Pinkerton.)

includes "scrub typhus," which assumed military importance in World War II. The etiologic agent, *R. tsutsugamushi,* is carried by the larval form of the tropical mite, *Trombicula akamushi.* Tsutsugamushi disease is an exanthematic febrile illness, often difficult to differentiate clinically from typhus and spotted fever. In most strains a necrotic lesion occurs at the site of attachment of the vector, together with regional lymphadenitis. The mortality without chemotherapy is high (20 to 60%). The disease has a reservoir in mice and other rodents and is readily trans-

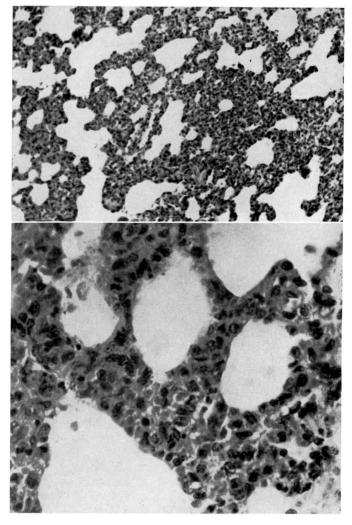

Fig. 7-3. Interstitial pneumonia in a case of tsutsugamushi disease

mitted to mice and guinea pigs by the injection of blood from human patients.

The pathologic changes are essentially like those in typhus and spotted fever, with the addition of mild rickettsial peritonitis, pleuritis, and pericarditis. Interstitial pneumonitis (Fig. 7-3), probably of rickettsial origin, is usually found but is often complicated by bacterial bronchopneumonia. The tendency for thrombosis to occur is much less than in typhus and spotted fever, and for this reason the rash does not become hemorrhagic and resembles more the eruption seen in measles. The cerebral and myocardial lesions resemble those of typhus and spotted fever.

Q fever. Australian Q fever, described in 1936, is probably identical with American Q fever and "Balkan grippe," which have been discovered more recently. The etiologic agent, *R.* (or *Coxiella*) *burneti*, has been isolated from ticks in Montana. Unlike other rickettsiae it passes through porcelain filters. Clinically there is usually no rash, but an atypical bronchopneumonia, discoverable at times only by x-ray examination, seems to be a constant finding. The mortality is low. The epidemiology is not yet clear. In Australia and the United States, slaughterhouse and stockyard workers have become infected, either directly or by the inhalation of tick feces. Epidemiologic studies of "Balkan grippe" suggested the inhalation of dust contaminated by animals rather than person-to-person transfer as the mode

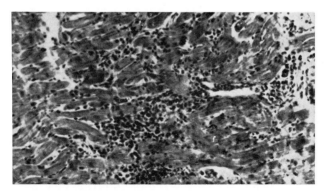

Fig. 7-4. Interstitial myocarditis in a case of tsutsugamushi disease.

of transmission. In fatal cases the lungs show firm consolidation and microscopically an interstitial pneumonia, with inflammatory cells in the alveolar walls, while the alveolar spaces contain fibrin with only a few mononuclear cells.

Diagnosis of rickettsial diseases. The Weil-Felix reaction, carried out much like the Widal reaction in typhoid, is of value in the diagnosis of typhus, spotted fever, and tsutsugamushi disease. The organisms used are strains of *Bacillus proteus* isolated from patients. Although this organism is unrelated to the etiologic rickettsiae, agglutination occurs frequently in high titers for some unknown reason. In typhus, agglutination in high titer with *B. proteus* OX19 is characteristically obtained, while in tsutsugamushi disease, the principal agglutinins are against *B. proteus* OXK. In Rocky Mountain spotted fever, agglutinins for both of the foregoing strains, as well as for OX2, are commonly present. Q fever is not associated with agglutinins for *B. proteus.*

Injection of guinea pigs with blood from suspected cases is often necessary for the accurate diagnosis of sporadic cases of typhus, spotted fever, and Q fever. After the strain has been established in guinea pigs, cross-immunity tests with known strains are carried out. Complement-fixation tests are also valuable.

Vaccination. Although the rickettsiae refuse to grow on cellfree bacteriologic media, vaccines of undoubted value have been prepared against typhus, spotted fever, and Q fever. Of the various sources of rickettsiae, the infected yolk sac membrane of the developing chick embryo has proved most suitable for largescale production of vaccine. The rickettsiae grow freely in the cells lining the yolk sac and are readily freed from their host cells and from the yolk to form the emulsion used for vaccination.

BARTONELLOSIS (CARRIÓN'S DISEASE)

Carrión's disease is of considerable importance in Peru, Ecuador, Chile, and Colombia but has not been reported elsewhere. It is caused by a rickettsia-like organism, *Bartonella bacilliformis*, which is carried by sandflies. It occurs in two stages: an acute febrile anemia (Oroya fever) and a nodular cutaneous eruption (verruga peruana). The anemic stage is caused by the growth of the organism in the red blood cells. In severe cases the red cell count falls rapidly and death occurs in a few days. The cutaneous eruption occurs during convalescence from the

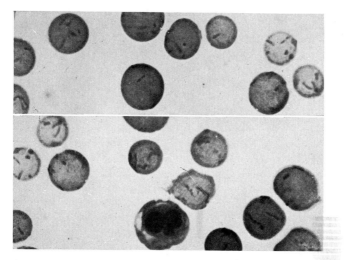

Fig. 7-5. Oroya fever, showing bacillary and coccoid forms of *Bartonella bacilliformis* in the erythrocytes. (Giemsa-stained blood film.)

anemic stage or may occur in persons who have passed through a mild anemic stage without clinical illness or with only mild illness.

The organism, which grows in special cell-free media, is found in proliferating endothelial cells of the cutaneous lesions as well as in the red blood cells. In fatal cases not only the red cells but the reticuloendothelial cells in almost all organs are filled with organisms. The cutaneous lesions microscopically resemble rapidly growing hemangioendotheliomas, but eventually they heal without leaving scars. Diagnosis is made by finding the organism in red blood cells in Giemsa-stained blood smears (Fig. 7-5) or by blood culture.

VIRAL DISEASES

Several of the larger viruses are nearly as large as rickettsiae and some of the smaller bacteria, whereas the smaller viruses approach molecular size (8 mμ). Nucleic acid (RNA or DNA) appears to be the infectious heart of the virus particle and is concentrated in the interior, within a protein exterior part. This simple form, however, may be modified in some viruses. The inner core may consist of a nucleoprotein (nucleic acid combined with protein), as in the influenza virus; and the protein coat in more complex animal viruses may be surrounded by an envelope consisting of lipid, protein, and sometimes carbohydrate.

In association with many viral infections, *inclusion bodies* are seen in the infected cells. The bodies occur either in the nucleus or in the cytoplasm. They vary considerably in shape and size but usually are roughly spherical, and their average size is about that of the erythrocyte. They usually are eosinophilic with ordinary staining methods, but may be basophilic or amphophilic, and they tend to be surrounded by a clear zone in the nucleoplasm or cytoplasm in which they are embedded.

The inclusion bodies of several of the larger viruses, such as those of smallpox, are clusters of small rickettsia-like structures known as *elementary bodies.* Such inclusions are granular in appearance when suitably stained. The inclusion bodies associated with the smaller viruses are homogeneous or coarsely vacuolated. They may be aggregates of elementary bodies, too small to be seen as individuals, or they may arise from the damaged cytoplasm or nucleoplasm of cells. It has been suggested that in the early stages, inclusion bodies are basophilic because of the presence of nucleic acid in the viruses, and in the later stages they become eosinophilic because they lack infectious viruses and represent only the altered site they once occupied.

The important properties of viruses are as follows: (1) Viruses grow only within cells, often only within certain types of cells and in certain species of animals (cell and host specificity). They cannot be cultivated in cell-free media. They can be grown only in media containing living cells or in the membranes of the developing egg embryo. (2) There may be a formation of inclusion bodies (see previous discussion). In many viral diseases, however, these structures are not seen. (3) Many viruses lie dormant in tissues for long periods of time (latent infection), producing neither symptoms nor lesions. Under certain circumstances the infection may flare up. Latent infections may be established in utero and may remain so for a long time after birth. It is not certain what causes this latency, but contributing factors may be the presence of antibodies or other viral inhibitors (e.g., *interferon,* a protein produced by viral-infected cells). (4) Viruses are sensitive to environmental conditions (e.g., temperature, radiation, nutritional changes, etc.), which affect intracellular enzyme functions. (5) Viral infections tend to pave the way for bacterial infection, which is often the true cause of death. (6) Immunity of high degree and long duration characteristically follows viral infections. Exceptions to this are the common cold, influenza, and herpes simplex. (7) Many viruses are transmitted to man by insect vectors. (8) Viral infections in general do not respond to usual antibacterial chemotherapeutic agents such as the sulfonamides, chloramphenicol, tetracyclines, and penicillin. This is probably because of their intracellular location and metabolic dependence on their host cells.

The microscopic changes produced by viral infection are almost as varied as those produced by bacteria, including degeneration and necrosis of cells; inflammatory cell reaction, chiefly mononuclear; fusion giant-cell formation; and hyperplasia. Sometimes, cellular inclusion bodies accompany these lesions. Of particular interest is the fact that certain tumors of lower animals are apparently caused by viruses, notably the Rous chicken sarcoma, the Shope rabbit papilloma, leukemia in fowl and mice, and Lücke's carcinoma of the frog kidney. In the latter tumor nuclear inclusions are seen. The possible relationship of viruses to human cancer is under investigation. Certain viruslike particles have been identified in human leukemic cells, but some investigators claim these are mycoplasmas and not viruses.

For the isolation of viruses the intracerebral or intranasal injection of mice and the intranasal injection of ferrets have proved particularly successful, but in certain viral diseases the monkey is the only animal that has been successfully infected. The propagation of viruses in tissue cultures and on the chorioallantoic and yolk sac membranes of the chick embryo has also been of great value. In tissue cultures, cytopathogenic agents have been isolated that are not yet associated with specific diseases. Growth of viruses on mammalian cells cultivated in vitro has been an important technique in the recent increase of knowledge of viruses and viral infection.

The classification of viruses is based upon the chemical composition, morphologic features, and antigenicity of the mature virus particle *(virion)*. Generally two major groups are considered, depending on the nucleic acid content—RNA or DNA viruses. These are further subclassified as to size of the virion, morphologic features of the subunits *(capsomeres)* of the protein coat *(capsid)*, presence or absence of an envelope, and antigenic types. The following viral diseases will be grouped according to the system of the body in which the chief clinical manifestations are seen.

Viral diseases of central nervous system

General considerations. The viral diseases of the central nervous system form a group of great clinical importance. In addition to those in which a viral etiology has been proved by transmission to experimental animals, there are several conditions of probable viral etiology.

Viruses produce a diffuse inflammation of brain or cord substance (encephalitis or myelitis) or cause lesions in both brain and cord (encephalomyelitis). Meningitis is a common accompanying feature and in some cases may be the predominant lesion (e.g., lymphocytic choriomeningitis). For the most part, the viruses develop within ganglion cells of the brain and cord and in neuroglial cells. Nervous tissue responds to the necrosis of these cells by an inflammatory reaction, essentially like that in other tissues but with certain special features. Since the lesions produced by different viruses have many histologic features in common, certain general types of lesions may first be described. Capillary congestion and petechial hemorrhages into the perivascular spaces and surrounding brain substance are common to most viral infections. Accumulations of lymphocytes and plasma cells around blood vessels (perivascular cuffing) is another common type of lesion. Early degenerative changes in ganglion cells are difficult to recognize, but nuclear degeneration, especially when accompanied by the accumulation of large mononuclear phagocytes around the damaged cells, is clear evidence of cell death. This phenomenon is called *neuronophagia*. The mononuclear phagocytes are derived from the microglial cells, which are believed to be of mesenchymal origin and members of the reticuloendothelial system.

Focal collections of neuroglial cells (glial nodes) appear to be an attempt at repair and correspond to fibroblastic proliferation outside of the nervous system. Swelling, sometimes with proliferation, of capillary endothelium occurs much as it does in inflammatory lesions elsewhere but rarely is accompanied by thrombosis. Focal areas of demyelinization and encephalomalacia may be seen, but extensive demyelinization is likely to occur only in so-called postinfection encephalomyelitis.

Rabies. Rabies is a viral disease, always fatal when untreated, which is usually acquired by the bite of a dog. Rabies has been found in bats, and human infection has been caused by the bite of a bat. The disease has also been recognized in wolves, foxes, skunks, squirrels, and other animals that may transmit it to humans. The virus is introduced into the wound with the saliva and travels slowly along the peripheral nerves to reach the brain. The long incubation period in most cases (often several months) allows time for preventive vaccination. When a dog suspected of having rabies has bitten a human being, the dog should be captured alive. If the dog has rabies, death will occur in a few days, and a positive diagnosis can be made by finding the characteristic inclusion bodies (Negri bodies) in the ganglion cells of the brain. Intracranial injection of emulsified dog brain into mice may give a positive diagnosis in some cases in which Negri bodies cannot be found. Staining tissue from the brain or salivary glands of the dog with fluorescent antibody is regarded as a reliable diagnostic technique.

Clinically the disease is manifested by muscular spasm, excitement, generalized convulsions, and eventual coma. The pathologic lesions are confined to the brain and spinal cord. Grossly no striking changes are seen. Microscopically there may be areas of petechial hemorrhage, perivascular accumulations of lymphocytes, and ganglion cell degeneration with the accumulation of phagocytic cells (neuronophagia). In the ganglion cells are found the pathognomonic, eosinophilic, intracytoplasmic Negri bodies. Often, however, the inflammatory reaction is minimal, and the only evidence of the disease is the presence of these Negri bodies. Goodpasture believed that the Negri bodies are composed largely of degeneration products of the neurofibrillae, but other workers have thought that they are composed of elementary bodies. With ordinary staining methods the Negri bodies appear homogeneous or vacuolated rather than granular.

Poliomyelitis (infantile paralysis). Poliomyelitis is an acute viral infection in which the most important lesions are those involving the spinal cord. It is primarily a disease of children. The relative immunity of adults is probably the result of mild unrecognized or asymptomatic infections during childhood. During epidemics, which occur in the late summer and fall, many children who do not show paralysis suffer from mild upper respiratory or gastrointestinal symptoms, with or without minor neurologic findings. The virus may be isolated from the throat washings of such children. These mild or abortive cases are believed to be about six times as common as the cases with frank paralysis and probably play an important part in the epidemiology of the disease. There is some evidence that apparently healthy people may act as carriers of the virus.

Experimentally the disease may be transmitted to monkeys by intranasal injection of the virus, and some strains have been adapted to mice. The high concentration of the virus in human stools and its isolation from sewage suggest that under natural conditions the gastrointestinal route of infection may be important. The evidence suggests that the bloodstream is the principal route by which the virus reaches the central nervous system. Paralytic disease can be prevented by an antibody barrier in the bloodstream.

The cultivation of the virus in tissue culture has led to the development of a vaccine that has reduced the incidence of paralytic poliomyelitis.

Clinically the disease is characterized by fever, malaise, headache, vomiting, and occasionally by neck rigidity. Spinal fluid examination usually shows 10 to 200 cells per cubic millimeter, with lymphocytes predominating, although neutrophils may be more conspicuous in the early stages. Within two or three days flaccid paralysis of the arms and legs commonly occurs. This lower motor neuron type of paralysis is caused by necrosis of the ganglion cells in the anterior horns of the spinal cord. Involvement of the respiratory center leads to sudden death. In certain cases the brain is involved, giving a clinical picture suggesting encephalitis.

Grossly the spinal cord and, in the superior type, the brainstem and dentate nucleus may show edema and petechial hemorrhages. The microscopic lesion consists essentially of degeneration and necrosis of the ganglion cells, followed by inflammation, and is usually best seen in, but not limited to, the anterior horns of the spinal cord. Intranuclear inclusions are said to be present in the ganglion cells in the early stages, but they are difficult to find in human autopsy material. Such inclusions have been demonstrated in experimental infection in monkeys. The various changes occurring in the ganglion cells include swelling and chromatolysis (dissolution of Nissl substance); nuclear alterations such as displacement, loss of staining, fragmentation, pyknosis, and disappearance; and fragmentation and shrinkage of cells. Often the ganglion cells have largely disappeared. The various types of reaction described earlier—perivascular mononuclear-cell cuffing, petechial hemorrhage, neuronophagia, and glial nodes—are characteristically seen (Fig. 7-6). Neutrophils are usually present in considerable numbers, often in focal collections, and their presence is important in differenti-

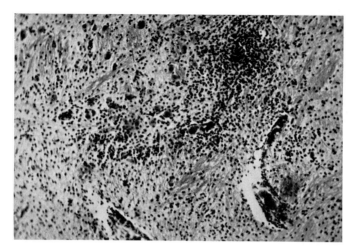

Fig. 7-6. Acute poliomyelitis. Focal and diffuse collections of inflammatory cells, some of which are perivascular in position.

ating the superior type from encephalitis lethargica, since the inflammatory cells are almost all mononuclears in the latter disease. In poliomyelitis a slight lymphocytic infiltration of the meninges commonly occurs. Also, lesions may be present in the cerebellum and cerebrum. Lesions sometimes seen outside the nervous system include parenchymatous degeneration of liver and kidneys, myocarditis, slight splenomegaly, and generalized lymphadenopathy (lymphoid hyperplasia).

In unrecovered cases the paralyzed muscles show atrophy and replacement by fatty tissue and connective tissue.

Encephalitis lethargica. Encephalitis lethargica (von Economo's disease) is a disease of unknown cause that was common after World War I but is now rarely diagnosed. The establishment of the viral origin of St. Louis encephalitis, Japanese B encephalitis, equine encephalomyelitis, and Australian X disease, all of which resemble epidemic encephalitis pathologically, is probably the most important reason for believing in the viral nature of the latter disease. The herpes virus has been suspected of causing encephalitis lethargica but is rarely recovered by animal inoculation, and on the whole the evidence is far from conclusive.

The clinical picture is variable and is characterized by various combinations of somnolence, excitement, diplopia, and reflex changes. The mortality during the acute stage is 20 to 40%. Lethargy may persist for many months. Dementia, permanent cranial nerve paralysis, and other neurologic symptoms may occur. Paralysis agitans, with slow speech, expressionless face, and pill-rolling tremor, is a common sequela, even when the initial attack is mild. The spinal fluid, in the acute stage of the disease, shows a normal or slightly increased cell count (lymphocytes), and neutrophils are absent.

The gross and microscopic lesions are seen in the cerebral cortex, basal ganglia, midbrain, and pons and are in general similar to those of poliomyelitis except for their different distribution, less severe degeneration of ganglion cells, and the absence of neutrophils, already commented on. Perivascular collections of lymphocytes are the most constant and conspicuous microscopic feature. Inclusion bodies have not been described.

St. Louis encephalitis. St. Louis encephalitis shows only minor clinical and pathologic differences from encephalitis lethargica but is readily transmissible to mice by the intracerebral injection of brain tissue from fatal cases. Unfortunately the virus cannot be recovered from spinal fluid by this method. Evidence of mosquito transmission of this type of encephalitis has been obtained. The usual transmission cycle in nature involves birds and mosquitoes, and man is an incidental host when bitten by an infected mosquito. The virus has been recovered from chicken mites. Lesions are most prominent in the midbrain and brain-stem, but they occur to a lesser degree in the cerebral cortex, cerebellum, and spinal cord. Microscopically they are similar to those of encephalitis lethargica, although meningeal infiltration by lymphocytes tends to be more striking in St. Louis encephalitis. Inclusion bodies have not been demonstrated. Serious sequelae of the type following encephalitis lethargica occur only rarely.

Equine encephalomyelitis. Equine encephalomyelitis is of particular interest as an example of a disease that was thoroughly studied in a lower animal (the horse) before there was reason to suspect its importance in human pathology. It occurs in two strains, the eastern and western, which only partially cross-immunize. The disease is immunologically distinct from St. Louis encephalitis and other known types of viral encephalitis. The pathologic lesions involve the brain and spinal cord and microscopically resemble those of encephalitis lethargica, but neutrophils are more prominent. The disease is almost certainly conveyed to man by mosquitoes. Inclusion bodies are not seen. The eastern form in man is more severe and has a higher mortality than the western form. Another equine disease, Venezuelan equine encephalomyelitis, is self-limited when it occurs in man and rarely is fatal.

Lymphocytic choriomeningitis. Lymphocytic choriomeningitis is characterized by headache, nausea, vomiting, and rigidity of the neck. In some cases the clinical picture resembles that of influenza. It has a low mortality, and the pathologic picture in man has not been sufficiently studied. In mice and guinea pigs, which are readily infected by the inoculation of spinal fluid from a human case, there is a severe lymphocytic reaction in the meninges, and interstitial pneumonia is also found. The infection occurs naturally in lower animals, particularly the mouse. Inhalation of dusts contaminated by secretions or excreta of infected mice may be the means of transmission of the disease to man. The possibility of arthropod vectors has been suggested.

Acute disseminated (postinfectious) encephalomyelitis. Acute disseminated encephalomyelitis occurs after certain infectious diseases (notably measles, mumps, smallpox, and chickenpox) and vaccination for smallpox or rabies. It also occurs spontaneously. Some workers believe that the viruses of the antecedent diseases, or introduced by vaccination, are etiologically involved, either directly or by inducing cerebral anoxia. The evidence for this is not conclusive, but in some instances the virus has been isolated from the brain or inclusion bodies have been demonstrated. The most widely held theory, however, is that an autoimmune mechanism is responsible for the disease.

Microscopically most of the lesions just described as characteristic of the viral encephalitides are inconspicuous, and the essential feature is extensive perivascular demyelinization, best demonstrated by the Weigert stain. This stain colors the normal myelin sheaths black, and areas of demyelinization stand out clearly.

Diagnosis of viral encephalitides. The various types of viral encephalitis are difficult to distinguish from one another and from certain types of noninfectious encephalitis on purely clinical grounds. Accurate diagnosis must therefore be based upon isolation of the virus or upon immunologic tests.

Unfortunately the isolation of the neurotropic viruses in animals is usually possible only by the injection of brain material obtained post mortem. This method is of value in determining the nature of the virus involved in an epidemic. When the virus has been transmitted to mice, guinea pigs, or other experimental animals, cross-immunity tests with known strains may be carried out. In isolated nonfatal cases, tests for neutralizing and complement-fixing antibodies are valuable. Diagnosis is based on a rise in titer during the course of the disease.

Respiratory viruses

General considerations. The lung, like the central nervous system, reacts to viral infections in a rather characteristic manner, so that the viral cause of a pulmonary lesion may be strongly suspected from histologic evidence alone. Viral pneumonias are of the interstitial type. Inflammatory cells are largely of the mononuclear variety and accumulate chiefly in the alveolar walls and in the peribronchial and septal connective tissue. The alveolar lining cells often undergo cuboidal metaplasia, and mitotic figures are seen in them. The alveoli either remain free from exudate or contain a serous or protein-containing exudate, with only a few inflammatory cells, chiefly mononuclear. Condensation of this exudate by inspired air often forms a hyaline eosinophilic membrane that lines the alveoli. These features, although suggestive, are not pathognomonic of viral infection, since they occur in infections with other intracellular parasites (*Rickettsia* and *Toxoplasma*) and probably in certain bacterial and allergic inflammations of the lung.

The damage inflicted by viruses often makes the lung susceptible to bacterial invasion. Secondary bacterial pneumonia, with its usual picture of exudation into the air spaces, is often present in fatal cases and may obscure the characteristic picture of the original viral pneumonia. There is evidence, for example, that a preceding infection of the lung with the influenza virus is of etiologic importance in certain epidemics of staphylococcal pneumonia.

Influenza. Influenza is numerically the most important of the viral diseases; it is estimated that about 500,000,000 cases with 15 million deaths occurred during the pandemic of 1918-1919. Smith, Andrews, and Laidlaw, in 1933, reproduced the disease in ferrets by the intranasal injection of filtered washings from the nose and throat of human cases, thus demonstrating the viral nature of the disease. Mice are also susceptible, and the virus may be propagated in the fertile egg. Several antigenically different strains are known. Vaccination against the disease is available but presents some problems because of strain differences and the short duration of immunity.

Clinically the disease is a respiratory infection with fever, prostration, and muscular pains. Clinical diagnosis is difficult in sporadic mild cases. Reliable laboratory diagnosis can be made by isolating the virus or by demonstrating antibodies in the blood of the patient. The serologic procedures commonly used are the hemagglutination-inhibition and complement-fixation tests. In its uncomplicated form the disease lasts for only two or three days and recovery is rapid. Fatalities are largely caused by bacterial pneumonia resulting from secondary infection with the influenza bacillus, pneumococci, streptococci, staphylococci, and other organisms. The conditions that initiate and terminate epidemics and pandemics are unknown.

Pathologically influenza is characterized by an acute inflammation of the nasopharynx, trachea, and bronchioles, with congestion, edema, and necrosis and desquamation of the epithelial lining cells. Mucosal epithelial cells may exhibit hyperchromatism and pleomorphism. Metaplasia frequently occurs. Grossly the lungs most frequently show patchy areas of firm deep red consolidation, giving the picture of hemorrhagic bronchopneumonia. Occasionally the picture is that of lobar pneumonia. Acute splenitis and other visceral changes characteristic of sepsis are seen. Alveolar emphysema is present in the less involved areas, and severe interstitial emphysema is occasionally seen, even spreading to the subcutaneous tissues in the neck (p. 477).

Microscopically the picture of viral pneumonia, as just described, is seen only in cases with early fatal termination and is usually obscured by a superimposed purulent bacterial pneumonia. Often, however, the viral type of pneumonia may still be seen in the less involved areas. The pneumonic lesions during the pandemic of 1918-1919 showed a striking tendency to heal by organization rather than by resolution, probably because of severe damage to the alveolar lining cells. Inclusion bodies are not found in association with either human or experimental influenza. However, electron microscopy has revealed aggregates of intranuclear particles and the presence of the same particles in the cytoplasm, the exact nature of which has not been determined.

Common cold. The common cold (coryza), like influenza, has been shown to be caused by a virus. Progress in the study of this disease has been slow because of the insusceptibility of laboratory animals other than the chimpanzee. Further similarity to influenza is seen in the fact that secondary bacterial invaders are responsible for the formation of mucopurulent exudate and for the distressing symptoms which appear after the first two or three days. Involvement is usually confined to the nasopharynx, pharynx, larynx, and trachea, and pneumonia is of rare occurrence. Immunity is of a very transient nature, perhaps partly because of the occurrence of immunologically different strains of the virus.

Pathologically one sees hyperemia and swelling of the involved mucous membranes, with an exudate which is at first serous but rapidly becomes mucopurulent with the advent of secondary bacterial infection. Hyperplasia and increased secretion of the mucous glands may persist for many weeks after recovery. Involvement of the mucosa lining the accessory nasal sinuses may prolong the infection because of the imperfect drainage of these cavities. No definite inclusion bodies have been described in association with the common cold.

Adenoviruses. Adenoviruses are a group of viruses that cause catarrhal inflammations of the pharynx and eye (pharyngoconjunctival fever, acute febrile pharyngitis, acute follicular conjunctivitis, and epidemic keratoconjunctivitis). Other members of the group have caused epidemic acute respiratory disease in military recruits. Characteristic intranuclear inclusions have been observed in the lungs of patients dying from severe adenovirus pneumonia. Adenovirus type 12 produces undifferentiated sarcoma when inoculated into newborn hamsters.

Viral pneumonias in infants and children. Several types of fatal pneumonia occur in infancy and childhood which have microscopic features that are so distinctive they suggest the etiologic diagnosis. One of these is *Adams' epidemic pneumonitis of infants,* characterized by interstitial pneumonia, often with syncytial giant cells, and with cytoplasmic inclusions in the epithelium of the bronchi, in lining cells of the alveoli, and in the giant cells. Unlike measles pneumonia, nuclear inclusions are not apparent. The etiologic agent has been identified as the respiratory syncytial (RS) virus, formerly named "chimpanzee coryza agent" because it was first isolated from chimpanzees with coryza.

Goodpasture and co-workers, in 1939, described a type of infantile pneumonia associated with intranuclear inclusions in the lungs. Today this is believed to have been *adenovirus pneumonia*. Other distinctive forms of pneumonia in infants and children are *measles giant cell pneumonia* and the pneumonia of *cytomegalic inclusion disease* (see discussion following).

Measles giant cell pneumonia. In 1910 Hecht described a distinctive type of pneumonia of infancy and childhood (Hecht's giant cell pneumonia). It is an interstitial pneumonitis, characterized by large, multinucleated giant cells formed by proliferation and fusion of cells that line alveoli, alveolar ducts, and bronchioles (syncytial giant cells). Intracytoplasmic and intranuclear inclusions are also present. Until recently the etiologic agent was not known. In 1959 Enders and colleagues isolated measles virus at autopsy from materials obtained from patients with typical giant cell pneumonia.

Cytomegalic inclusion disease. A virus in the salivary gland that probably infects many persons subclinically may cause an intrauterine infection that produces symptoms in early infancy. In fatal cases large, intranuclear inclusion bodies and occasionally

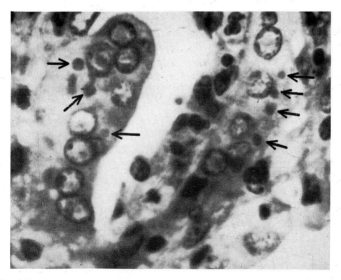

Fig. 7-7. Cytoplasmic inclusion bodies in multinucleated cells lining pulmonary alveoli. Several faintly stained nuclar inclusions are also present (from a case of giant cell pneumonia).

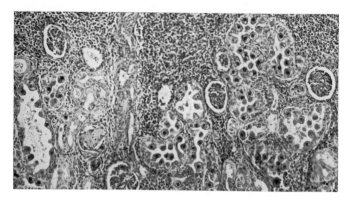

Fig. 7-8. Kidney. Cytomegalic inclusion disease of infancy showing intranuclear inclusion bodies.

smaller, less conspicuous intracytoplasmic inclusions may be found disseminated in many organs (Fig. 7-8). Interstitial inflammation (e.g., in the lungs and kidneys) is likely to be present, characterized by lymphocytic, plasma cell, and macrophagic infiltration. Intestinal ulcerations and encephalitis have also been reported. Periventricular calcification in the brain of infants may occur. The characteristic large inclusions may also be found incidentally in the salivary glands or various organs of children or adults who have been ill with other diseases. Obvious clinical evidence of the viral infection in older children and adults is not common. The inclusions have occasionally been recognized in renal epithelial cells contained in urinary sediment.

Primary atypical pneumonia. Primary atypical pneumonia is an epidemic disease with very low mortality, occurring chiefly in young adults. It has been of frequent occurrence in army camps. Clinically it is characterized by coryza, fever, sore throat, headache, and dry cough with little sputum. Leukopenia, rather than the leukocytosis that accompanies bacterial pneumonia, is the rule. Roentgenograms show consolidation of the lung, spreading outward from the hilus.

Grossly the lungs show patchy, deep red, firm consolidation. Microscopically the picture is that of an interstitial pneumonia, with accumulation of mononuclear cells in the alveolar walls and peribronchial connective tissue. Cuboidal metaplasia of the alveolar lining cells and hyaline membrane formation are seen in some cases. The etiology of this condition is not yet clear. The term *virus pneumonia* has been applied to the condition, but *atypical pneumonia* seems preferable at the present time. The relation of the disease to Q fever, to benign histoplasmosis, and to certain mild infections of the psittacosis group requires further study. Some cases are associated with the development of cold agglutinins and infection with *Mycoplasma pneumoniae,* the Eaton agent.

Cutaneous viruses

Smallpox (variola). The etiologic agent of smallpox is characterized by its affinity for the epidermis. Transmission is either by direct contact or by droplet infection from the respiratory tract. The skin lesions begin as papules, which later become vesicles, then pustules, and finally crusts. The lesions may be discrete, confluent, or hemorrhagic, the last type being almost always fatal. Healing with pitting of the skin is characteristic of the confluent form. A mild form of the disease, known as alastrim, or para-smallpox, is also recognized. The historic aspects of vaccination with cowpox (vaccinia) are too well known to require discussion here.

Clinically the disease is characterized by severe headache and high fever. The fever usually subsides with the appearance of the papular skin lesions but returns with the vesicular and pustular stages of the lesion.

The specific changes of smallpox are seen in the epithelial cells of the skin and mucous membranes. Typical inclusion bodies (Guarnieri bodies) are seen in the cytoplasm of these cells. These inclusions, originally believed by Guarnieri to be protozoa, are now known to consist of closely packed elementary bodies, each having a diameter of about 0.2μ. Intranuclear inclusion bodies also occur. As a result of the presence of the virus, the epithelial cells undergo swelling (ballooning degeneration) and necrosis. Vesiculation and pustule formation occur, but on mucous surfaces the lesions become punched-out ulcers rather than pustules, probably because of the lack of a horny layer.

A fatal outcome may result from secondary bacterial infection in the form of pneumonia, which may lead to septicemia, the etiologic agent being most often a streptococcus or a pneumococcus. It is probable that this bacterial pneumonia is preceded by pneumonia of the viral type. In some instances, however, signs of bacterial infection are not present, and death is believed to be caused by the overwhelming viral infection. Occasionally, acute disseminated encephalitis is a complication.

Chickenpox (varicella). Chickenpox is a mild viral infection of childhood characterized by a typical skin eruption. The disease is acquired either by direct contact or through the upper respiratory tract. The cutaneous lesions are most numerous on the face and trunk but eventually have a generalized distribution, often including the buccal and pharyngeal mucosa. They pass through macular and papular stages and become vesicular, with a surrounding bright red erythematous ring. Eventually crusts form, beneath which epithelial repair takes place. Fresh crops of lesions appear in the same skin areas on successive days, so that lesions in various stages of development may appear side by side. This is in contrast to the lesions of smallpox, which evolve simultaneously.

Microscopic examination of the lesions shows congestion and edema of the corium, with mononuclear cell infiltration. Vesicles containing fluid are found in the epidermis. Vesicle formation is preceded by ballooning degeneration and disruption of epidermal cells. Some of the affected cells become multinucleated. Nuclear inclusions are found in many of the epidermal cells, including the multinucleated ones.

The rare fatalities that occur are usually associated with disseminated infection, in which case similar inclusions are found in the viscera. Varicella pneumonia has been described in adults and may be fulminant and fatal. The complication of postinfection (acute disseminated) encephalomyelitis is a rare occurrence.

Herpes zoster. Herpes zoster (shingles) is characterized by the formation of an erythematous and vesicular eruption along the course of sensory nerves. The lesions occur on the trunk or face and are usually associated with pain, discomfort, fever, and malaise. Involvement of the eye (zoster ophthalmicus) may have serious results unless treated promptly.

The cutaneous vesicular lesions are microscopically similar to those of varicella and also show acidophilic nuclear inclusion bodies. The basic lesion, however, is degeneration in the posterior root ganglia with associated perivascular mononuclear infiltration. In the process of healing, portions of the ganglia may be converted into scar tissue. It is generally agreed that varicella and herpes zoster are different manifestations of an infection caused by a single virus, known as the varicella-zoster (VZ) virus.

Herpes simplex. Herpes simplex is the common "cold sore" or "fever blister," which occurs most often on the lips but may involve the mouth (herpetic stomatitis), the genital mucosa, the conjunctiva, the skin of the face, or other regions. It may occur spontaneously but most often appears during the course of some febrile illness. There is reason for believing that the virus often lies dormant in tissues and is stimulated to produce lesions by some unknown mechanism which commonly acts in the presence of fever.

If fluid from a human vesicular lesion is rubbed into the scarified cornea of a rabbit, a specific viral conjunctivitis is produced. The virus is relatively large and causes granular nuclear inclusion bodies, which usually fill but do not distend the nuclei. Intracranial injection in mice causes an encephalitis that may be serially transmitted. The histologic appearance of this lesion in mice resembles that of encephalitis lethargica. Rare cases of human encephalitis show nuclear inclusions resembling those of herpes, in which the herpes virus has been recovered from the brain.

Histologic examination of the cutaneous lesions shows epithelial degeneration and necrosis, with vesicle formation. The vesicles resemble those of varicella microscopically. The nuclear inclusions already described are present in many of the epithelial cells.

Recently it has become clear that "hepatoadrenal necrosis," a fatal infection of newborn infants, is generalized herpes simplex infection ("herpes simplex neonatorum"). Typical inclusions are found in the focal necroses in the liver and adrenal glands. The mothers of these infants usually show mild herpetic lesions of the vagina but are otherwise asymptomatic.

Measles (rubeola). For years it has been possible to transmit measles only to monkeys but not to other laboratory animals, and for this reason the study of its virus has been difficult. In recent investigations it appears that the measles virus has been adapted to suckling mice, and possibly to suckling hamsters. There are morphologic and immunologic similarities of measles in human beings and distemper in animals.

Measles is highly communicable and is spread chiefly by droplet infection through the upper respiratory tract. Clinically it is characterized by fever, cough, coryza, conjunctivitis, and a distinctive type of nonhemorrhagic macular rash, which is most severe on the face but involves the entire body. Koplik's spots, which are of early diagnostic significance, occur in the mouth, usually opposite the first molar teeth. They consist of minute white flecks, formed by necrotic epithelial cells and surrounded by a bluish areola, outside of which is a red areola.

The cutaneous lesions show vacuolar degeneration and eventual necrosis of the epithelial cells and considerable perivascular lymphocytic infiltration, with endothelial proliferation in the capillaries, arterioles, and venules. The capillaries are greatly congested and occasionally rupture to form minute areas of hemorrhage in the corium. Koplik's spots show an essentially similar picture.

In fatal cases death is usually caused by bronchopneumonia. It is difficult to separate the lesions caused by bacterial pneumonia from those produced by the initial viral infection. Most fatalities occur late in the course of the disease, and although the bronchopneumonia seen then is often of the interstitial type, it has no particularly characteristic features. In patients dying early in the course of the illness a peculiar type of pneumonia with giant cell formation and nuclear and cytoplasmic inclusions has been described (p. 169). In addition to bronchopneumonia, other bacterial infections may complicate measles, especially otitis media. Postinfection encephalitis is a rare and serious complication. Cytoplasmic and sometimes intranuclear inclusions, as well as multinucleated giant cells, have been demonstrated in the brains of some patients with fatal measles encephalitis.

In the lymphoid tissue of the tonsil and appendix large multinucleated cells have been observed in prodromal measles. These cells in lymphoid tissue, believed by some to be formed by fusion of lymphocytes and possibly plasma cells, are known as "Warthin-Finkeldey giant cells." Occasionally the finding of these giant cells in routine examination of surgically removed appendices has enabled the pathologist to make a diagnosis of measles before the appearance of the rash or Koplik's spots. Cytologic examination of nasal smears from children with catarrhal symptoms may enable early diagnosis by recognition of the giant cells of measles.

German measles (rubella). German measles is a mild exanthem affecting children and young adults. A macular rash develops rapidly on the head and trunk and disappears in a few days. The virus of rubella has recently been isolated and is presently being thoroughly studied.

The most important aspect of this otherwise rather trivial infection is the occurrence of congenital abnormalities in some

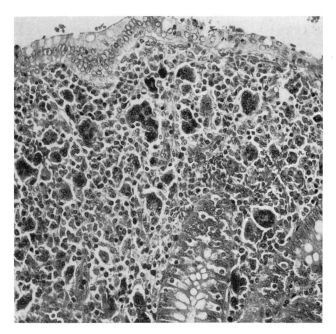

Fig. 7-9. Warthin-Finkeldey giant cells in the lymphoid tissue of the mucosa of the appendix in measles.

infants born of mothers who acquire the disease in the early months of pregnancy. The virus may interfere with normal fetal development, the most common defects being microcephaly, deaf-mutism, cardiac abnormalities, cataract, and dental defects. In one carefully conducted, prospective study it was noted that *major* defects occurred in 15% of children of mothers who had rubella during the first sixteen weeks of pregnancy and that *minor* abnormalities were seen in an additional 16% of children.

Molluscum contagiosum. Molluscum contagiosum is a benign skin disease characterized by the occurrence of raised, umbili-cated, waxy cutaneous nodules. These lesions may be multiple, in which case the diagnosis is usually made clinically, or single, in which case the lesion may be suspected of being neoplastic and is often excised for diagnosis. The lesions heal spontaneously, usually after a few months, and are not associated with con-stitutional symptoms. The prickle cells of the epidermis undergo hyperplasia and degeneration, with the development of rounded hyaline masses (molluscum bodies) in their cytoplasm. These eosinophilic (sometimes basophilic) inclusion bodies are aggregations of the minute elementary bodies of the virus.

Miscellaneous viral infections

Mumps. The virus of mumps has an affinity for the salivary glands and the testis (or ovary). The outstanding symptom is painful swelling of the parotid gland. Orchitis is rare before puberty but occurs in about one fifth of the cases in male adults. The infection may be transmitted serially in monkeys by the injection of saliva directly into Stensen's duct and has been cultivated in embryonated eggs.

Histologically the parotid gland shows severe congestion and edema, catarrhal inflammation of the excretory duct, degenerative changes in the glandular epithelium, and leukocytic infiltration of the tubules and interstitial tissue. Repair takes place without permanent obstruction of the ducts or formation of scar tissue. In the testis one finds a similar acute inflammatory reaction, probably dependent on primary injury to the tubular epithelium. Repair may be associated with a reduction in size of the affected testicle. Impotence and sterility are rare, since the condition is usually unilateral and, even when bilateral, does not often cause enough permanent damage to interfere with normal function. Sterility may occur in bilateral disease if testicular atrophy is severe enough.

Meningoencephalitis may occur during or after parotitis or even in the absence of symptoms of salivary gland disease. Oophoritis, pancreatitis, and subacute thyroiditis are other possible manifestations of mumps. Characteristic inclusion bodies have not been observed in tissues of patients with mumps.

Yellow fever. Yellow fever is a highly fatal, mosquito-borne viral disease of great clinical importance in the tropics, particularly in Africa and South America. The outstanding clinical features are fever, severe jaundice, hematemesis, hemorrhage into the gastrointestinal tract, hematuria, and evidences of severe renal damage, including uremia in fatal cases. Unfortunately the control of the mosquito vector, *Aedes aegypti*, while it has greatly reduced the disease, has not completely eradicated it, since there is a reservoir in monkeys and perhaps other wild jungle animals from which forest mosquitoes, particularly of the genus *Haemagogus*, may transmit the infection to man. The endemic form of the disease in South America is called "jungle yellow fever." Human vaccination is carried out by injecting virus that has been modified by cultivation in media containing minced mammalian embryonic tissue.

Liver disease is the key feature of yellow fever and is manifested by abnormalities of serum bilirubin and a prothrombin deficiency. The degree of prothrombin deficiency and its rate of recovery indicate the extent and duration of the hepatic lesion. A hemorrhagic tendency, caused by the prothrombin deficiency, may result in a secondary lesion of hemoglobinuric nephrosis. Death may result either from severe liver damage or from renal failure.

Postmortem examination shows hemorrhage into the gastrointestinal tract, a yellow liver often mottled with red areas, pale swollen kidneys, and a friable dark red spleen. Microscopically there is extensive necrosis of liver tissue with fatty infiltration that at first has a midzonal distribution but later becomes more diffuse. The damaged liver cells appear swollen, eosinophilic, and finely granular, with intracytoplasmic hyaline areas (Councilman bodies). Nuclear inclusions, less prominent and less easy to recognize than those of other viral infections, are occasionally found in human liver and almost constantly in fatal yellow fever in the monkey. This type of inclusion ("Torres body") forms a small irregular diffuse eosinophilic mass adjacent to or partially surrounding the nucleolus. The necrosis of liver cells is so extensive that one might expect repair by fibrous tissue, but hepatic cirrhosis as a sequela of yellow fever has not been reported. In the kidneys severe hemoglobinuric (lower nephron) nephrosis is found. Other lesions that have been described include myocardial degeneration, and petechial hemorrhages in the brain, as well as on serous surfaces.

Viral hepatitis. *Infectious hepatitis* and *serum hepatitis* are similar but immunologically distinct viral infections, characterized clinically by fever, nausea, tenderness of the liver, splenomegaly, and in severe cases by jaundice. The mortality is low. Infectious hepatitis is common and may be endemic or epidemic. It is usually acquired through the oral route, but occasionally may follow inoculation. Serum hepatitis occurs as the result of parenteral injection of human blood products, originating from latently infected donors. It has a longer incubation period (sixty to one hundred and sixty days) than infectious hepatitis (fifteen to forty days). Microscopically in nonfatal, transient disease, hepatic cells show hydropic degeneration ("balloon cells"), hyaline degeneration (cytoplasmic "acidophilic bodies"), and necrosis (individual cells or focal), associated with infiltration by lymphocytes and macrophages, most prominent in the portal areas but extending into the lobules. The reticulum is intact, and bile canaliculi contain bile pigment. In more severe disease, submassive or massive necrosis and collapse of reticulum occur, producing the picture of so-called subacute or acute yellow atrophy. These patients die or subsequently develop postnecrotic cirrhosis. Inclusion bodies are not found in viral hepatitis. The kidneys show cholemic nephrosis as a result of jaundice. Animal transmission has not been definitely accomplished. (See also p. 493.)

Phlebotomus fever. Phlebotomus fever clinically resembles dengue but is transmitted by the sandfly *Phlebotomus papatasii.* The disease exists in the areas of Europe, Asia, and Africa between 20° and 45° north latitude where conditions are favorable for breeding of the vector. A rash does not occur in this disease. It has not been transmitted to animals, and nothing is known concerning its pathologic features.

Coxsackie viral infections. Viruses of the Coxsackie group belong to the larger group of enteroviruses. They have been isolated from throat washings and feces in a variety of human diseases, as well as from asymptomatic persons. The thirty types fall into two groups, A and B.

The study of these viruses is incomplete. Strong evidence indicates, however, that group A viruses cause *herpangina,* a mild febrile illness of infancy characterized by vesicular and ulcerative lesions on the soft palate and in the faucial areas. Group B viruses apparently cause *epidemic pleurodynia* (Bornholm disease), a febrile illness in which the outstanding symptom is severe pain in the abdomen and chest, with painful respiration. The disease is of short duration and has never been fatal. Both of these diseases have been recognized clinically for many years. There is some evidence that certain strains of group A and group B Coxsackie viruses may cause a nonfatal type of aseptic meningitis. Coxsackie viruses, especially group B, also cause myocarditis of the newborn and acute nonspecific pericarditis.

ECHO viruses. The ECHO (enteric cytopathogenic human orphan) viruses became recognized when tissue cultures were used for isolation from stools. More than twenty types have been identified. Some types have been recognized as causing epidemics of diarrheal disease in infants and children. Other types appear to cause an aseptic meningitis without paralysis or sequelae. A variety of other clinical effects have been attributed to these viruses. Little is known about the pathologic features of diseases caused by the ECHO viruses because fatalities are rare.

Epidemic hemorrhagic fever. Epidemic hemorrhagic fever, described by Japanese workers in 1943 and probably recognized 10 years earlier by the Russians, first appeared in United States troops in Korea in 1951. The cause is not known but is generally believed to be a filtrable agent, despite the failure of all attempts to isolate the agent. Some evidence suggests a mite as the vector and a rodent (field mouse) as the reservoir.

The clinical picture is dominated by fever, hemorrhage, and severe renal involvement, with associated changes in fluid balance. Early deaths have been ascribed to shock, and late deaths (up to the thirtieth day of illness) to renal failure.

The characteristic pathologic features are (1) hemorrhagic lesions, particularly in the renal medullae, right atrium, and gastrointestinal submucosa; (2) a peculiar type of necrosis in the renal medulla, anterior lobe of the pituitary, and adrenal glands; and (3) mononuclear infiltration of the heart, pulmonary alveoli, pancreas, spleen, and liver. The renal lesions, because of the areas of coagulative necrosis and hemorrhage, somewhat resemble infarcts grossly. Microscopically the changes include those of lower nephron nephrosis, but the total picture in the kidney is almost pathognomonic of the disease. The basic change appears to be increased vascular permeability with edema, serous transudates, and hemorrhages.

PSITTACOSIS-LYMPHOGRANULOMA VENEREUM AGENTS

As mentioned previously, the group of obligate intracellular parasites causing such diseases as psittacosis, lymphogranuloma venereum, trachoma, and inclusion conjunctivitis are no longer considered to be viruses. These agents are intermediate between the rickettsiae and the viruses and are named the *Bedsoniae* or *Chlamydiae*. Cat-scratch disease is included in this section because it is generally believed to be caused by one of these agents, although the organism has not been isolated. Its possible relationship to atypical mycobacteria is noted.

Psittacosis. Psittacosis is acquired by inhalation of a rickettsia-like agent *(Bedsonia)* present in dried urine and feces from infected birds. It has recently been shown that several birds other than those of the parrot family, including pigeons and the fulmar petrel (a sea gull), may harbor the agent and cause

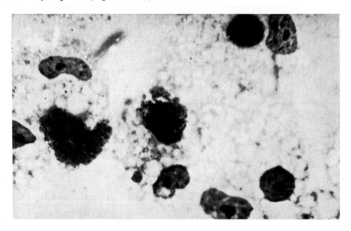

Fig. 7-10. Psittacosis. Three deeply stained granular cytoplasmic inclusions composed of closely packed elementary bodies.

human infection. Since the causative agent has been isolated from different species of birds, the more general name *ornithosis* has been proposed for the disease.

Clinically psittacosis is an acute febrile illness, with intense headache and physical signs of an atypical pneumonia. Leukopenia, instead of the leukocytosis that accompanies bacterial pneumonia, is an important diagnostic feature.

Pathologically one finds splenomegaly and congestion and cloudy swelling of the viscera, as in any acute infection, but the characteristic changes are in the lungs. Here we find patchy pneumonic consolidation. Microscopically the picture is that of a pneumonia in which mononuclear cells rather than neutrophils, predominate. At first an alveolar exudate, with fibrin and leukocytes, is prominent, but during resolution an interstitial component of the inflammation is apparent. The alveolar lining cells are stimulated and appear to have become cuboidal in type with frequent mitoses.

Spherical clusters of minute coccoid elementary bodies of rather characteristic appearance are found with great difficulty in sections of human lungs, but they are very conspicuous in the brain tissue of mice after intracerebral injection of the agent, and they may also be found in mononuclear cells in the lung during the early stages of experimentally induced pneumonia.

Lymphogranuloma venereum. Structurally and antigenically the agent producing lymphogranuloma venereum is like that of the other *Bedsoniae.* The disease is discussed in Chapter 8 (p. 200).

Trachoma. The agents causing trachoma and inclusion conjunctivitis are similar and are referred to as TRIC agents. In film preparations from the infected conjunctiva, spherical clusters of coccoid elementary bodies are commonly found in the cytoplasm of the epithelial cells. The cytologic picture somewhat resembles that seen in psittacosis and lymphogranuloma venereum. Trachoma can be reproduced in the monkey. The lesion is characterized by subepithelial congestion, newly formed capillaries, and focal collections of lymphocytes and macrophages with lymphoid follicle formation, causing granular elevations of the conjunctiva. Necrosis and scarring of the lesions may occur. A serious complication is corneal involvement with necrosis and ulceration.

Inclusion conjunctivitis (swimming-pool conjunctivitis). Inclusion conjunctivitis initially is similar pathologically to trachoma, but recovery takes place without necrosis and other complications. The reservoir of infection is in the genitourinary tract. Newborn babies are infected during passage through the birth canal, and adults are infected by bathing in unchlorinated pools or lakes.

Cat-scratch disease. Cat-scratch disease is a self-limited type of granulomatous and suppurative lymphadenitis, possibly caused by an agent of the psittacosis-lymphogranuloma venereum group, although attempts to isolate the agent have been unsuccessful. Recently it has been suggested that atypical mycobacteria may be responsible, since photochromogenic acid-fast bacilli have been isolated from lymph nodes of patients diagnosed as having cat-scratch disease. In recent years it has been definitely associated with contact with cats. A transient papule occurs at the site of entry (usually on the hand or arm), and the regional lymph nodes become greatly swollen. Fever is variable. Over a period of weeks or months the lesions slowly subside, with or without suppuration. In excised lymph nodes one finds focal areas of suppuration, or cores of necrotic debris containing relatively few neutrophils, surrounded by wide bands of epithelioid cells, with a few giant cells. The picture resembles that of lymphogranuloma venereum and may even be mistaken for chronic tularemia or tuberculosis. A specific cutaneous test with antigen prepared from purulent material of patients known to have the disease is helpful in establishing the diagnosis.

Chapter 8

Spirochetal and venereal diseases

S SYPHILIS

Syphilis, caused by a spirochete, the *Treponema pallidum,* is the most important of the venereal diseases. It causes disability and death mainly from involvement of the heart, blood vessels, and nervous system, but any organ may be affected. The clinical manifestations are extremely variable, and latent periods occur in which there are no clinical signs other than positive serologic reactions. The course of the disease is described in three stages. The characteristic lesion of the primary stage (chancre) is a hard ulcer that develops at the point of entrance of the organisms, and hence is usually on the genitalia. The secondary stage, developing about six weeks after the chancre, is characterized by maculopapular skin rashes, mucous patches on the oral mucosa, and generalized slight lymph node enlargement. Tertiary lesions develop after a latent period of months or years. They may be localized areas of specific, granulomatous inflammation with gummy necrosis (gumma) or a chronic nonspecific inflammation with gradual destruction of tissue and development of fibrosis. This latter type of reaction is more common. Penicillin is effective in the treatment of early syphilis (primary and secondary lesions).

In contrast with the varied clinical and gross manifestations of syphilis, the microscopic features are relatively simple and constant but rarely pathognomonic. Lesions of the skin in any stage of syphilis may show considerable and irregular epithelial hyperplasia and sometimes, as in certain gummatous ulcers, may simulate a cancerous change (pseudocarcinomatous hyperplasia). The inflammatory cells in syphilitic lesions are predominantly lymphocytes and plasma cells, situated around small blood vessels and later more diffusely spread throughout the tissue. Fibroblastic proliferation and fibrosis accompany the process. Small blood vessels in syphilitic lesions exhibit changes, frequently an intimal thickening (endarteritis) and luminal narrowing or obstruction. In addition to the factor of hypersensitivity, this vascular change and consequent ischemia probably contribute to the necrosis of the gumma. Final proof of the syphilitic nature of a lesion depends upon demonstration of the spirochete. Spirochetes are numerous in primary and secondary lesions but are scarce in tertiary lesions.

The *Treponema pallidum (Spirochaeta pallida)* is a slender organism, 5 to 15 μ in length, i.e., usually about once or twice the diameter of a red blood cell. It is characterized by its thinness and by the closeness and regularity of its corkscrewlike spirals, which average about twelve in number. It is stained only with great difficulty and is best demonstrated in smears from syphilitic lesions by dark-field examination or against a black background of India ink. In tissues it may be demonstrated by Levaditi's method, or some modification of it, in which the spirochete is impregnated with silver. Methods for their staining in tissues are technically difficult and uncertain.

Primary stage of syphilis. The *chancre,* or primary syphilitic lesion, appears at the point of inoculation of the spirochete after an incubation period of one to four weeks. An abrasion of the skin or mucosa facilitates entry of the organism but probably is unnecessary for penetration of the genital mucosa. The chancre is on the genitalia in more than 90% of cases, the next most common location being the lips or mouth. In 20% or more of cases no primary lesion develops, or it is hidden in the urethra or vagina and passes unnoticed. Syphilis has been transferred by blood transfusion, the spirochete being directly inoculated with the donor's blood. In such cases there is no primary lesion.

Very soon after penetration the organisms spread to the regional lymph nodes, and then by way of the bloodstream become widely distributed in tissues of the body. Hence prophylactic treatment must immediately follow exposure.

After an incubation period of about three weeks the chancre begins as a thickening and hardening of the surface tissue. The epithelium of this area becomes necrotic and sloughs off, leaving a shallow ulcer a few millimeters to a centimeter in diameter. The ulcer is single, round, and characterized by painlessness and hardness. The induration extends to form a flat hard mass, which exudes clear serum but no pus. Secondary infection may occur and change the characteristic features. Histologically the lesions show fairly dense granulation tissue with many small vessels and an infiltration of lymphocytes and plasma cells. These chronic inflammatory cells at first surround the small blood vessels but

Table 8-1. *Spirochetal diseases*

Disease	Spirochete	Morphology of spirochete	Main features of disease
Syphilis	*Treponema pallidum*	5 to 15 μ long, about 12 slender, tightly wound regular coils	Venereal; widespread
Yaws (frambesia)	*Treponema pertenue*	Resembles *T. pallidum*	Nonvenereal; lesions and stages similar to syphilis
Pinta	*Treponema carateum*	Indistinguishable from *T. pallidum*	Nonvenereal; bluish pigmented and depigmented areas of skin
Relapsing fever	*Borrelia recurrentis Borrelia duttonii*	7 to 20 μ long, easily stained, 5 to 10 loosely wound, wavy spirals	Spread primarily by lice and ticks; organism found in blood smears during febrile period
Spirochetal jaundice (Weil's disease) Spirochetosis icterohaemorrhagica	*Leptospira icterohaemorrhagiae*	6 to 15 μ long, fine tightly wound spirals enclosing axial filament, prolonged to form straight or hooked ends	Hemorrhages in various organs, particularly lungs; degeneration and necrosis in liver and kidney; spirochetes excreted in urine
Vincent's angina	*Borrelia vincentii*	5 to 10 μ long, 3 to 8 irregular shallow spirals; constantly found with long fusiform bacilli (*B. fusiformis*)	Symbiotic infection, associated with gangrenous and sloughing lesions of mouth, throat, and respiratory tract
Ratbite fever (sodoku)	*Spirillum minus*	2 to 5 μ long, broad spiral organism, regular spirals, blunt ends with flagella	Febrile infection caused by bite of infected rat; primary lesion at point of inoculation; recurring chills and fever; spirochete sometimes demonstrated in blood but better isolated by injection of blood into mice

later spread out and become diffuse. The hardness of the lesion results from connective tissue formation and the accumulation of inflammatory cells. Necrosis is absent except on the surface. Secondary infection may change the histologic picture. There is nothing absolutely characteristic about the lesion, and certain diagnosis depends on demonstration of the abundant spirochetes.

The chancre heals in three to eight weeks. The induration disappears, the area is recovered by epithelium, and healing leaves only slight fibrosis or scarring. The serologic tests for syphilis usually become positive about one or two weeks after the appearance of the chancre.

With development of the chancre the regional lymph nodes (usually inguinal) become enlarged, firm, and shotty, but are not painful. In the enlarged nodes there is hyperplasia of the cells lining the sinuses, which are filled with mononuclear cells. Small areas of focal necrosis may occur, but there is no tendency for the glands to suppurate.

Secondary stage of syphilis. Secondary lesions appear six to ten weeks after the development of the chancre and are characterized by simultaneous appearance over the whole body, insignificant tissue reaction with little tissue destruction, and richness in organisms. Serologic tests for syphilis are almost invariably positive and are most dependable during this stage.

During the incubation period and the period of the chancre, spread has occurred throughout the whole body by lymphatics and bloodstream. Multiplication in these new foci results in the breaking out of innumerable lesions. On the skin they most commonly take the form of a flat, red (macular) or raised (papular) rash, but any type of skin eruption may be imitated. Sore throat is common, and elevated, white "mucous patches" involve the oral mucosa. There is a generalized slight lymph node enlargement, the glands being hard, discrete, and shotty. Histologically the lymph nodes may show marked follicular hyperplasia, simulating giant follicular lymphadenopathy. Flat condylomas (condyloma latum) develop in moist areas about the genitals or anus. These are broad lobulated elevations in which epithelial overgrowth is a marked feature.

In all secondary lesions the histologic change is essentially a perivascular accumulation of lymphocytes and plasma cells, with varying amounts of vascular dilatation and congestion. In macular lesions cells are few in number. In papular lesions cells are numerous in deep layers of the epithelium and in the

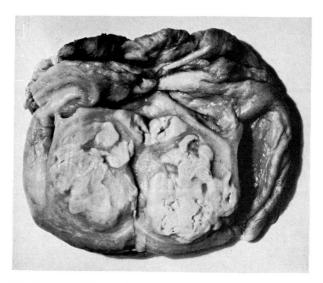

Fig. 8-1. Gumma of the testis.

corium. Focal epidermal abscesses occur in pustular lesions, but ulceration is not particularly common. The epithelium shows little change except in the condylomas, where papillomatous overgrowth may be marked. Healing occurs without scars. Milder recurrences of secondary lesions, separated by latent periods of apparent health, are the usual course.

Tertiary stage of syphilis. Between secondary and tertiary lesions there occurs a latent period of a few months to five or as long as twenty years. During this period the person appears well, and the presence of active syphilis is recognizable only by serologic tests. Nevertheless, during this period there progresses a slow, mild, chronic inflammation in various invaded tissues, particularly the cardiovascular system or nervous system. This slow destruction and fibrosis may lead to eventual functional breakdown or may be evident only by gross or microscopic examination after the death of the individual.

Gumma is a less common type of tertiary lesion, characterized by great destruction of tissue and relatively few organisms. The gumma may be found in almost any organ or tissue. It is usually a solitary nodule of necrotic tissue, varying from microscopic size to a diameter of several centimeters. The opaque necrotic

Table 8-2. *Differential features of gummas and tubercles*

	Gumma	*Tubercle*
Giant cells	Less frequent	Common
Epithelioid cells	Less numerous	More numerous
Lymphocytes and plasma cells	More numerous	Less numerous
Tissue structure	Often still visible	Completely obliterated
Fibroblasts	May be found in center of gumma	Absent from necrotic area
Blood vessels	Sometimes present	Absent
Size	May be several centimeters in diameter	Rarely large
Number	Frequently single	Rarely single

material has an elastic or "gummy" consistency. Microscopically it presents features of coagulation and caseation necrosis, because in areas, "ghost" or "shadow" forms of underlying tissue architecture can be seen, and elsewhere amorphous, granular debris is evident. About the necrotic material is a margin of lymphocytes and mononuclear cells. Multinucleated giant cells are less frequent than in tuberculosis. Proliferation of connective tissue cells encapsulates the lesion, and vascularized connective tissue may extend a considerable distance into the necrotic center. Differences between gummas and tubercles are outlined in Table 8-2, but histologic differentiation of single lesions is not always possible without demonstration of organisms. The history of associated lesions usually must be considered in diagnosis.

When a gumma involves skin or the mucous membrane, there is sloughing of necrotic material, so that an ulcer results. Gummatous ulcers have irregular sharp walls, a punched-out appearance, and an irregular base. The palate is a common site and may be completely perforated. Gummas heal with absorption of the necrotic material and formation of dense fibrous distorting scars. The distortion is particularly well seen in the liver, where deep contracted scars produce a peculiar irregular lobed appearance *(hepar lobatum)*.

Occasionally there is involvement by numerous miliary gummas, which begin as the usual perivascular involvement, but in which necrosis is slight or never complete. Healing occurs with diffuse and irregular fibrosis of the tissue.

As syphilis may affect practically any organ or tissue, only the more important are considered here.

Circulatory system. The aorta is involved more commonly than any other organ, probably in every case of active syphilis. It is especially the ascending aorta and arch that are affected, parts that possess a particularly rich lymph supply. This distribution is in contrast to that of atherosclerosis, which very considerably involves the lower abdominal portion. All layers are affected. The adventitia shows perivascular collections of lymphocytes and plasma cells and later is scarred and thickened. The most important damage is to the media, in which destruction of elastic fibers and muscle and scar formation so weaken the wall as to allow aneurysmal bulging. The intima is involved by an irregular fibrous thickening, which appears as an irregular wrinkling and pitting. The resulting "tree-bark" appearance (linear furrowing) is grossly characteristic but not pathognomonic. More distinctive are the small, puckered stellate fissures, which are the result of underlying medial scars. The intimal change causes little functional damage, except when it involves the sinuses of Valsalva, where it may result in narrowing or occlusion of coronary openings, an important complication of syphilitic aortitis. Similar syphilitic lesions, also with aneurysm formation, less commonly involve other arteries. Proximal portions of the coronaries may be stenosed or obliterated by syphilitic endarteritis.

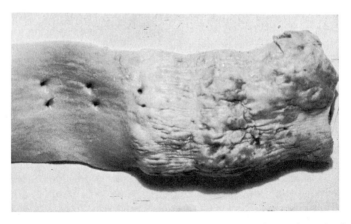

Fig. 8-2. Syphilitic aortitis. Note the longitudinal striation and tree-bark appearance.

Heart. Syphilis may involve the region of the aortic valve and probably the myocardium. Changes in the aortic valves may be dilatation of the aortic ring, thickening and shortening of the cusps of the valve, and separation of the cusps at the commissures. These three types of change, which may occur singly or in combination, all produce insufficiency of the aortic valve. The extra burden of diastolic regurgitation into the left ventricle causes a work hypertrophy of that part.

The myocardium may be affected by narrowing or occlusion of the proximal portions or openings of the coronaries. The resultant myocardial ischemia may cause angina pectoris and myocardial fibrosis. Granulomatous myocarditis with formation of gummas occurs rarely. There is a dispute as to whether a primary nonspecific myocarditis is caused by syphilitic organisms that is characterized by interstitial infiltration of lymphocytes and plasma cells, followed by fibrosis. Conducting bundles may be involved by any of the myocardial lesions associated with syphilis and give rise to heart block.

Nervous system. Syphilitic involvement of the nervous system may appear as meningeal and/or vascular lesions, general paresis (dementia paralytica), or tabes dorsalis (locomotor ataxia). Also a gumma may develop in any part of the brain and simulate a tumor in its manifestations.

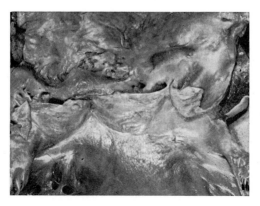

Fig. 8-3. Narrowed coronary ostia in syphilitic aortitis. (From Scotti, T. M.: Heart. In Anderson, W. A. D., editor: Pathology, ed. 5, St. Louis, 1966, The C. V. Mosby Co.)

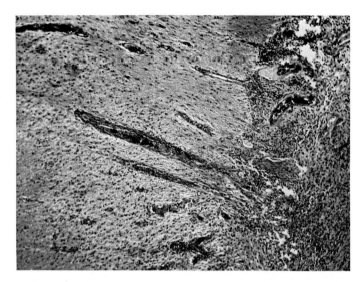

Fig. 8-4. Syphilitic meningitis. The inflammatory exudate of the meninges is extending into cerebral tissue, particularly around vascular spaces.

MENINGEAL INVOLVEMENT. The meningeal involvement is usually chronic and, rarely, acute meningitis. The usual form is associated with considerable thickening and adherence of all layers. The tissues are infiltrated with lymphocytes, plasma cells, and macrophages. The blood vessels are involved, and perivascular infiltration and fibrosis give rise to the meningeal thickening. Varying degrees of degeneration of underlying nerve cells accompany the meningitis. The meningeal changes may involve the cranial nerves or produce obstructive hydrocephalus. Narrowing of the cerebral vessels (syphilitic endarteritis) may lead to cerebral atrophy or arterial thrombosis and infarcts of the brain (meningovascular syphilis).

GENERAL PARESIS. General paresis is usually a late manifestation of syphilis. Treponemas have been demonstrated in the involved tissue. The disease is manifested by dissolution of mental powers and balance and, finally, complete insanity. Varying degrees of atrophic change affect the cerebral convolutions, the ventricles are dilated, and there is usually some accompanying meningeal involvement, with thickening and adhesions. Micro-

Table 8-3. *The course of syphilis*

Stage	Time	Lesions	Pathologic background	Result
Incubation period	Average 3 weeks	No clinical signs	Reproduction of organisms locally at site of inoculation, and widespread distribution throughout body	Development of chancre
Primary	6 weeks	Chancre; local lymph node enlargement	Hard ulcerative lesion at point of inoculation, with many organisms; serologic tests for syphilis become positive	Heals spontaneously with slight scarring
Secondary	1 to 3 years; latent periods and recurrences	Eruptive lesions on skin and mucous membranes; generalized lymph node enlargement	Localized areas of congestion with perivascular round cell infiltrations; minimal tissue destruction; lesions rich in spirochetes and highly infective; serologic tests for syphilis positive	Heals spontaneously with minimal scarring
Latent periods	6 months to 20 years	Present but not evident clinically	Progressive destruction of parenchymatous tissue and replacement by scar tissue, producing eventual functional breakdown; serologic tests for syphilis may be positive or negative	Partial healing with fibrosis, producing functional and anatomic disturbances of organs
Tertiary	Lasts for remainder of life	Chronic destructive fibrosing lesions and/or gummas may involve any organ; aortitis with aortic valve involvement and regurgitation, coronary ostial narrowing, aneurysm, meningitis, meningovascular, general paresis, tabes dorsalis		

scopic changes include degeneration and reduction in number of nerve cells and fibers in the cerebral cortex, especially in the frontal region, and proliferation of cortical neuroglia. Collections of plasma cells and lymphocytes are present about blood vessels. Storage in the microglia of a large amount of iron-containing substance, which gives a Prussian blue reaction, is a most characteristic finding.

TABES DORSALIS. Tabes dorsalis (locomotor ataxia) is characterized by a degeneration of the posterior roots and posterior columns of the spinal cord as a result of syphilis. The reason for the degenerative process is not clear. Injury to the nerve fibers has been attributed to meningitis about the dorsal roots, to direct inflammation in the dorsal root ganglia, to a toxin, or to the presence of the spirochete itself. Varying degrees of meningeal inflammation and thickening accompany the cord changes. The changes are usually most pronounced in the lumbar portion of the cord. The posterior columns are shrunken and retracted and pale gray on the cut surface. In these degenerated areas axons and myelin sheaths have disappeared, and there is increased neuroglial tissue (gliosis). In the posterior roots there are also demyelinization and a decrease in number of nerve fibers. Frequently the optic nerve is also involved. Occasionally there is a round-cell infiltration where the posterior roots penetrate the arachnoid.

Congenital syphilis. Syphilis is frequently congenital, but it is not hereditary. Placental and fetal tissues are a particularly good soil for growth of the spirochete, and congenital infection probably occurs whenever the mother has active syphilitic infection. The maternal infection may be old and clinically latent, or it may have been acquired just before or during pregnancy. Infection of the fetus may result in death in utero and abortion, in premature labor and stillbirth, or in a live child with active syphilitic lesions. In some cases the child appears well at birth but later develops evidence of syphilis (lues tarda). The fetus probably does not become infected before the fifth month of pregnancy. The Langhans layer of cells of the placental villi, which does not disappear until after sixteen weeks, apparently protects against intrauterine infection until that time.

Placenta. The placenta of a syphilitic infant is abnormally large. It often shows changes caused by the infection, but infrequently so great as to be diagnostic. Thickening of the intima and adventitia of the vessels of the placenta and umbilical cord and the enlargement of the villi by new connective tissue formation about the central blood vessels have been ascribed to syphilis.

Skin lesions. Syphilitic infants frequently show mucocutaneous lesions. These are usually in the form of a maculopapular rash, blebs or bullae on the hands and feet, and desquamation. Rhinitis, with snuffles, and fissures about the lips and anus (rhagades) may occur. The infant appears small and undernourished, but the liver and spleen are enlarged.

Organ involvement. The main changes are delayed, or there is faulty development of organs, which appear enlarged, dense, and fibrous. The lung, liver, spleen, pancreas, and kidney are frequently involved. The change in the lung is commonly called white pneumonia (pneumonia alba). The pulmonary alveoli are not fully developed, being lined by cubical epithelial cells, and their walls are greatly thickened by fine connective tissue and

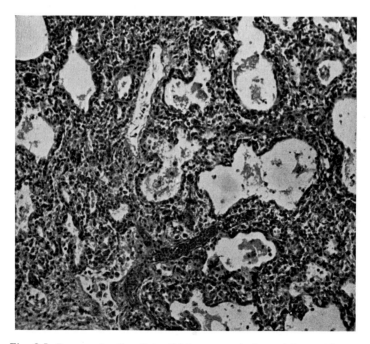

Fig. 8-5. Pneumonia alba. Interstitial pneumonia in an infant with congenital syphilis. Note the cuboidal cells lining the glandlike alveolar spaces.

small round mesoblastic cells. An interstitial infiltration by mono-nuclear cells also occurs. In the enlarged liver there is an increase of connective tissue, particularly around portal areas, but gener-ally extending diffusely throughout the liver. Focal areas of gummatous necrosis and many focal collections of small, round, dark, blood-forming cells may be seen. Similar excess hemato-poietic activity is evident in the spleen. Fibrosis or undifferenti-ated mesoblastic tissue is also prominent in the pancreas and kidney. In the latter organ a prominent neogenic zone at the outer edge of the cortex indicates the delayed develop-ment.

Osteochondritis. Osteochondritis is the most constant lesion of congenital syphilis. It may be the sole lesion and is a valuable aid in roentgenologic diagnosis. In long bones the line of ossifica-tion between cartilage and bone is wide, irregular, yellowish, and opaque, instead of a normal thin, even, gray translucent line. There is irregular and incomplete ossification in this area, with development of a cellular granulation tissue. Osteoblastic activ-ity is diminished, with disturbance of normal resorption and alteration in the growth of cartilage. Periostitis with thickening frequently accompanies the osteochondritis, but it seldom occurs alone.

Other effects. Later forms of congenital syphilis produce various scars and deformities, some of which are characteristic stigmas of the disease. These include gummatous destruction of the nasal bones (saddle nose), bulbous or tapered incisors with a notch in the center of the biting edge *(Hutchinson's teeth)*, *interstitial keratitis* producing corneal opacity, and *saber shin* resulting from periostitis. Lesions of the central nervous system are not uncommon, but cardiovascular lesions are rare.

OTHER SPIROCHETAL DISEASES

Yaws (frambesia). Yaws is a tropical disease closely similar to syphilis and caused by a spirochete, *Treponema pertenue,* which is almost indistinguishable from the syphilitic spirochete. In yaws the serologic tests for syphilis are positive, and treatment with penicillin or arsenicals is effective. Yaws is not a venereal disease; it spreads by direct contact, mainly to children. An initial primary lesion develops at the point of inoculation, usually on a leg or arm, which at first is a papule and then develops into a larger papillomatous lesion (raspberry-like, thus the term *frambesia*). It may heal or persist and ulcerate. Weeks later this is followed by generalized scattered scaly macules. These go on to the development of papules and frambesiform, papillomatous lesions. The initial lesion has severe epithelial hyperplasia, with lymphocytes and plasma cells in the dermis. Usually the spirochete is found only in the epidermis. The predominant involvement of the epidermis in yaws is in contrast to syphilis, in which the main changes and the spirochetes are found in the corium. In the scaly macular lesions, epithelial proliferation is slight and cellular infiltration is scanty. Late tertiary lesions may ulcerate and show epithelial hyperplasia. Histologic differentiation of the cutaneous and subcutaneous lesions of yaws and syphilis is unreliable. In addition to skin ulcers, destructive lesions of the bones occur in the tertiary stage.

Yaws differs from syphilis in that (1) the initial lesion is extragenital, (2) the infection is acquired most often in childhood but is never congenital, (3) the usual absence of mucous membrane lesions in the secondary stage, and (4) macular eruptions (roseola), iritis, and alopecia are uncommon. A long latent period between secondary and late manifestations is unusual in yaws, but the tertiary lesions are similar to those of late syphilis. Skeletal involvement is common, with a high incidence of osteoporosis. Yaws is a milder disease than syphilis, and there is a less frequent involvement of cardiovascular and nervous systems. *Gangosa* (a destructive nasopharyngitis), *goundou* (an exostosis of nasal bones), and *juxta-articular nodes* have been considered sequelae of yaws.

Pinta (carate, mal de los pintos). Pinta is a nonvenereal infection due to a spirochete, *Treponema carateum (Treponema herrejoni),* morphologically indistinguishable from the spirochete of syphilis. It is common among dark-skinned peoples of Central and South America, particularly in Mexico and Colombia. The exact method of transmission is undetermined, but probably it is by direct contact. Insect transmission also has been suggested. The serologic tests for syphilis are positive in most cases, especially in the late stages, and penicillin and arsenicals are effective in therapy.

The initial lesion is a persistent nonulcerating papule, followed in five or more months by secondary lesions (pintids) in the form of macules and papules. At first they are red, then they show varying degrees of pigmentation, some of them being of a slatyblue color. The terminal stage is a disfiguring white area of complete depigmentation. The lesions tend to be symmetrically

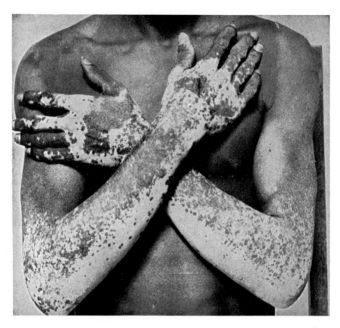

Fig. 8-6. Pinta. (Courtesy Dr. Howard Fox; from Sutton, R. L., and Sutton, R. L., Jr.: Diseases of the skin, ed. 10, St. Louis, The C. V. Mosby Co.)

arranged and usually are on the extremities. Except in the terminal stage, spirochetes are demonstrable by dark-field examination in lymph extracted from the lesions and in the epidermis by silver impregnation of histologic sections.

The earlier lesions of the skin show a thickened epidermis with elongated papillary processes, edema, infiltration of lymphocytes, and scanty basal pigment. The corium shows an abundant perivascular leukocytic infiltration, mainly plasma cells and lymphocytes, and numerous melanophores. The late lesions are characterized by epidermal atrophy with absence of basal pigment, with many melanophores and lymphocytic accumulation in the corium. The final stage is one of epidermal atrophy with loss of papillae, complete absence of pigment, and fibrosis of the corium. There are lymph nodal lesions similar to those of syphilis, but with the constant presence of melanin pigment.

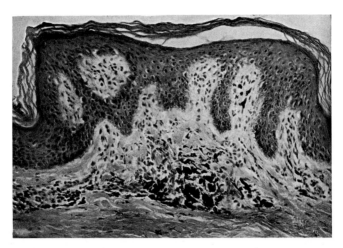

Fig. 8-7. Pinta. Microscopic lesion of the skin before the final stage, showing epidermal thickening, absence of basal pigment, melanophores, and inflammatory cells in the corium. (Courtesy Dr. Howard Fox; from Sutton, R. L.,, and Sutton, R. L., Jr.: Diseases of the skin, ed. 10, St. Louis, The C. V. Mosby Co.)

Aortitis and cerebrospinal fluid changes similar to those of syphilis have been described clinically in some cases.

Weil's disease (spirochetosis icterohaemorrhagica). Weil's disease (spirochetal jaundice) is a severe prostrating infection caused by a spirochete, *Leptospira icterohaemorrhagiae,* and characterized by sudden onset, fever, jaundice, hemorrhagic tendencies, muscular pain, and renal involvement. Spread occurs to man principally from rats, although other animals may harbor the organisms (e.g., mice, dogs, pigs, and horses). The organism is excreted in the rat's urine, and human infection occurs through the skin. The condition occurs mainly in crowded communities living under damp, unhygienic conditions, as in trenches during war. Laboratory diagnosis is most easily made by inoculation of blood into guinea pigs. Generalized jaundice is usually but not invariably present.

Damage to capillaries is shown by widely distributed minute hemorrhages. The liver is slightly enlarged and bile stained. Microscopically one sees biliary stasis in central portions of the lobule, dissociation of hepatic cords, and degeneration of hepatic cells. Focal necrosis may be present. Regeneration of hepatic cells, particularly late in the disease, is also noted. The kidneys exhibit degeneration and necrosis in convoluted tubules and interstitial lymphocytic infiltration. Degenerative, inflammatory, and reparative changes are common in muscle fibers, particularly those of the calf or pectoral region.

Similar but much rarer leptospiral diseases are canicola fever, caused by *Leptospira canicola,* and Fort Bragg or pretibial fever, caused by *Leptospira autumnalis.*

Fusospirochetosis. A symbiotic infection caused by a spiro-chete, *Borrelia vincentii,* and a long fusiform bacillus, *Bacillus fusiformis,* is often referred to as Vincent's infection. The mouth is most commonly affected (trench mouth), with the production of necrotizing lesions, particularly on the pharyngeal or tonsillar areas or gums. The same organisms are often associated with gangrenous bronchial and pulmonary lesions and may be found in lung abscesses probably as secondary invaders. Genital fuso-spirochetal lesions also occur, particularly in persons with low resistance to infections. The genitalia and perineum are involved by ulcerative and destructive lesions, which give rise to intense local pain and foul discharge. The genital lesions are commonly considered to be venereal in nature, but there is some doubt about this. Most of the cases are probably the result of auto-inoculation.

Relapsing fever. Relapsing fever is a widespread acute spiro-chetal disease, characterized by recurring paroxysmal attacks of fever and prostration and disseminated by lice and ticks. The louse-borne type, caused by *Borrelia recurrentis,* is spread in epi-demic fashion from man to man by *Pediculus humanus.* Usually there are one to three febrile relapses, each lasting four to six days. Spirochetes are numerous in the peripheral blood. The mortality is low in otherwise healthy persons, but it has reached 50% in epidemics during periods of famine. The tick-borne form of relapsing fever is epizootic among rats and other rodents, and the causative spirochete, *Borrelia duttonii,* may be trans-mitted incidentally to man by the bite of a tick of the genus *Ornithodoros.* There are usually four or more febrile relapses, lasting two to four days. During febrile periods spirochetes are demonstrable in the peripheral blood, and the mortality is very low.

There are no very characteristic pathologic changes. Around the malpighian bodies the spleen shows zones of hemorrhagic congestion and infiltration of neutrophilic leukocytes and mononuclear cells. Foci of necrosis are also present. Spirochetes are abundant and easily demonstrated by silver stains. The liver, kidneys, and heart show degenerative changes, and the liver also exhibits focal necrosis.

Ratbite fever (sodoku). Ratbite fever is usually the result of a bite by a wild rat in which the organism *Spirillum minus* is commonly parasitic. Dogs, cats, and mice have also been reported to transmit the infection. A primary lesion develops at the portal of entry, followed by recurring attacks of chills and fever, a cutaneous eruption, lymph node enlargement, leukocytosis, muscular pains, and prostration. The organism may sometimes be demonstrated in blood smears, but it is more commonly isolated from blood by inoculation of mice. The condition responds to treatment with arsenicals. A clinically similar condition that also may follow a rat bite is caused by *Streptobacillus moniliformis* (Haverhill fever).

NONSPIROCHETAL VENEREAL DISEASES

Chancroid (soft chancre). Chancroidal infection, caused by *Haemophilus ducreyi*, is an acute venereal disease characterized by soft genital ulcers, which often are followed by enlargement and suppuration of inguinal lymph nodes. Microscopically the primary ulcer shows a superficial layer of necrotic debris, neutrophils, fibrin, and red blood cells, fringed by a zone rich in plasma cells, macrophages, and neutrophils. Small, newly formed vessels show severe endothelial swelling and proliferation in this zone. Fibroplastic proliferation is slight. The underlying deepest zone shows dense infiltration by lymphocytes and plasma cells.

Gonorrhea. See pp. 417 and 742.

Granuloma inguinale. Granuloma inguinale (granuloma venereum) is a chronic ulcerative granulomatous infection involving the skin and subcutaneous tissues of the external genitalia and the inguinal region, but occasionally occurring on other parts of the body. The spread is probably by venereal means. Small intracellular coccobacillary forms *(Donovania granulomatis),* called Donovan bodies, are present in the lesions and apparently represent the causative agent. They have been cultivated in the yolk of developing chick embryos. The lesions show luxuriant granulation tissue, massively infiltrated by macrophages and plasma cells, with only a few lymphocytes and neutrophilic leukocytes. The pathognomonic cell in the lesion is a large mononuclear cell, 25 to 90 μ in diameter with

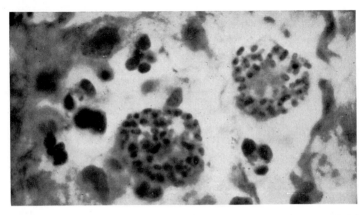

Fig. 8-8. Donovan bodies of granuloma venereum (inguinale). (×1900.) The Donovan bodies within macrophages are stained with silver. (From Torpin, R., Greenblatt, R. B., and Pund, E. R.: Amer. J. Surg. **44**:551, 1939.)

many intracytoplasmic clear areas filled with the deeply staining round or rodlike Donovan bodies. These bodies stain intensely with silver salts, giving a closed safety-pin appearance because of their ovoid shape and intense bipolar staining. Nonspecific regional lymphadenopathy sometimes occurs. In lesions with severe fibroblastic reaction, interference with lymphatic drainage may result and lead to elephantiasis of the genitalia. Rarely lesions may develop in more distant sites as a result of hematogenous spread.

Lymphogranuloma venereum. Lymphogranuloma venereum (lymphogranuloma inguinale, lymphopathia venereum) is an infection of worldwide distribution and is quite common in America, particularly among the Negro race. The causative agent is not a virus, as formerly thought, but is an agent similar to that responsible for psittacosis, an organism *(Bedsonia)* intermediate between rickettsiae and viruses. Venereal spread is probably most common. An evanescent and often unnoticed primary lesion is followed later by a variety of manifestations, such as inguinal lymph node enlargement (buboes), genital elephantiasis, rectal stricture, and warty polypoid growths about the anus, vulva, urethra, and in the rectum or the vagina. The disease has a marked predilection for lymphatic structures, with

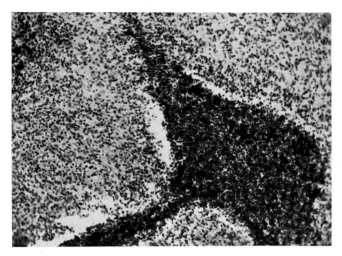

Fig. 8-9. Lymphogranuloma inguinale. Characteristic stellate abscess in a lymph node. The irregular necrotic center containing neutrophilic leukocytes is surrounded by mononuclear cells.

resulting lymph stasis, elephantiasis, and ulceration. Constitutional symptoms are common in the acute stage. An immunologic skin test (Frei test) and a complement-fixation test are valuable diagnostic aids.

Lymphatic spread from the primary lesions leads, in males, to the formation of inguinal buboes. In females lymphatic drainage from deeper parts of the vagina and the cervix is to pararectal and parasacral glands, and this commonly leads to inflammatory stricture of the rectum. This is the most serious manifestation of lymphogranuloma venereum. Some investigators disagree with the lymphatic theory of origin of proctitis and rectal stricture in the female and suggest other possible modes of development of these lesions: (1) anal coitus; (2) infection by way of the anal canal resulting from spillage of infected material from the vulva during coitus; and (3) direct spread of the causative organisms from the posterior wall of the vagina to the rectum. In males, rectal stricture is uncommon but may occur as a result of anal coitus.

Acute changes in the inguinal lymph nodes are characteristic. Minute miliary abscesses may be evident grossly. Microscopically

Table 8-4. *Differential features of chancre, soft chancre, lymphogranuloma venereum, and granuloma inguinale*

	Etiology	Diagnostic tests	Inguinal nodes	Gross features	Microscopic pathology
Chancre	Syphilis *Treponema pallidum*	Demonstration of spirochete Serologic tests for syphilis + one to two weeks after appearance of chancre	Slight enlargement, discrete, shotty	Hard, painless ulcer	Not pathognomonic; certain diagnosis depends on demonstration of spirochetes
Soft chancre chancroid	*Haemophilus ducreyi*	Intradermal test + after third week	Large, suppurative	Soft, ulcerative lesion, often multiple	Not pathognomonic; but three ill-defined zones are present
Lymphogranuloma venereum	Psittacosis-lymphogranuloma venereum agent (*Bedsonia*)	Frei test	Large focal necrosis appears after primary lesion has subsided	Primary lesion is small, painless, nonindurated, and papular; later there may be elephantiasis and secondary ulceration and rectal stricture, especially in females	Lymph nodes show multiple stellate abscesses surrounded by mononuclear cells, including macrophages of epithelioid type
Granuloma inguinale	Donovan bodies, bacilli (*Donovania granulomatis*)	Demonstration of Donovan bodies in smear or tissue section	Ulceration may involve inguinal region (nonspecific regional lymphadenopathy sometimes occurs)	Irregular spreading areas of ulceration (scarring may cause obstruction of lymphatics and elephantiasis of genitalia)	Specific large, mononuclear cell, with intracytoplasmic clear spaces and Donovan bodies

there are circumscribed masses of large mononuclear cells, the centers of which become necrotic with the formation of irregular or stellate-shaped abscesses containing many neutrophilic leukocytes and surrounded by densely packed mononuclear cells. Among the latter cells are macrophages that resemble epithelioid cells and tend to be arranged in palisade fashion. An occasional Langhans giant cell may be seen. In vulvar elephantiasis (esthiomene) the essential change is a thrombotic lymphangitis, with chronic edema and sclerosing fibrosis resulting in induration and enlargement of involved parts. Similar lymphangitis is present in rectal stricture, with the addition of miliary infiltrations of the muscularis by lymphocytes and plasma cells and ulceration of the mucosa. Rarely systemic lesions have been described, apparently caused by hematogenous dissemination.

On transmission of the causative agent to mice by the intracranial route, clusters of elementary bodies similar to those of psittacosis may be seen in mononuclear cells composing the exudate in the meninges and in the substance of the brain. The infective agent may be grown in the yolk sac of the chick embryo, smears from which show the elementary bodies.

Chapter 9

Mycotic, protozoan, and helminthic infections

F **MYCOSES**
ungi are cellular filamentous plants belonging to a division
called thallophytes. Because of the absence of chlorophyll, they
must obtain food from organic material already synthesized. They
may be saprophytic or parasitic; i.e., they may obtain their
food from dead organic material or a living organism. Fungous
infections are not rare in man and are frequently serious. Yeasts
and fungi may be stained prominently in tissue sections by means
of the periodic acid–Schiff stain, methenamine silver stain, mucin
stains (for capsules of some organisms, e.g., cryptococci), and
acridine orange fluorescent stain. Superficial involvement of
skin or mucous membrane is a common type of fungous infection, as in athlete's foot and thrush. The more serious types of
parasitic fungi produce widespread chronic destructive lesions.
Fungi that are ordinarily saprophytic, such as *Aspergillus,*
Mucor, and *Candida,* are producing infection with increasing
frequency in patients receiving antibiotic or steroid therapy.

Actinomycosis. Actinomycosis is a chronic suppurative infection caused by *Actinomyces bovis* (principally in cattle) and *A.*
israeli (common in man). In cattle the disease is known as
"lumpy jaw." *Actinomyces* are normally present in the mouth.
Although these organisms are related to the true bacteria, they
also exhibit some features similar to those of the higher filamentous fungi. The organism grows in the tissues in colonies
composed of a tangled, felted mass of filaments, surrounded by
radiating projections known as "clubs" (hence the term *ray*
fungus). Club formation occurs only in tissues, and not in culture, and is thought to be a reaction on the part of the organism to the surrounding tissues. A protein substance encasing
the terminal clubs makes them eosinophilic. When pus from a
lesion is spread in a thin layer on a glass slide, the actinomycotic
colonies may be seen grossly as yellow "sulfur granules." In-

fections caused by the aerobic, partially acid-fast *Nocardia asteroides* are relatively rare but result in a similar disease. A granulomatous nocardiosis caused by an intracellular organism has been described.

Some break in skin or mucous membrane is apparently necessary to allow entrance of the organism into the body. A direct contagion has not been proved. The infection is geographically widespread. The region of the mouth, jaws, or face is most commonly affected. The intestinal tract, particularly the ileocecal region and appendix, is next in frequency. Here it may be mistaken clinically for chronic appendicitis, and after operation it may leave a chronic sinus. The liver often becomes involved in any type of abdominal actinomycosis. Occasionally the fallopian tubes are infected. Pulmonary actinomycosis may simulate a chronic abscess, caused by ordinary pyogenic bacteria, or tuberculosis.

The characteristic lesions are chronic abscesses resulting from progressive penetration and destruction of tissue. Many leukocytes are present in the zone of suppuration, surrounded by a wall of granulation tissue containing many mononuclear cells and occasional giant cells. In older areas there is distinct connective tissue formation. Histologic diagnosis depends on finding the ray fungus in the abscesses.

In the cervicofacial type the lesion usually starts in the gums and spreads to the submaxillary region. where there may be tumorlike masses or soft suppurating lesions and chronic sinuses from which pus escapes. Occasionally the primary lesion is in the skin. Intestinal involvement produces a chronic inflammatory mass and may lead to suppurating sinuses. Spread to the liver by the portal bloodstream results in multiple, small, ragged abscess cavities. The thoracic type begins in the bronchioles and subsequently involves the parenchyma and pleura, with eventual perforation of the chest wall. Spread is rarely through lymphatics but is usually by direct extension or the bloodstream. Actinomycotic septicemia may result in metastatic abscesses in various organs and tissues.

Mycetoma pedis (**Madura foot**). Mycetoma pedis is a chronic suppurative infection of the foot caused by a variety of fungi or funguslike organisms, which may be differentiated by cultural studies. Granules representing colonies of the organism are found in the tissues and in discharged pus. About half the cases are caused by certain of the actinomycetes, such as *Nocardia* *brasiliensis, N. caviae,* or *Streptomyces sp.* (actinomycetoma), and the remainder are caused by a variety of true fungi, e.g., *Madurella mycetomi, M. grisea,* or *Monosporium apiospermum* (maduromycosis or Madura foot).

Aspergillosis. Most members of the genus *Aspergillus* are saprophytic and nonpathogenic. Some are found as harmless invaders of the external auditory canal, nasal sinuses, and external genitalia and as secondary invaders in lung abscesses. In involvement of the ear the external auditory canal may be partly filled with foul moist material spotted with black granules. The lung appears to be the most common site of important infection. The pulmonary lesion may be in the form of a bronchopneumonia, abscesses, small infarcts (resulting from thrombosis caused by vascular invasion by organisms), or a mass of *Aspergillus* mycelia ("fungus ball") in a cavity. The latter may be newly formed or it may be a preexisting inflammatory (e.g., tuberculous) or carcinomatous cavity. Chronic granulomatous reaction to the organisms in the lungs has also been reported. A primary fatal disseminated infection is uncommon, but aspergillosis as a secondary complication is more frequent and tends to occur in patients with debilitating disease who have received steroid or antibiotic therapy. Aspergillosis in other tissues or organs is characterized by abscesses, necrotizing lesions, and sometimes chronic granulomatous inflammation.

Candidiasis. *Candida* species include yeastlike organisms, or Fungi Imperfecti, of which the chief pathogenic member is *Candida albicans,* the cause of thrush in children. This lesion is seen most often in debilitated infants and children as white patches or false membranes on the mucosa of the tongue, gums, lips, cheeks, esophagus, or pharynx. It occasionally occurs in diabetics and in leukemia patients or following antibiotic therapy. Vulvovaginitis also may occur. Candidial endocarditis has been reported in drug addicts and as a complication following cardiac surgery.

Phycomycosis. Phycomycosis is an uncommon infection of the lungs, ears, nervous system, or intestinal tract caused by a fungus that is more commonly encountered as a saprophyte or contaminant. The lesions may show an intense necrotizing and suppurative inflammatory process in which the irregularly branching coenocytic or nonseptate filaments of the fungus are seen. Although this infection is commonly called "mucormycosis," there are several species of Phycomycetes that may be

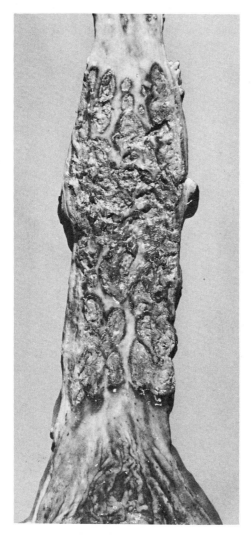

Fig. 9-1. Esophageal candidiasis in a patient with leukemia. (Courtesy Dr. J. F. Kuzma.)

causative, including *Mucor, Rhizopus,* and *Absidia.* These fungi have a tendency to invade vessels, causing thrombosis and infarction. Phycomycosis is especially seen in patients with uncontrolled diabetes mellitus, leukemia, and other debilitating diseases and in those receiving antibiotics, corticosteroids, chemotherapeutic agents for cancer, and irradiation.

Histoplasmosis. Histoplasmosis (reticuloendothelial cytomycosis) is an infection with an oval, yeastlike organism (2 by 4μ), *Histoplasma capsulatum.* The disease was discovered and named by Darling in 1906; the causative organism was recognized as a yeast by Rocha-Lima in 1912 and was cultured by DeMonbreun in 1933. Widespread occurrence of the disease and prevalence in the United States have been recognized only in recent years with the development of a skin test (histoplasmin), which indicates past or present infection, and with specific serologic tests that indicate active disease. Positive diagnosis depends on finding the organisms in cultures of the sputum, blood, or bone marrow or in biopsied tissue such as lymph nodes.

The infection is not spread between individuals but appears to be from soil contaminated by fecal material of chickens, pigeons, starlings, other birds, and bats. In South Africa most of the recognized benign pulmonary infections seem to have been acquired from contaminated caves (cave disease). Endemic areas of histoplasmosis have been found in many parts of the world, particularly near large rivers and where there is high humidity with warm temperatures. In some endemic areas of the United States, histoplasmin skin tests have indicated that 70 to 85% of the population have had an infection. Fewer than one in 1,000 develop active progressive disease, perhaps from endogenous reinfection. The lungs are believed to be the usual portal of entry of the organisms.

From developing knowledge of the disease it appears that histoplasmosis can be roughly categorized into four forms: (1) acute pulmonary, (2) chronic pulmonary, (3) acute disseminated, and (4) chronic disseminated. The acute pulmonary form is most common. It is mild, benign, and often is undiagnosed or is considered a "flulike" or viral pulmonary infection. In endemic areas it is considered a common cause of unexplained fever in children. Chronic pulmonary histoplasmosis is progressive, forming granulomatous inflammation with caseation necrosis and cavitation, and is frequently misdiagnosed as pulmonary tuberculosis, or it may occur in association with tuberculosis. It is seen most commonly in middle-aged and elderly men and has a poor prognosis. Localized, nonfatal, pulmonary granulomatous lesions with caseation necrosis, calcification, and fibrotic borders may occur. A solitary pulmonary nodule may appear as a "coin" lesion in a chest x-ray film. Healed, calcified lesions in the lung and regional lymph nodes may resemble the healed primary complex of tuberculosis. The acute disseminated disease may be either benign or progressive, the latter being fatal, and may occur at any age, but particularly in the young and elderly. The spleen, lymph nodes, and liver are enlarged. There is a septic-type fever, with anemia and

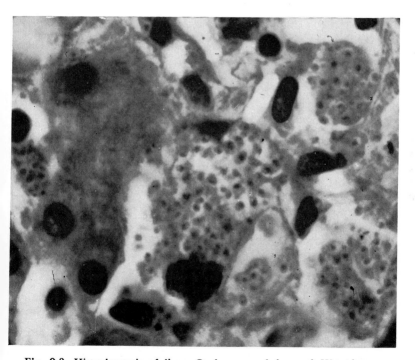

Fig. 9-2. Histoplasmosis of liver. Oval or round form of *Histoplasma capsulatum* in reticuloendothelial cells (Kupffer cells, macrophages). From fatal case of progressive systemic histoplasmosis in infant. (From Baker, R. D.: Fungus infections. In Anderson, W. A. D., editor: Pathology, ed. 5, St. Louis, 1966, The C. V. Mosby Co.)

leukopenia. Bone marrow smears may reveal the organisms or granulomas, and sometimes the organisms may be found in mononuclear cells in blood smears. The chronic disseminated form occurs mainly in elderly people and is usually fatal.

The characteristic pathologic change in disseminated forms is a widespread reticuloendothelial hyperplasia, with a large number of the encapsulated organisms within phagocytic cells. Organs most commonly involved are the spleen, liver, lymph nodes, lungs, bone marrow, oral mucosa, adrenals, and intestines. Hyperplasia of endothelial cells lining small blood vessels may lead to partial or complete occlusion of their lumina. Ulcerations of the colon, tongue, larynx, and pharynx and a patchy pneumonitis are also common. Vegetative endocarditis has occurred. In certain organs, particularly the adrenal glands, caseation necrosis may occur. Organisms in these necrotic areas are often atypical, being distorted and larger than the usual *Histoplasma*. Adrenal involvement has eventuated in Addison's disease.

Cryptococcosis. Cryptococcosis (torulosis, European blastomycosis) is a mycotic disease caused by *Cryptococcus neoformans (C. hominis, Torula histolytica),* a budding, yeastlike, nonmycelial fungus characterized by a mucinous capsule. Although not a frequent infection, it is geographically widespread, affects all ages (two thirds of cases are between 30 and 60 years), and is the commonest cause of mycotic meningitis. The meninges, brain, and lungs are most often involved, but skin, mucous membranes, and other organs are occasionally affected. Nervous system involvement is usually fatal, whereas a localized lesion elsewhere may be amenable to surgical excision. *C. neoformans* has been isolated from soil and pigeon droppings. The portal of entry into the body is not apparent but is believed to be usually the respiratory tract from which the organisms make their way to the central nervous system and to other sites.

Meningeal cryptococcosis is characterized by pale, grayish, mucoid, translucent nodules or a diffuse exudate. In about half the cases there are intracerebral lesions. The basal ganglia and the midbrain as well as the cortex may be involved. There is little cellular reaction to the infection, particularly in the nervous system, where the organisms are in small cystlike spaces filled with the mucoid material of the capsular polysaccharide. Less common are granulomatous lesions. In the lungs there may be widespread involvement or localized lesions. Histiocytic cells may be numerous, and the organisms may be within macrophages or may be extracellular. Older lesions may be more granulomatous, with some giant cells and fibrosis. Skin lesions are usually the result of systemic infection, but sometimes they are isolated, suggesting that the organisms may occasionally

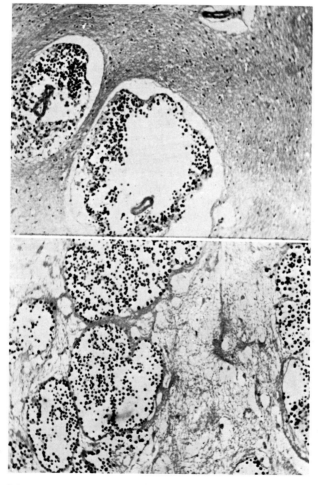

Fig. 9-3. Cerebral cryptococcosis. Cystic areas in cerebral tissue contain the numerous small round parasites.

enter the body through the skin. These lesions may remain localized or spread to the central nervous system. Systemic cryptococcosis may develop as a terminal infection in patients with leukemia or malignant lymphoma.

The *Cryptococcus* organism appears in tissues as a spherical or ovoid budding cell, 5 to 10μ in diameter, with a mucinous capsule up to five times the diameter of the cell proper. The capsule, which fails to stain by usual histologic methods and appears as a clear halo, may be stained by mucicarmine or by certain stains for acid mucopolysaccharides. No mycelia are formed. In pulmonary and meningeal infections the organisms may be found in fresh unstained preparations of sputum and spinal fluid, and the capsule may be rendered prominent by mixture with India ink.

North American blastomycosis (Gilchrist's disease). Infection with *Blastomyces dermatitidis,* a yeastlike organism, is largely restricted to the North American continent. It most commonly involves the skin and lungs but also may be more widely systemic. The primary site of the infection is almost always pulmonary. The cutaneous type forms a chronic or subacute ulcer. Systemic blastomycosis may have widespread involvement of the lungs, subcutaneous tissue, nervous system, internal organs, bones, and joints.

Blastomycetes are round or oval unicellular organisms, are about 20μ in diameter, and have a thick refractile double-contoured cell wall. Reproduction takes place in the tissues by budding.

The cutaneous lesions are most frequently on the face, hands, and legs. They begin as papules, which slowly ulcerate and extend at the margin. Minute abscesses, frequently showing individual organisms within them, are present in and beneath the epidermis, and the surrounding tissue is infiltrated by lymphocytes, plasma cells, macrophages, fibroblasts, and neutrophilic leukocytes. Giant cells are often present and may contain organisms in their cytoplasm. Certain diagnosis depends on seeing the organisms in the tissue. The epidermis often undergoes pronounced hyperplasia with irregular extensions downward into the dermis, simulating carcinoma (pseudoepitheliomatous or pseudocarcinomatous hyperplasia). Pulmonary disease is characterized by chronic suppurative and granulomatous inflammation, sometimes with foci of caseation necrosis. Blastomycetes are found within and outside of giant cells. South American blastomycosis (paracoccidioidal granuloma) is similar to the North American blastomycosis, but the organisms in the tissues show multiple buds, and lesions of lymph nodes and mucous membranes are prominent.

Coccidioidomycosis and coccidioidal granuloma. Infection with the fungus *Coccidioides immitis* is endemic in southwestern United States, particularly California, but a few cases have been reported in other parts of the Americas. Warm, dry, and dusty areas apparently are suitable for spread of the infective arthrospores. The portal of entry is the respiratory tract, but in exceptional cases abrasions of the skin are believed to have been the site of entry of the organisms. In most cases the infection is focalized in the lungs, is self-limited, and is asymptomatic. More severe but self-limited infections may be manifested by an acute respiratory illness (influenzal or pneumonic form). This is the form sometimes referred to as Valley fever or San Joaquin fever. Sensitivity to the fungus, as manifested by a skin test with coccidioidin, develops ten to forty days after infection, and transient humoral antibodies (precipitins and complement fixation) may be detectable. The allergy as shown by reaction to coccidioidin remains, and the patient, after recovery, is highly resistant to reinfection. In a few cases manifestations of erythema nodosum or erythema multiforme develop.

In a small proportion of infections, instead of arrest there is a progressive or disseminated coccidioidomycosis (coccidioidal granuloma), and in such cases the mortality is high. The lungs, skin, bones, and lymph nodes are most frequently involved. The central nervous system also may be affected. The condition is easily mistaken for tuberculosis or blastomycosis. Diagnostic proof depends on demonstrating the fungus either by culture and animal inoculation or microscopically in tissue. In tissues the organism may be found free or in giant cells as a rounded body, 5 to 70μ in diameter, with a highly refractile, double-contoured capsule and containing endospores. Reproduction of endosporulation differentiates the organisms from blastomycetes, which reproduce by budding.

Morphologically the lesions in the lungs resemble those of tuberculosis, with tubercle-like foci and varying degrees of caseation necrosis. Although predominantly granulomatous, a suppurative reaction with microabscesses is often a concomitant feature. Organisms may be seen in the lesions, some of which show endospores. Fibrocaseous foci may undergo cavitation.

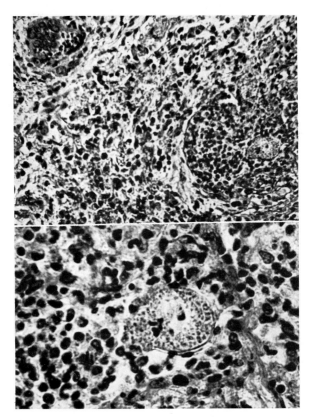

Fig. 9-4. Coccidioidomycosis of the lung. Note the endosporulating organism and multinucleated giant cell.

Pleural involvement and regional lymphadenopathy occur. Healed or arrested disease is evidenced by residual nodules in the lung and mediastinal lymph nodes, similar to the primary complex of tuberculosis, or by a single solid parenchymal lesion (coccidioidoma), or by a thin-walled cavity. In progressive disease the active lesions in the lungs become more widespread, and with dissemination, abscesses and granulomatous foci (tubercle-like lesions) appear in many organs. These lesions may simulate those of blastomycosis, but differentiation is possible by recognition of the endosporulating organisms. In the skin

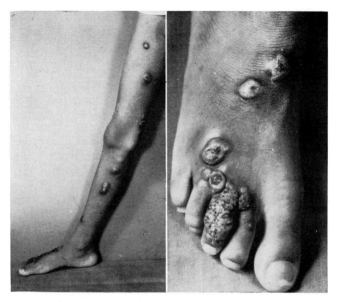

Fig. 9-5. Sporotrichosis.

lesion, as in blastomycosis, pseudoepitheliomatous or pseudo-carcinomatous hyperplasia of the epidermis occurs.

Rhinosporidiosis. Rhinosporidiosis is a chronic infection with *Rhinosporidium seeberi,* an endosporulating organism that produces polypoid or pedunculated tumorlike masses on the nasal mucosa. The condition is rare in the United States and is reported most commonly from Ceylon and India.

Sporotrichosis. The fact that sporotrichosis, an uncommon fungous infection, occurs mainly in farmers and nurserymen suggests that spread may be from plants. The primary lesion is usually on the skin of the arms or hands, and apparently it is related to a minor puncture wound, such as a thorn prick. The inflammation is a combined granulomatous and suppurative type. The skin lesions are usually multiple, ulcerative, and easily mistaken for gummas. Frequently they are situated along the course of the lymphatics, which become thickened. The fungus appears in the involved tissue as a small, spindle-shaped, single-celled gram-positive organism. Only rarely does dissemination occur throughout the body to cause visceral lesions. In the disseminated forms it is possible that the respiratory and intestinal tracts are portals of entry. The causative organisms are few and difficult to demonstrate in the tissues in the usual case of human sporotrichosis, but tend to appear in large numbers and are more readily demonstrated in lesions of human disseminated disease, as well as in the experimental disease in mice.

Chromoblastomycosis. Relatively uncommon but occurring in widely distributed areas, chromoblastomycosis is an infection by moldlike pigmented fungi belonging to the genera *Hormodendrum* and *Phialophora*. It occurs mainly in farmers or persons having contact with vegetation and affects the skin, usually of an extremity, producing a verrucous dermatitis. It does not become systemic. The lesions may be papular, verrucous, or ulcerative. Microscopic diagnosis is made by finding the brown, thick-walled, rounded septate cells of the fungus in the lesion. Epithelial proliferation, sometimes pseudoepitheliomatous, may

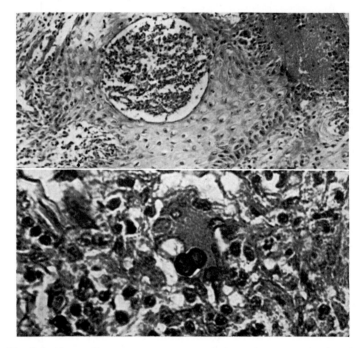

Fig. 9-6. Chromoblastomycosis. Note the dark, thick-walled organisms in a tiny epidermal abscess (top) and in a giant cell (bottom).

be prominent, and a cellular reaction with plasma cells, macrophages, and multinucleated giant cells commonly occurs. Microabscesses are frequently present also.

PROTOZOAN INFECTIONS

The main protozoan diseases in man are amebiasis, caused by *Entamoeba histolytica;* malaria, caused by sporozoa of the genus *Plasmodium;* trypanosomiasis; and leishmaniasis.

Amebiasis. The pathogenic *Entamoeba histolytica* is an actively motile and phagocytic organism 20 to 30μ in diameter. It has a single, delicate, barely distinguishable nucleus. The trophozoite (not the cyst) form penetrates the tissue of the large intestine, causing characteristic chronic ulcers. Its presence may or may not be associated with the clinical symptoms of amebic dysentery. Metastasis of the amebae through the portal vein to the liver results in liver "abscess."

Human infection results from ingestion of mature amebic cysts, usually in contaminated food or water. After ingestion the cysts pass through the stomach, unchanged, into the small intestines. Excystation of the cysts, which begins in the terminal ileum, is followed by development of a colony of trophozoites in the cecum and their establishment throughout the colon. It is possible that trophozoites may remain as commensal organisms in the lumen of the intestines without giving rise to clinical disease, although some investigators believe that in all cases there is tissue penetration by the trophozoites, associated with varying degrees of clinical and pathologic manifestations. According to the latter view, asymptomatic cases may occur in which the lesions are too small to be detected. Some of the trophozoites become encysted in the lumen of the colon. At first the cysts are immature and contain one nucleus, but by successive nuclear division the cysts become quadrinucleated, and it is the latter, mature form that is transmissible to man.

When trophozoites invade the mucosa of the intestine, they produce lysis of the tissue. At first the lesions are minute, almost pinpoint sized. The amebae then penetrate the submucosa and extend laterally, producing large, characteristically undermined and flask-shaped ulcers. The ulcers have shaggy, yellowish brown edges and a floor formed by submucous or muscular coats. Initially there is very little inflammatory cell infiltration, except for a few mononuclear cells. Secondary bacterial infection from the intestine is usual, and this results in further tissue destruc-

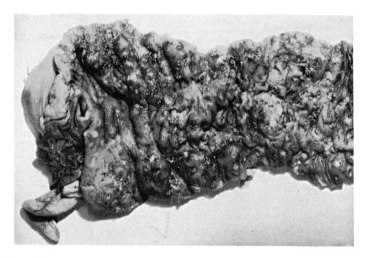

Fig. 9-7. Amebic colitis. Note the shaggy and irregular areas of ulceration.

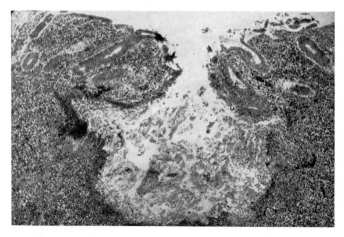

Fig. 9-8. Amebic ulcer of the colon. Note the undermining of edges and the characteristic shape. (AFIP.)

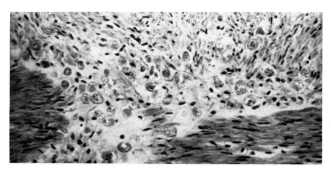

Fig. 9-9. Amebae in submucosa and invading muscularis, amebic colitis. Note the absence of any significant tissue reaction. (AFIP.)

tion and leukocytic infiltration. Granulation tissue appears later in the bases of the ulcers. A fibrinous serositis may be caused by amebae migrating through the wall of the colon to the serosal surface. In severe cases there may be perforation of muscular and serous coats and general peritonitis or adhesions to neighboring structures. The cecum, flexures, and rectum are common sites, but any portion of the large bowel, including the appendix may be involved. The small intestine is rarely affected. Occasionally a localized mass of granulation tissue may occur in the wall of the colon, secondary to amebic ulceration. Such a lesion, known as "amebic granuloma" or "ameboma," may be mistaken for carcinoma of the colon clinically, or when in the cecum, it may simulate simple appendicitis. Microscopically the ameboma consists of fibrous tissue, lymphocytes, plasma cells, and eosinophils.

Liver "abscess" is the most frequent complication. It may be single or multiple and have a diameter of a few millimeters or many centimeters. The lining is rough and shaggy, and in older "abscesses" there is a connective tissue wall. The contents are grumous, semifluid, and yellowish red or chocolate colored. Microscopically the amebae are found in the edge of living tissue and in the adjacent necrotic material. True pus is not present, unless secondary bacterial infection occurs; but the term *abscess* is commonly used for these liquefied, necrotic, amebic lesions. Occasionally transportation of the organisms by hepatic veins results in a similar lung "abscess." However, the most frequent cause of these pulmonary lesions is direct extension of hepatic "abscess" through the diaphragm.

Balantidium coli infections. See p. 626.

Malaria. Malaria is an infection with a protozoan parasite, which has an asexual cycle in a man and a sexual cycle in the *Anopheles* mosquito. The parasite is a sporozoan, and three common species infect man, causing three types of the disease: *Plasmodium vivax* (tertian malaria), *P. malariae* (quartan malaria), and *P. falciparum* (estivoautumnal, or malignant tertian, malaria). A rare fourth type is that caused by *P. ovale*. They differ in the interval of time required for the completion of a cycle in man, with paroxysms of chills occurring at the time of sporulation.

Life cycle. The parasite is injected into man by the bite of an infected *Anopheles* mosquito. After an exoerythrocytic phase of seven to ten days, the parasite reaches the bloodstream and invades a red blood cell, where it enlarges and matures, producing a characteristic large form (schizont), which can be identified by appropriate stains of the blood. The intracellular parasite makes use of the hemoglobin in the red cell, using up the protein fraction and leaving the "heme" portion as a brownish, granular "malarial" pigment, which is a form of hematin, and not melanin. By intracellular division the large form breaks up into a number of small forms (merozoites). Rupture of the red cell releases the pigment and merozoites into the bloodstream. Each of these attacks a new red cell, and the asexual cycle (schizogony) is repeated. The time taken for completion of this cycle is quite uniform and constant for the particular type of parasite. Consequently large numbers mature and rupture into the bloodstream at about the same time and produce the characteristic malarial chill, which recurs at regular intervals.

A few of the intracellular parasites develop sexual forms, called microgametocytes and macrogametocytes, instead of the asexual sporozoites. These forms, when released into the bloodstream, do not reenter new red cells but perish unless taken into the stomach of an anopheline mosquito along with its blood meal. Here they undergo maturation into microgametes and macrogametes during the early phase of the sexual cycle (sporogony). Subsequently the microgametes and macrogametes fuse to produce a motile fertilized form (zygote), which penetrates the wall of the stomach and forms a cyst (oocyst). Large numbers of spores develop within this cyst, eventually reach the salivary glands of the mosquito, and are ready to infect the next person bitten.

General pathology. Pathologic changes in malaria are dependent on the following factors: (1) Large numbers of red cells are parasitized and destroyed, with the production of a secondary anemia. (2) The malarial pigment (hematin) is a peculiar breakdown product of hemoglobin and is produced in large amounts. It does not occur normally in the body and is not an intermediate product in the breakdown of hemoglobin and the formation of bile pigment. The pigment is taken up by phagocytic cells of the reticuloendothelial system. The resulting reticuloendothelial hyperplasia contributes to enlargement of the spleen and liver. The deposited pigment imparts a slaty gray or grayish black color to the enlarged spleen and to a lesser extent discolors the liver. (3) Obstruction of small blood vessels is probably the most important factor in the pathology of malaria. This is seen particularly in *P. falciparum* malaria and is mainly caused by the formation of small agglutinated masses of parasitized and pigmented erythrocytes. An undue stickiness of the surfaces of the parasitized red blood cells is apparently responsible for the agglutination; and the malarial pigment may be a factor in the pathogenesis of this process. The vascular obstructions result in insufficient blood supply to various tissues. In certain organs (e.g., the brain) this ischemia may result in dysfunction or even the development of small areas of necrosis.

Lesions in individual organs. In addition to the following characteristic changes in the organs in malaria, one may demonstrate the plasmodia in properly stained sections of tissues, e.g., in the parasitized erythrocytes in capillaries and in phagocytic cells of the spleen, liver (Kupffer cells), bone marrow, and other organs.

SPLEEN. The spleen may be greatly enlarged and is discolored a slaty gray or grayish black. Microscopically an enormous amount of pigment is seen in phagocytic cells.

LIVER. The liver is usually only slightly enlarged and discolored. Microscopically pigment is seen in the Kupffer cells lining the sinusoids. Occasionally, small focal areas of necrosis are present.

BONE MARROW. In the bone marrow some hyperplasia and retention of pigment are evident microscopically.

NERVOUS SYSTEM. Tiny areas of hemorrhage and focal necrosis with softening may be found in the brain and cord. Cerebral involvement occurs particularly with severe *P. falciparum* infections. Small blood vessels here, as in other tissues, appear congested and obstructed with agglutinated masses of parasitized red cells. In cases not too rapidly fatal the so-called "malarial granuloma" of Dürck may be found. Around a central occluded capillary is an area of necrotic tissue, surrounded in turn by a zone of extravasated red cells and proliferating neuroglial cells. The necrotic material is removed, and a cellular nodule of neuroglial cells remains. The effects of cerebral lesions in malaria depend on their position and extent.

KIDNEY. Usually no gross changes are evident in the kidney. Mild microscopic changes occur constantly. These are mainly tubular degenerations and blockage of tubules by casts. In certain cases, as in the complication called blackwater fever, the renal changes are severe.

Blackwater fever develops in certain cases of malaria. It is characterized by sudden, massive intravascular hemolysis. There is an intense hemoglobinuria with the passage of red or reddish black urine. This complication is usually fatal. The reason for its development in certain cases is unknown. The kidneys show marked degeneration, particularly of the convoluted tubules, and many tubules contain pigment casts. The renal changes are similar to those of hemoglobinuric nephrosis (p. 385).

Leishmaniasis. Leishmaniasis is a tropical condition caused by protozoan parasites with a complex life cycle. Transmission is by the *Phlebotomus* fly (sandfly). The three main types of *Leishmania* are morphologically indistinguishable.

Leishmania donovani produces the disease kala-azar (visceral leishmaniasis), prevalent in India and in parts of China, but also occurring in the Mediterranean region. The organism can be seen in phagocytic cells of the reticuloendothelial system. The intracellular parasites in tissue sections resemble *Histoplasma* but can be differentiated by the presence of the kinetoplast and the lack of a capsule. The spleen is greatly enlarged.

Leishmania tropica produces the oriental sore (cutaneous leishmaniasis), a chronic granulomatous ulcer, prevalent in the Mediterranean region and in Central and South America.

Leishmania brasiliensis (American leishmaniasis, mucocutaneous leishmaniasis) results in chronic granulomatous ulcers similar to the oriental sore. There is a distinct tendency to involvement of the skin and mucosa of the mouth, nose, and

larvae of the dog and cat hookworm, *A. brasiliense,* can penetrate the human skin. It produces an irritating skin lesion (creeping eruption or cutaneous larva migrans) but does not proceed to maturity. This must be distinguished from the form of visceral larva migrans caused by ingestion of embryonated eggs of *Toxocara canis* (an ascarid of dogs and cats). In this condition the larvae penetrate the small intestine and migrate throughout the viscera, producing fever, eosinophilia, hepatomegaly, pulmonary symptoms, and allergic granulomas in various organs.

Strongyloidiasis. *Strongyloides stercoralis* is a nematode that may have a free-living direct cycle in soil or a parasitic indirect cycle. In the latter, noninfective rhabditiform larvae, passed in the stools to the soil, develop into infective filariform larvae, which penetrate the skin or buccal mucosa, enter vessels, and reach the lungs, undergoing some maturation, and later reach the intestinal tract by swallowing. A focal acute colitis may result, with areas of reddening and swelling of the mucosa and submucosa (Fig. 9-11). The female worm deposits eggs in the mucosa where they hatch and produce rhabditiform larvae. The latter are passed in the stool but occasionally can transform to

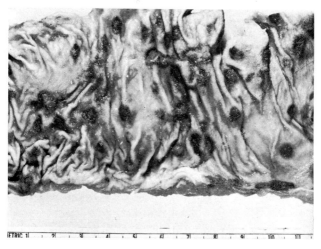

Fig. 9-11. Lesions of intestinal mucosa associated with strongyloides infection.

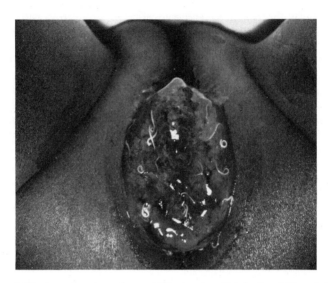

Fig. 9-12. Rectal prolapse in a child, showing *Trichuris trichiura* infection.

filariform larvae in the colon, so that reinfection can take place by penetration of the infective larvae into the colonic mucosa.

Trichuriasis. *Trichuris trichiura,* or whipworm, is one of the commonest intestinal parasites. Infection is acquired by swallowing eggs that have matured in the soil. The larvae are hatched in the small intestine, where they are attached to the mucosa and undergo maturation, then descend to the cecum to become adults. The adult worms are found in the cecum and colon, sometimes in tremendous numbers. The mucosa may be congested or may show small focal areas of inflammation. Eosinophilia is a frequent accompaniment.

Filariasis. The filariae are roundworms that live in the lymphatics or tissues of man. The infective filariform larvae are injected into the skin by a biting insect, and the larvae mature to adults in the appropriate site. The most widespread is *Wuchereria bancrofti,* found in parts of Central and South America, Africa, India, Asia, and various Pacific islands. At one time there was a focus of cases in South Carolina. The adult worms live in the lymphatics of man, mainly in the pelvic region and in the genitalia in the male, causing an obliterative

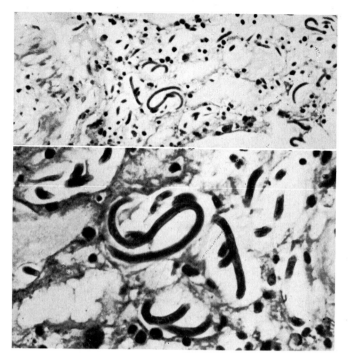

Fig. 9-13. Microfilariae of *Wuchereria bancrofti* in the epididymis.

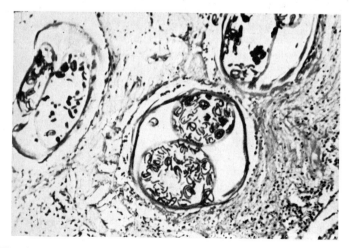

Fig. 9-14. Onchocercoma; adult worm, containing many microfilariae, embedded in an inflammatory nodule.

granulomatous lymphangitis. Eventually this may result in lymphatic obstruction and consequent elephantiasis of the scrotum or limbs. About a year after infection, larvae (microfilariae) appear in the blood, usually with nocturnal periodicity. The microfilariae, when taken up by various culicide and anopheline mosquito vectors, develop into infective larval forms. Infections with *Brugia (Wuchereria) malayi* are similar, although the microfilariae are somewhat different.

Onchocerca volvulus is a nematode causative of onchocerciasis. It is found in circumscribed areas of Guatemala and Mexico (at elevations of 1,100 to 5,000 feet) and in West Africa. Spread is by the gnat or black fly, *Simulium*. The adult worms are found in localized inflammatory fibrous nodules (onchocercomas), most common in American onchocerciasis in subcutaneous tissue of the head region. Microfilariae are found in superficial parts of the skin and are particularly abundant near the nodule, but also at a distance. An erysipeloid dermatitis, eosinophilia, and ocular disturbances are common manifestations. Invasion of the eye by microfilariae frequently produces visual disturbances and blindness.

Trichinosis. *Trichinella spiralis* has been found to have infected 15% or more of bodies examined at autopsy in various parts of the United States. With the consideration of this high incidence, clinical symptoms are uncommon. The infection is common in rats, from which pigs and other flesh-eating mammals may become infected. Pigs, however, are more commonly infected by eating uncooked garbage containing infected pork scraps. Ingestion by man of partially cooked or raw pork containing the larvae in muscles frees the encysted larvae in the small bowel. Here they mature in the intestinal mucosa; the adults copulate and the fertilized females give birth to larvae, which invade tissues, penetrate blood vessels, and reach the voluntary muscles, in which they become encysted. The extraocular, masseter, tongue, larynx, diaphragm, cervical, and intercostal muscles are most frequently and heavily involved. Sites of tendinous insertions especially are affected. Occasionally a massive encystment in muscles is accompanied by myositis, with swelling, pain, and tenderness. Muscle fibers degenerate, and focal inflammatory reactions occur about the larvae. After a time the encysted larvae die and become calcified. Interstitial myocarditis, with infiltrations of neutrophilic and eosinophilic leukocytes, is common in trichinosis, although the larvae almost never encyst in

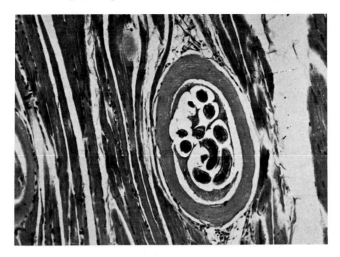

Fig. 9-15. Encysted trichina in voluntary muscle.

the muscle of the heart. Inflammatory and hemorrhagic foci may be found also in the central nervous system. Clinical trichinosis may have allergic manifestations.

Flukes

The trematodes, or flukes, are nonsegmented flatworms that live in the blood or tissues and have complicated life cycles. Those most important in man are the blood flukes (schistosomes), the liver flukes (*Clonorchis sinensis* and *Fasciola hepatica*), and the lung fluke *(Paragonimus westermani)*.

Schistosomiasis (bilharziasis). The male and female blood flukes live in various parts of the portal bloodstream, and the eggs are excreted with feces or urine. The eggs hatch in fresh water, and the resulting free-swimming organisms (miracidia) attack and infect appropriate species of snails. After a period of development and multiplication in the molluscan host, forktailed, free-swimming forms (cercariae) are discharged and can penetrate human skin coming into contact with the infected water. Transient local irritation or an urticarial rash may appear at the site of entry in the skin. Having penetrated peripheral venules, or lymphatics of the dermis, the larvae are carried in the bloodstream, and those that reach the portal circulation survive and mature. The important lesions that develop are caused by the deposition of eggs in the liver, the walls of the bowel and urinary bladder, and other tissues.

Schistosoma haematobium is most prevalent in Africa. The pelvic veins, particularly the vesiculoprostatic plexus, are the frequent location of the parasites, and the terminal-spined ova are deposited in the wall of the bladder and passed in the urine. The irritation of the ova in the bladder wall gives rise to cystitis, hematuria, and sometimes carcinoma of the bladder. The rectal wall also may be affected.

Schistosoma mansoni infections are widely distributed in Africa, northern South America, and the Caribbean region. The mature worms locate mainly in the lower colonic and rectal branches of the portal veins. The lateral-spined eggs extruded into the intestinal wall cause a chronic inflammatory reaction. Pseudotubercles and small abscesses form around the ova, and fibrosis and thickening of the bowel wall eventually develop. Many ova are carried by the portal stream to the liver and deposited around portal spaces, where they cause formation of pseudotubercles and fibrous nodules. Eventually this may lead to a progressive "pipe-stem" cirrhosis, with obstruction of the portal circulation, splenomegaly, and ascites (p. 505).

Schistosoma japonicum infections are common in the Far East, particularly in the Yangtze Valley of China and in areas of Japan, Formosa, and the southern Philippines. The adult worms are most commonly in branches of the superior mesenteric vein draining the small intestine. The eggs, which have only a small rudimentary lateral spine, are extruded through the wall of the small bowel, in which they cause much irritation, dysenteric symptoms, chronic inflammation, and fibrous thickening. Many eggs are carried to the liver, in which they cause pseudotubercle formation, periportal fibrosis, portal obstruction, splenomegaly, and ascites.

Nonhuman varieties of schistosome cercariae have caused severe dermatitis (swimmer's itch) in some areas of the United States, although the parasites are incapable of developing to maturity in man.

Tapeworms

A tapeworm is a long, hermaphroditic worm consisting of a series of proglottids and a small head provided with suckers or hooklets or both. Each mature proglottid may produce a large number of eggs. With the exception of the dog tapeworm

(Echinococcus) and sometimes the pork tapeworm *(Taenia solium)*, man harbors the mature worm, and larval forms occur in an intermediate host.

Hymenolepis nana (dwarf tapeworm). *Hymenolepis nana* is the smallest human tapeworm and the commonest in the United States. The adults are 10 to 40 mm. long and may be numerous in the upper ileum. Infection is chiefly in children and is usually acquired by ingestion of eggs from human or rodent sources.

Taenia saginata (beef tapeworm). Living cysticerci (larval forms) of *Taenia saginata* are ingested with insufficiently cooked beef. It is the second most common tapeworm in the United States. Maturation of the larva takes place in the intestine after it has attached itself to the mucosa. The adult worm has a small pyriform head with four lateral suckers and a body with 1,000 to 2,000 proglottids, extending for many feet. Symptoms may be slight and are caused by irritations from their large size.

Taenia solium (pork tapeworm). In *Taenia solium* infection the intermediate host is the hog. The worm is 8 to 12 feet long, has a small globular head with four sucking discs and a number of hooklets, and has about 1,000 proglottids. While uncommon in the United States, the pork tapeworm is particularly important because the larvae as well as the adult can develop in man. Hence, when infection is present, precautions to prevent ingestion of eggs are essential. Intestinal infection in man occurs by ingestion of living cysticerci (larvae) in poorly cooked pork that attach themselves to the mucosa and become adult worms. If eggs are ingested by man, embryos (oncospheres) liberated by action of gastric juice migrate into the body tissues and become encysted larvae, or cysticerci *(cysticercosis)*. The brain, eye, muscles, heart, liver, and lungs have been involved by the cysticerci, with disturbances resulting from the space that they occupy and the surrounding inflammatory reaction.

Diphyllobothrium latum (fish tapeworm). *Diphyllobothrium latum*, also known as *Dibothriocephalus latus*, undergoes two stages intermediate between man, a procercoid larval stage in a cyclops and a plerocercoid larval stage in fresh-water fish. Infection in man occurs by ingestion of raw fish containing the plerocercoid larvae, which mature in the intestine. The adult worm is long and has a almond-shaped head with two lateral sucking grooves but no hooklets.

Echinococcosis (hydatid disease). In the case of *Echinococcus granulosus*, the adult worm is found in the dog and doglike animals and other mammals. Dogs acquire the infection from eating carcasses of sheep, cattle, and hogs in endemic areas. The adult worm is small, measuring 3 to 5 mm. in length. The head is distinctive with four sucking discs and a circle of hooklets. Three proglottids constitute the body. Man may be infected by swallowing the ova in dust, food, or water contaminated by the feces of an infected animal, usually a dog, or by hand-to-mouth transmission after close contact with (e.g., petting) an infected dog. Oncospheres (embryos) are liberated in the intestine, penetrate the wall into blood vessels, and pass to the liver and other organs. Lodged in an organ, they form cystic structures known as unilocular hydatid cysts, which vary up to 20 cm. or even more in diameter. The cysts have a white outer layer and a granular inner germinal layer. From this inner layer new cysts develop, and scolices, or heads, of new worms are formed. These can be recognized by seeing the row of hooklets. Eventually the larvae die out, and the cyst becomes converted into a puttylike mass with calcification of the capsule. This capsule, seen in liver but not bone cysts, is the result of fibrosis accompanying the host's inflammatory response to the cyst. Material from hydatid cysts, used as antigen, results in a skin reaction (Casoni test). This intradermal reaction and also a complement-fixation test may be helpful in clinical diagnosis. In addition to this form of hydatid disease caused by *E. granulosus,* there is a more serious type,

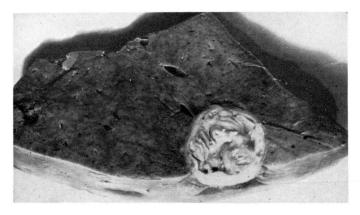

Fig. 9-16. Echinococcus cyst of the liver. Note the convoluted membranous content.

characterized by invasive, alveolar or multilocular cysts (echinococcosis alveolaris), which is produced by *E. multilocularis.* The alveolar cyst, appearing most frequently in the liver, consists of a spongy mass of minute, irregular cavities. It is not encapsulated, tends to grow peripherally into the adjacent tissue, often undergoes necrosis, and evokes a granulomatous inflammatory response in the tissue. The adult tapeworm of *E. multilocularis,* which is similar to that of *E. granulosus,* is found in the fox, dog, and cat; and the chief sylvatic intermediate hosts are the microtine rodents. Hydatid disease caused by *E. granulosus* is not commonly acquired by man in the United States, only a few indigenous cases being reported. It is more frequent in occurrence in northwestern Canada and Alaska. A high incidence is present in Australia, New Zealand, Uruguay, Argentina, northern and southern Africa, and in parts of Europe. Alveolar cysts of *E. multilocularis* are prevalent in Central Europe, Russia, Siberia, and Alaska.

Chapter 10

Chemical poisons, radiation injuries, and nutritional disturbances

CHEMICAL POISONS

Poisons are chemical agents which injure tissues by their reaction with them. With many poisons the effects depend on the quantitative factor of dosage, and many substances which are innocuous or even necessary to the body in small doses are harmful when concentrated or in large quantities. Although use of poison is an ever-popular method of suicide, more than 50% of poisonings appear to be accidental and less than 1% homicidal. Many chronic poisonings are the result of industrial hazards (e.g., lead poisoning and silicosis) and, as such, form an important group of diseases.

Poisons may be classified as follows:

Corrosives—acids and alkalies, including such common poisons as sulfuric acid, lye, phenol, and formaldehyde; these destroy cells at the point of contact—mouth, esophagus, stomach, etc.

Metals—mercury, arsenic, lead, phosphorus, etc. commonly produce damage of the kidney, liver, and other organs.

Gases—chemical asphyxiants such as carbon monoxide, irritants, and "war gases."

Volatile organic poisons—alcohols, cyanides, chloroform, and carbon tetrachloride; these have variable effects.

Nonvolatile organic poisons—barbiturates, alkaloids, petroleum products, etc.

Industrial poisons—beryllium, fluorides, silica, aniline dyes, chromates, DDT, and other pesticides.

Bacterial toxins and food poisons—tetanus, staphylococcal, and botulinus toxins and mushroom poisoning.

Animal venoms—poisons from snakes, spiders, jellyfish, scorpions, etc.

Antibiotics and other drugs—sulfonamides, penicillin, etc. may cause injury either from individual allergic sensitization or from local effects on the tissues.

When poisoning is suspected at an autopsy, the stomach and its contents, portions of small and large intestine, and part of the liver and kidneys should be preserved in chemically clean, wide-mouthed, glass bottles with glass tops. These should be sealed by wax with some special imprint or seal and submitted to the toxicologist with indication of the poisons suspected from the clinical and pathologic findings.

The two poisons most frequently found in fatal cases are carbon monoxide and barbiturate compounds, which together account for a large proportion. Mercuric chloride and methyl alcohol are also relatively common. Table 10-1 gives an indication

Table 10-1. *Clinical symptomatology of common poisons**

Symptoms	Death in a few minutes	Death in a few hours	Death in 24 hours	Death in several days
None (rapid death)	Carbon monoxide Cyanide Nicotine Strychnine			
Coma		Carbon mon-oxide Morphine	Alcohols Barbiturates	
Gastroin-testinal		Arsenic Phosphorus Fluoride Oxalate	Heavy metals Phosphorus	Heavy metals
Central nervous system			Camphor Methyl salicylate	Alcohols Barbiturates Lead
Respiratory			Nitrogen oxides Phosgene	
Hepatotoxic				Carbon tetra-chloride Chloroform Phosphorus
Renal fail-ure				Mercury Glycols Chromate
Blood (met-hemoglo-binemia)				Chlorates Nitrates Acetanilid

*Adapted from Adelson, L.: Amer. J. Clin. Path. **22:**509, 1952.

of the survival time of the patient and the symptomatology caused by some common poisons.

Corrosive poisons. The chief effect of corrosive strong acids and alkalies is local destruction of tissues. Sulfuric, nitric, and hydrochloric acids produce rapid destructive effects on mucous membranes when ingested. Similar effects may be produced by contact with the skin. Corrosive action is often evident on the mucosa of the lips, mouth, and pharynx as well as esophagus and stomach. The lesions are reddish brown or black from sulfuric acid, grayish white from hydrochloric acid, and yellowish brown from nitric acid. In the stomach and intestine the crests of mucosal folds are most severely affected. With sulfuric acid the stomach may be intensely red or have a black tarry appearance (carbonization). The stomach wall feels hardened, rough, and dry. With nitric acid there is no hardening, but extensive ulceration and sloughing of the mucosa occur. With hydrochloric acid the tissue is reddened or blackened and shriveled. The strong acids acting on blood form acid hematin, with widespread brownish black discoloration.

Ingestion of a corrosive alkali such as lye produces softening, swelling, and often ulceration of the mouth, esophagus, and stomach. The stomach feels soapy. If the poisoning is not fatal, healing occurs with marked fibrosis, severe stricture of the esophagus being a common result.

Phenol (carbolic acid) produces fixation and partial detachment of mucosa. These areas are whitish and of leathery consistency. The characteristic odor of phenol aids in identification.

Mercury. Corrosive sublimate (bichloride of mercury) has effects which depend on dosage and length of survival time. In the acute cases there is corrosion of the stomach and duodenum, the mucosa of which appears white and opaque. In the colon there is an intense hemorrhagic and membranous inflammation. If there is survival for a few days or weeks, severe destruction of renal tubular epithelium occurs, with calcium deposition in the necrotic tubules. In such cases death usually results from anuria. It is apparent that the lesions are produced in the sites where the metal is absorbed (upper gastrointestinal tract) and excreted (colon and kidneys).

Arsenic. Inorganic arsenic, such as in arsenical insecticides, may produce acute poisoning with effects on the stomach, nervous system, and vascular endothelium elsewhere. Chronic arsenic poisoning may be characterized by skin pigmentation and hyperkeratosis of plantar surfaces of hands and feet, peripheral nerve degeneration, and hepatic damage.

Lead. Acute lead poisoning is rare, but chronic lead poisoning (plumbism) appears commonly as an industrial disease where lead or compounds of lead are used. Poisoning also may occur from drinking water carried in lead pipes and from bat-

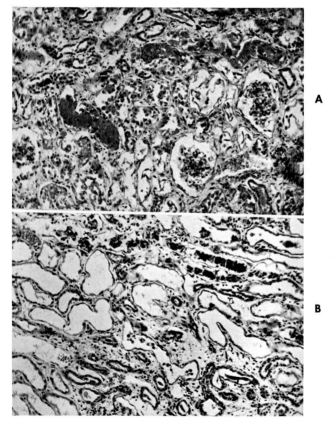

Fig. 10-1. Kidney, mercury bichloride poisoning. **A,** Kidney seven days after the ingestion of poison. Note the destruction and desquamation of tubular epithelium. **B,** Kidney on the eleventh day. Note the loss of tubular epithelium, flattened tubular lining, and dark calcium masses deposited on necrotic debris in the tubular lumina.

tery casings burned as fuel. Characteristics of lead poisoning are intestinal colic, weakness of extensor muscles, secondary anemia with reticulocytes, polychromasia and basophilic stippling prominent in the blood smears, a blue line on the gums, and mental disturbances. Lead becomes deposited chiefly in bones as a lead phosphate, apparently by a mechanism similar to that causing calcium deposition. Parathyroid hormone will mobilize the lead from the bones. Lead can also be demonstrated in the brain, liver, and kidneys.

The most constant lesions due to lead are the blue line of the gums and the anemia with stippling of red cells. Other findings frequently present are degeneration of anterior horn cells, a chronic muscular atrophy and fibrosis, degeneration of male gonads, and blue patches on the mucosa of the intestine. Acid-fast intranuclear inclusion bodies may be found in the liver cells and tubular epithelium of the kidneys.

Phosphorus. Acute phosphorus poisoning causes death by failure of the circulation. Fatty degeneration and necrosis develop in the liver, and milder fatty changes develop in the heart and kidney. Chronic phosphorus poisoning produces necrosis of the jaws, particularly around infected teeth.

Cadmium. Inhalation of cadmium fumes is an occasional industrial hazard. It may produce an acute pneumonitis, which is sometimes fatal. Repeated short exposures may result in severe emphysema.

Carbon monoxide. Carbon monoxide poisoning is due to inhalation of illuminating gas, exhaust of automobiles, or gas from a defective stove or heater. The carbon monoxide has a much greater affinity for hemoglobin than has oxygen, so that death is due to asphyxia. The blood and congested tissues have an unusually bright red color. Fatal cases may show symmetric areas of softening or small hemorrhages of the brain, often involving lenticular nuclei or globus pallidus. These lesions are the delayed result of anoxemia. In some instances the anoxemia may produce changes elsewhere in the brain, including focal degeneration, demyelinization or necrosis, edema, dilated blood vessels, and perivascular hemorrhages.

Nitrogen dioxide. *Silo-filler's disease* is a fibrosing and obliterating bronchiolitis due to inhalation of irritating fumes from freshly filled silos. The toxic agent appears to be nitrogen dioxide, some of which is partially polymerized to nitrogen tetroxide.

Alcohol. *Methyl alcohol* (wood alcohol or methanol) causes

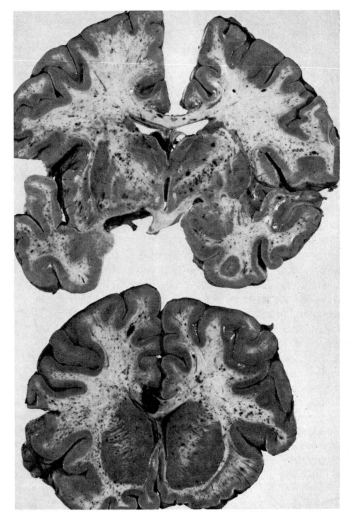

Fig. 10-2. Carbon monoxide poisoning with petechial hemorrhages in cerebral tissue.

poisoning by oxidation to formic acid, injuring particularly the highly specialized tissues of the retina, brain, liver, and kidneys. If there is recovery from acute poisoning, blindness may follow due to atrophy of optic nerves. Repeated ingestion of small quantities of methyl alcohol in denatured alcohol apparently causes no permanent injury.

Alcoholism due to *ethyl alcohol* may be of either acute or chronic form. In *acute alcoholism* death is frequently due to some complication of the intoxication, such as trauma or suffocation, rather than the result of alcoholism itself. The stomach has a hyperemic mucosa with small petechial hemorrhages or erosions. The brain is wet and edematous, and the cerebrospinal fluid appears to be in excess. *Chronic alcoholism* is associated with several pathologic changes, although few are specific effects of the alcohol per se. The gastric mucosa is involved by a mild chronic catarrhal inflammation. One of the most constant findings is enlargement or marked fatty metamorphosis of the liver. Portal cirrhosis of the liver is present in 5 to 8% of alcoholic addicts, and 50 to 60% of patients with cirrhosis have a history of alcoholism. It seems certain that chronic alcoholism is a factor in many cases of cirrhosis, although the relationship is not a direct one (p. 500). Many alcoholics suffer nutritional deficiencies, a possible factor in hepatic changes and in another common complication, peripheral neuritis. Resistance to infection appears to be lowered. Retrograde changes in the myocardium have been attributed to the direct effect of alcohol (alcoholic cardiomyopathy).

Cyanides. *Hydrocyanic acid* and *cyanides* cause very rapid death without leaving diagnostic morphologic changes. The characteristic odor of peach kernel or bitter almonds assists in detecting the poison. Cyanides are respiratory enzyme poisons.

Chloroform. Chloroform in excess may produce degeneration and necrosis in the liver. Carbon tetrachloride similarly damages the liver and also produces a severe acute tubular degeneration of the kidney which may cause death from renal failure.

Petroleum products. Petroleum products such as kerosene, gasoline, and lighter fluid produce central nervous system depression and pulmonary lesions. The latter are often more serious with the development of a bronchopneumonia in which a mononuclear leukocytic infiltration and hyaline membranes are prominent features.

Beryllium. Exposure to beryllium dusts or fumes may occur in the manufacture of fluorescent light materials and beryllium alloys of copper, and it has resulted in distinctive pulmonary disease (berylliosis). In the acute form there is extensive pulmonary consolidation with exudate of fluid and mononuclear cells in alveolar spaces and of lymphocytes and plasma cells in alveolar walls. The chronic form is an extensive irregular and nodular pulmonary fibrosis, with granulomas having a center of fibrinoid or granular debris surrounded by zones of mononuclear cells, with fibrosis and some lymphocytes and plasma cells. Multinucleate giant cells similar to those of tuberculosis and also basophilic "conchoidal" bodies may be present in the granulomas. The extensive pulmonary fibrosis may lead to marked dyspnea and right-sided heart failure. Berylliosis has been noted to cause more bronchiolar and vascular damage than seen

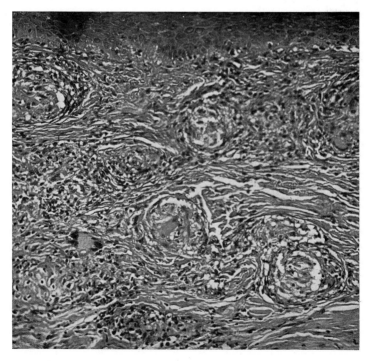

Fig. 10-3. Beryllium granuloma of the skin.

in sarcoidosis, from which differentiation is difficult. Demonstration of beryllium in involved tissue may be necessary for definite diagnosis.

Similar granulomatous lesions may occur in the skin following local injury by breaking of fluorescent lamp tubes. These nodular lesions are extremely chronic and persistent, and permanent healing may result only when the tissues containing the foreign material are excised.

Fluorine. Chronic fluoride intoxication occurs among certain cryolite workers and, in mild degree, in areas where drinking water contains more than one part per million of fluorides. Such content in water is found in many parts of the United States, but especially in southern and western areas. The earliest and main effect of this is a hypoplasia of the enamel of the teeth called *mottled enamel*. The permanent teeth are affected during their process of calcification, i.e., during the first 8 or 9 years of life. The fluorine has a direct local action on enamel-forming cells. The teeth show grayish white blotchy or chalky areas on their surfaces, with some irregular pitting. It has been estimated that a daily intake of 0.1 to 0.15 mg. fluorine per kilogram of body weight is sufficient to produce mottled enamel. There is evidence that in geographic areas where mottled enamel is common the incidence of dental caries is decreased. Fluorine appears to have a definite action in protection of teeth from caries, although the mechanism of this is not established. Fluorides in larger dosage cause a diffuse *osteosclerosis* of bones. Such changes have been described in cryolite workers.

Food poisoning. Whereas poisons such as arsenic are sometimes added to food by accident or design, food poisoning usually refers to the effects of pathogenic bacteria growing in the food or to poisons in plant tissues, such as in certain mushrooms. A number of infections by bacteria and worms may be spread by food, but food poisonings with acute gastrointestinal symptoms are mainly due to infection of the food with organisms of the paratyphoid B *(Salmonella)* group. Local superficial inflammatory lesions develop in the intestine. *Botulism* is the toxemia resulting from the ingestion of the exotoxin of *Clostridium botulinum* with food, and its principal effects are on the nervous system. Proper cooking of food will destroy the toxin. Ingestion of preformed enterotoxin, produced by staphylococci growing in certain foods, is another cause of food poisoning.

Mushroom poisoning is due most commonly to *Amanita*

phalloides, ingestion of which causes acute gastrointestinal symptoms and a high mortality (45 to 70%). Fatty degeneration in the liver, heart, kidneys, and voluntary muscles is the most prominent autopsy finding. Some gastroenteritis and also degenerative changes in the brain may be present.

Poisonous fish may be harmful in several ways: through their bite or sting, through bacterial contamination or allergens, or through specific toxic effects of their flesh, liver, or roe (ichthyosarcotoxism). Certain species, e.g., barracuda, appear to be toxic in certain seasons or geographic areas. The fish family Tetraodontidae (blowfish, toadfish, puffer, etc.) appears to be inherently poisonous, and death may occur in less than an hour or up to twenty hours after ingestion (mortality 60%). The nature of the poison, tetraodontoxin, is unknown.

Arachnidism. The venom of the female *Latrodectus mactans* (black widow spider) is a potent poison which appears to be a toxalbumin. Apparently it acts on nerves or nerve endings, producing painful muscular contractions. Fatal cases have shown an acute hemorrhagic nephritis, and in experimental animals areas of necrosis in the liver, kidneys, spleen, and adrenals have been seen.

Sulfonamide compounds. Administration of sulfonamide drugs is complicated in some cases by deleterious effects on many organs, but most serious are the injuries to the kidney and blood-forming tissues. All the sulfonamides have caused damage, but serious effects seem most frequently to follow the use of sulfathiazole. The sulfonamides act as mild irritants and foreign bodies when precipitated in tissues or placed in serous cavities. Many of the more serious reactions to the sulfonamides give evidence of being of allergic nature, particularly the skin rashes and the effects on blood vessels, myocardium, and hematopoietic tissues.

In the urinary tract there occurs the additional complication of obstruction due to precipitation of acetylated derivatives of the sulfonamides in the renal tubules, ureters, and bladder.

Penicillin. Penicillin may result in hypersensitivity reactions when administered. Although the incidence is small in relation to the number of doses administered, it has been said to head the list of drugs causing reactions in frequency, diversity, and severity. When it results in death, it is usually because of an immediate anaphylactic reaction, rather than a delayed urticaria or serum sickness.

Penicillin itself does not act as an antigen, but its degradation products can serve as a haptene to combine with protein to form an antigenic haptene-protein complex.

INJURY BY IONIZING RADIATION

All living cells are damaged by ionizing radiation and may be destroyed by sufficient dosage, but the degree of susceptibility varies. Radiation has its main therapeutic usefulness in the treatment of malignant tumors (p. 262). Radiosensitivity and radioresistance of various cells and tissues are only relative. Immature or poorly differentiated cells and those undergoing mitosis are radiosensitive. The most radiosensitive cells are those of lymphoid tissue, blood-forming organs, intestinal epithelium, and germ cells. Less sensitive are the cells of dermal epithelium, vascular endothelium, salivary glands, growing bone and cartilage, the eye, and collagen and elastic tissue. Least radiosensitive (i.e., radioresistant) are cells of the kidneys, liver, thyroid, pancreas, adrenals, mature bone and cartilage, muscle, and nervous tissue. The effect on cells does not appear to be recognizable as of a specific type, but is a degeneration that, if sufficiently severe, leads to death of the cell.

Effects of radiation on surviving cells include mutations or permanent alterations in their physiologic capabilities. An important delayed or late effect is a tendency of cells injured by radiation to undergo malignant change. Cancers of skin and of bone have been the most frequent neoplasms produced by localized radiation, and leukemia has been the most frequent malignancy following whole body radiation.

The *effects of whole body radiation* depend on dosage, and on whether it is a single large exposure or repeated doses. A single large dose of total body radiation (e.g., atomic bomb exposure) causes depletion of cells, particularly in tissues where the cell population is normally renewed by continued cell division and maturation. Intestinal epithelium, bone marrow, and the testes are particularly affected. Early loss of intestinal epithelium leads to diarrhea, with dehydration and loss of body sodium. A lesser dose with survival for several days shows effects on hematopoietic tissues, with depletion of leukocytes, platelets, red blood cells, and lymphocytes. Purpuric and hemorrhagic manifestations develop, with decreased resistance to infections. An increased incidence of leukemia has been noted in atomic bomb victims who survived the immediate effects. The effects of low-dosage whole body radiation that is repeated or spread out over a long time are under intensive investigation. The important effects may be in carcinogenesis and genetic changes.

NUTRITIONAL DISTURBANCES

Adequate dietary intake is necessary for maintenance of health. Not only is an adequate caloric content necessary, but certain proteins, minerals, and vitamins also are essential. Slight deficiency may be difficult to recognize pathologically, as well as clinically. The problem is further complicated by the rarity in man of pure deficiencies such as may be produced in carefully controlled experimental animals. Inadequate diets for human beings often lack several essentials so that the resulting lesions are a mixture. The role of dietary inadequacies in the pathogenesis of atherosclerosis, cirrhosis of the liver, and other diseases is discussed elsewhere.

Vitamins are organic compounds essential in the diet for normal growth and maintenance of life. They are active in the regulation of metabolism and tranformation of energy but do not themselves furnish energy or building material, and they are effective in small amounts. Several vitamins, particularly thiamine, riboflavin, and nicotinic acid, are closely concerned with intracellular respiration, providing chemical groupings essential for intracellular oxidations and reductions.

Vitamin A

Vitamin A is a fat-soluble, unsaturated alcohol and has as its precursor certain vegetable pigments known as carotenes. Deficiency results in night blindness, dermatosis, and xerophthalmia.

One of the diagnostic features of vitamin A deficiency is subnormal dark adaptation. Vitamin A is an essential constituent of retinal pigments used to register visual stimuli. When it is deficient, the regeneration of visual purple is delayed and dark adaptation is poor.

The primary effect of vitamin A deficiency is on epithelium, which undergoes atrophy and replacement by a keratinizing type of epithelium. In man the specific lesions are found in the eyes, conjunctiva, lining epithelium of various organs and ducts, and skin with its appendages. The commonest and earliest appearance of metaplastic squamous epithelium is in trachea and bronchi, and next in the pelvis of the kidney. The eye changes

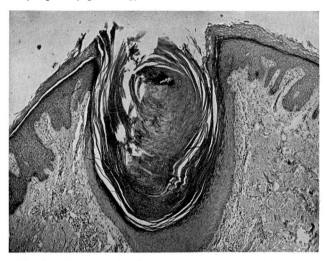

Fig. 10-4. Hyperkeratosis of hair follicle in vitamin A deficiency. (Courtesy Dr. Chester N. Frazier; from Sutton, R. L., and Sutton, R. L., Jr.: Diseases of the skin, ed. 10, St. Louis, The C. V. Mosby Co.)

are also a metaplasia of the corneal and conjunctival epithelium, followed by corneal infection. The skin is rough, scaly, and dry because of hyperkeratosis of skin and hair follicle epithelium, and metaplasia of sweat gland epithelium.

Vitamin A can be demonstrated in microscopic sections by fluorescence microscopy. Ultraviolet light is used, the vitamin A exhibiting a fading greenish fluorescence in the dark field. By this method vitamin A has been found distributed in the lipids of the epithelial and Kupffer cells of the liver; epithelial cells of the adrenal cortex; tubular and Leydig cells of the testicle; granulosa, theca, and stroma cells of the ovary; fat cells; gland cells of the lactating breast; and in kidneys with abnormal glomerular permeability.

Hypervitaminosis A. Hypervitaminosis A has been reported in a few cases, mainly in infants. The vitamin A concentration in the blood is increased. Bones are affected by roentgenologically evident cortical thickening, and the infants have pain and swelling over the long bones. Excessive vitamin A may inhibit bone growth in children and cause premature closure of epiphyses.

Vitamin B complex

Vitamin B has been found to contain a number of specific factors. The chemical nature of most of them being known, they are more properly designated by their correct chemical names rather than referred to as B_1, B_2, etc. The factors in the B complex include thiamine hydrochloride, riboflavin, nicotinic acid, pantothenic acid, pyridoxine hydrochloride, etc. The B complex is found in yeast, whole grain cereals, wheat germ, rice polishings, etc.

Thiamine hydrochloride (B_1). Thiamine is a water-soluble vitamin, the deficiency of which results in beriberi. The main clinical features are loss of appetite, peripheral neuritis with muscle tenderness and changes in reflexes, tachycardia, cardiac failure, and edema. Thiamine is important in the intracellular metabolism of glucose, the pyrophosphate of thiamine acting as a coenzyme (with carboxylase) in the breaking down of pyruvic acid. Thiamine deficiency is believed to be a factor causing *Wernicke's disease.*

Beriberi. Beriberi occurs in acute and chronic forms. The findings in chronic forms when seen at autopsy are usually complicated by an infection. The more acute and uncomplicated forms are characterized by dilatation and moderate hypertrophy of the heart, generalized edema, hydrothorax, hydropericardium, and congestion of viscera. Microscopically the heart shows edema, with hydropic degeneration of muscle fibers. Microscopic nerve lesions are most frequent in nerves supplying the lower extremities; cranial and vagus nerves are also frequently affected. There is vacuolar degeneration of Schwann cells, followed by fragmentation of axis cylinders and myelin sheath degeneration.

Riboflavin (B_2 or G). Deficiency of riboflavin (ariboflavinosis) is said to produce in man a lesion called *cheilosis,* characterized by superficial cracks or fissures at the angles of the mouth. A nasolabial seborrheic skin lesion, glossitis, and circumcorneal congestion also may be present. Riboflavin appears to be important in tissue respiration, for combined with phosphoric acid it unites with specific proteins to form enzymes which act as dehydrogenases.

Pantothenic acid and pyridoxine hydrochloride. The role of these factors of the B complex in human pathology is still uncertain. Pyridoxine-deficient monkeys have been shown to develop atherosclerosis, and the possibility has been suggested that pyridoxine deficiency may be a factor in the pathogenesis of some instances of atherosclerosis in man.

Nicotinic acid (P-P). Considerable evidence indicates that deficiency of nicotinic acid is an important factor in pellagra, although probably in most cases multiple deficiencies are present. Nicotinic acid is an essential component of the pyridine-protein intracellular enzyme systems, important in carbohydrate metabolism.

Pellagra. Pellagra is characterized by brown, scaly, patchy skin eruptions and by soreness of the mouth, redness of the tongue, indigestion, diarrhea, and nervous disturbances. The skin lesions tend to appear particularly in areas exposed to sunlight.

Pathologic changes are found in the skin, gastrointestinal tract, and nervous system. The skin lesions begin with edema of papillae, dilatation of papillary blood vessels, and degeneration of connective tissue of the superficial part of the corium. This is followed by epidermal hyperplasia and hyperkeratosis with an increase in pigment. The lesions are similar to sunburn or x-ray dermatitis. In late stages the epidermis is thin and atrophic, and the corium is fibrosed. The oral mucosa may be affected in a similar fashion.

The intestinal lesions are more characteristic. The colon is thick walled, reddish, and may have a patchy pseudomembranous change in the mucosa. The mucosa may be infiltrated by chronic inflammatory cells, but most pathognomonic is a cystic dilatation of the crypts of Lieberkühn.

The nervous lesions appear late and are more prominent in the central nervous system than in peripheral nerves. Patchy degeneration may be present in the cerebrum, and in the spinal cord irregular patches of myelin degeneration most commonly involve posterior columns.

Ascorbic acid (vitamin C)

Ascorbic acid is a water-soluble vitamin, a deficiency of which leads to scurvy. This vitamin is essential for the production and maintenance of intercellular substances of mesenchymal origin, i.e., collagen of fibrous tissue, the matrices of bone, dentine, and cartilage, and the intercellular cement substance of vascular endothelium. Mesenchymal tissues (fibroblasts, osteoblasts, etc.) grow in the absence of vitamin C, but they cannot produce intercellular substance. Hemorrhages and changes in bone are the prominent features of scurvy. In vitamin C–deficient animals fractured bones cannot be restored to functional integrity. The broken ends are united by fibroblasts, but neither collagen nor osseomucin is produced. There is little evidence that excess of vitamin C promotes healing of wounds or fractures, but deficiency of vitamin C appears to have serious effects and prevents formation of scars of normal strength. Deficiency of vitamin C interfers with the production of acid mucopolysaccharides, which occurs in the early stages of normal wound healing.

Excretion of excess ascorbic acid in the urine may be quantitatively determined by the dichlorphenol indophenol indicator. The ascorbic acid content of the white cell–platelet layer of centrifuged blood is the most significant indicator of the vitamin C status of the body. Scurvy does not occur until this is entirely depleted.

Scurvy. Human scurvy is more common in children (Barlow's disease) than in adults. The essential features are hemorrhages, changes in bones and teeth, and anemia.

The hemorrhages may be in any organ or tissue and vary from small petechiae to massive hematomas. Any injury or trauma to a tissue predisposes to hemorrhage, which is due to changes in the intercellular substance between capillary endothelial cells. Petechial hemorrhages in the skin are most prominent clinically. In infants very painful subperiosteal hemorrhage is common.

The skeletal lesions are most prominent at the costochondral junctions, the ends of the femurs and tibias, and at the wrists. Grossly there is a curved, yellowish, widened zone at the junction of the diaphysis and cartilage. Microscopically this zone shows evidence of disordered growth and interruption of the process of ossification. Fragile connective tissue fibers are formed, a watery zone appears about the osteoblasts, and osteoid tissue is defective. Elsewhere in the bones also new bone formation is lacking, whereas bone resorption goes on at a normal rate. The result is rarefaction of bone, similar to that which occurs in senility.

Lesions in the teeth may occur before skeletal lesions are prominent. The gums become swollen and bleed easily. The teeth tend to loosen and may even fall out as a result of rarefaction of alveolar bone. Degenerative and atrophic changes develop also in the substance of the teeth themselves.

Vitamin D

Vitamin D (calciferol, D_2, and 7-dehydrocholesterol, D_3) is a fat-soluble vitamin which not only is available in food but also may be formed from ergosterol in the skin by ultraviolet irradiation. It is important in calcium and phosphorus metabolism, the part which it plays being to increase calcium absorption from the intestine or to increase phosphorus retention and

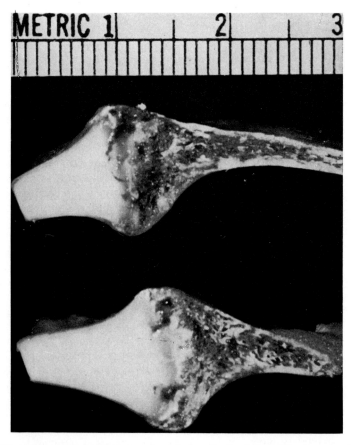

Fig. 10-5. Costochondral junction of the ribs in rickets. The junctional zone is wide and irregular in contrast to the normal appearance of a narrow sharp line of ossification.

in turn calcium retention. Thus, for action of this vitamin, adequate mineral intake is essential.

Rickets. Deficiency of vitamin D leads to rickets in growing children. In adults the corresponding condition is osteomalacia. Rickets is most common in infancy, but an adolescent form also occurs. Adequate mineral intake and solar radiation, as well as dietary vitamin D, are important in the prevention of rickets.

Rickets is fundamentally a deficient calcification of osteoid tissue and an abnormal cartilage involution in growing bones. Endochondral bone growth is disturbed. The excess of uncalcified osteoid tissue results in unusual softness of the bones, which become bent and deformed near the joints. Such deformities are common about the knees (bowlegs), costochondral junctions (rachitic rosary), and thorax (pigeon breast). The most significant gross changes are seen on the cut surface of an epiphysial region. The tissue is softened, and the normally sharp narrow line of ossification is replaced by a wide irregular zone of soft gray tissue. Histologically the area shows great disorder of growth with excess osteoid tissue and failure of its calcification. In all parts of the bones there is an excess formation of bone matrix, which remains uncalcified or eventually is poorly calcified. The bone marrow becomes fibrous.

Teeth suffer from the same lack of calcification as occurs in bones. The lesions are in the permanent dentition. Dimpling of the enamel, furrows, and other types of defects may result.

Hypervitaminosis D. Vitamin D overdosage is known to result in deleterious effects. A very large intake is necessary in man before damage is caused. In experimental animals the main effects are skeletal osteoporosis, due to osteoclastic resorption, and calcium deposition in soft tissues, particularly in arteries and in the kidney.

Vitamin E (alpha-tocopherol)

Little is known about the pathology of vitamin E deficiency in man. In experimental animals vitamin E deficiency leads to degenerative and atrophic changes in the testes and also to severe degenerative changes in skeletal muscles, accompanied by marked cellular infiltrations.

Vitamin K

Vitamin K is necessary for the formation of prothrombin, an essential in the clotting mechanism. Absorption of vitamin K from the intestine is favored by the presence of bile salts. Lack of vitamin K causes a hemorrhagic tendency, as noted in obstructive jaundice and in the hemorrhages of newborn infants.

Kwashiorkor

A nutritional deficiency of infancy and childhood prevalent in West Africa and elsewhere has been called kwashiorkor and other names. It appears to be a protein deficiency, although it is inexactly known whether it results from deficiency of protein as a whole or of certain specific amino acids. Deficiency of certain minerals, such as magnesium, may also be important. The affected children develop rashes and ulcerations of the skin, edema, an enlarged fatty liver, and sometimes hepatic necrosis. Acinar atrophy and apparent relative fibrosis of the pancreas are prominent findings. Infections are important as a precipitating factor and as a cause of death.

Chapter 11

Disturbances of growth

The process of growth of cells, tissues, organs, and of the body as a whole presents unsolved problems of great complexity. The disturbances in growth of the body as a whole (i.e., dwarfism, giantism, etc.) are hormonal, metabolic, or congenital developmental disturbances and are considered elsewhere (p. 827). The repair of tissue after injury and replacement of tissue lost through normal wear and tear are processes which proceed continuously. The cells and tissues which are least highly organized and differentiated in function and structure (e.g., connective tissues) are most easily replaced. Highly organized structures, such as renal glomeruli or ganglion cells of the central nervous system, are irreplaceable. Between these extremes are all gradations in capacity for regeneration, repair, and response by growth to normal or abnormal stimuli.

Hypertrophy is an increase in the size of an organ or a cell. *Hyperplasia* is an increase in the number of cells. Enlargement of an organ may be by increase in the size or in the number of its component cells or structures. Enlargement of the heart is practically always brought about by an increase in the size of the muscle fibers, which do not become more numerous. Enlargement of a kidney may be accomplished by an increase in the size of the component nephrons (glomeruli and their tubules), but their number cannot be increased. On the other hand, organs such as the liver, endocrine glands, and lymphoid tissues have little power to increase the size of their cells, but they enlarge by the process of hyperplasia.

Hypertrophy of cells and organs occurs in a variety of physiologic and pathologic conditions. Examples of physiologic hypertrophy are the enlargement of voluntary muscles by exercise or of the uterus during pregnancy. Compensatory hypertrophy is the enlargement of the residue of an organ or tissue when a portion is removed or destroyed; e.g., if one kidney is removed, the remaining kidney, if normal, enlarges because of an increase in the size of the individual nephrons (renal counterbalance).

The necessity for increased function appears to be the basis of enlargement of an organ, and the term *work hypertrophy* is frequently justifiable. The heart undergoes hypertrophy when greater work is thrown on it by increased peripheral resistance (hypertension) or by abnormality of valvular function. The final details of the mechanism by which hypertrophy is accomplished are not known, but a sufficient blood supply appears to be a necessity. Increased hormonal activity also may be a cause of hypertrophy. Excess of growth hormone of the pituitary brings about hypertrophy of various organs, e.g., the abdominal organs and heart. In the case of the hypertrophy and hyperplasia of the breasts during menstrual cycles and in pregnancy, endocrine stimulation by hormones from the ovary appears to be the controlling mechanism.

Metaplasia is a change from one type of cell to another. It may be the result of chronic inflammation or irritation, impairment of nutrition and function, or demand for altered function. A common example is a change from columnar or secretory epithelium to a flattened or squamous type. This change may be observed in bronchial mucosa, the gallbladder, or the endocervix, as a result of chronic inflammation. Vitamin A deficiency produces a similar metaplasia (p. 247). Metaplasia is common also in cells of the connective tissue type, with the appearance of cartilage or bone in unusual situations such as scars, arteriosclerotic blood vessels, injured and sightless eyes, or degenerated areas of a goiter.

Anaplasia is a reversion or transformation of cells into a more primitive, embryonic, or undifferentiated type. Such cells have a greater faculty for growth and multiplication but less capacity for specialized function. Anaplasia is an important feature of tumor growth, and in general its degree parallels that of the malignancy of the neoplasm.

TUMORS

Willis has defined a tumor or neoplasm as "an abnormal mass of tissue, the growth of which exceeds and is uncoordinated with that of the normal tissues, and persists in the same excessive manner after cessation of the stimuli which evoked the change."* Berenblum has given the following statement which epitomizes

---

*From Willis, R. A.: Pathology of tumours, St. Louis, 1953, The C. V. Mosby Co.

our present knowledge of the nature of a tumor: "A tumor is an actively-growing tissue, composed of cells derived from one that has undergone an abnormal type of irreversible differentiation; its growth is progressive, due to a persistent delay in maturation of its stem cells."* Although the essential nature of the differentiation is still unknown, it is to be distinguished from regenerative, reparative, and inflammatory processes. Considerable evidence has accumulated that the cancerous change in a cell is not necessarily irreversible but that a reversion to normal may occur. Tumors are composed of cells and intercellular substances such as may be found in embryonic or mature tissues. Growth activity predominates over function, although the latter is not necessarily lacking. In certain tumors, such as those from endocrine glands, functional activity may be an important feature. Endocrine activity also occurs in some tumors of nonendocrine origin. Tumors act as parasites, absorbing nourishment from the blood, growing with enhanced vitality at the expense of normal tissues, and yet performing no useful work for the body.

Benign tumors are those which grow slowly and expansively, and unless they are in some vital spot or interfere with an important organ they are well tolerated and do not necessarily interfere with the person's well-being or shorten his life. They are composed of well-differentiated mature types of tissue.

Malignant tumors are more rapidly growing, will infiltrate and extend into normal structures and, unless effectively treated, interfere with health and eventually cause death. They are usually composed of more embryonic or poorly differentiated cells. Another term for a malignant tumor is *cancer*.

Classification of tumors

Neoplasms are classified according to structure and origin, as etiology is too uncertain to form a satisfactory basis. No grouping seems entirely satisfactory, but the simplest and most common classification divides tumors into the following varieties:

Tumors of mesenchymal origin
    Benign
    Malignant—sarcoma

---

*From Berenblum, I. In Florey, H.: General pathology, ed. 3, Philadelphia and London, 1962, W. B. Saunders Co., p. 538.

Tumors of epithelial origin
   Benign
   Malignant—carcinoma
Mixed tumors and teratomas
   Benign
   Malignant

In the first class (tumors of mesenchymal origin) are included not only fibroblastic tumors but also those of cartilage, bone, fat, blood vessels, lymphatic tissue, mesothelium, muscle, and blood-forming tissues. The mixed tumors are those arising from multipotential cells and containing more than one type of tissue. Teratomas arise from totipotential cells, often contain representatives of all three germ layers, and show attempts at organ formation.

The tumors of particular organs are considered with the other lesions of those organs, where details of classification and structure are presented.

Characteristics of benign tumors

Benign tumors do not endanger life unless they are so situated as to interfere with some vital organ or function. They grow slowly and after reaching a certain size may remain stationary. Their growth is expansive; they push aside normal tissues but do not invade, and hence they appear as circumscribed, well-demarcated, and even encapsulated growths. They do not metastasize; i.e., secondary tumors are not formed in other organs. Necrosis and ulceration are less frequent than in malignant tumors. Local removal is usually successful and not followed by recurrence. Histologically they are composed of a well-differentiated, mature type of tissue closely imitating the normal tissue of their origin. Rarity of mitoses reflects their slow growth. No sharp line separates benign and malignant tumors, and differences are often a matter of degree. Borderline cases are quite common and often difficult to classify.

Characteristics of malignant tumors

Malignant tumors are those whose unhindered progression invariably leads to death of the person. They often grow rapidly, infiltrating and invading surrounding tissues, so that they are unencapsulated and poorly demarcated. Metastases develop in distant organs. Local removal of a malignant tumor, unless absolutely complete, is followed by recurrence at the same site.

They are more prone to degeneration and ulceration than are benign tumors. They may produce cachexia and anemia. Histologically they are composed of embryonic, primitive, or poorly differentiated cells. They exhibit *anaplasia,* a structural derangement of the component cells. There tends to be polymorphism and unsuccessful imitation of their tissue of origin. Relative frequency of mitosis reflects their rapid growth, and abnormal forms of mitotic nuclei may be present. Malignant cells have nuclei and nucleoli of larger average size than in corresponding nonmalignant cells.

Estimation of malignancy and prognosis

The factors which must be considered in estimating the result of a cancer include (1) the type of tumor, (2) its situation, (3) the duration, size, spread, and presence or absence of metastasis, (4) the age and condition of the patient, (5) the rate of clinical growth, (6) the histologic structure, and (7) the radiosensitivity of the tumor.

The *type of tumor* is important, since cancers vary in their degree of malignancy and course. Certain tumors, such as the basal cell carcinoma of the skin, grow slowly and rarely metastasize. At the other extreme are tumors of rapid growth and early extension, such as myeloma of bone and lymphosarcoma.

The *situation* of a tumor influences the outcome because it may interfere with vital structures or may be such as to make operative removal impossible, e.g., in the case of gliomatous tumors of the brain or of carcinoma of the esophagus.

The *duration* of the tumor influences prognosis, as it allows time for spread. Thus, a tumor which is easily curable in an early stage may be hopeless later. *Extensive local spread* or *metastasis* in other organs suggests an earlier and more inevitable end. On the other hand, long duration of a tumor with only slight increase in size and no metastasis suggests slow growth, low malignancy, and a relatively favorable outcome.

Age is of some importance, in that certain tumors seem to progress more rapidly in younger persons. *Pregnancy and lactation* cause more rapid growth in cancer of the breast.

Radiosensitivity of a tumor is often important in determining how long life may be prolonged or if cure is possible.

Histologic structure is of importance in indicating the type of tumor, rapidity of growth, and degree of anaplasia or differentiation. Systems of histologic grading have been evolved.

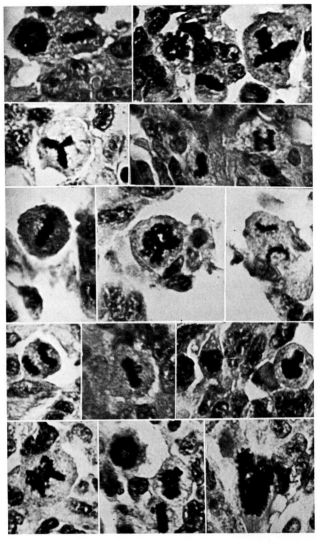

Fig. 11-1. Mitotic nuclei: typical and atypical forms from a rapidly growing carcinoma.

Microscopic grading of cancer. Many factors other than histologic structure influence the degree of malignancy; but among tumors of the same type and arising at the same site, there are variations in malignancy which can be correlated roughly with the degree of anaplasia or undifferentiation. Such microscopic grading of the malignancy of a tumor, if put on a numerical and standardized basis, is helpful in predicting the course of the disease when used in conjunction with the other factors noted above, such as size, degree of extension, etc. It may also be of help in determining the type of treatment likely to give the best results. In general, the greater the anaplasia of a tumor (i.e., the higher the microscopic grade of malignancy), the greater is the radiosensitivity. Numerical systems of histologic grading, if used alone, may have limited prognostic value for individual cases.

Broders originated and popularized a method of grading according to which tumors are divided into four grades of malignancy, as follows:

Grade I—tumors showing a marked tendency to differentiation, with three fourths or more of their cells differentiated

Grade II—three fourths to one half of the cells differentiated

Grade III—one half to one fourth of the cells differentiated

Grade IV—one fourth to none of the cells differentiated*

While this system of grading is generally useful, it is often extended and modified in the case of tumors of certain organs, e.g., cervix uteri or rectum. The various modifications are noted later as these tumors are considered. Statistics regarding the duration of life in untreated cancer (i.e., the natural history of the disease) must be known to evaluate methods of therapy.

Clinical stage classification of cancer. The clinical staging of cancer is the division of cases of cancer into groups according to a plan based on extent of the disease. One such plan, known as the TNM system, uses three components: the size or extent of the primary tumor (T), the involvement of regional lymph nodes (N), and the presence or absence of distant metastasis (M). Increasing involvement of each element may be denoted by combining the letter with a number from 0 to 4, so that a shorthand system of designating extent of a cancer of a particular site may be used. Categorization into stages may then be according to classification agreed upon for each site.

---

*From Broders, A. C.: Surg. Clin. N. Amer. **21:**947, 1941.

Effects of radiation on tumors

The effects of roentgen rays and radium on tissues are similar. Only the gamma rays are used in therapeutic work. The alpha and beta rays, which are more destructive but less penetrating, are excluded by screening. All tissues, normal and neoplastic, are affected by radiation so that radiosensitivity is a relative term. Cells which are actively proliferating or which are of primitive type are more sensitive than normal tissues, so that there is usually a considerable margin between the doses which are damaging to neoplastic and to normal tissue, respectively.

The effects of gamma rays on growing cells vary with the intensity and duration of exposure and consist of (1) destruction of some cells, (2) inhibition of imminent mitosis, followed by abnormal mitosis and disruption of the cells, and (3) damage to resting cells so that continued proliferation fails. Cells in a premitotic phase are believed to be particularly susceptible, although this has been questioned.

Radiation may also have effects which are not directly on the cells. Action on blood vessels supplying tumor tissue may be of importance. An early effect of radiation is extreme hyperemia due to distention of capillaries, and this may be followed by thrombosis or rupture. Larger blood vessels may be completely obliterated. The effect on the tumor bed contributes to the effects of radiation on tumor tissue.

Radiosensitivity of tumors. Since all tumors can be affected by radiation, the terms *radiosensitivity* and *radioresistance* are but relative. Radiosensitivity does not necessarily imply curability by radiation. Some highly radiosensitive tumors, such as lymphosarcoma, are rarely curable by radiation. Other tumors, which are radioresistant, may be curable. Easy accessibility and tolerance of surrounding structures are important factors in curability. Radiation may be valuable in relief of pain, e.g., in skeletal metastasis from carcinoma of the breast, even though not curative.

Radiosensitivity varies with the reproductive activity of the tissue (law of Bergonié and Tribondau) and increases with increasing anaplasia and embryonal quality of tumor cells. The tumor bed is also important; a bed of slight vascularity or of fat, bone, or cartilage is unfavorable. Tumor recurrences tend to be more resistant than was the original tumor. The presence of infection in the tissue appears to decrease sensitivity.

Lymphomatous tumors are examples of radiosensitive tumors

which are affected by relatively low dosage of radiation without appreciable damage to adjacent normal tissue. Radioresponsive tumors, such as basal cell carcinoma of the skin and carcinoma of the uterine cervix, require a larger dose for similar regression. Radioresistant tumors, such as malignant melanoma and osteogenic sarcoma, require high dosage for response, so that damage to normal tissue may equal or exceed that done to the tumor.

Spread and metastasis of tumors

Malignant tumors spread by direct invasive growth into surrounding tissues and by the formation of secondary tumors not connected with the original neoplasm. This latter process, which is called metastasis, is due to extension by lymphatics, by the bloodstream, and by implantation. The distribution of metastatic tumors appears to be determined by the number of tumor emboli which reach and lodge in various organs and tissues, as well as by differences in suitability of different tissues for the growth of tumor cells. Metastatic tumors are most common in lungs, liver, bones, kidneys, and adrenals. Spleen and skeletal muscle are relatively infrequent sites of metastasis.

The characteristic invasiveness of malignant tumors may be associated with a reduced mutual adhesiveness of cancer cells, which may be dependent in part on an abnormally low calcium content. Of uncertain or speculative importance in the mechanism of invasion are such factors as rapidity of growth of the tumor, motility of the tumor cells, phagocytic properties of the tumor cells, and elaboration of lytic products by the tumor cells. The old hypothesis of Ribbert that there is a loss of growth restraint on the part of the surrounding tissues has little to support it.

Lymphatic metastasis. This is the common method of spread of carcinoma. Tumor cells grow into lymphatic channels and are broken off and carried as *emboli* to a lymph node. Here the tumor cells lodge and can often be seen in the subcapsular space or peripheral sinus. Thus a secondary tumor is started, which may eventually overwhelm the node, break through the capsule, and spread locally as well as onward in the lymphatic system.

There also may be lymphatic spread by *permeation,* i.e., by direct and continuous growth along a lymphatic channel. While lymphatic permeation probably occurs, lymphatic embolism appears to be more common.

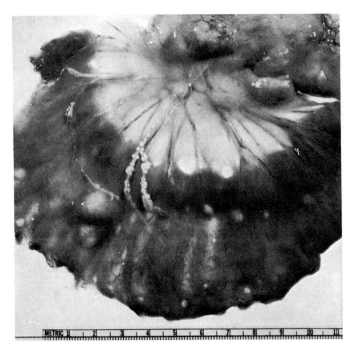

Fig. 11-2. Lymphatic extension of a carcinoma in mesentery with metastasis in the lymph nodes.

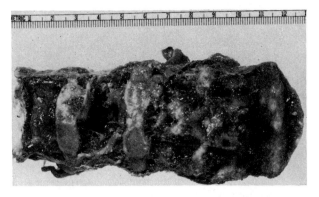

Fig. 11-3. Metastatic carcinoma from the breast in the vertebral column. Grayish masses of tumor are present in the bodies of vertebrae, some of which are collapsed or cystic.

Lymph nodes draining the area of a primary carcinoma occasionally contain granulomas of a tuberculoid or sarcoidlike appearance, apparently stimulated by irritant materials absorbed from the neoplastic area. Intracellular asteroid bodies or other inclusions may be present. The draining lymph nodes may contain paramyloid material or may show marked sinusoidal and follicular histiocytic change.

Metastasis by the bloodstream. This is the common method of spread of sarcoma, but many carcinomas spread in this fashion as well. Tumor cells penetrate the thin wall of a vein, are broken off, and are carried away as emboli. Tumor emboli that enter branches of the portal vein lodge in the liver, and that organ is the common site for metastasis from tumors of the intestinal tract. Tumor emboli from systemic veins tend to lodge in the lung or, carried by the paravertebral venous system, reach the bones of the vertebral column, shoulder girdle, and pelvis. Undoubtedly some tumor cells reach the arterial circulation directly or by passage through pulmonary capillaries. Probably many tumor emboli fail to survive. The tissues in which the emboli lodge must be capable of rapidly supplying adequate blood or nourishment for the tumor tissue.

Metastasis by implantation. This type of metastasis occurs when tumor cells involving a serous or mucous membrane become detached and are later implanted on other areas. Carcinoma of the ovary commonly spreads throughout the peritoneal cavity in this fashion. When cancer involves a serosal surface, considerable fluid is usually present in the cavity and often

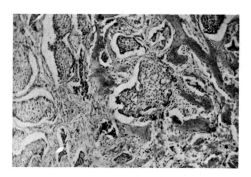

Fig. 11-4. Metastatic carcinoma from the breast in bone marrow.

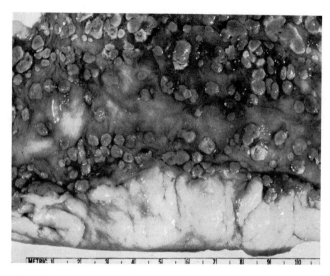

Fig. 11-5. Carcinomatous nodules on the peritoneal surface of the colon.

is of a hemorrhagic character. Tumor cells may be demonstrable in such fluids by centrifuging and making smears and paraffin sections of the cellular material thus thrown down. Implantation of malignant cells may also occur in operative wounds and along the track of a needle puncture.

Metastatic tumors are uncommon in certain tissues, such as voluntary muscle, heart, and spleen. Blood-borne metastasis involves mainly liver, lung, and bone. Metastatic tumors of the brain are most commonly from the lung, breast, stomach, prostate, and adrenal. Those tumors which metastasize to bone with particular frequency are hypernephroma of the kidney and carcinomas of the prostate, lung, ovary, breast, testis, and thyroid.

Cachexia

Wasting of marked degree and severe anemia are common in late stages of malignant disease but are far from an invariable occurrence. Cachexia is often influenced by starvation, in the case of tumor in the alimentary tract, and by infection. There is no evidence of a specific toxin or poison from cancer tissue.

Remote manifestations of cancer. Apart from cachexia, anemia, and formation of metastases, cancers occasionally are associated with various types of remote manifestations. Migratory thrombophlebitis is sometimes associated with carcinoma of the body or the tail of the pancreas or, less frequently, with cancer of other viscera. Hypertrophic pulmonary osteoarthropathy may occur with tumors of the lung. Pigmented verrucous lesions of the skin (acanthosis nigricans) in adults occurs in association with some intra-abdominal cancers. Familial intestinal polyposis may be associated with melanin deposits in the lips, skin of the face, and digits (Peutz-Jeghers syndrome). The malignant carcinoid syndrome (p. 648) and other remote effects of secretory activity of neoplastic cells are common with tumors of endocrine organs. Large fibrogenic tumors may be associated with hypoglycemia. A small proportion (about 17%) of cases of dermatomyositis are in individuals who have a malignant tumor. Other remote manifestations include increased serum acid phosphatase from prostatic carcinoma, the occasional occurrence of Cushing's syndrome, peripheral neuropathy or excess antidiuretic hormone in patients with bronchogenic carcinoma, and the presence of hypercalcemia with various cancers.

Multiple malignant neoplasms

The occurrence of more than one cancer in an individual is not uncommon. Such an event may be in one of the following classes: (1) multiple cancers developing due to proneness to malignant change in a single abnormal tissue, e.g., multiple cancers of the bowel in association with familial multiple polyposis or multiple cancers of the skin in xeroderma pigmentosum; (2) multiple neoplasms arising in paired endocrine organs, e.g., ovary or adrenal; (3) apparent multiple tumors arising under circumstances where there could be spread by seeding, e.g., discrete tumors of the same type involving renal pelvis, ureter, and urinary bladder; and (4) true, independent multiple cancers of different types and in different organs.

Estimations indicate that about 4% of patients with cancer develop multiple malignant tumors. The evidence suggests that the presence of one cancer does not confer immunity but that, on the contrary, there is greater proneness to another cancer.

Causes of death in malignant diseases

The immediate cause of death in cancer is most commonly a pulmonary disorder, such as pneumonia, embolism, abscess, atelectasis, etc. Cachexia appears to be a frequent contributing cause and is particularly common with cancer of the breast, stomach, and colon. Renal failure is common with carcinoma of the cervix, bladder, and prostate. Tumors of the alimentary tract may cause death by obstruction. Intracranial tumors cause death by pressure effects within the rigid casing of the nervous system.

Cytologic diagnosis of malignancy

Papanicolaou demonstrated, in smears made from vaginal secretions, that cells shed from the cervix, endometrium, and vagina showed characteristics which reflected hormonal, inflammatory, and neoplastic conditions of the tissue from which the cells originated. Of particular importance was the finding that early carcinoma of the cervix, at a stage when its visual examination might reveal no abnormality, could be detected by microscopic study of the cells.

The recognition of malignant cells from the cervix is based on nuclear characteristics, which are enlargement, variations in size, shape, and structure, and hyperchromasia. Less frequently macronucleoli and mitoses are important features. These nuclear alterations are found also in cancer cells shed from other tissues. The certainty of identification as malignant cells increases with the number of distinguishing features which are recognized. The presence of two or more characteristics is necessary to safely identify a cell as a cancer cell. Interpretation of the presence of cancer is also more accurate when based on the changes in many cells, although under some circumstances a few seriously altered cells may be of great significance.

In addition to the morphologic characteristics of the nucleus of the malignant cells, the application of cytochemical methods for evaluating increased DNA and RNA characteristic of rapidly growing cells is being tested.

Nuclear enlargement or increase of the nucleocytoplasmic ratio is an important characteristic of malignant cells, although it also may be found in cells with certain degenerative changes and in cells of benign proliferative reactions. Change in nuclear size can best be appreciated when it can be compared to a normal, nonmalignant cell of the same origin. *Variation in nuclear size also* is observed in the cells of some malignant tumors, and is more significant when of marked degree. *Variations in nuclear shape* may be related to cellular shape or may be unrelated.

Observed in many malignant cells, and more commonly associated with rapidly growing cancers, it may be seen as bizarre or lobulated nuclear forms, or other abnormal configurations.

Alterations in nuclear structure as compared with the chromatin pattern of the normal interphase nucleus characterize many malignant cells. The chromatin may be aggregated in coarse masses, or may vary from one site to another in the nucleus. Many and varied aberrations of chromatin pattern are encountered on examining many different cancer cells. *Hyperchromasia,* an increase in intensity of nuclear staining, may be due to an increase in the amount of chromatin material or to a change in its character. Although an important feature of malignant cells, it may be simulated by overstaining, so it is important to compare with normal cells in the same preparation.

Macronucleoli are enlarged, circumscribed, acidophilic nuclear bodies, one or more of which are found in some malignant cells. Abnormality of shape of the nucleoli in addition to enlargement is of added significance. Large basophilic intranuclear

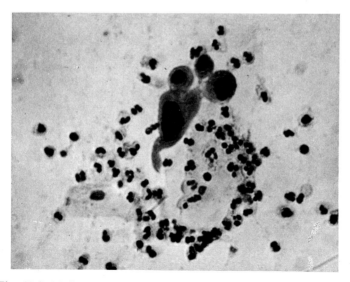

Fig. 11-6. Malignant cells in a vaginal smear from a carcinoma of the uterine cervix. Leukocytes are present also.

masses may occur, but also are seen in the nuclei of cells from benign proliferative processes.

Mitosis is uncommonly seen in isolated tumor cells, but the occurrence of an abnormal cell division is significant.

The importance of cytologic diagnosis lies in its ability to detect cancer in an organ at an early stage. Because of anatomic location, most organs are not accessible for cytologic examinations in a practical screening or case-finding procedure for the detection of early cancer. Most useful for the uterine cervix, cytologic examination may be applied also to endometrium, mouth, lung, urinary tract, prostate, and skin. Obtaining suitable cells from the stomach or other parts of the intestinal tract requires special methods or instruments, but cytologic examination may be a diagnostic aid in patients with symptoms related to these areas.

The original Papanicolaou method involved examination of cells obtained by vaginal aspiration. For detection of cancer of the uterine cervix, smears of cells obtained by direct scraping of the region of the squamocolumnar junction of the cervix have been found to be more advantageous. Papanicolaou divided his cytologic findings into five groups. This classification, which has been rather widely used, is as follows:

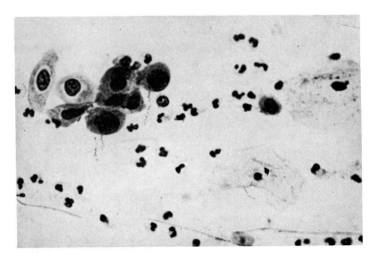

Fig. 11-7. Cells from a cervical cancer as seen in a vaginal smear.

Class I—absence of atypical or abnormal cells
Class II—atypical cytology but no evidence of malignancy
Class III—cytology suggestive of malignancy but not conclusive
Class IV—cytology strongly suggestive of malignancy
Class V—cytology conclusive for malignancy

Estimating the degree of malignancy of a cancer, as is frequently attempted in grading tumors by histologic examination, is not done on cytologic examinations.

Cytologic evidence of malignancy should be confirmed whenever possible by biopsy and histologic examination.

Experimental study of tumors

The chief advances of experimental cancer research hinge on three discoveries: (1) that certain tumors are transplantable from animal to animal within a given species, (2) that malignant tumors can be initiated by the use of chemical "carcinogenic" agents, and (3) that certain tumors, e.g., the chicken sarcoma of Rous, can be transferred by means of a cell-free filtrate or extract and are apparently of viral etiology. Further facts have been gleaned by observation of tumors grown in tissue culture, and breeding experiments with animals have thrown light upon hereditary and other factors in tumor incidence. Study of cellular metabolism, particularly of the biochemical function and ultrastructure of the cell nucleus, has been a promising field of recent cancer research.

The transplantability of tumors in mice and rats was discovered early in the century by Loeb and Jensen. Transplantability varies greatly in different tumors and is usually successful only with animals of the same species. Only the intact tumor cells grow, and in the new host the tumor cells are direct descendants of the original malignant cells; i.e., no new tumor is formed and the process is comparable to metastasis. Although ordinarily there is resistance to heterotransplantation of tumors, some tumor transplants may continue to grow within resistant animals if inoculated into the brain or the anterior chamber of the eye. Greene has suggested that the successful growth of human tumors in guinea pig eye may be correlated with poor prognosis of the tumor in the original host. Resistance to heterotransplantation has been broken down by various artificial means, including cortisone treatment of the recipient animals.

The production of cancer by chemical irritation or stimulation was achieved by Yamagiwa and Itchikawa, who found that repeated painting of the skin of rabbits with tar resulted in carcinoma. Previous knowledge of occupational cancers suggested that such a result might be expected. Paraffin on tar-workers and chimney sweeps were known to be peculiarly subject to the development of squamous cell carcinoma of the skin. Isolation of the chemicals in tar responsible for the carcinogenic action was the work of Kennaway and his associates. The potent carcinogens were found to be polycyclic hydrocarbons, among the most powerful of which are 1:2:5:6 dibenzanthracene, methylcholanthrene, and 3:4 benzpyrene. These compounds have a chemical relationship to certain naturally occurring substances, such as deoxycholic acid, estrogen, and sterols. There is some evidence that endogenous cancer-producing agents may exist. Carcinogenic extracts have been obtained from human tumors, but the nature of the agent is as yet unknown. Among agents that have been proven carcinogenic for man are radiation, betanaphthylamine, arsenic, chromates, and benzol. The time period that elapses between the first exposure to a carcinogenic agent and the appearance of a tumor is about 10 to 15% of the biologic life span (5 to 15 years in man).

Other substances (cocarcinogens) may augment the effect of the known carcinogenic agents, even though alone they may have little or no carcinogenic activity. Croton oil acts as an effective cocarcinogen in producing tumors of the skin by painting with tar. This and other experimental studies have suggested a two-stage hypothesis of carcinogenesis: an initiating stage, in which the cells undergo irrreversible change into latent or dormant tumor cells, and a promoting stage, during which there is a change to progressive growth.

Feeding azo dyes produces carcinomas of the liver in experimental animals, but the carcinogenic effect may be prevented by riboflavin. Other remotely acting carcinogens, such as 2-acetyl aminofluorine, have been discovered.

Hormonal imbalance has been effective in producing certain types of tumors in experimental animals. Estrogen administration may produce tumors of the mammary gland, uterus, pituitary, testis, and thymus. In human pathology there is considerable evidence of an important role of hormonal imbalance in some carcinomas of the endometrium and prostate and in some tumors of the thyroid.

Rous discovered a sarcoma, the causative agent of which could be transmitted to chickens by means of a cell-free and bacteria-free filtrate. It is well established that the Rous sarcoma and other similarly transmissible tumors of fowls are of viral origin. Other tumors of fowls and a mammalian tumor, a papilloma of the skin of rabbits discovered by Shope, are of viral origin; but there appears to be no direct evidence that viruses are etiologic agents in human tumors.

The biologic mechanism of tumor development as a result of the action of carcinogens, viruses, or hormonal imbalance is still unknown. One hypothesis is that of "somatic cell mutation." This theory postulates a gene mutation in a somatic cell as the specific cellular change responsible for tumor induction. This would conveniently explain the irreversibility of the neoplastic change, the great variety of tumors, and the frequency of nuclear abnormalities.

Heredity as a factor in cancer has been suspected from the high incidence in certain families. Breeding experiments with mice, in which there were strains produced having a very high incidence of cancer of the breast, pointed in the same direction. However, extrachromosomal factors also are at work here, for the incidence is influenced by estrogenic hormones and by a "milk factor," i.e., a substance in the mother's milk which has many properties of a virus and influences the development of breast cancer. Experimentally, heredity has been shown to be important in influencing the type and site of cancer and the age at which it occurs.

Causation of cancer

Cancer should be regarded, not as a single disease, but as a group of diseases in which there may be etiologic multiplicity. The etiology of cancer has to be considered as a separate problem for each organ. Many causative factors and carcinogenic agents are known, but a single ultimate cause of all forms of cancer has so far eluded discovery.

Three main hypotheses. In the development of knowledge about the causes of cancer, three main hypotheses have had a vogue. These are the irritation hypothesis, the embryonal or maldevelopment hypothesis, and the microbic, parasitic, or viral (infection) hypothesis. It is evident that each one of these factors plays some part in the causation of some cancers, and at the present time no single final cause is known which is applicable to all cancers.

The hypothesis that cancer may be caused by chronic, prolonged, or repeated irritation is based upon the observation of their frequent association, as in old burn scars or in a gall-bladder containing stones. But chronic irritation is regularly associated with the development of cancer only when the source of the chronic irritation has some special cancer-producing (carcinogenic) properties. This is the case in the occupational occurrence of certain tumors, such as cancers of the skin in workers having prolonged contact with tar, pitch, soot, or mineral oils; cancers of the urinary bladder in aniline dye workers; cancers of the lung in chromate workers; and cancers of bones in workers with luminous paints containing radioactive materials. The situation is similar in the cases of pioneer workers with roentgen rays, who from prolonged and repeated overexposure to radiation developed irritative lesions of the skin which eventually became cancers.

Conheim developed a classic theory of etiology of tumors based upon *"rests" of fetal cells*. According to this theory misplaced or superfluous embryonic cells failed to proceed to full development, remained dormant for a period, and then with recommencement of growth resulted in a tumor. The theory was extended by Ribbert who suggested that the misplacement of the cells put them beyond the normal controls of growth, thus allowing their lawless proliferation. These theories seem applicable to certain tumors such as chordomas, pituitary craniopharyngiomas, and to certain tumorlike developmental abnormalities (hamartomas), but their general applicability is doubtful. Displacement of tissue will not in itself result in a tumor.

Parasites as a cause of certain tumors in animals appear to act by causing chronic irritation. There is little evidence that parasites or bacteria are important in human cancer. An exception to this is that *Schistosoma haematobium,* a parasite common in Egypt, produces chronic irritation in the urinary tract and a high incidence of cancer of the bladder.

Viruses are established as a cause of some neoplasms in animals, but there is as yet no proof that any human cancer is caused by a virus. Electron microscopic studies of human cancer cells have so far failed to provide clear evidence of causative viral particles. Theories that have been proposed are that a causative virus acts by induction of somatic mutation or by the carrying of specific genetic traits to a new host cell. New stimulus in research on a possible role of viral infection in human cancer has been given by the demonstration that viruses are nucleoproteins with one type of nucleic acid. Evidence that viruses change the genetic code of the cells which they infect, reproducing by metabolism of the cells from genetic material within the cells, suggests new theories and direction for investigation. Studies on a distinctive childhood lymphomatous tumor with a certain geographic occurrence in Africa has given new stimulus to a search for infective origin.

Trauma or a single mechanical injury often seems to have some relationship to development of tumors, especially in the testis, bone, or breast. However, it is not established that it can cause cancer in a healthy tissue. Usually the injury only calls attention to a cancer which is already present but unrecognized.

Excessive exposure to sunlight (ultraviolet wavelengths shorter than 3,200 Å) is an important causative factor in many cancers of the skin. These occur after many years of overexposure and chronic sunburn, and so are seen mainly in sailors or farmers in sunny southern areas. Fair-skinned persons are more susceptible to this injury.

Heredity is demonstrably important in certain specific types of tumors, such as neuroblastoma (retinoblastoma) of the eye and multiple polyposis of the colon. In other specific tumors of certain sites, e.g., carcinoma of the stomach, the evidence of increased incidence among relatives suggests a hereditary influence. There probably is no general overall hereditary predisposition to cancer, but such hereditary tendencies toward cancer as may exist operate independently for different tumor types.

Mesenchymal tumors

The benign mesenchymal tumors are named according to their type of tissue, e.g., fibroma (fibrous connective tissue), lipoma (fat), and myoma (muscle). The malignant connective tissue tumors, or sarcomas, may be undifferentiated; or they may be so well differentiated that their tissue of origin is recognizable, e.g., fibrosarcoma and liposarcoma. Various forms of connective tissue tumors are listed in Table 11-1 for purposes of description.

Fibroma. Fibromas are derived from and composed of fibrous connective tissue and are of wide distribution. Most commonly they are found in connection with skin, subcutaneous tissue, fascia, or tendons, but also in certain organs, such as the ovary, kidney, breast, and intestine. With slow and expansive growth,

Table 11-1. *Mesenchymal tumors*

Origin or type of cell	Benign form	Malignant form
Fibrous connective tissue	Fibroma	Fibrosarcoma
Peripheral nerve sheaths	Neurofibroma	Neurogenic sarcoma
	Schwannoma	Malignant schwannoma
Fatty tissue	Lipoma	Liposarcoma
Myxomatous tissue	Myxoma	Myxosarcoma
Cartilage	Chondroma	Chondrosarcoma
Bone	Osteoma	Osteogenic sarcoma
Muscle	Myoma	Myosarcoma
Smooth	Leiomyoma	Leiomyosarcoma
Striated	Rhabdomyoma	Rhabdomyosarcoma
Notochord	Chordoma(rare)	Chordoma
Lymphocytic tissue		Lymphosarcoma
Serous linings		Mesothelial sarcoma
Blood or lymph vessels	Angioma	Angiosarcoma
Neuroglia	Glioma	Gliosarcoma
Cell origin undetermined		Undifferentiated sarcoma
		Small round cell sarcoma
		Large round cell sarcoma
		Mixed cell sarcoma

they tend to encapsulation. Microscopically they are composed of interlacing bundles and fibers of collagenous connective tissue.

Desmoid is a fibroma rising in musculoaponeurotic structures, particularly frequent in the lower anterior abdominal wall. Trauma seems to be a predisposing factor, and most cases have occurred in women who have borne children. There may be local infiltration of muscle, but sarcomatous transformation and metastases do not develop.

Keloid is an excessive formation of a fibrous scar, resulting in a tumorlike mass resembling a fibroma. Certain persons, particularly among the Negro race, are prone to this excessive fibrosis following injuries of the skin. Microscopically the keloid consists of dense bundles of collagenous and hyalinized connective tissue (p. 822).

Fibrosarcoma. Fibrosarcoma is a malignant tumor tending to differentiate in the direction of fibrous connective tissue. It occurs at any age, but the highest incidence is in the fifth and sixth decades. The most common site of origin is in the extremities, particularly the lower, but the origin may be from connective tissue in any region. Fibrosarcoma appears as a

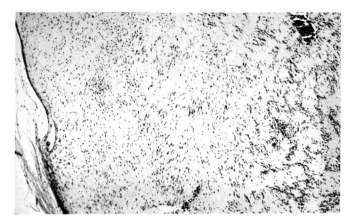

Fig. 11-8. Neurilemoma; palisading of nuclei is evident on the right.

rounded, lobulated tumor, often appearing circumscribed or encapsulated, and either hard and fibrous or soft and friable, depending on the amount of collagenous tissue which has been formed. Areas of degeneration, necrosis, myxomatous change, or cyst formation may be present. Simple excision is often followed by recurrence. Following repeated recurrences, death may result from visceral metastasis or from infection and hemorrhage of the ulcerating tumor. The degree of malignancy tends to be proportional to the number of mitotic nuclei and tumor giant cells and to the scarcity of collagen fibers. Tumors composed of two or more mesenchymal derivatives that ordinarily are not found together in a single tumor have been called *mesenchymomas*. With rare exceptions, such tumors are malignant.

Large fibrous tumors, particularly of the abdomen, pelvis, retroperitoneal area, and thorax, are occasionally associated with attacks of hypoglycemia. The hypoglycemic episodes, which simulate hyperinsulinism, cease on removal of the tumor. Insulin is not demonstrable in the tumor tissue, and the mechanism of the hypoglycemia is not known.

A benign growth, possibly granulomatous in nature, which simulates a sarcomatous lesions, has been called pseudosarcomatous fasciitis or fibromatosis. It grows rapidly, usually in subcutaneous tissues, and affects children as well as adults. The bulk of the tumor is composed of myxoid fibroblastic proliferation, with many capillaries, and some lymphoid and histiocytic cells. Typical mitoses may be numerous. There is lack of encapsulation, and irregular extension occurs into adjacent tissues.

Neurofibroma and neurilemoma. Neurofibromas and neurilemomas *(Schwannomas)* arise from the sheaths of cranial or peripheral nerves. Of the cranial nerves the eighth is the most commonly involved, the tumor being found in the cerebellopontine angle (acoustic neurinoma). The exact origin of the peripheral nerve sheath tumors (e.g., from the sheath of Schwann, endoneurium, perineurium, etc.) has been a subject of discussion in recent years, and the terminology used has varied depending on the favored theory.

Von Recklinghausen's disease is a familial form of *multiple neurofibromatosis.* Neurofibromas are found on branches of the

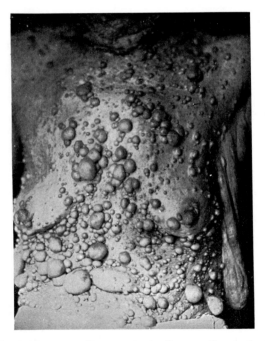

Fig. 11-9. Multiple neurofibromatosis (molluscum fibrosum). (Courtesy Dr. Emil Theilman; from Sutton, R. L., and Sutton, R. L., Jr.: Diseases of the skin, ed. 10, St. Louis, The C. V. Mosby Co.)

cutaneous nerves and along nerve trunks of the thorax, brachial and lumbar plexus, and extremities. Cranial nerves and spinal nerves within the spinal canal are sometimes involved as well. Coffee-colored areas of skin pigmentation are common stigmas of this disease. The tumors are benign nonencapsulated focal lesions or may diffusely involve the nerves from which they grow. In a small proportion of cases one or more of the tumors may become malignant. A loose wavy arrangement of fibrils, sometimes with formation of whorls, is characteristic of neurofibroma. Mucoid degeneration of the collagen of the tumor is common. In addition to this multiple form, neurofibromas sometimes are seen as *solitary lesions* (e.g., in the skin).

Neurilemomas, which are often included in the general family of neurofibromas, may be single or multiple, but they do not develop into a generalized condition such as Von Recklinghausen's neurofibromatosis. Palisading of nuclei is characteristic, and often a double palisade encloses a space (Verocay body). Malignant change in a neurilemoma does not occur or is very rare. In contrast to neurofibromas, the neurilemomas are encapsulated.

Neurogenic sarcoma (neurogenous sarcoma). Sarcomatous tumors of soft tissue may be found in distinct relation to nerves. More often such relationship is not demonstrable, and in such cases the features suggesting a neurogenous origin are (1) arrangement of the cells in definite bundles with an interlacing pattern of the herringbone type; (2) wavy, fine, elongated nuclei which tend to line up in parallel fashion to form rows (palisading); and (3) fibrils, demonstrable by silver stains, distributed in pericellular fashion.

The proportion of sarcomas of skin and subcutaneous tissues which are of neurogenous origin is a matter of debate. Ewing and others have held that the majority of such spindle cell sarcomas arise from peripheral nerves. From a practical standpoint the criteria of degree of malignancy and the prognosis are the same for neurogenic sarcoma and fibrosarcoma, varying with the number of mitoses and tumor giant cells and the scarcity of fibers. It may be difficult to determine whether a neurogenic sarcoma is derived from fibroblastic elements of the sheath (neurofibrosarcoma) or from Schwann cells (malignant *Schwannoma* or malignant neurilemoma).

Lipoma. Lipomas are benign, circumscribed masses of an adult type of fat tissue. They occur in many situations, but especially in the subcutaneous tissues of the back or shoulder region. In some cases they are multiple, grow to a large size, and appear to have a familial factor in their causation. In certain rare instances they show a connection with nerves and are painful. Microscopically they are composed of fat cells of the usual type found in adipose tissue, although of a larger average size. *Hibernoma* is a rare type of fatty tumor which arises from a structure in human beings, homologous to the so-called hibernating gland of animals, and which develops from persistent brown multilocular fat.

Liposarcoma. Liposarcoma is composed of embryonic fat cells containing small fat globules in their granular cytoplasm. Much of the tumor may be undifferentiated and highly cellular. In some areas mature types of fat cells may be found.

There are two types of liposarcoma. One variety, the adult form, is composed of granular cells resembling those found in chronic inflammation of fat tissue. Trauma to fatty tissue often seems to precede this type of tumor. The second type is an embryonal liposarcoma (myxoliposarcoma). This tumor contains many tiny proliferating blood vessels, mucus-producing cells, and some embryonal fat tissue. Liposarcomas of an extremity often have a significant myxomatous component.

Liposarcomas occur most often around the buttocks, lower limbs, and in the retroperitoneal spaces. They occur as a relatively common type of soft tissue tumor in infancy and childhood and are quite radiosensitive.

Myxoma. Myxoma is a mesenchymal tumor in which a mucoid intercellular substance (probably hyaluronic acid) separates stellate embryonic connective tissue cells so as to resemble in appearance primitive mesenchyme or the tissue of the umbilical cord. A pure myxoma is rare, but a myxomatous change or degeneration in a portion of some other type of connective tissue tumor is not uncommon.

Myxosarcoma. Myxosarcoma is likewise very rare as a pure tumor.

Tumors of bone. *Chondroma, chondrosarcoma, osteoma,* and *osteogenic sarcoma* are tumors which usually arise in connection with skeletal structures and are considered in Chapter 24.

Muscle tumors. The benign tumors are of two types: *rhabdomyoma,* an extremely rare tumor of striated muscle, and *leiomyoma,* a very common tumor composed of smooth muscle. Leiomyomas are most frequent in the uterus, where they have an abundant fibrous stroma and are commonly called "fibroids" (p. 757). They also occur in many other situations where smooth muscle is normally found, as in the intestinal tract. Malignant transformation of a uterine myoma to a *leiomyosarcoma* may occur. A pure *rhabdomyosarcoma* is relatively uncommon, but striped muscle fibers are sometimes found in malignant mixed tumors such as those of the kidney (p. 409) and uterus (p.

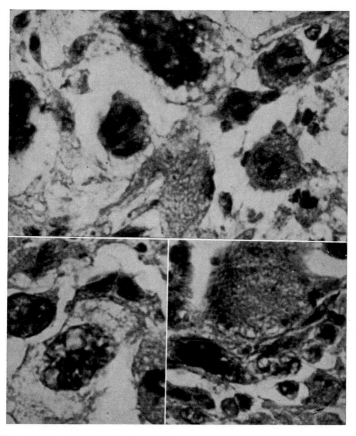

Fig. 11-10. Liposarcoma; giant lipoblasts with large bizarre pyknotic nuclei and foamy or vacuolated cytoplasm. (From Haukohl, R. S., and Anderson, W. A. D., editors: Pathology seminars, St. Louis, 1955, The C. V. Mosby Co.)

762). Pleomorphic rhabdomyosarcomas occur mainly in the extremities of older persons. An alveolar type of rhabdomyosarcoma has been described in adolescents and young adults. Embryonal or botryoid rhabdomyosarcomas occur chiefly in infants or young children and are located mainly in the orbital region or the urogenital tract.

The so-called *granular cell myoblastoma* is an uncommon tumor which has been interpreted as derived from primitive myoblasts. Most examples have been found in the tongue, but some have appeared in skin, skeletal muscle, and other sites. They are composed of large polyhedral cells with small nuclei and an abundant, pale granular cytoplasm. Cross striations and structures resembling myofibrils have been observed in some cases. The tumor may be encapsulated, but in most instances it is locally infiltrative. It is benign but often is associated with pseudocarcinomatous hyperplasia of the overlying epithelium.

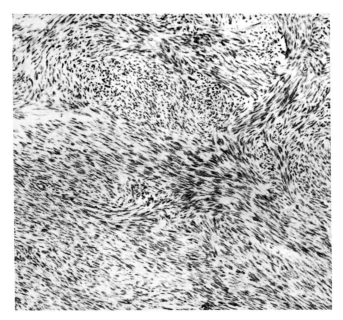

Fig. 11-11. Leiomyoma. The intertwining bundles of smooth muscle fibers run in various directions, and some are cut transversely.

The so-called "organoid" variety most often arises in the upper thigh. Its true nature is debatable, but it is a distinctly different tumor, and a neurogenous or paraganglionic rather than a myoblastic origin has been suggested. Because of uncertain histogenesis, others have referred to this tumor by the noncommittal term of "alveolar soft-part sarcoma." The tumor is very slow in its growth but may metastasize by the bloodstream to the lung, brain, or elsewhere.

Chordoma. Chordoma is a rare tumor which arises from notochordal remnants at the upper or lower ends of the vertebral column. It is composed of large, clear, closely packed cells having a vacuolated cytoplasm (p. 874).

Lymphomatous tumors. *Lymphocytic lymphosarcoma, reticulum cell sarcoma,* and other tumors of lymphoid, reticuloendothelial, and blood-forming tissues are considered in Chapter 16. Plasma cell tumors occur as solitary or multiple tumors of bone marrow (myeloma) and also as extramedullary tumors, mainly in the nasopharyngeal region.

Mesothelioma. Mesothelioma is a primary tumor arising from serous surfaces such as the pleura, pericardium, and peritoneum (p. 483).

Angioma. Tumors composed of endothelial cells tending to form blood or lymphatic channels consist of both benign and malignant forms. Specialized varieties are glomus tumors and hemangiopericytomas. They are considered on p. 315.

Glioma. The gliomas are tumors arising from the neuroglial or supporting cells of the central nervous system (p. 874).

Undifferentiated sarcoma. Many of the malignant mesenchymal tumors fail to differentiate into recognizable types of cells. They are often given descriptive designations such as small round cell sarcoma, large round cell sarcoma, mixed cell sarcoma, and spindle cell sarcoma, although there may be little practical advantage in such labels. Mitoses are numerous in these highly malignant growths.

Small round cell sarcoma arises in a variety of sites and tends to be rapid in growth and metastasis. It forms a fairly well-demarcated, pinkish white, fleshy mass in which areas of degeneration and hemorrhage are common. Microscopically it is composed of small, round, uniform cells, among which are abundant thin-walled blood vessels. The *large round cell sarcomas* are similar grossly but are composed of cells that are larger, are less uniformly round, and have more abundant cytoplasm. Many of the tumors designated as small and large round cell sarcomas are in reality lymphosarcomas and reticulum cell sarcomas. The *mixed (polymorphic) cell sarcomas* are made up of cells having variable size and shape, often with bizarre tumor giant cells.

Spindle cell sarcoma shows some differentiation toward recognizable fibroblastic cells. The tumor is somewhat harder in the gross, less prone to degenerative changes, and less malignant than the round cell forms. It is composed of bundles of elongated spindle-shaped cells with oval nuclei. When the elongated cells are cut transversely, they appear rounded and show but scanty cytoplasm.

General characteristics of sarcoma. Malignant mesenchymal tumors are more prone to occur at any age throughout life than are carcinomas. During the first few decades of life they have a much higher relative frequency than malignant epithelial tumors. They tend to be soft and of fleshy appearance and consistency, except in the highly differentiated types. Hemorrhages and degenerative changes are common in the tumor tissue. They usually have abundant, thin-walled blood vessels, which are intimately associated with the tumor cells, whereas in epithelial tumors the blood vessels are contained in the stroma which separates groups of tumor cells. The thinness and intimacy of vessels in sarcomas readily enable the tumor cells to grow through their walls. Hence they commonly metastasize by way of the bloodstream, the lung being the most frequent site for secondary tumors. Lymph node metastasis also occurs in 5 to 10% of sarcomas.

Epithelial tumors

Tumors derived from and made up of epithelial tissues may be classified into two groups, the benign and the malignant (carcinoma). An epithelial tumor, like normal epithelial tissue, has a connective tissue stroma which supports the epithelium and in which are contained blood and lymphatic vessels. Insufficiency of this stroma, on which nutrition depends, results in degenerative changes and necrosis in the tumor. On the other hand, the stroma may progress equally with the growth of the epithelial elements or even exceed it, producing fibroepithelial tumors (e.g., fibroadenoma of the breast) or, in the case of carcinoma, scirrhous tumors.

Benign epithelial tumors

Benign epithelial tumors are of two main types: papilloma, which grows outward from an epithelial surface, either cutaneous or mucous, and adenoma, which is derived from and imitates glandular epithelium. The benign tumors progress slowly. By their expansile growth they compress surrounding tissue but do not infiltrate and never form metastases. The cells tend to conform closely to a normal appearance.

Papilloma. In a papilloma the tumor cells are situated externally, elevated from the surface, and arranged around a central core of connective tissue containing blood vessels. The surface of a papilloma is exposed to injury by pressure or friction, so that ulceration, infection, and inflammatory changes are common. The main feature distinguishing them from carcinoma is that the tumor cells do not penetrate the underlying tissues.

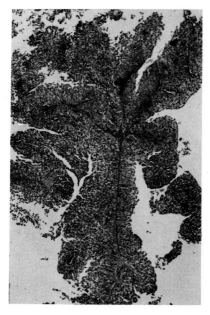

Fig. 11-12. Papillomatous tumor of the urinary bladder. The central, branching stromal stalk is covered by irregular layers of neoplastic cells.

Papillomas may originate from skin, mucous surfaces, or the lining of cysts. Cutaneous papillomas may be true tumors, but a group of inflammatory growths of the skin are also loosely called papillomas. The latter include venereal warts (condylomas), the common warts of children (verruca vulgaris), which are of infectious origin, and pyogenic granulomas, or excessive growths of granulation tissue.

The true papilloma of the skin is a hard rough tumor with a broad base which may be several centimeters in diameter. The surface is rough and fissured, often with marked keratinization of the superficial cells. When keratinization is excessive, these may be called cutaneous horns.

Some papillomatous tumors of the skin are pigmented and may be confused with true melanomas. They have the structure of an ordinary cutaneous papilloma, but there is abundant melanin in the epidermal cells.

Papillomas from mucous surfaces often have long delicate processes attached around a thin central stalk. This type is seen in its typical form in the bladder. Another variety consists of a single, thick, fingerlike process. This type characteristically occurs in the intestine, sometimes in large numbers. Papillomas of mucous surfaces are often called polyps. Multiple polyposis of the large intestine is a familial or hereditary condition in which a malignant change in one or more of the tumors eventually occurs.

Intracystic papilloma, in which the projection of the tumor is into the cavity of a cyst, is seen particularly in cystic lesions of the ovary and of the breast.

Adenoma. An adenoma is a benign tumor derived from glandular or secretory cells. It usually has a slow rate of growth and a well-defined margin; it quite accurately reproduces the tissue from which it is derived. The tumor cells may function and produce a secretion similar to, or the same as, that produced by the normal glandular tissue. Thus mucin tends to be produced in intestinal growths, colloid in thyroid adenomas, and bile in liver adenomas. In the case of adenomas made up of endocrine tissue, excessive secretory activity may result in clinical evidence of hyperactivity of the particular endocrine gland. Distention with secretory material and cyst formation is also a common result of functional activity (cystadenoma).

Since any glandular tissue may give rise to tumor, adenomas are of extremely varied structure. Those which grow within the

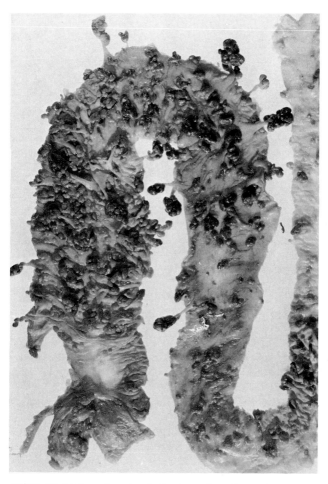

Fig. 11-13. Multiple polyposis of the large intestine. (Courtesy Dr. J. F. Kuzma.)

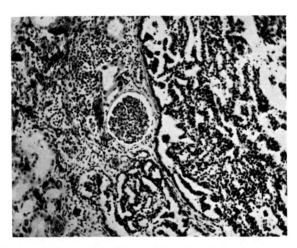

Fig. 11-14. Adenoma of the kidney. The edge of the tumor is shown so that a glomerulus and tubules are evident in the left half of the illustration.

substance of a gland tend to be rounded and encapsulated. Those which grow from the secretory cells of a mucous membrane, such as endometrium, tend to be polypoid and pedunculated.

Malignant epithelial tumors

Carcinoma. Malignant epithelial tumors form a most important group because of their numerical frequency and serious effects. They vary widely in rate of growth, in degree of anaplasia or differentiation, and in gross and microscopic appearance. They are distinguished from benign epithelial tumors in that they invade and destroy normal tissue and usually will spread by metastasis.

Carcinomas differ in the degree to which they imitate their tissue of origin. In some cases the resemblance to normal tissue is very close, with well-formed glands, tubules, or lining epithelium. At the other extreme there may be so much anaplasia or reversion to an embryonic type of tissue that the origin of the tumor or even its epithelial nature is difficult to determine.

The stroma likewise is variable. Invading carcinoma cells utilize the existing stroma of the destroyed tissue. When the

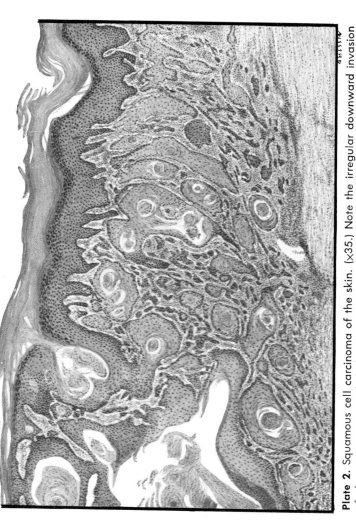

Plate 2. Squamous cell carcinoma of the skin. (×35.) Note the irregular downward invasion of the squamous epithelial cells, which are fairly well differentiated and are forming numerous keratin "pearls." (From McCarthy, L.: Histopathology of skin diseases, St. Louis, The C. V. Mosby Co.)

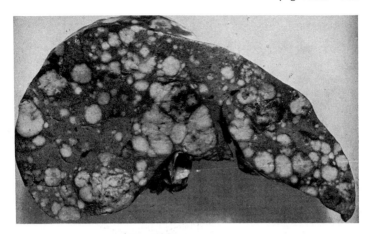

Fig. 11-15. Metastatic carcinoma of the liver. Primary tumor in the stomach.

tumor growth is rapid, the connective tissue and blood vessels are often inadequate to support and nourish the tumor, so that degeneration and death of tumor cells result. Other tumors (scirrhous) tend to stimulate the growth of the connective tissue stroma, sometimes to exceed the development of the epithelial elements.

A number of terms are used in the classification and description of carcinomas. *Squamous cell carcinoma* arises from surface epithelium such as skin, mouth, lip, or cervix, and it is made up of squamous epithelial cells. It may also arise from the esophagus, anus, larynx, nose, sinuses, renal pelvis, ureters, bladder, and bronchi. It is most easily identified by the presence of prickle cells or keratinization. *Adenocarcinoma* is a tumor with cells having a glandular arrangement or origin. The terms *scirrhous, medullary,* and *mucoid* or *gelatinous,* as used here, refer to gross and microscopic appearance. A *scirrhous carcinoma* is hard and fibrous because of abundant stroma. A *medullary carcinoma* is soft and brainlike in consistency because it has little connective tissue stroma. *Mucoid* or *gelatinous carcinomas* are soft and translucent as a result of an accumulation of a mucoid or colloid material. Carcinomas are frequently not uniformly scirrhous, medullary, or mucoid throughout their whole substance. *Carcinoma simplex* is a carcinoma of glandular tissue in which the cells are arranged in solid cords and masses.

Mixed tumors and teratomas

Most tumors are composed of cells of one type, e.g., glandular epithelium as in simple adenoma. However, there are tumors in which tissues of different character occur together in the same growth, and these are classified as mixed tumors or teratomas.

Hamartomas. Hamartomas are tumorlike malformations composed of an abnormal mixture of the normal constituents of an organ or tissue. The constituents may be abnormal in amount, in arrangement, in degree of maturation, or in all these respects. These developmental masses lack the capacity of true neoplasms for limitless proliferation.

Embryonic tumors. Embryonic tumors arise in early life from tissues that are still undifferentiated and which continue to proliferate at the embryonic level. They include Wilms' tumor of the kidney (nephroblastoma), retinoblastoma (retinal neuroepithelioma), embryonic tumors of the liver, and embryonic sarcomas of the urogenital organs of children.

Mixed tumors. Mixed tumors are derived from pleuripotential cells, i.e., cells capable of differentiation into more than one type of tissue. Such tumors are often embryonic tumors which show differentiation into tissues which are not normally seen in the same adult organs, but which can be derived from immature mesenchyme. In such tumors of the kidney (Wilms' tumor or embryoma, p. 409) and liver both epithelial and connective tissue elements are commonly present, but organ development is not found. Mixed tumors containing a mixture of tumor forms derived from mesenchyme have been termed *mesenchymomas*. They are most frequent in the urogenital tract (uterus, p. 762) and breast, but they also occur in other soft parts.

Teratomas. A teratoma is a tumor containing organs or distinct fetal structures representing all three primitive layers of blastoderm. They are derived from totipotential cells, i.e., cells capable of differentiation into an organ or tissue foreign to the part. They arise from immature tissues which have the neoplastic power of progressive independent growth. The malignant examples may continue to proliferate at the embryonic level and produce tissues of all degrees of immaturity.

Teratomas may arise from either (1) the totipotential cells of the ovary or testicle or (2) an undeveloped "rest" of cells of the morula prior to the differentiation of the primitive layers. They most often arise in the ovary or testicle. It has commonly been considered that from some unknown stimulus one of the unfertilized cells begins to grow and attempts to form a new individual, but the correctness of this theory is unproved. In the ovary these tumors are common and usually are cystic (dermoid cysts) but may be solid.

Those teratomas which arise from "rests" of undifferentiated tissue are most common near the growing ends of the body, in the sacrococcygeal region or at the base of the skull. They may, however, arise in almost any situation. This type of teratoma is closely related to the various types of joined twins and parasitic fetuses. Sacrococcygeal teratoma appears to be associated frequently with twins or a family history of malformations. It occurs predominantly in females, arising between the rectum and sacrum, and is usually detectable at birth. Teratomas are comparatively frequent also in the anterior mediastinum.

Teratomas may be benign or malignant. Occasionally one type of cell in a teratoma becomes malignant, and metastases are made up of this type of cell alone.

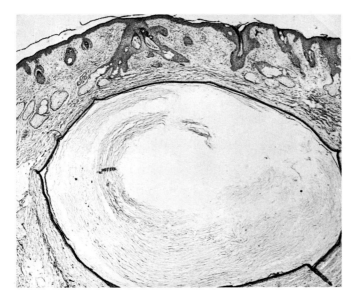

Fig. 11-16. Epidermal cyst of skin, lined by a thin layer of squamous epithelium and filled by a layered mass of keratin.

CYSTS

A cyst is a cavity containing fluid and surrounded by a definite wall. There is usually a lining of cells (e.g., epithelial, mesothelial, etc.).

Classification of cysts

The many varieties of cyst can be fitted into the following classification:

Retention cysts—due to blockage of ducts or tubules, with cystic distention of the proximal portion. Cysts of the kidney and pancreas are usually of this type. Some cysts of the skin may be of this type, and some may be of traumatic origin (inclusion cysts).

Cysts due to developmental errors—those arising from the branchial clefts, thyroglossal duct, and from remains of the wolffian duct (hydatids of Morgagni). Also of developmental origin are some sebaceous cysts of the skin, cystic hygromas (p. 317), and the cysts associated with spina bifida (p. 886).

Cystic tumors or cystomas (cystadenomas)—those which arise very commonly from the ovary, thyroid, and other organs.

Cysts from serous cavities—those which arise by outpouchings from bursae and tendon sheaths (e.g., "Baker's cyst" of the knee).

Parasitic cysts—those due to the *Echinococcus granulosus* (hydatid cysts) and amebiasis.

Pseudocysts—those formed as a result of hemorrhagic material (hematoma) which has become encapsulated. Also to be included here are the cystlike spaces formed as a result of mucinous degeneration.

Chapter 12

The cardiovascular system

The circulatory system, which includes the heart, blood vessels, and lymphatics, is concerned with the essential nutrition of tissues. Disease of this system is a major cause of illness and disability and is the leading cause of death in the United States.

DISEASES OF BLOOD VESSELS AND LYMPHATICS

Generally speaking, lesions of blood vessels are important in proportion to the degree to which they reduce circulation to vital tissues. Such an effect is most commonly produced by a hardening and thickening of arterial walls, referred to as arteriosclerosis. Arteries and veins are also subject to inflammations (arteritis and phlebitis), dilatation (aneurysm and varicosity), and neoplasm (angioma). Thrombosis, embolism, and hemorrhage are important accompaniments of vascular diseases.

Structure of arteries

Arterial vessels are composed of three coats: intima, media, and adventitia. The *intima,* or inner layer, consists of a lining layer of endothelial cells, beneath which are a few muscle and connective tissue fibers. The *media* is formed by muscular and elastic tissue. A condensation of the elastic tissue at the inner margin of the media forms the internal elastic lamella. This inner elastic band frequently appears wavy because of postmortem contraction of the vessel. A less definite outer condensation of elastic tissue sometimes forms an external elastic lamella. The *adventitia,* or outer wall, contains a loose network of connective tissue and elastic fibrils, carrying blood vessels (vasa vasorum) and nerves to supply the vessel wall.

The vascular supply to the wall of blood vessels is richer and more extensive than was previously suspected. Small vessels supplying arterial walls are much more numerous in older persons and in the presence of atherosclerosis. Intimal vasa vasorum are common in atherosclerotic vessels, but their presence in a normal intima is disputed.

Arteries may be divided into three main classes according to size and structural variations: elastic arteries, muscular arteries, and arterioles. The group of elastic arteries includes the largest vessels, the aorta, and its immediate branches. In this group the vessel wall contains elastic tissue in greatest proportion. Elastic recoil of these vessels maintains blood flow and pressure during diastole. The second group, the muscular distributing arteries, are the medium-sized vessels, such as the brachial, radial, and femoral arteries. In these vessels elastic tissue is present in smaller amount, and muscular tissue is greater. The third group, the arterioles, includes the small arteries of organs down to the size of capillaries. In these vessels muscular tissue is most abundant and elastic tissue is relatively slight. Their contraction is important in regulation of blood pressure and flow.

Arteriosclerosis

The term *arteriosclerosis* literally means "hardening of the arteries" and is sometimes used synonymously with "atherosclerosis." However, according to present usage, arteriosclerosis is a generic term that includes three diseases of the arterial tree: (1) atherosclerosis, (2) Mönckeberg's medial sclerosis, and (3) arteriolosclerosis. In the first disease the principal change is in the intima; in the second it is in the media; and in the third the intima, the media, or both may be involved.

Atherosclerosis. Intimal thickening and regressive changes are the characteristic features of atherosclerosis. It affects mainly the large elastic vessels, the aorta being most severely involved. It also affects the coronary, renal, and cerebral arteries and the larger arteries of the extremities. The intimal lesions range from small, slightly raised, longitudinal yellow streaks ("fatty streaks") to larger, pearly gray or gray-yellow nodules or plaques, containing lipid and hyalinized connective tissue ("fibrous plaques"), and advanced lesions with ulceration, thrombosis, hemorrhage, and calcification ("complicated lesions").

Several theories have been advanced as to the nature of the primary change in the *pathogenesis* of atherosclerosis: (1) The earliest change consists of fatty streaks resulting from lipids in the intima (present in smooth muscle cells and foam cells, the latter being considered by some to be macrophages and by others to be modified smooth muscle cells). The lipids filter through the endothelium along with plasma, either as free molecules or carried in macrophages (foam cells), and the larger lipoprotein complexes are trapped in the intima. Prior damage to the intima is not apparent, but excess lipids in the plasma, nutritional disturbances, or hormonal factors may enhance lipid infiltration. (2) An alteration of acid mucopolysaccharide, elastic tissue, and fibroblasts in the intima results from some form of injury (hemodynamic, endocrine, or metabolic). An increase in mucopolysaccharide and connective tissue precedes lipid deposits, which are derived from the plasma or are locally synthesized. (3) Mural thrombi occur on the endothelium that become organized and incorporated into the intima and then are infiltrated by lipid.

It is generally agreed that, no matter what the primary event is, the presence of lipid in the vessel wall stimulates fibrous tissue

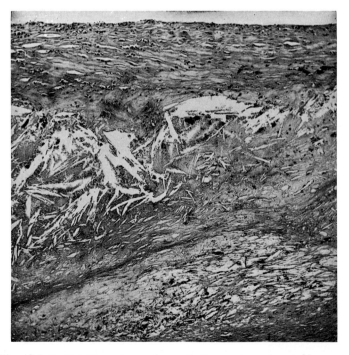

Fig. 12-1. Section through an advanced atheromatous plaque. Numerous cholesterol clefts are seen in the pale central part. The small dark spots are caused by calcium deposits. (Courtesy Dr. E. M. Hall.)

proliferation and is important in the development of athero-sclerotic lesions. The intramural fatty deposits, in the early lesions, have a similar lipid composition as the blood plasma, suggesting lipid infiltration from the plasma. It is probable that intramural enzymes break down the lipid, releasing cholesterol and fatty acids, which incite fibrous tissue proliferation. With progression of the lesions, lipid-laden, fibrous plaques form. In larger lesions the central portion is frequently soft, containing degenerated and necrotic tissue, free fat, and visible cholesterol crystals. Microscopically the cholesterol appears as clear, elongated, fusiform clefts because the crystals have been dissolved out in preparation of the section. The soft yellow nodule is an atheroma ("porridgelike" mass). In advanced lesions, ulceration of atheromas and superimposed thrombi may be seen. The internal elastic lamina is frayed and fragmented, and in places it may be absent. Calcium salts become deposited in the atheromatous lesions and form thin, brittle, calcified plates, which may crack easily. When an atheromatous plaque is large, it may encroach upon and cause thinning of the media. Progressive loss of elasticity accompanies atherosclerosis, but much of this may be an aging effect.

The atheromatous lesions are much more prevalent in the abdominal than in the thoracic aorta. Their distribution is patchy; they are eccentrically placed, as a rule; and they are found at points of stress, e.g., on the posterior wall of the aorta, especially about orifices of the intercostal and lumbar arteries, and at the point of branching of major vessels. Atherosclerosis may be superimposed upon syphilitic lesions in the thoracic aorta.

Complications of atheromatous plaques include: (1) narrowing of the lumen, resulting in ischemia; (2) thrombosis over the plaque, producing occlusion of the lumen, or in the case of small thrombi, they may organize, become incorporated into the intima, and contribute to growth of the plaque; (3) hemorrhage into the plaques, which in some instances (e.g., coronary artery) may contribute to luminal occlusion and also may initiate thrombosis; (4) rupture of soft atheromatous material into the lumen, which may cause occlusion at the site (in a small vessel), give rise to an embolus, or initiate thrombosis; (5) formation of an aneurysm because of thinning and weakening of the media adjacent to the large plaque.

Obstruction of small vessels, caused by the plaque itself or one of its complications, may lead to serious ischemic effects, e.g., sudden death or myocardial infarct with involvement of the coronary arteries, infarct of the brain in cerebral atherosclerosis, and hypertension with renal arterial disease. The Leriche syndrome, occurring chiefly in men and characterized by ischemic effects in the lower limbs (e.g., pallor, coldness, cramps, claudication), an inability to maintain a penile erection, and impotence, is the result of a progressive atheromatous thrombotic occlusion of the abdominal aorta at or above its bifurcation.

Etiology. The etiology of atherosclerosis involves a complex interrelationship between multiple factors, both endogenous and environmental. The actual cause or causes are unknown, but there are various *predisposing* or *contributing factors.* In recent years the role of *plasma* and *dietary lipids* has been emphasized. There is evidence that an increase in serum beta-lipoproteins, hypercholesterolemia and an increased cholesterol-phospholipid ratio in the blood are significant in the development of atherosclerosis. The role of triglycerides is presently under investigation. People whose diet contains large amounts of saturated animal fat and cholesterol have a higher serum cholesterol level and an increased incidence of coronary atherosclerotic heart disease than those whose diet is low in these fats. It is interesting to note that some birds who do not have animal fats in their diet (e.g., certain species of pigeons) develop spontaneous atherosclerosis similar to that in man. Certain diseases associated with hypercholesterolemia, such as *diabetes mellitus, hypothyroidism,* and *familial hypercholesterolemia,* are frequently associated with atherosclerosis. *Hereditary predisposition* is a factor, but it is not certain whether or not this is related to familial patterns of lipid metabolism.

Cholesterol feeding in rabbits is a well-known experimental method of producing atherosclerosis. Similarly atherosclerosis has been produced in the dog, rat, mouse, and other animals, but, in certain of these, other procedures are necessary, e.g., the use of antithyroid drugs or surgical removal of the thyroid gland. In monkeys atherosclerosis can be produced by pyridoxine deficiency without any special fat diet. Hyperlipemia also appears to increase the tendency to thrombosis. Heparin, in addition to its anticoagulant effect, helps to correct the abnormal lipoprotein pattern often found in atherosclerotic patients.

The influence of *sex* is evident in the observation that atherosclerosis is much less likely to occur in women before the menopause, although the incidence increases progressively after the menopause. The protective factor premenopausally may be estrogen. *Hormonal* effect is also noted in women who have castration of the ovaries; they develop coronary atherosclerosis more often and at an earlier age than those with intact ovaries. The incidence and severity of this disease are less in men treated with estrogens for carcinoma of the prostate than in nontreated men. It has been demonstrated that hormones tend to lower serum cholesterol-lipoprotein concentrations, including, in addition to estrogen, growth hormone, ACTH, corticoids, thyroid preparations, and androsterone. *Age* is considered by some investigators to be important; but it should be noted that atherosclerosis is not a disease limited to advanced age. Proponents of the aging theory point out that there is a progressive intimal thickening in the arteries from the time of birth, although this may be related to continued intravascular mechanical stress. It has also been suggested that intimal plaques are essentially compensatory phenomena in response to underlying medial weakness resulting from degenerations associated with aging. *Emotional stress, physical inactivity,* and *smoking* are other possible contributing factors. *Local hemodynamic forces* in the bloodstream (e.g., turbulence of flow and sites of increased wall tension) are undoubtedly important in the development of atherosclerosis. This is suggested by the fact that atheromatous plaques are most prevalent at or just beyond the orifices or bifurcations of arteries and at points where vessels are relatively fixed. *Hypertension* is apparently not a primary cause of atherosclerosis but may aggravate the lesion by accentuating the local hemodynamic factors; or when hypercholesterolemia exists in a hypertensive patient, the high intravascular pressure probably accelerates infiltration of lipid through the arterial wall.

Medial sclerosis (Mönckeberg's sclerosis). Medial sclerosis occurs particularly in the medium-sized muscular arteries, such as the femoral, radial, and temporal, usually in the elderly. There are degeneration, swelling, and fragmentation of medial muscle fibers, followed by calcium deposition. Occasionally bone is formed in the vessel wall. The vessels become hard and tortuous, so that palpable vessels such as the radial artery can be felt as rigid tubes. The medial changes alone do not narrow the lumen and have little effect on the circulation. However, the medial sclerosis may be associated with intimal atheromatous lesions that could interfere with blood flow. Vasotonic influences may be causative factors. In experimental animals, similar lesions are produced by the administration of epinephrine, nicotine, or other agents that produce prolonged spasm of the vessels.

Arteriolosclerosis. There are two types of arteriolar change characterized by thickening of the vessel wall and narrowing of the lumen: hyaline arteriolosclerosis and hyperplastic arteriolosclerosis, both of which are characteristic but not pathognomonic of hypertension.

In *hyaline arteriolosclerosis* the wall is thickened and hyalinized as a result of deposition of a hyaline material in the intima and media, with obliteration of the underlying cellular details. There is a controversy as to the origin of the vascular hyalin. Some investigators have demonstrated by electron microscopy that the hyalin is deposited primarily in intimal spaces, possibly derived

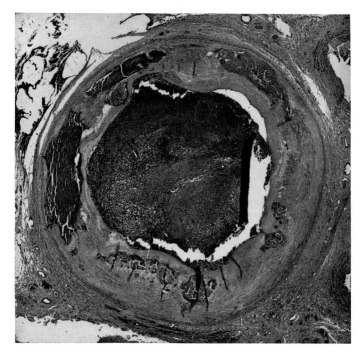

Fig. 12-2. Mönckeberg's medial sclerosis. Note the dark calcified plaques in the media. A recent thrombus fills the lumen. (Courtesy Dr. E. M. Hall.)

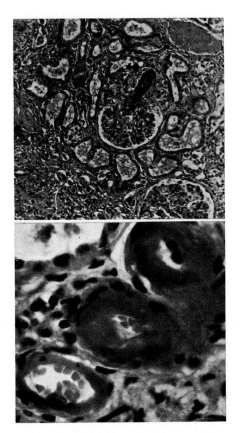

Fig. 12-3. Hyaline arteriolar sclerosis of the kidney. Note the severe involvement of the entering arteriole of a glomerulus. From a case of essential hypertension.

from excessive infiltration of plasma proteins, and that larger deposits tend to infiltrate the adjacent elastic tissue and media. Others interpret the ultrastructural features of hyaline areriolosclerosis as evidence that the hyaline material is derived from increased basement membrane substance of endothelial and smooth muscle origin. Hyaline arteriolosclerosis is especially seen in the kidneys and other organs in patients with benign hypertension.

Hyperplastic arteriolosclerosis usually affects larger arterioles and is associated with severe hypertension, particularly with accelerated (or malignant) hypertension. It is characterized by cellular proliferation of the intima, hypertrophy of the muscle cells of the media, and fibrosis of the adventitia. The intimal change consists of concentric lamellae of fibroblasts and elastic fibers ("onionskin" appearance) associated with luminal narrowing. Recently in one electron microscopic study it was concluded that the increased cellularity of the intima results from the presence of smooth muscle cells migrating from the media and that there is a proliferation of smooth muscle cells in the media.

Both forms of arteriolosclerosis may coexist in a tissue, e.g., in a patient who has had benign hypertension for years and then suddenly develops acceleration of the hypertension. Fibrinoid necrosis of the arterioles ("necrotizing arteriolitis") may also be noted in arteriolosclerosis, particularly in cases of malignant hypertension.

Endarteritis obliterans. The use of the term *endarteritis obliterans* is not really correct, since it implies an inflammatory process, which is not present in the conditions so designated. The term applies to a localizing process affecting small arteries that is characterized by intimal thickening and narrowing or obliteration of the lumen. Such may be seen in atherosclerosis involving the muscular arteries of the lower extremities, often associated with superimposed thrombosis. Known as "arteriosclerosis obliterans," this may interfere with the flow of blood and, if collateral circulation is inadequate, may cause serious ischemic changes. Intimal proliferative thickening may be seen in small arteries in areas of chronic inflammation, e.g., adjacent to tuberculous cavities of the lung or in the base of a peptic ulcer. It also develops in the blood vessels of a region where active circulation is no longer needed, i.e., as an involutionary change in vessels whose capillary beds have been reduced by tissue atrophy. Hence it occurs in the hypogastric arteries and ductus arteriosus after birth, in the arteries of the uterus and ovaries in old age, and in involution of uterine arteries after pregnancy.

Inflammation of arteries

Acute nonspecific arteritis. Acute inflammation of an artery may arise from local *bacterial infections,* which spread to involve vessel walls. It may also result from intravascular spread of infections, as in septicemia or embolism. Complications of infec-

Fig.
12-4

Fig.
12-5

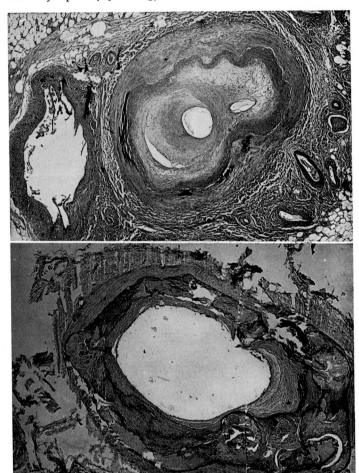

Fig. 12-4. Arteriosclerosis obliterans. Significant intimal proliferation ("endarteritis") of the anterior tibial artery. Organized thrombus surrounds the larger luminal opening. Dry gangrene of the great toe in a 73-year-old Negro woman. (From Gore, I.: Blood and lymphatic vessels. In Anderson, W. A. D., editor: Pathology, ed. 5, St. Louis, 1966, The C. V. Mosby Co.)

Fig. 12-5. Arteriosclerosis obliterans. Note the excessive medial calcification of the tibial artery. Gangrene and cellulitis of the great toe and dry gangrene of the fourth and fifth toes in an 82-year-old white man. (From Gore, I.: Blood and lymphatic vessels. In Anderson, W. A. D., editor: Pathology, ed. 5, St. Louis, 1966, The C. V. Mosby Co.)

tious arteritis include thrombosis, rupture with hemorrhage, and aneurysmal formation (so-called "mycotic" aneurysms). Other microorganisms, e.g., *rickettsiae,* and noninfectious agents, e.g., *trauma* and *chemicals,* may also produce acute nonspecific arteritis.

Chronic arteritis. Chronic arteritis of the granulomatous type may be seen in *tuberculosis* and *syphilis.* The important lesion in syphilis is aortitis, characterized mainly by a chronic necrotizing and fibrosing inflammation, although small gummatous granulomas are sometimes seen.

Necrotizing arteritis. Acute arteritis associated with necrosis of the vascular wall, usually of the fibrinoid type, is a characteristic of certain hypersensitivity reactions (as with sulfonamides, other drugs, and foreign serum). A similar type of vasculitis may be seen in the group of so-called "collagen diseases," in which altered immunity plays a role, e.g., in rheumatic fever, systemic lupus erythematosus, polyarteritis nodosa, and rheumatoid arthritis. In the last-named disease, in addition to acute arterial and arteriolar lesions, there may be an aortitis with aortic in-

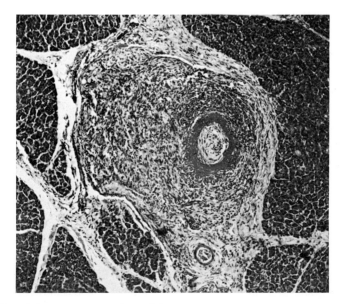

Fig. 12-6. Polyarteritis nodosa of the pancreas.

sufficiency similar to that seen in syphilis, particularly in cases of "rheumatoid" ankylosing spondylitis.

Polyarteritis nodosa. Polyarteritis nodosa (periarteritis nodosa) is an acute inflammation with degeneration and necrosis involving the walls of medium-sized and small arteries. Various organs and tissues may be involved, but most frequently affected are the kidneys, heart, liver, gastrointestinal tract, muscles, and peripheral nerves. These tissues may be involved together or successively. The variety of organ involvement produces clinical pictures, which are of great variability and are difficult to diagnose. Biopsy of a nodule from skin or muscle frequently enables clinical recognition. The condition may occur at any age. It is estimated that in about 10% of cases there is recovery.

The etiology has been variously ascribed to a specific virus, rheumatic fever, streptococci, and allergy. Frequent association of the condition with asthma or other allergic states and similarity to vascular changes in known hypersensitivity reactions favor the hypothesis that it may be a severe manifestation of hypersensitivity.

The inflammatory changes have been thought in some instances to begin in the adventitia and in other cases in the intima or innermost part of the media. Acute, subacute, chronic, and healed stages have been described. The earliest, or acute, phase is characterized by fibrinoid necrosis, usually beginning in the media. In the subacute stage there is cellular exudation. Eosinophils are the most characteristic cells of the inflammatory reaction, but lymphocytes, plasma cells, and neutrophilic leukocytes may be present. The occurrence of plasma cells, in view of their role in antibody production, may be evidence of the hypersensitivity mechanism. Exudation is followed by proliferative changes around the vessel, and also of the intima. Thrombosis often occurs. Occlusion of the lumen and infarction are common results. In the chronic phase granulation tissue develops and healing begins. Absorption of exudate and fibrosis result in the final healed condition. When various organs are involved successively, the several stages may be evident in the different organs.

Yellowish red nodules, which occur on the affected vessels, are usually caused by small localized dilatations or aneurysms at points of degeneration, inflammation, and weakening of the vessel wall. Nodules may be formed also by the localized cellular infiltration and proliferation. Rupture of one of the aneurysmal nodules may result in serious hemorrhage.

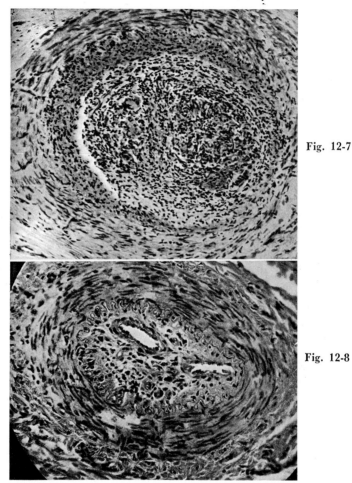

Fig. 12-7

Fig. 12-8

Fig. 12-7. Thromboangiitis obliterans (Buerger's disease) in the digital artery of the finger. Early proliferative phase in the organization of a thrombus. Note the presence of giant cells. (From Gore, I.: Blood and lymphatic vessels. In Anderson, W. A. D., editor: Pathology, ed. 5, St. Louis, 1966, The C. V. Mosby Co.)

Fig. 12-8. Thromboangiitis obliterans (Buerger's disease). Canalization of an organized thrombus. Lymphocytes, fibroblasts, and endothelial cells are present in the central mass. Note the characteristic wavy internal elastic membrane. Gangrene and ulceration of the thumb in a 30-year-old white man. (From Gore, I.: Blood and lymphatic vessels. In Anderson, W. A. D., editor: Pathology, ed. 5, St. Louis, 1966, The C. V. Mosby Co.)

Temporal arteritis. Temporal or cranial (giant cell) arteritis is a granulomatous inflammatory process affecting mainly temporal or other cranial arteries. It occurs chiefly in older age groups, is usually self-limited, and has a better outlook than that in polyarteritis nodosa, but it may be complicated by blindness in one or both eyes because of involvement of the retinal arteries. The affected vessels show an inflammatory infiltrate, chiefly lymphocytes, in the intima and inner part of the media and a disruption of the internal elastic lamina associated with multinucleate giant cells. Eosinophils are usually absent from the exudate. There may be patchy necrosis of the media. Fibrous healing of the inflammation causes luminal narrowing. Thrombosis may occur.

Thromboangiitis obliterans. Buerger introduced the term *thromboangiitis obliterans* to describe an inflammatory condition of the vessels of the extremities, in which thrombosis and later fibrosis interfere with the blood supply to the limbs. The condition occurs almost exclusively in males who are tobacco smokers. The etiology is uncertain. By some it has been considered a specific infection, and others believe that allergy to tobacco plays an important role. Buerger's disease usually begins before 35 years of age and appears unrelated to the occurrence of arteriosclerosis. It may affect arms as well as legs, produces severe pain in the involved extremities, and is closely correlated in its progression with a continuation of smoking or in lack of progression with abstinence from smoking. Small and medium-sized vessels of upper and lower extremities are segmentally involved. Evidence of atherosclerosis is usually lacking.

An acute lesion has been described as a fresh or incompletely organized thrombus containing multiple tiny abscesses (microabscesses). These are foci of neutrophilic leukocytes, usually surrounded by mononuclear epithelioid cells and sometimes multinucleated giant cells. Later the neutrophilic leukocytic foci disappear, although the epithelioid cell nodules may remain.

In this early stage an inflammatory infiltrate may involve all coats of a segment of a deep artery and adjacent vein. There is rarely any necrosis in the vessel wall. The inner elastic lamina is intact. The process advances to a proliferative stage with organization and healing by fibrosis. Usually arteries, veins, and nerves become bound together in a dense fibrous scar. Some recanalization of the lumen often develops. Venous valves are damaged and disrupted by the inflammation and organization of thrombi.

The early acute phase may give little clinical evidence of its presence. Following thrombosis and organization, insufficient blood supply to the extremity may result in pain on exercise (intermittent claudication) or even gangrene of the ischemic tissues. The degree of circulatory disturbance is largely influenced by the amount of collateral circulation that can be established.

Neurogenic arterial disease

Raynaud's disease. Raynaud's disease or syndrome is characterized by symmetric pallor of both hands (rarely the feet), accompanied by numbness, tingling, and burning sensations, caused by functional vasospasm of the arterioles. Cyanosis, redness, and even ischemic necrosis may ensue. The disease occurs chiefly in young women; the cause is unknown but exposure to cold and emotional stimuli may initiate the attacks.

Raynaud's phenomenon. Raynaud's phenomenon, in which there are similar symptoms caused by vascular spasm, is secondary to known diseases or conditions, e.g., Buerger's disease, arteriosclerosis obliterans, trauma (in typists, pianists, pneumatic hammer operators), Sudeck's bone atrophy, cervical rib syndrome, progressive systemic sclerosis (generalized scleroderma), systemic lupus erythematosus, ergotism, polyarteritis nodosa, etc.

Aneurysm

An aneurysm is a localized abnormal, persistent dilatation of a vessel, usually an artery. The dilatation, resulting from a weakness of the vessel wall, may be saccular, fusiform, or cylindrical. In the typical aneurysm all layers of the vessel wall are included. Certain lesions, called false aneurysm and arteriovenous aneurysm, are not true aneurysms in the sense of the foregoing definition. A dissecting aneurysm is not a typical aneurysm, in that there is not a dilatation including all layers of the vascular wall, but there is some distention of the outer portion of the wall. The *causes* of arterial aneurysms include atherosclerosis, syphilis, cystic medial necrosis, acute bacterial infections, congenital weakness of the wall, and trauma. The aorta is the most common site of aneurysms. Aneurysms may also arise in the heart wall, usually the left ventricle, as a result of a myocardial infarct.

Atherosclerotic aneurysm. Today atherosclerotic aneurysm is the most common form of aortic aneurysm because of the lowered incidence of syphilis (formerly the commonest cause)

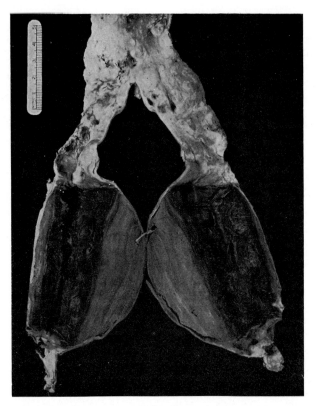

Fig. 12-9. Atherosclerotic aneurysm of the abdominal aorta. Aorta and aneurysm have been bisected lengthwise to show the laminated thrombus almost filling the sac. Note the channel kept open by force of the bloodstream. (From Gore, I.: Blood and lymphatic vessels. In Anderson, W. A. D., editor: Pathology, ed. 5, St. Louis, 1966, The C. V. Mosby Co.)

and because of the increasing age of mankind. It occurs most commonly in men, usually in the sixth or seventh decade or beyond. Aneurysms result when the atheromatous lesions are severe enough to produce destruction and weakening of the underlying media. They are usually of the fusiform type, less frequently saccular, and often contain laminated thrombi. The thrombus may not completely obstruct the lumen of a large vessel such as the aorta, although it may occlude the ostia of its

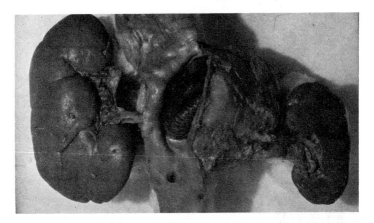

Fig. 12-10. Saccular aneurysm of the aorta obstructing the renal artery. Note the laminated thrombus in the aneurysmal sac, atrophy of the right kidney, and hypertrophy of the left kidney. The aortic intima above the aneurysm shows the characteristic "tree-bark" roughening of syphilitic aortitis.

branching vessels; but it may obstruct the lumen of a small artery (e.g., popliteal artery), affected by an aneurysm. By far the commonest site of an atherosclerotic aneurysm is the abdominal aorta, especially the infrarenal segment, although the thoracic aorta and other arteries (e.g., popliteal artery) may be other sites. The serious complications include compression of adjacent structures and rupture with hemorrhage and, in some instances, thrombotic occlusion and thromboembolism.

Syphilitic aneurysm. Syphilitic aneurysm, a late manifestation of syphilis, usually involves the first portion or the arch of the aorta, although the abdominal aorta or other vessels are occasionally affected. The localized dilatation is caused by weakening of the media by destruction of the elastic tissue. Disruption and loss of elastic fibers are evident microscopically in the wall of the aneurysm. The media of the vessel is partially replaced by connective tissue. The saccular variety is most common. It increases progressively in size, causing atrophy and erosion of any structure on which it impinges, including bony tissue. Thrombosis in successive layers occurs in the aneurysmal sac. This serves to strengthen the wall to some extent, although there is little organization of the thrombus. Aneurysms have little direct effect

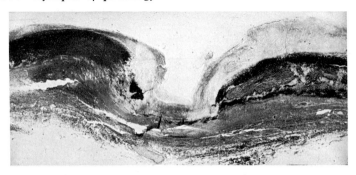

Fig. 12-11. Syphilitic aortitis with beginning aneurysm. Elastic tissue (stained black) of the media is destroyed in a local area, with bulging at the weakened point.

upon the heart or circulation, and symptoms usually result from the pressure and erosion of adjacent structures. The outcome is commonly perforation and death from hemorrhage.

Dissecting aneurysm. Dissecting aneurysm is produced by penetration of circulating blood into the wall of a vessel and its subsequent extension for varying distances along its length. It is simply a hemorrhage into the vessel wall itself, which by its force splits, or "dissects," the wall, causing a widening of the vessel. The aorta is the vessel commonly involved.

The dissection is through the media of the vessel, at the junction of the outer one third and inner two thirds, and extends for short or long distances proximally or distally. At the end of its dissection it may rupture externally by tearing through the outer portion of the wall. Less commonly it perforates again into the lumen. Sudden death results from perforation externally into surrounding tissues or into the pericardial sac (producing cardiac tamponade) when the first portion of the aorta is involved. Rupture back into the lumen occasionally leads to recovery, either through lining of the channel by endothelium or more rarely by thrombosis, organization, and fibrous obliteration of the channel.

About 70% of dissecting aneurysms begin in the ascending aorta. The primary intimal tear at this point is usually transverse, irregular, and 1 or 2 cm. in length. Dissection distal to the primary tear is longer than that proximal to the rupture, although some proximal dissection almost always occurs. In a few instances a primary intimal tear is absent. Since a large proportion of primary tears are 1 or 2 cm. above the aortic valve, the frequency of rupture into the pericardial sac is easily understood. Dissection distally may progress to the aortic bifurcation and beyond. Extension of the dissection into the origins of the branching arteries may cause obstruction of these vessels. If the hemorrhage ruptures back into the original aortic lumen, it does so through a secondary intimal (reentry) tear.

The underlying cause of dissecting aneurysm is some degenerative change or defect of the media. The medial changes have been described as a fatty degeneration and atrophy of muscle fibers, hyaline and mucoid degeneration of connective tissue, and swelling, fragmentation, and loss of staining power of elastic fibers. Peculiar areas of necrosis and mucoid degeneration are found in the media *(idiopathic cystic medionecrosis of aorta)*. These degenerative changes are without inflammatory reaction but are associated with necrosis and small cystlike spaces between the elastic fibers. Medial degenerative changes have been described in hypothyroidism. Syphilis is not an etiologic factor in dissecting aneurysm, but hypertension is present in a very high proportion of cases. Aortic dissection occurs most commonly in the fifth and sixth decades. One fourth of the cases occur before the age of 40 years and sometimes with pregnancy. There is also an association with Marfan's syndrome and with coarctation of the aorta.

The exciting cause is usually a sudden increase of blood pressure because of mental or physical stress; trauma is rarely a factor, although dissecting aneurysm is an occasional complication of carotid arteriography. The primary tear of the intima may start at an atheromatous ulcer, but this is unusual. Most investigators believe that rupture of the vasa vasorum in the weakened media is the initial event causing intramural hemorrhage and that the primary intimal tear is secondary to this.

Mycotic aneurysm. Aneurysms may occur in small arteries in which localized inflammation has produced sufficient weakening of the vessel wall. Such a process produces nodules in polyarteritis nodosa. When the vascular inflammation is caused by bacterial infection, the resultant aneurysm is called "mycotic." In mycotic aneurysm the inflammation is usually caused by the lodgment of an infected embolus or by infection of the wall by way of vasa vasorum. Occasionally extension of infection from inflamed aortic valves affects the sinuses of Valsalva or adjacent portions of the aorta, producing a mycotic aneurysm in that area which is often referred to as an "erosive aneurysm."

Congenital aneurysm. Congenital aneurysms occur particularly on superficial cerebral vessels, sometimes in miliary fashion. They are caused by a muscular defect in the media at points of bifurcation, a small saccular ("berry") aneurysm developing in the angle. In addition to the muscular defect, degeneration of the internal elastic membrane as a result of continued overstretching from blood pressure is necessary before aneurysm develops. The muscular defect, and not the aneurysm itself, is congenital. Rupture of such an aneurysm is an important cause of subarachnoid hemorrhage. Congenital aneurysms occasionally occur in the aorta, e.g., in the sinus of Valsalva.

Traumatic aneurysm. Weakening of the arterial wall caused by a penetrating or blunt injury may result in an aneurysm, usually saccular. The commonest site is the thoracic aorta, frequently related to the compression chest injuries sustained in automobile accidents.

False aneurysm. False aneurysm is an organized hematoma that communicates with the lumen of a blood vessel; i.e., the wall of the aneurysm is not composed of elements of the blood vessel wall. It occasionally follows a traumatic rupture of a small vessel, as by a knife or bullet.

Arteriovenous aneurysm. Arteriovenous aneurysm is really a fistula, or an abnormal communication, between an artery and a vein. Its usual cause is traumatic penetration of an adjacent artery and vein. It may arise from a rupture of an arterial aneurysm (e.g., aorta) into an adjacent vein (e.g., superior or inferior vena cava). Less commonly it may be a developmental anomaly or occur in a vascular neoplasm (glomus tumor). If vessels of a considerable size are involved, the direct arteriovenous shunt produces disturbance in circulation that may lead to cardiac hypertrophy. The artery and vein proximal to the fistula may become dilated.

Phlebitis

Inflammation of veins is often an extension of a local infection to involve their walls. Such an event is common in the infected puerperal uterus, or as a complication of appendicitis (pylephlebitis, or inflammation of the portal vein). Thrombosis usually develops in the infected veins, and spread of the infection may thus occur by infected emboli as well as directly along the vein wall. Phlebitis occasionally complicates acute systemic infectious diseases. Acute noninfectious phlebitis may also occur in hypersensitivity angiitis and as a result of trauma or chemical injury. Chronic nonspecific and granulomatous forms of phlebitis exist. Idiopathic phlebitis also occurs. An obliterative endophlebitis of small hepatic veins (veno-occlusive disease of the liver), probably caused by the ingestion of *Senecio* alkaloids, has been reported in Jamaica and elsewhere.

Venous thrombi. A thrombus may form in a vein as a result of phlebitis (*thrombophlebitis*) or may be caused by factors other than inflammation (*phlebothrombosis*). Obstruction of a major vein may cause chronic venous insufficiency. In a lower limb this may result in edema, induration, sometimes ossification, eczematous dermatitis, pigmentation, and ulceration. A rare complication, and one that occurs only when there is massive venous obstruction, is gangrene. Frequent, recurrent formation of thrombi in the same segment of a vein or, more often, in widely scattered areas of the body or the extremities is known as "thrombophlebitis migrans" (as occurs in thromboangiitis obliterans) or "phlebothrombosis migrans" (such as that related to visceral cancer). The association of visceral carcinoma with thrombosis in one or more major veins or with phlebothrombosis migrans is referred to as the *Trousseau syndrome*. The release of thromboplastin or proteolytic enzymes from the cancer site is regarded as the cause of thrombosis in this syndrome.

Varicose veins

Abnormally tortuous and dilated veins (*varicose veins* or *varicosities*) are produced by increased intravenous pressure and weakness of the vein walls. The condition is seen most frequently in the veins of the lower extremities, the hemorrhoidal veins, or the veins at the lower end of the esophagus.

Varicosities of the lower extremities, involving principally the superficial veins, are either *primary*, developing as a result of inherent weakness of the wall of veins and a relative increase in intravenous pressure, or *secondary* to venous obstruction (e.g., thrombosis or extrinsic pressure by tumors). Heredity may play a role in the incidence of varicose veins. Defects of venous valves are not usually the primary cause, except in rare cases of congenitally absent valves. Distortion of valves in thrombophlebitis may be contributory. Loss of supporting perivenous tissues (as in emaciation or advanced age) may contribute to varicosities. Thrombosis and chronic venous insufficiency are possible complications of varicose veins in the lower limbs.

Hemorrhoids are varicosities of hemorrhoidal veins. Varices at the lower end of the esophagus are common where there is obstruction in the portal circulation, as in cirrhosis of the liver. Rupture of one of these distended vessels with hemorrhage is a common terminal event in cirrhosis of the liver.

Superior vena cava obstruction

Obstruction of the superior vena cava interfering with the return flow of blood to the heart results in elevated venous pressure in the upper extremities and thorax, delayed circulation time in the upper half of the body, cyanosis and edema of the face, neck, and upper extremities, and distention of collateral venous channels (azygos, internal mammary, lateral thoracic and vertebral collateral routes) in the upper portion of the body. The obstruction is caused most frequently by intrathoracic neoplasms, lymphomas, and aortic aneurysms. Bronchogenic carcinoma is a relatively frequent basis of the obstruction caused by invasion of the venous wall by the tumor.

Lymphangitis

Inflammation of the lymphatics may appear in infections, and spread may occur from a local area along the lymphatics to the lymph nodes. When such inflammation is superficial, e.g., on the arm, the lymphatic involvement may be seen as reddish, painful streaks, and the lymph nodes of the axilla become enlarged and tender (see lymphadenitis, p. 543).

Lymphatic obstruction

Obstruction of lymphatic flow from an area results in retention of fluid in the part, which becomes enlarged and hard. Marked degrees of the enlargement are called elephantiasis and are commonest when the lymphatic obstruction is caused by filariae, although a similar effect is produced by inflammatory destruction of lymphatics. Idiopathic lymphedema (noninflammatory) occasionally occurs; it may be congenital or may develop later in life. Operative procedures may interfere with normal lymph drainage, and in the case of radical amputation of the breast an enlargement and brawny edema of the arm may result. Lymphangiosarcoma may complicate a severe prolonged lymphedema, of either idiopathic or postoperative origin.

Tumors of blood and lymphatic vessels

Angiomas are tumors made up of blood or lymph vessels (hemangiomas or lymphangiomas). They are often congenital and probably arise from embryonic rests of mesodermal tissue. Some may be simply vascular malformations, but many are true neoplasms. Angiomas are common in childhood. Lindau-von Hippel disease is a hereditary developmental defect in which hemangiomas occur in the brain, retina, and elsewhere. Also frequently found in this condition are cystic lesions of the kidneys and pancreas and hypernephroma of a kidney.

Hemangioma. There are several types of hemangiomas. *Capillary hemangioma* is composed of well-differentiated, thin-walled capillaries. It may appear as a dark red, elevated mass ("strawberry nevus") of the skin in infants, which tends to disappear spontaneously in later childhood, or it may show up as the typical "port wine stain," especially of the face and neck. *Cavernous hemangioma,* in which the vascular spaces are dilated, engorged blood sinuses, also occurs in the skin and is the common type in

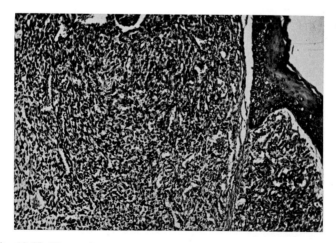

Fig. 12-12. Hemangioma of the skin. The squamous epithelial surface is evident on the right. The tumor is composed of tiny, thin-walled blood channels and proliferating endothelial cells.

internal organs such as the liver. *Hemangioendothelioma* is a form of capillary hemangioma in the young that consists of solid masses of proliferating endothelial cells, with only a few patent vessels. This type is seemingly locally invasive in its growth and may be misdiagnosed as a malignant tumor. *Sclerosing hemangioma* is a blood vessel tumor in which there is overgrowth of the collagenous connective tissue framework of the tumor. This results in occlusion of the vessels and breakdown of trapped red cells. Phagocytes containing hemosiderin pigment may be sufficiently numerous to give the tissue a brownish color. Other macrophages contain lipoid material. A few giant cells are usually present. The tumor must be differentiated from a melanoma or a xanthoma. *Kaposi's idiopathic hemorrhagic sarcoma* is considered on p. 817.

Lymphangioma. The three main types of lymphangioma are the simple, or *capillary,* the *cavernous,* and the *cystic (hygroma).* The capillary and cavernous types are similar to the corresponding hemangiomatous tumors but differ in the absence of red cells in their channels and in the frequent presence of lymph follicles and lymphocytes.

The cystic type of lymphangioma or hygroma occurs in the neck or axilla and is designated respectively as *hygroma colli*

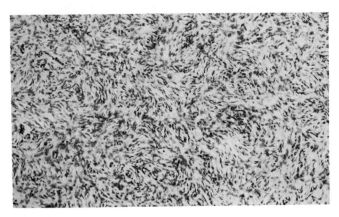

Fig. 12-13. Xanthofibroma (sclerosing hemangioma) of the skin. Elongated cells form a characteristic irregular curled pattern with many small vascular channels.

cysticum and *hygroma axillare*. Originating from lymphatic nests which retain embryonic power of irregular growth, they grow to be large, multilocular cystic tumors. Their cavities are lined by endothelium and contain straw-colored fluid. Lymphoid tissue is often abundant in the cyst walls.

Glomus tumor (angiomyoneuroma). The glomus is an arteriovenous anastomosis, found normally in the skin and concerned with temperature regulation. The glomus tumor, or angiomyoneuroma, arising from this structure occurs in the extremities and is characterized clinically by intense pain and

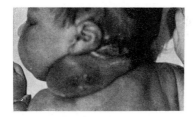

Fig. 12-14. Cystic hygroma of the neck.

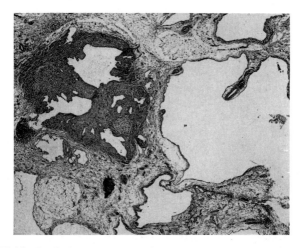

Fig. 12-15. Cystic hygroma. Irregular channels and cystic spaces containing lymph have a connective tissue stroma, which is mainly loose, but with denser areas and occasional accumulation of lymphocytes.

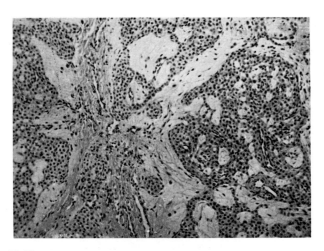

Fig. 12-16. Glomus tumor.

tenderness. Vasomotor phenomena and atrophic changes in the involved extremity are sometimes associated.

The tumors are composed of a tangled mass of blood vessels enclosed within a capsule. In the vessel walls are masses of peculiar cuboid or rounded glomus cells, probably derived from pericytes, and smooth muscle cells. Bundles of myelinated nerves are recognizable in or near the capsule of the tumor, from which slender, nonmyelinated fibers pass among the glomus cells and become continuous with their cytoplasm.

Hemangiopericytoma. Hemangiopericytoma is a vascular tumor composed of endothelial tubes surrounded by rounded or elongated cells believed to be derived from pericytes, as are the epithelioid cells of the glomus tumor. Pericytes, described by Zimmerman, are contractile cells wrapped about capillaries, which function in changing luminal size. Most examples have been benign, but local invasion and even metastases have been reported.

Angiosarcoma. In contrast to the benign angiomatous tumors, angiosarcomas are rare. Malignant hemangioendotheliomas occur mainly in adults, and relatively few cases have been reported in childhood. Lymphangiosarcoma is practically unknown in children. In adults, lymphangiosarcoma may develop in an area of severe persistent lymphedema of an extremity. This may occur as a rare complication of radical mastectomy for cancer of the breast.

DISEASES OF THE HEART
Cardiac failure

Cardiac failure is a clinical state in which the heart is unable to maintain an adequate circulation for bodily needs. It may be acute or chronic. *Acute heart failure* may be the result of sudden failure of the myocardium because of infarction, rapid pericardial hemorrhage (cardiac tamponade), obstruction to outflow as in massive pulmonary embolism, or inadequate venous return to the heart (as in various forms of shock). In acute failure caused by myocardial injury or massive pulmonary embolism there is a sudden reduction in cardiac output, the cardiac chambers dilate, and acute venous congestion ensues (acute congestive heart failure). In acute heart failure associated with shock the fall in cardiac output is evident, but acute venous congestion is not a manifestation, except in cardiac shock caused by myocardial injury (e.g., infarction), in which acute congestive failure may also be present.

Chronic (congestive) heart failure is the consequence of progressive diseases that weaken the heart directly or cause an increased demand on the heart, occurring most commonly in association with atherosclerotic coronary heart disease, hypertensive cardiopathy, and valvular deformities. The clinical picture is related to hemodynamic changes, namely those concerned with blood flow and pressure relations throughout the cardiovascular system, and disturbances in the body fluids and electrolytes.

To explain the development of the manifestations of congestive heart failure, two mechanisms have been suggested in the past that are known as "backward failure" and "forward failure." According to the *backward failure* theory, there is an increase in diastolic pressure within the failing ventricle or ventricles, followed by a rise in atrial pressure that is transmitted backward, producing an elevated pressure in the veins. In *forward failure* the manifestations result from failure of the heart to pump a sufficient output, causing a diminished flow of blood to the tissues, particularly to the kidneys. Actually these two mechanisms do not function independently of each other, since in a continuous circulation one does not occur without the other. Whenever the cardiovascular system makes sufficient adjustments to maintain adequate output, a state of *compensation* is reached. The principal compensatory phenomena are tachycardia, cardiac dilatation, and cardiac hypertrophy. When the adjustments are inadequate, a state of cardiac *decompensation* is said to exist.

Heart failure may involve either side of the heart separately or the entire heart, but in the latter the features frequently are predominantly those of right-sided heart failure. In *left-sided heart failure* the major manifestations are those associated with passive congestion and edema of the lungs. In more severe cases, pulmonary hypertension results, leading to failure of the right side of the heart. *Right-sided heart failure* is frequently combined with that of the left, although there are instances in which it is isolated. The manifestations of right-sided heart failure include subcutaneous edema (particularly in the dependent parts of the body), hydrothorax, ascites, passive congestion of the liver and spleen, generalized venous congestion, cyanosis, and usually, increased blood volume. The cardiac output in typical congestive heart failure is usually reduced, although in some patients at rest it may be normal. Cardiac failure associated with diminished output is called "low output heart failure." Cardiac failure associated with hyperthyroidism, arteriovenous shunts (including arteriovenous fistulas and the vascular shunts in the bones in Paget's disease, or osteitis deformans), and severe anemias may be accompanied by an elevated cardiac output; thus it is given the designation "high output heart failure."

The pathogenesis of edema in cardiac failure is an intriguing problem that has held the interest of investigators for a long time but is still not completely solved. For many years the edema has been explained as a consequence of increased venous pressure, leading to a rise in capillary blood pressure, increased filtration, and edema. Although increased venous pressure plays a part in the development of edema, the emphasis today is upon the importance of retention of sodium and water in the body. The role of intrinsic renal mechanisms and hormonal or neural factors (e.g., reduction in glomerular filtration rate, enhanced renal tubular reabsorption of sodium, hypersecretion of aldosterone or a decrease in the rate of inactivation of aldosterone by the liver, and an increased release of antidiuretic hormone) has been discussed in Chapter 4.

Congenital heart disease

Congenital malformations of the heart are usually either (1) abnormalities of the great vessels or their valves, (2) failure of completion of the septa between atria or ventricles, or (3) anomalies of the size or position of the heart. Frequently two or more cardiac anomalies occur in association. In 10 to 15% of patients with congenital heart disease, anomalies exist in other parts of the body. Defects that cause a shunt of blood from the venous to the arterial side (i.e., from right to left) are commonly associated with cyanosis. The main factor in the cyanosis is the admixture of venous and arterial blood in the peripheral circulation. The oxygen deficiency gives rise to a compensatory increase both in the number of red cells in the blood (polycythemia) and in their average size. Clubbing of the ends of fingers and toes is also common in such cases. Other manifestations of congenital heart disease are dyspnea on exertion, poor feeding, lack of weight gain, and cardiac murmurs. Serious complications include congestive heart failure, bacterial endocarditis, paradoxical embolism, cerebral abscess (even in the absence of bacterial endocarditis), pulmonary tuberculosis, rupture of the aorta or cerebral arteries, cerebral embolism and infarction, and sudden death.

Congenital heart disease occurs in about five per 1,000 live births. Most cardiac anomalies have their inception during the fifth to eighth weeks of embryonic life. Intrinsic factors of faulty germ plasm or hereditary tendencies are important etiologically in some cases. Marfan's syndrome (arachnodactyly) is frequently associated with abnormalities of the great vessels or heart. In mongolism and Turner's syndrome, both related to chromosomal aberrations, cardiovascular anomalies are often seen. Extrinsic factors such as viral infections and the ingestion of certain drugs by the mother appear to be etiologically important in other cases. German measles in the mother during the first two months of pregnancy is associated with a significant incidence of congenital cardiac effects. Thalidomide, taken during the early weeks of pregnancy, is associated with cardiac septal defects as well as with phocomelia, a deformity of the limbs.

An anatomic classification of congenital heart disease (modified from Abbott) is as follows:

Anomalies of the heart as a whole
   Ectopia cordis
   Dextrocardia
   Congenital idiopathic hypertrophy
   Endocardial fibroelastosis
   Congenital rhabdomyoma

Defects of atrial and ventricular septa
    Patent foramen ovale
    Defects of atrial septum
    Persistent ostium atrioventriculare commune
    Localized defects of ventricular septum (maladie de Roger)
        Eisenmenger's complex
    Congenital aneurysms of ventricular septum
Truncus arteriosus or anomalous development of the great vessels
Transposition of the arterial trunks
Pulmonary stenosis and atresia
    Tetralogy of Fallot
Aortic and mitral atresia with rudimentary left ventricle
    Tricuspid atresia with rudimentary right ventricle
Anomalies of chordae and endocardium
    Chiari's network
    Fenestration of semilunar valves
    Subaortic stenosis
    Bicuspid aortic valve
Patent ductus arteriosus
Coarctation of the aorta
Anomalies of the coronary arteries

The following include some of the commonest forms of clinical congenital heart disease and are amenable to surgical treatment.

Pulmonary stenosis. Isolated pulmonary stenosis is usually valvular and associated with an intact ventricular septum. Less frequently there is stenosis of the infundibulum of the right ventricle. The right ventricle becomes hypertrophied, and there often is poststenotic dilatation of the pulmonary trunk. If a patent foramen ovale or an atrial septal defect is present, a right to left shunt and cyanosis may develop. Sometimes a defect of the ventricular septum or a patent ductus arteriosus may be associated with pulmonary stenosis. An uncommon cause of obstruction to the flow of blood from the right ventricle is stenosis of the main pulmonary artery or its branches.

Patent ductus arteriosus. Normally during fetal life, blood passes from the pulmonary artery through the ductus arteriosus to the aorta, thus bypassing the lungs. Obliteration of the channel occurs a few weeks after birth. When it remains open, it is often associated with other defects, such as pulmonary stenosis or patent septa. The abnormal left to right shunt at the ductus level causes increased work of the left ventricle and hypertrophy of that chamber, as well as enlargement of the pulmonary artery and its branches. If pulmonary hypertension develops, there results hypertrophy of the right ventricle, a reversed shunt (right to left), and cyanosis.

Aortic stenosis and coarctation of the aorta. Narrowing of the aortic opening (valvular, subvalvular, or supravalvular) is less common than pulmonary stenosis and causes left ventricular hypertrophy. Narrowing of the aorta beyond the valve (coarctation of the aorta) occurs in infantile and adult types. In the infantile type there is a narrowing of the aorta between the origin of the left subclavian artery and the insertion of the ductus arteriosus. This narrowing is an exaggeration of the normal fetal condition. This form is associated with other cardiovascular anomalies and is fatal early in infancy. In the adult type there is a sharp constriction of the aorta, just proximal, at, or immediately distal to the insertion of the ductus arteriosus. This form is compatible with long life. Compensatory collateral circulation develops through internal mammary and intercostal vessels, and the left ventricle hypertrophies. In some cases the ductus arteriosus may be patent.

Atrial septal defects. It is frequently found that the foramen ovale has remained open but with a competent although unfused valve. In such cases no important transseptal leakage occurs. However, with a widely patent, inadequately guarded foramen ovale, a shunt of blood from left to right occurs, with enlargement of the right atrium, the right ventricle, and the pulmonary artery. The left ventricle remains relatively small. Other types of atrial septal defects are a persistent ostium primum in the lower end of the septum, a defect high in the septum (sinus venosus type), or an absence of the entire atrial septum. When a septal defect is complicated by pulmonary hypertension, the shunt may be reversed (right to left). An atrial septal defect combined with mitral stenosis (acquired or congenital) is known as Lutembacher's syndrome.

Ventricular septal defects. Patency of the ventricular septum, usually in its upper membranous portion, is a common anomaly. Small defects may cause little disturbance. Large defects cause hypertrophy of the left and right ventricles as a result of a left to right shunt. The defect may be associated with cyanosis if pulmonary hypertension and reversal of the shunt occur as a result of increased pulmonary vascular resistance. In some instances it is believed that the pulmonary vascular resistance is caused by an abnormal persistence of the fetal vascular pattern rather than by increased pulmonary blood flow.

Tetralogy of Fallot. The tetralogy of Fallot is a common association of defects that includes (1) a patent ventricular sep-

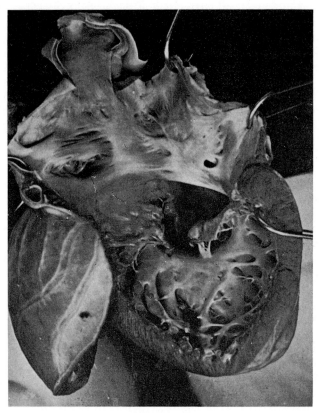

Fig. 12-17. Congenital defect of the ventricular septum (ostium atrio-ventriculare commune). (Courtesy Dr. V. Moragues.)

tum, (2) pulmonary stenosis (infundibular or valvular), (3) relative displacement of the aorta to the right so that it tends to lie above the patent part of the ventricular septum, and (4) hypertrophy of the right ventricle. Depending on whether the pulmonary stenosis is severe or mild, the patient may be cyanotic or acyanotic. Pulmonary artery atresia may be present in some cases. In severe pulmonary stenosis or pulmonary artery atresia, collateral circulation to the lungs is through the bronchial arteries or other aortic branches. A patent ductus arteriosus may be present.

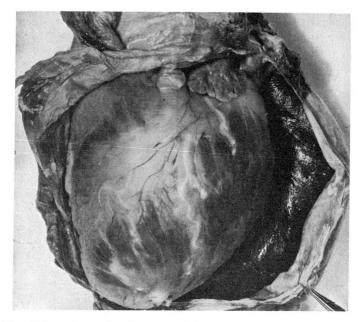

Fig. 12-18. Hemopericardium caused by the rupture of an aneurysm into the pericardial sac.

Lesions of the pericardium

Abnormalities of the pericardium are frequently secondary to diseases elsewhere; but they may be primary.

Serous atrophy of pericardial fat. In any chronic disease with severe emaciation, the subepicardial fat may be reduced in amount, and it acquires a watery, translucent gelatinous character.

Hydropericardium. The pericardial sac normally contains about 30 to 50 ml. of fluid. The presence of more than 100 ml. is called hydropericardium, and amounts as large as 1 or 2 liters may accumulate. The usual cause is cardiac failure. It also occurs in the nephrotic syndrome, in hypoproteinemic states, and as a result of mediastinal lesions obstructing pericardial venous circulation. Large amounts present some interference with the heart's action and reduce inflow by pressure on incoming veins.

Hemopericardium. Petechial hemorrhages of the pericardium are common in many toxic, infectious, and asphyxial conditions.

Actual hemorrhage into the pericardial sac (hemopericardium) may result from cardiac rupture after infarction, rupture of a saccular or dissecting aneurysm of the aorta into the pericardium, or trauma of the heart and great vessels. The effect depends upon the rate of hemorrhage as well as on the amount. Acute hemorrhage with rapid accumulation in the sac of 200 or 300 ml. may interfere with cardiac action and cause death from acute heart failure (cardiac tamponade). The hemorrhage causes a rapid rise of pressure outside the heart that, when it exceeds the venous pressure, prevents the heart's filling in diastole. At autopsy the pericardial sac and the great veins are distended with blood, but the heart is contracted and empty. Slow leakage of a liter or more of blood into the sac may interfere less with the heart's action.

Acute pericarditis. Acute pericarditis may be caused by rheumatic fever, pyemia, certain infectious diseases, and spread from adjacent inflammations of pleura, lung, mediastinum, and myocardium. Mild pericarditis is usual over myocardial infarctions, and sometimes occurs in uremia. These various causes usually produce a fibrinous or serofibrinous exudate, except for pyogenic infections which tend to produce fibrinopurulent or purulent pericarditis. When the exudate is predominantly fibrinous, movements of the heart form the fibrin into cords or villi, and the surface of the heart and parietal pericardium have a peculiarly shaggy appearance. This is often referred to as "bread-and-butter" appearance. Frequently encountered in clinical practice is acute nonspecific (or "benign") pericarditis, which is usually serofibrinous. In most cases the cause is undetermined; some are attributed to a viral origin.

Tuberculous pericarditis. Tuberculous pericarditis is usually caused by an extension from adjacent lung, pleura, or mediastinal lymph nodes. It is a chronic serofibrinous pericarditis, characterized by very distinct thickening of visceral and parietal layers. Tuberculous granulomatous lesions are seen in the thick pericardial walls at the base of the exudate. Organization of the latter often results in firm pericardial adhesions; but localized pockets of fluid or liquefied caseous debris may be present.

Chronic pericarditis and pericardial scars. True chronic pericarditis does exist but more commonly seen are the scars or adhesions of a previous acute pericarditis. The scars are usually whitish irregular areas of fibrosis on the anterior surfaces of the ventricles and often are called "soldier's spots" or "milk plaques."

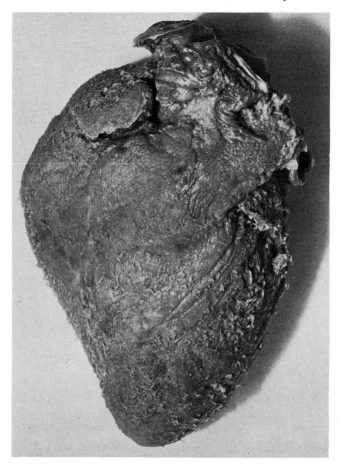

Fig. 12-19. Acute fibrinous pericarditis. Note the shaggy coat of fibrin covering the surface of the heart.

They represent areas of organized and scarred pericardial exudate.

Adhesions between visceral and parietal layers of pericardium may vary from just a few bands to complete obliteration of the sac. *Adherent pericardium* (so-called "chronic adhesive peri-carditis") seldom, if ever, causes embarrassment or hypertrophy of the heart, except possibly in some instances where prominent

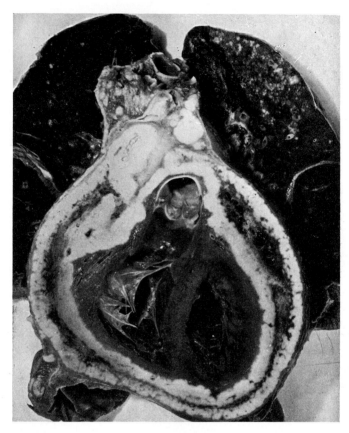

Fig. 12-20. Tuberculous pericarditis. Note the tremendous thickening of the visceral and parietal pericardium, the massive caseation of the mediastinal lymph nodes, and the tuberculous areas in lung tissue.

adhesions extend to adjacent structures, e.g., mediastinum and thoracic cage ("chronic mediastinopericarditis"). *Chronic constrictive pericarditis* (Pick's disease) is a condition in which fibrous thickening of the pericardium mechanically interferes with the heart action and the circulation. Entering veins are constricted, and increased systemic venous pressure, chronic hepatic congestion, ascites, and hydrothorax develop. Similar progressive hyaline thickening and adhesions may involve the serosa over the spleen, liver, and undersurface of the diaphragm.

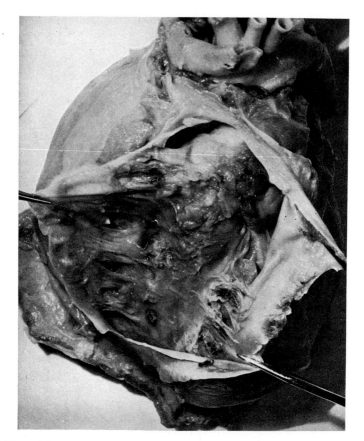

Fig. 12-21. Adhesive pericarditis. The pericardial sac has been opened, and the fibrous bands joining the visceral and parietal pericardium are evident.

The cause in most cases is unknown (idiopathic), but often it is tuberculous or purulent pericarditis. Polyserositis of unknown cause (Concato's disease) is characterized by large effusions into the various serous cavities, including pericardium. It may terminate in constrictive pericarditis.

Rheumatic fever

Rheumatic fever is a systemic, poststreptococcic, nonsuppurative inflammatory disease that seriously affects the heart and also involves arteries, joints, tendons, subcutaneous tissues, and nervous system. It is usually acquired in childhood (especially 4 to 15 years of age) and is widespread in temperate zones but less common in warm climates. It is the chief cause of heart disease in persons under 40 years of age.

Etiology. The cause of rheumatic fever is still not completely solved. It is generally agreed that it occurs after infection (frequently nasopharyngitis) with Group A beta-hemolytic streptococci. The lesions of rheumatic fever are not the result of direct infection by these organisms but represent an allergic or hypersensitivity reaction. Experimental cardiac lesions similar to those of rheumatic fever have been produced by sensitization of animals to foreign proteins. The human disease occurs usually after a latent period of two or three weeks after the streptococcal infection, and elevated titers of antibodies to antigens of Group A beta-hemolytic streptococci can be demonstrated. The prevalent view is that the organisms have the ability, in some way, to stimulate production of antibodies in the host that react with its own tissue (autoantibodies). Certain investigators have suggested that a virus or a virus acting in synergy with streptococci may be the cause of rheumatic fever. In addition to age and climate, mentioned previously, there are other predisposing factors that may play a role in increasing the incidence of rheumatic fever, including poor socioeconomic conditions (overcrowding, poor nutrition) and possibly hereditary susceptibility.

Characteristic lesions. Characteristic lesions of rheumatic fever are innumerable minute foci of injury to interstitial and supporting tissues, i.e., collagen and its supporting ground substance throughout the body. The heart and blood vessels especially are susceptible. In the early phases the inflammatory reaction is exudative (edema and increased acid mucopolysaccharide), but there may follow a degenerative and proliferative type of reaction. In the most severe foci of injury there occurs a degenerative change in connective tissue (swelling and fragmentation of collagen, fibrinoid degeneration) and proliferation of histiocytic cells, forming a "submiliary" granuloma. In their characteristic form, as may be seen in the myocardium, each of these minute nodules of proliferative inflammation is known as an Aschoff body. The eventual result is fibrosis.

Rheumatic heart disease. Death may occur during the acute phase of rheumatic fever, but most deaths occur years after the acute attack and are caused by valve deformities. The cardiac involvement is a *pancarditis;* i.e., pericardium, myocardium, and endocardium are injured. *Pericarditis* is important mainly in acute phases; it is a fibrinous, sometimes serofibrinous, sterile form. Healing results in fibrous adhesions with partial or complete obliteration of the pericardial cavity. The *myocarditis* is characterized by the presence of specific Aschoff bodies, widespread damage to the interstitial collagen framework of the myocardium, and the development of areas of fibrosis. Foci of nonspecific myocarditis and of necrosis of muscle fibers may also be seen in the active disease. The myocardial fibrosis partly results from the involvement of coronary vessels, as well as from fibrous change in Aschoff nodules, producing a weakened heart muscle. The *endocarditis* very commonly leads to mitral stenosis and often to aortic stenosis, but only occasionally does it deform the tricuspid or pulmonary valve. These serious valvular deformities along with myocardial involvement result in a failure of the circulation.

The Aschoff body, as it occurs in the myocardium, is an oval or elongated nodule of microscopic size, situated interstitially between muscle fibers and often adjacent to a small blood vessel. Swelling, degeneration, and fragmentation of collagenous fibers and the presence of Aschoff cells are characteristic features. The Aschoff cells are large, elongated, and irregular, often have multiple vesicular nuclei, and have granular basophilic cytoplasm. These proliferative cells are usually considered to be derived from cardiac (Anitschkow) histiocytes or primitive resting mesenchymal cells, although certain investigators have suggested that they may be derived from injured myocardial fibers. Lymphocytes, plasma cells, or even neutrophilic leukocytes also may be present in acute phases. Gradual replacement of the Aschoff cells by fibroblasts results in a tiny fibrous scar in which lymphocytes may persist for many months. Aschoff bodies occurring in the heart elsewhere than in the myocardium are composed of the same elements but are less regularly arranged and are of a different shape and distribution; hence they are less easily recognized. Granulomatous foci in extracardiac lesions may be suggestive of, but should not be confused with, Aschoff bodies.

Rheumatic endocarditis. The mitral valve is involved most frequently; the mitral and aortic valves combined, next; the aortic valve alone, less frequently; and still less commonly, the tricuspid and pulmonary valves. The earliest changes are in the

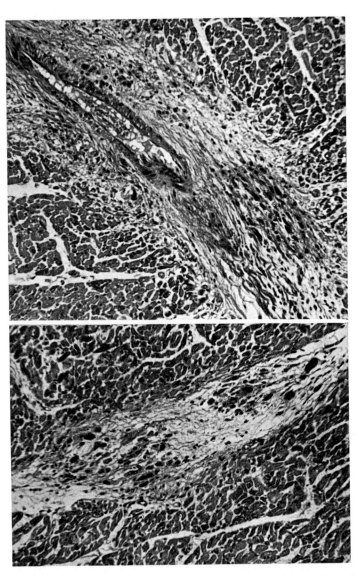

Fig. 12-22. Aschoff bodies in the myocardium. Note the perivascular position in the upper figure and the characteristic large dark cells.

subendothelial layers, with degeneration of connective tissue and proliferative activity. The inflammation spreads throughout the whole valve substance, and histologically it shows edema, alteration of collagen, fibrinoid change, an exudate of macrophages, plasma cells, and lymphocytes, with occasional neutrophils and the formation of young capillaries. Aschoff cells may be seen, but rarely well-formed Aschoff bodies. The endothelium is destroyed. Vegetations form at the line of contact of the leaflets (i.e., areas of trauma), usually 1 to 5 mm. from the free margin. These vegetations are multiple, firm, small, smooth, warty masses, which consist mainly of platelets and fibrin; bacteria are absent. Being firm and not crumbly, they do not give rise to emboli. Areas of hyalinization and necrosis develop within the inflamed tissue. Healing of the inflammation results in a thick, distorted, retracted, and insufficient valve. Severe degrees of stenosis are a particularly common result in the mitral valve. Bacterial endocarditis or nonbacterial thrombotic endocarditis may be superimposed on healed valvular lesions. These complications, as well as mural thrombi in the left atrium or its appendage (especially in mitral stenosis), may give rise to emboli. Frequently the mural endocardium is also involved. The endocardium of the left atrium, just above the posterior leaflet of the

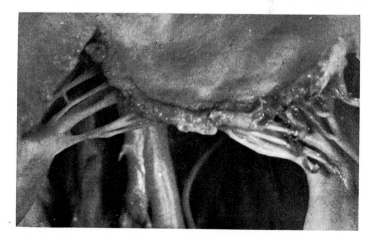

Fig. 12-23. Rheumatic vegetations on the mitral valve. (Courtesy Dr. V. Moragues.)

mitral valve, is often thickened and irregular (MacCallum's patch). The microscopic picture is similar to that seen in the valves. Chordae tendineae also are involved and eventually become shortened and fibrous. Biopsy of the left atrial appendage at the time of surgical valvulotomy for mitral stenosis frequently shows Aschoff bodies, even in cases that clinically have not appeared to be active.

Extracardiac rheumatic lesions. "Growing pains," a frequent minor manifestation of rheumatic fever in children, result from synovitis of the hamstring tendons. Heel pain is caused by synovitis of the bursa of the Achilles tendon. Fibromyositis also occurs. Small subcutaneous nodules are often present and consist of a central necrotic area with fibrinoid change, surrounded by histiocytes and fibroblasts in a radial, palisade arrangement.

In joint involvement (rheumatic polyarthritis) the synovial membranes are swollen and hyperemic. The increased fluid in the joint is cloudy but not purulent. Degenerative and necrotic changes and granulomatous formations are present in deeper structures; these are somewhat similar to Aschoff bodies. Ankles, knees, and wrists are most often affected.

Involvement of the nervous system, clinically called Sydenham's chorea (Saint Vitus' dance), is a diffuse meningoencephalitis, which is rarely fatal. Aschoff bodies are not found in the nervous system, but one sees congestion and thrombosis of small vessels, endothelial proliferation, and perivascular round cell infiltration.

Pleural involvement is very common in rheumatic fever. Rheumatic pleurisy is usually associated with effusion of sterile, serofibrinous fluid. Sometimes the exudate is highly fibrinous and heals with fibrous pleural adhesions. The lung may have characteristic rheumatic involvement of small blood vessels, but a specific rheumatic pneumonia also has been described (p. 466).

Cardiac lesions in rheumatoid disease. Rheumatoid arthritis may be accompanied by cardiac lesions. Focal granulomatous nodules with fibrinoid necrosis may be found in the pericardium, valve leaflets, or myocardium. These nodules resemble those seen in the subcutaneous tissue in this disease and in rheumatic fever. In ankylosing "rheumatoid" spondylitis, one may see aortitis with aortic valvulitis, simulating syphilitic cardiovascular disease.

Syphilitic heart disease

Syphilitic heart disease is described on pp. 188 and 189.

Bacterial endocarditis

Bacterial infections of endocardium, which are in reality involvements of cardiac valves, form two groups of conditions that differ in their bacterial etiology, pathogenesis, clinical effect, and pathologic anatomy. They are commonly called acute and subacute bacterial endocarditis. The acute variety usually runs a rapid course of less than six weeks. The course of the subacute

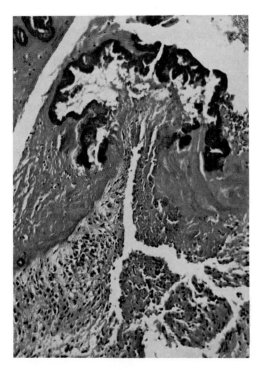

Fig. 12-24. Vegetation on the mitral valve in subacute bacterial endocarditis. Dark masses of bacteria at the top are partially embedded in fibrin. The thickened valve leaflet (below) is diffusely infiltrated by large mononuclear cells and is involved by the necrosis. Few neutrophilic leukocytes are seen in the fibrin. (From Scotti, T. M.: Heart. In Anderson, W. A. D., editor: Pathology, ed. 5, St. Louis, 1966, The C. V. Mosby Co.)

form is less severe and more prolonged, for even without treatment its duration is a matter of months.

Subacute bacterial endocarditis. Subacute bacterial endocarditis (endocarditis lenta) is caused by *Streptococcus viridans* in most cases (70 to 90%) but may be caused by other organisms, e.g., enterococci, *Haemophilus influenzae*, *Brucella* organisms, staphylococci, etc.

The focus of infection from which the organisms reach the heart usually is not obvious. Bacteremia is believed to occur by the entrance of organisms from such foci as infected teeth or tonsils. Such mild and transient bacteremias are probably quite common, and other factors are necessary for the localization of the organisms on the valves. Previous damage to a valve and certain congenital cardiac abnormalities are important predisposing factors. Subacute bacterial endocarditis is most often superimposed on an old rheumatic valvular injury, or it affects congenitally bicuspid aortic valves. Other congenital anomalies that are sites for infection include ventricular septal defects, pulmonary stenosis, and subaortic stenosis. Patency of the ductus arteriosus and coarctation of the aorta also appear to predispose to endothelial infection ("bacterial endarteritis").

The organisms may gain a foothold directly on the valves that have been injured by preexisting disease or may do so by localizing in nonbacterial vegetations (degenerative verrucal

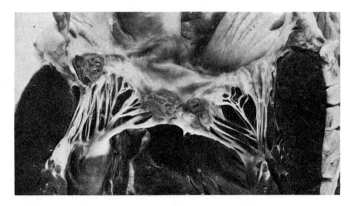

Fig. 12-25. Pneumococcal endocarditis. Large vegetations on the mitral valve.

endocardiosis), which have been found to occur in a variety of conditions, including old rheumatic heart disease. The valvular vegetations form a suitable medium for the multiplication of the organisms.

Cardiac lesions. The tendency to affect injured valves has already been emphasized. The mitral valve is most commonly involved; the aortic valve is next in frequency, with tricuspid and pulmonary lesions occurring relatively rarely. Vegetations form on the valves as warty or polypoid friable masses, from which portions are easily detached. They are more friable and detachable than rheumatic vegetations, but they are firmer and have less tendency to ulceration and valve destruction than the vegetations of acute endocarditis. Aneurysm of a valve cusp or perforation can occur. The vegetations are likely to extend, so as to involve mural endocardium and chordae tendineae. From the mitral valve the vegetations may spread up on the left posterior wall of the atrium. Microscopically the vegetations consist of masses of necrotic tissue with some fibrin, platelets, and leukocytes covered by a layer of bacteria, lying on granulation tissue and possessing a fibrous base, which merges with underlying endocardium. Fibrin usually forms a protective mantle on the surface of the vegetation. Healing occurs by invasion of the base of vegetations by fibroblasts and capillaries, endothelialization of the surface, formation of a capsule, and calcification of the necrotic center. Viable bacteria may persist for long periods in the middle of healing vegetations.

Changes in the myocardium are usually slight and inconstant. In some cases there are minute inflammatory foci in the myocardium, called Bracht-Wächter bodies. Subpericardial hemorrhages are quite common.

Extracardiac lesions. Pathologic changes in organs other than the heart result from breaking away of small portions of the friable valvular vegetations. The effects of embolism give rise to a varied symptomatology. Embolism is evidenced in the kidney by hematuria and infarcts, in the spleen by pain caused by infarction, in the skin by petechiae, in the retina by hemorrhages and blindness, in the brain by hemiplegia or other evidences of cerebral infarction, and in blood vessels themselves by the formation of mycotic aneurysms. Because of the low virulence of the organisms, a suppurative reaction is uncommon in the embolic lesions.

The renal lesion associated with subacute bacterial endocarditis (focal necrotizing glomerulonephritis) usually has definite peculiarities. The smooth surface of the slightly swollen kidney is covered by punctate hemorrhages so that they have been called "flea-bitten kidneys." Microscopically the focal nature of the change is characteristic; only certain glomeruli are involved and the rest are normal (p. 372). This lesion is thought to be an immunoallergic, rather than an embolic, phenomenon.

While bacteremia is usually demonstrable throughout the disease and is a useful feature in diagnosis, bacteria-free periods may occur even though there are repeated emboli to various organs.

Acute bacterial endocarditis. Acute bacterial endocarditis (ulcerative endocarditis) is caused by virulent organisms, most often by *Staphylococcus aureus* (60 to 82% of cases), also by gram-negative bacilli, and less commonly by hemolytic streptococci, pneumococci, gonococci, and other organisms. The endocarditis and septicemia, while rapidly fatal, are often only a complication of another serious condition, such as lobar pneumonia. Thus, unlike the subacute form, the primary focus of the infection is usually obvious.

The mitral and aortic valves are most commonly affected. Frequently, previously normal valves are involved, but old rheumatic valvulitis or congenital defects may precede the bacterial infection. The vegetations on the valves tend to be dense, large, friable, and with a tendency to ulceration and destruction of the valve. Actual perforation of a valve may occur. Spread to involve mural endocardium is less frequent than in the subacute type of endocarditis. The vegetations consist of masses of fibrin, platelets, necrotic valvular tissue, neutrophils, and clumps of bacteria. The underlying valve is necrotic and heavily infiltrated by neutrophils. Abscesses may be seen. Abscesses of the myocardium and the valve rings occur in acute bacterial endocarditis. The extracardiac complications are similar to those of subacute bacterial endocarditis except that embolic lesions, which are often numerous, tend to be suppurative, and focal necrotizing glomerulonephritis is less frequent.

Noninfective endocarditis

Rheumatic endocarditis. Rheumatic endocarditis is discussed on p. 331.

Atypical verrucous endocarditis (Libman-Sacks). Warty mural and valvular vegetations, which represent neither the rheumatic nor bacterial types of endocarditis, have been described by Libman and Sacks. It is found associated with 40 to 60% of cases of disseminated lupus erythematosus (p. 807). The vegetations often occur on both valve surfaces, and also in the valve pockets. Embolic phenomena are not a characteristic feature. The essential change is a hyaline swelling of subendothelial collagen with fibrinoid degeneration, followed by an inflammatory reaction with macrophages, plasma cells, capillary proliferation, and later fibrosis. *Hematoxylin-staining bodies* that are remnants of the nuclei of mesenchymal cells may be present.

Nonbacterial thrombotic endocarditis. Nonbacterial vegetations, forming along the line of closure of valves, occur in various conditions. Swollen collagen and fibrinoid change in the underlying valve are present, but inflammatory cells are not conspicuous, thus the condition is often called "degenerative verrucal endocardiosis." Former terms, "cachectic" or "terminal" endocarditis, are not appropriate. These vegetations may give rise to embolism; they also may serve as a nidus for the development of bacterial endocarditis.

Lambl's excrescences, small filiform processes on the noduli Arantii of the aortic cusps, may represent healed vegetations of this nonbacterial type.

Valvular deformities

Deformities of cardiac valves result from a healed or chronic valvulitis, or occasionally they are congenital malformations. The results of inflammation in the valves are seen as thickening, adhesions, retraction, and shortening of the leaflets. There may be a narrowing of the valve opening (stenosis), or closure of the valve may be insufficient so that leakage (regurgitation) occurs through it. Valvular insufficiency and stenosis may be produced by the same deformity. Valve deformities are common on the left side of the heart (aortic, mitral) but are uncommon on the right side (tricuspid, pulmonary). *Chiari's network* is a mesh of fine or coarse fibers in the right atrium, originating about the margins of the eustachian and thebesian valves and attaching in the area of the crista terminalis or the floor of the right atrium. It is uncommon and represents developmental vestiges of the right valvula venosa and the septum spurium. Rarely, thrombi develop in the network and give rise to pulmonary embolism.

Aortic stenosis. Aortic stenosis may occur as a pure lesion, but frequently it is associated with aortic insufficiency. Noncalcific valvular stenosis is usually caused by rheumatic fever. Congenital valvular and subaortic stenosis also occur. Bicuspid aortic valve is sometimes associated with aortic stenosis. Calcific aortic stenosis is attributed mainly to rheumatic fever; but when it occurs in advanced age, particularly in the absence of lesions in other valves, it is regarded as atherosclerotic in origin (Mönckeberg's aortic sclerosis). Healed bacterial endocarditis, especially related to *Brucella* organisms, is a possible cause. Left ventricular failure, hypertrophy, and dilatation result from the stenosis. Sudden death may occur.

Aortic insufficiency. Regurgitation through the aortic valve during diastole may result from dilatation of the aortic ring or from changes in the leaflets themselves. Dilatation of the ring may accompany dilatation of the rest of the heart, or it may result from spread of syphilitic aortitis. Changes in the leaflets are commonly caused by syphilis or rheumatic fever. The leaflets may be simply affected or distorted at the commis-

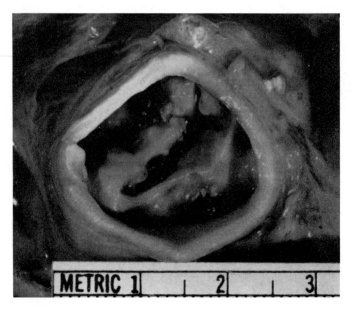

Fig. 12-26. Aortic valve, showing calcific stenosis.

sures, but often the whole leaflet is thickened, with rounded edges and distinct shortening and retraction. Diastolic regurgitation through the aortic valve is accompanied by a significant fall of systemic diastolic pressure and hence a high pulse pressure. Severe hypertrophy and dilatation of the left ventricle result from the extra work. Fibrosis of the endocardium, with formation of endocardial "pockets," caused by the regurgitating blood is a characteristic feature.

Mitral stenosis. Mitral stenosis is one of the commonest valve deformities and almost invariably is caused by rheumatic inflammation. Thickening, adhesions, and retraction of valve leaflets and chordae tendineae may produce all degrees of stenosis. The orifice may be narrowed to a tiny slit, or "buttonhole." The rigidity and retraction usually cause some insufficiency of the valve as well. Calcification is frequently present.

Increased work of the left atrium will compensate for a mild mitral stenosis. A more severe uncompensated stenosis results in increased pressure and stasis in the pulmonary circulation and increases the work of the right ventricle. Thus left atrial dilatation, chronic passive congestion of the lungs, and right ven-

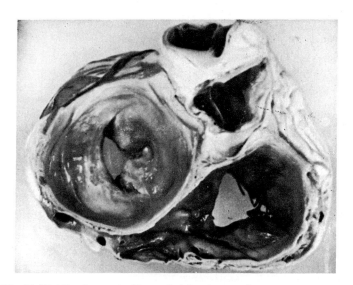

Fig. 12-27. Mitral stenosis; "buttonhole" valve opening.

tricular hypertrophy constantly accompany any great degree of mitral stenosis. In pure stenosis the left ventricle is normal or small in size.

Mitral insufficiency. Regurgitation through the mitral valve is most often a relative insufficiency resulting from the dilatation of the mitral ring accompanying a dilatation of the left ventricle, but insufficiency also may be caused by shortening and retraction of the leaflets and chordae tendineae. If regurgitation is severe, one finds atrial dilatation, severe hypertrophy of the right ventricle, and moderate hypertrophy of the left ventricle.

Tricuspid stenosis. Tricuspid stenosis is uncommon but may result from rheumatic inflammation or congenital disease.

Tricuspid insufficiency. Tricuspid insufficiency is usually caused by dilatation of the right ventricle, with associated dilatation of the valve ring. Fibrous thickening may occur from excess serotonin in the carcinoid syndrome (p. 649).

Pulmonary stenosis. Pulmonary stenosis is most often caused by congenital deformity of the valve rather than inflammatory scarring. It results in right ventricular hypertrophy. It also may occur as part of the carcinoid syndrome (p. 649).

Pulmonary insufficiency. Leakage through the pulmonary valve is very rare. It is usually caused by dilatation of the right side of the heart.

Endocardial fibroelastosis

Endocardial fibroelastosis is an endocardial thickening resulting from the proliferation of collagenous and elastic tissue elements. It is commonly generalized but is most prominent in the left ventricle and sometimes involves valves. Most cases are seen in infancy, with evidence of cardiac dysfunction or failure, but in some cases the cardiac disability is not present until childhood or adult life. Mural thrombosis with thromboembolism is more characteristic of the adult form of the disease.

The heart is usually greatly enlarged, chiefly because of hypertrophy and dilatation of the left ventricle. In addition to the thickened endocardium there may be a patchy myocardial fibrosis, which in some cases has been attributed to a thickening and narrowing of thebesian vessels.

The disturbance of function and production of symptoms may be related to interference with normal contraction by the thickened endocardium, interference with the vascular supply of the underlying myocardium producing anoxia, or impairment of

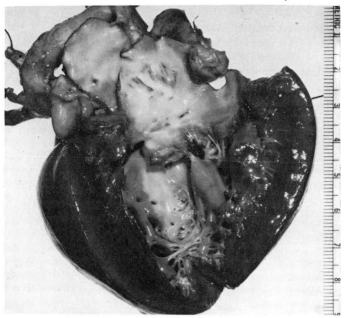

Fig. 12-28. Endocardial fibroelastosis.

conduction. The etiology is obscure. Infantile endocardial fibroelastosis is congenital in origin and probably is a developmental
abnormality. Other theories incriminate intrauterine endocardial
anoxia, congenital metabolic disturbance, lymph stasis, organizing
endocardial fibrin deposits, and mechanical stress. The cases
in which symptoms develop after adult life is reached, usually
have a lesser degree of endocardial thickening and probably
also are of congenital origin. Histochemical changes similar to
those of collagen diseases have been described. Some investigators consider impairment of cardiac lymph flow to be important
in the pathogenesis.

Endomyocardial fibrosis

In some areas, particularly in Africa, this idiopathic disease
is a relatively frequent form of cardiac disturbance, with circulatory failure and death. It consists of a massive, destructive, scarring process involving one or both ventricles, usually in the
apices and the inflow tracts. Dense, white fibrous tissue replaces

the endocardium and adjacent myocardium. In contrast to endocardial fibroelastosis, there is little or no increase of elastic tissue. The papillary muscles and chordae tendineae are affected and fused; the posterior leaflet of the atrioventricular valve often is sealed to the mural endocardium. Mural thrombi may be evident. The atria may be involved. Cardiac hypertrophy may or may not be present. Theories concerning etiology include viruses, malnutrition, and autoimmunity as possible causative factors.

Coronary heart disease

Coronary circulation. Right and left coronary arteries supply the heart, taking their origin from a protected position in the aortic sinuses of Valsalva. Tiny accessory openings occasionally occur adjacent to the main openings. The right coronary artery curves to the right in the atrioventricular groove as the right circumflex artery and then descends in the posterior interventricular sulcus as the posterior descending branch. The right coronary artery supplies the posterior half of the interventricular septum, a portion of the posterior part of the wall of the left ventricle, the posterior wall and almost all of the anterior portion of the right ventricle, and the right atrium. The left coronary artery early divides into circumflex and anterior descending branches. The circumflex branch supplies the left atrium and the left margin of the left ventricle, including part of its posterior wall. The anterior descending branch of the left coronary artery runs toward the apex in the anterior interventricular sulcus and supplies the anterior wall of the left ventricle, the immediately adjacent part of the anterior wall of the right ventricle, and the anterior half of the interventricular septum.

In normal hearts anastomotic communications between coronary vessels are small and are probably of little functional significance. However, when the coronary supply is interfered with by atherosclerotic narrowing or occlusion, anastomotic channels develop and enlarge where needed, and they may measure as much as 200μ or more. Such anastomotic development may provide some compensation for arteriosclerotic changes. The size (circumference) of the main coronary arteries in proportion to the weight of the heart provides a rough index of the functional capacity of the myocardium.

The thebesian veins are minute channels, which open directly into the cardiac chambers. Under abnormal circumstances, flow in these channels may be reversed, and they may assist in nutrition of the myocardium. Their assistance possibly contributes to the comparative rarity of infarction of the muscle of atria or the right ventricle, which are relatively thin walled.

Coronary sclerosis. Arteriosclerosis involving coronary vessels is of the atherosclerotic intimal type (p. 294). Intimal fibrous thickening, lipoid deposits, and often calcium deposition, all of which narrow the lumen of the vessel, are the main features. The larger vessels on or near the surface of the heart are particularly involved. Small arteries within the myocardium rarely show significant sclerosis. The left coronary artery is usually more severely affected than the right coronary artery.

The intima of normal coronary arteries is without demon-

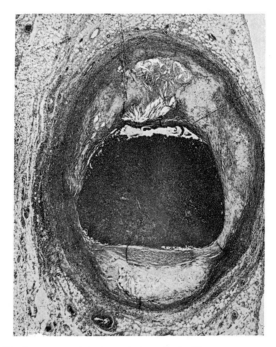

Fig. 12-29. Coronary sclerosis and thrombosis. The intima is irregularly thickened and the media thinned because of advanced atheromatosis. (From Scotti, T. M.: Heart. In Anderson, W. A. D., editor: Pathology, ed. 5, St. Louis, 1966, The C. V. Mosby Co.)

strable vasa vasorum, but in and around atherosclerotic lesions may be found capillaries, which take their origin from the intimal endothelium of the artery or from the medial vasa vasorum. The importance of hemorrhage from these delicate channels, in the initiation of coronary thrombosis, has been emphasized.

The *etiology* of coronary atherosclerosis is obscure. Heredity, sex, and race are factors of importance. In general, men are more susceptible to the disease than women. In women of young and middle age, coronary disease is seldom severe, and in women under 40 years of age it is infrequent except in association with obesity, hypertension, or hyperlipemia. In diabetic women over 40 years of age, significant coronary disease has as high an incidence as in diabetic men. Also in American Negroes the prevalence of coronary atherosclerosis and the extent of the lesions tend to be less than in white persons, except perhaps, in Negro women compared to white women. However sex difference is not significant among Negroes as it is among whites. Other possible etiologic factors have been discussed previously in the section describing atherosclerosis (p. 297).

Complications of coronary atherosclerosis are (1) narrowing of the arterial lumen by progression of the plaque, (2) thrombosis, (3) intimal hemorrhage, (4) rupture of an atheromatous plaque, and (5) rarely, aneurysmal formation.

Coronary arterial occlusion is most often caused by an atherosclerotic plaque itself or by one of its complications, particularly thrombosis. Intimal hemorrhage (into a plaque), in a few cases, causes complete occlusion of the lumen; it also may predispose to thrombus formation, as already mentioned. Rupture of the plaque may cause occlusion at the site, form an embolus, or initiate thrombosis. Another important cause of occlusion is narrowing of the coronary ostia by lesions of syphilitic aortitis. Less commonly other lesions produce coronary occlusion, such as embolism, polyarteritis nodosa, other forms of arteritis, and dissecting aneurysm.

Diseases of the coronary arteries in themselves are not necessarily accompanied by clinical or morphologic evidence of heart disease. However, when a sufficient degree of myocardial ischemia is produced to disturb the metabolism and performance of the heart, manifestations occur. The result is *ischemic* or *coronary heart disease*. Coronary heart disease, especially the atherosclerotic type, is the chief form of fatal cardiac disease in the United States. The effects of coronary artery disease include angina pectoris, myocardial fibrosis, myocardial infarction, congestive heart failure, cardiac hypertrophy and dilatation, and sudden death. A significant factor that may modify these effects, or may even prevent the development of myocardial ischemia, is an adequate collateral circulation through anastomotic channels.

Angina pectoris is characterized by paroxysmal pain in the chest provoked by an increase in the demands of the heart (e.g., by exertion, emotions, etc.) and is relieved by a decrease in the work of the heart. A transient myocardial ischemia (acute coronary insufficiency) is the cause, brought on by a disproportion between the oxygen requirements of the myocardium and the coronary arterial blood flow. The underlying coronary disease is usually coronary atherosclerosis with narrowing or occlusion of one or more branches of the coronary arteries. Other diseases causing angina pectoris, by reducing coronary blood flow or increasing the oxygen needs of the heart, are syphilitic coronary ostial narrowing, aortic stenosis or insufficiency, cardiac hypertrophy, and severe anemias.

Sudden death may be the termination of coronary artery disease in patients who have experienced anginal attacks, or it may occur in persons who appear healthy and have had no previous symptoms of cardiovascular disease. Commonly these patients have severe coronary atherosclerosis, with or without old organized thrombi, or recent coronary thrombosis may be the cause. The mechanism of sudden death is thought to be cardiac arrest or ventricular fibrillation.

Fibrosis of the myocardium, focal or diffuse, characteristically occurs in patients with a chronic, progressive type of myocardial ischemia, as in severe coronary atherosclerosis and stenosis of the coronary ostia. The myocardial lesion is usually found in patients who have had a history of attacks of angina pectoris or who died suddenly as a result of coronary insufficiency without myocardial infarction. The lesions are considered to represent fibrous replacement of atrophic muscle fibers, but some writers attribute them to healing of minute infarcts. If sufficient myocardial damage occurs, cardiac insufficiency, hypertrophy, and dilatation may ensue.

Myocardial infarction. A consequence of sudden myocardial ischemia, such as that which follows coronary thrombosis, is myocardial infarction, although this does not always happen. Muscle necrosis may be prevented if collateral circulation is ade-

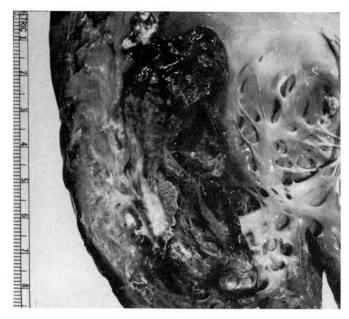

Fig. 12-30. Myocardial infarct, left ventricle, with attached mural thrombus.

quate; or the patient may die too soon after the coronary occlusion for visible changes of an infarct to develop. Conversely, infarction of the myocardium can occur in the absence of sudden occlusion. In such instances old atherosclerotic lesions with luminal narrowing or old organized atherosclerotic thrombi may be found, and it is assumed that the acute myocardial ischemia is the result of coronary insufficiency brought on by factors that increase the demand of the myocardium for more oxygen. Nevertheless, the usual cause of myocardial infarction is coronary atherosclerosis, with or without thrombosis. The vessel most frequently occluded is the anterior descending branch of the left coronary artery; next in frequency, the right coronary artery; and least often, the left circumflex artery. The occlusion is usually within 3 or 4 cm. of the ostia of the coronary arteries.

Myocardial infarction is usually accompanied by prolonged substernal oppression or pain, shock, electrocardiographic changes, fever, leukocytosis, increased transaminase activity of the serum, and increased sedimentation rate. The pathologic changes in an infarct of the myocardium have much in common with infarcts elsewhere, but certain features are peculiar because of the nature and function of the heart. The relative infrequency of infarction involving the atria or the right ventricle has been mentioned.

There is a characteristic *position* occupied by the myocardial changes after coronary occlusion. Occlusion of the anterior descending branch of the left coronary artery produces an infarct of the anterior part of the interventricular septum and of the apical and anterior part of the wall of the left ventricle. Obstruction of the circumflex branch of the left coronary artery affects the wall of the left ventricle in its lateral portion or in its posterolateral aspect. Obstruction of the right coronary artery produces an infarct that involves the posterior half of the interventricular septum and a portion of the posterior wall of the left ventricle.

While these are the usual and typical areas of myocardial infarction, the location of the coronary occlusion and the site of infarction do not always have a constant relationship. Blumgart and his colleagues have demonstrated "infarction at a distance," i.e., an infarct caused by sudden obstruction of an artery that had been supplying anastomotic channels and adequate nutrition to the affected area, which formerly was supplied by another coronary artery that had undergone gradual occlusion in the past. It has also been shown that ventricular infarcts show patterns similar to the known patterns of cardiac muscle bundles. Thickness of an infarct appears to be related to the complications of aneurysm and rupture of the myocardium.

The *appearance* of an infarct of the myocardium varies with its age. A visible infarct does not have time to develop if death rapidly follows coronary thrombosis. In early stages an infarcted area may be dark red or hemorrhagic in appearance. Later there appears a mottling of the yellowish opaque areas of necrotic muscle in the dark red tissue. Microscopically the necrotic muscle fibers appear swollen, hyaline, and lacking their striations and nuclei. Leukocytes abundantly infiltrate the area. The infarcted area undergoes softening (myomalacia cordis), which results in weakening of the area and sometimes rupture. Rupture is most common in the first week and is rare after the third week. Localized pericarditis is present over the area of infarction, and

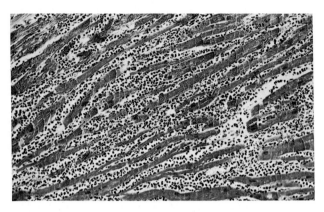

Fig. 12-31. Myocardial infarct. The muscle fibers are necrotic, and there is an abundant leukocytic infiltration.

mural thrombi form on the injured endothelium lining the region of infarction.

The *healing* of myocardial infarcts is by scar tissue, replacing the destroyed muscle, which does not regenerate. Necrosis of muscle and leukocytic infiltration are predominant features of the first week. In the second week one sees removal of necrotic muscle and replacement by connective tissue. This is evident grossly as a zone of red, depressed tissue surrounding pale brown areas of necrotic muscle. The new connective tissue lays down increasing amounts of collagen until the area is converted into a firm, grayish, fibrous scar. This process appears to be complete in five to eight weeks, depending on the size of the infarct.

In very early myocardial infarcts, before any gross or microscopic alterations are recognized by conventional methods of examination, certain chemical, histochemical, and electron microscopic changes can be demonstrated. Decreased enzyme activity within the myocardium seems to be a finding that is useful in the detection of early myocardial infarcts.

The *complications* and *causes of death* include (1) cardiac failure, left and/or right ventricular; (2) coronary failure or episodes of acute coronary insufficiency, while convalescing from the recent infarct; (3) cardiac shock; (4) mural thrombi with thromboembolism; and (5) rupture of the heart with hemopericardium (cardiac tamponade). Sudden death may be related

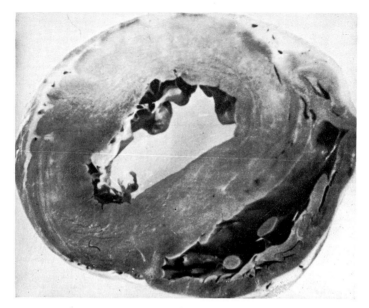

Fig. 12-32. Hypertrophy of the left ventricle, chronic hypertension. Note the excessive thickening of the wall of the left ventricle as compared with the wall of the right ventricle. The heart has been cut transversely through the ventricles.

to cardiac rupture, to massive pulmonary embolism, or to coronary failure. Ventricular aneurysms or calcification may develop in healed infarcts (so-called sequelae).

Hypertrophy and dilatation of the heart

Increase in size of the heart is the result of increased work thrown upon the organ and an enlargement of the individual muscle fibers and not the result of an increase in their number. Hyperplasia and regeneration of muscle fibers do not occur in the adult heart.

The average normal male heart weighs 300 grams, and the female heart weighs 250 grams. Normal heart weight appears to be expressed most easily in terms of the height of the person. The left ventricle averages 10 to 12 mm. in thickness, and the right ventricle averages 3 to 4 mm. In cases of great hypertrophy, weights may range from 700 to 1,000 grams.

When an unusual amount of work is thrown upon the heart muscle, it attempts to compensate by enlarging the muscle fibers. The portion of the heart that hypertrophies is determined by the location of the circulatory stress or burden imposed on it. Hypertrophy of the left ventricle results from (1) hypertension, either primary or secondary, such as that associated with chronic glomerulonephritis; (2) aortic regurgitation or stenosis; (3) mitral regurgitation; and (4) coronary sclerosis. Hypertrophy of the right ventricle is caused by (1) mitral stenosis; (2) pulmonary stenosis or regurgitation; (3) increased resistance in the pulmonary circulation (cor pulmonale), perhaps from emphysema or severe pulmonary arteriosclerosis; and (4) coronary sclerosis. Also, failure of the left ventricle throws increased work on the right ventricle and may cause hypertrophy.

Often dilatation of the cardiac chambers precedes and accompanies hypertrophy. One form of dilatation results from toxic effects on the myocardium, as in the degenerative cardiomyopathies and various types of myocarditis. Another form occurs

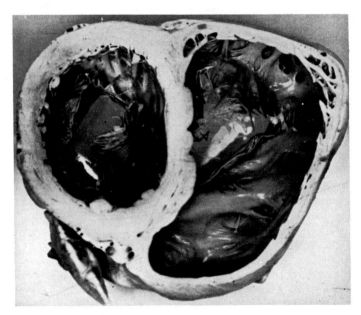

Fig. 12-33. Dilatation of the ventricles.

when there is an excessive demand imposed on the heart by structural defects (e.g., valvular disease) or increased peripheral resistance (hypertension). A localized dilatation may occur in a weakened area of infarction.

Cases of hypertrophy without obvious cause ("idiopathic cardiac hypertrophy") are seen in young adults, as well as in infants and children. A variant of this lesion is "familial cardiomegaly," in which a familial tendency extends over several generations. Usually the hypertrophy and dilatation affects all chambers. In some patients there is a localized area of unusually severe hypertrophy in the outflow tract of the left ventricle, producing manifestations of subaortic stenosis (so-called "familial muscular subaortic stenosis"). Other forms of idiopathic hypertrophy of the heart have already been mentioned, i.e., endocardial fibroelastosis and endomyocardial fibrosis.

In the past the diagnosis of "idiopathic hypertrophy" was made loosely and included such entities as glycogen-storage (Pompe's) disease and Fiedler's myocarditis.

Hypertensive heart disease

Peripheral hypertension produces hypertrophy of the left ventricle because of its increased load. The hypertension is a disturbance of peripheral arterioles, however, and the cardiac effects are secondary (p. 373). Coronary atherosclerosis or other cardiac lesions are not infrequently associated. Eventually the heart may be unable to cope with its increased work so that dilatation and congestive circulatory failure result. Congestive heart failure causes a considerable proportion of deaths from hypertension.

Cor pulmonale

Cor pulmonale or pulmonary heart disease is a condition in which the right side of the heart is subject to excessive strain and fails because of some abnormality of the pulmonary circulation or lesion of the lungs. Acute cor pulmonale may result from a massive pulmonary embolism that obstructs a major portion of the pulmonary circulation and is characterized by rapid dilatation of the pulmonary trunk, conus, and right ventricle. Multiple smaller emboli with organization may lead to chronic cor pulmonale. Other common causes of chronic cor pulmonale are chronic bronchitis with chronic obstructive emphysema and widespread pulmonary fibrosis arising from a variety of conditions. Primary pulmonary arteriosclerosis is a rare cause of cor pulmonale. The mechanism of production of chronic cor pulmonale appears to involve not only an obstruction in the pulmonary circulation but a failure of oxygenation, which induces a reflex vasoconstriction and rise of pulmonary blood pressure. In chronic obstructive emphysema a pulmonary insufficiency results from disturbed gas exchange because of ineffective alveolar ventilation and abnormal alveolar perfusion. Dyspnea, cyanosis, and polycythemia are common clinical accompaniments. The right ventricle becomes hypertrophied, and there may be some dilatation. With right-sided failure, hypertrophy of the right atrium may occur.

Myocarditis

Acute myocarditis is frequently associated with bacterial endocarditis, and other bacterial infections may be associated with direct invasion of the myocardium by pathogenic organisms. The nonspecific acute inflammation may be predominantly interstitial with little parenchymal damage; or degeneration and necrosis of muscle may be prominent with only slight interstitial inflammation being in evidence. Abscesses occur in pyogenic infections. Granulomatous myocarditis is seen in tuberculosis, brucellosis, and tularemia. Myocardial abscesses may also be present in brucellosis. Sarcoidosis produces tuberculoid granulomatous lesions in the heart and may even be a cause of sudden death. Rare gummatous lesions occur in tertiary syphilis. Fibrosis associated with narrowing of the coronary ostia in syphilis is sometimes mistaken for "chronic myocarditis." The same applies to the myocardial fibrosis associated with coronary sclerosis. Myocarditis also occurs in rickettsial infections such as typhus fever and in parasitic infections such as Chagas' disease *(Trypanosoma cruzi)*. In trichinosis a severe myocarditis may be present, although the larvae cannot encyst in the myocardial fibers. Fungous infections produce lesions of the myocardium similar to those seen in other tissues and organs. Certain drugs or poisons cause toxic effects upon the myocardium (degenerations and focal necrosis), followed by nonspecific inflammation. Serum sickness has been reported to have an associated myocarditis. Interstitial myocarditis with prominent eosinophils may follow sulfonamide administration (p. 245). Certain collagen diseases, including rheumatic fever, are associated with myocarditis. Rheumatoid arthritis is frequently accompanied by valvular and myocardial lesions similar to those of rheumatic heart disease or to the granulomatous lesions in subcutaneous rheumatoid nodules. Adhesive pericarditis is also common with rheumatoid arthritis.

In some instances pheochromocytomas are associated with myocardial lesions, which may be patchy areas of degeneration and necrosis of myocardial fibers followed by nonspecific inflammation and fibrosis. Presumably caused by secretion from the pheochromocytoma, the change has been called "norepinephrine myocarditis." It may be associated with unexpected death from myocardial failure.

Isolated, primary, or Fiedler's myocarditis is a severe myocarditis of unknown etiology that occurs unassociated with a disease process elsewhere to which it might be secondary. There may be either a diffuse infiltration of the interstitial tissue of the heart by lymphocytes, plasma cells, eosinophils, or focal granulomatous lesions with destruction of muscle fibers.

Other myocardial diseases

Fatty degeneration, fatty infiltration, glycogen infiltration, and *basophilic (mucoid) degeneration* of the myocardium have been mentioned previously in Chapter 2. *Atrophy* of the heart and the cardiac involvement in *hemochromatosis* have also been discussed (pp. 18 and 50).

Amyloidosis of the heart occurs as a feature of primary systemic amyloidosis and of amyloidosis associated with multiple myeloma. It also occurs as a distinctive type in elderly patients, in their seventh to ninth decades, with amyloid deposits largely restricted to the heart; and since it seems to be a manifestation of senescence, it is often referred to as "senile cardiac amyloidosis."

Nutritional disturbances also affect the heart. *Beriberi,* induced by a lack of vitamin B_1 (thiamine), is characterized by cardiac enlargement chiefly caused by dilatation, especially of the right ventricle. Excessive intake of alcohol may produce a similar nutritional disturbance, but it can also cause direct effect upon the myocardium, resulting in degenerative changes and fibrosis—so-called *alcoholic cardiomyopathy.*

Endocrine disturbances are seen in *hyperthyroid heart disease, hypothyroidism* (myxedema heart), and *acromegaly* (cardiac hypertrophy). The effect of *catecholamines* ("norepinephrine myocarditis") has been mentioned. *Carcinoid heart disease* is associated with the "carcinoid syndrome." In metastasizing

carcinoids of the intestine the increased serum levels of serotonin (5-hydroxytryptamine), or possibly other substances, cause
typical fibrotic lesions of the endocardium of the heart—chiefly
affecting the right side, and especially the pulmonary and tricuspid valves. The most common effects are pulmonary stenosis
and tricuspid regurgitation.

Myocardial lesions have been reported in patients dying suddenly and unexpectedly, who had been receiving treatment with
tranquilizers (phenothiazine compounds). The lesions consisted
of foci of myocardial degeneration, associated with hyperplastic
changes in arterioles and increased acid mucopolysaccharide in
and about these vessels.

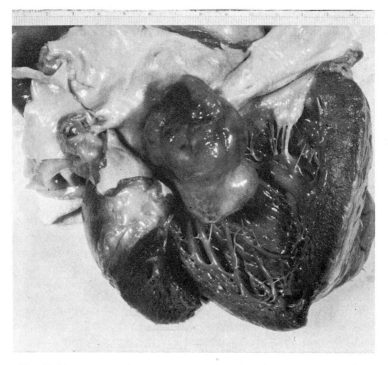

Fig. 12-34. Myxoma of heart. Note smooth glistening tumor attached to
septal wall of left atrium and partly blocking mitral orifice. (From
Scotti, T. M.: Heart. In Anderson, W. A. D., editor: Pathology, ed. 5,
St. Louis, 1966, The C. V. Mosby Co.)

Tumors and cysts of the heart

Both primary and secondary tumors of the heart are uncommon. The commonest primary tumor of the heart is the *myxoma*, a polypoid mass arising from the endocardium of one of the atria, particularly the left. This benign lesion, which occurs predominantly in adults, must be differentiated from edematous mural thrombi. A congenital, benign striated muscle tumor *(rhabdomyoma)* is seen chiefly in infants, often in association with tuberous sclerosis. The myocardial fibers forming the tumor-like nodules are distended with glycogen. While some regard

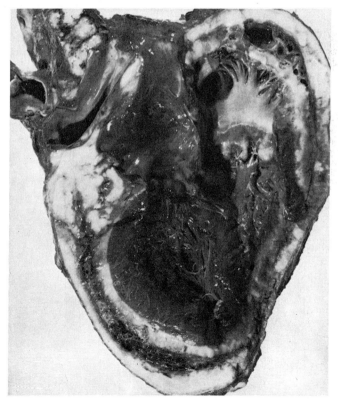

Fig. 12-35. Metastasis of bronchogenic carcinoma to the heart. There is extensive invasion of the pericardium and myocardium.

this lesion as the commonest primary tumor of the heart in infants and children, others believe that it is a developmental anomaly or hamartoma. Other benign, but infrequent, intra-cardiac and pericardial tumors include *fibroma, lipoma,* and *angioma*. Primary malignant neoplasms also originate in the heart or pericardium, such as *rhabdomyosarcomas* and *other intracardiac sarcomas* and *pericardial mesotheliomas* and *fibro-sarcomas*. Among *metastatic tumors* of the heart the most fre-quent originate from bronchogenic carcinoma, malignant lym-phoma, leukemia, and malignant melanoma.

In addition to these tumors, various types of cysts may occur in the heart and pericardium. *Blood cysts* are minute, round, red-brown nodules in the valves of infants, appearing chiefly on the atrial surfaces of the mitral and tricuspid valves. They are believed to result from blood being pressed into crevices on the surface of the cusps, followed by fusion of the mouths of the crevices. *Pericardial cysts* and the rare *intramyocardial epithelial cysts* are forms of congenital malformations, which may be found in persons of all age groups.

Chapter 13

The kidneys, urinary tract, and male genitalia

KIDNEY

Cardiovascular renal disease is a term used broadly to include the vascular and inflammatory disorders of the kidneys, the associated vascular lesions of other organs, and the effects on the heart and brain. Collectively this group of conditions causes about one third of all deaths and is the cause of death in one half of persons over 50 years of age.

The kidneys play an essential part in this group of conditions. The renal lesions are of two main types: (1) inflammatory, with primary involvement of glomeruli (glomerulonephritis) or interstitial tissue (pyelonephritis); and (2) vascular, with primary involvement of arterioles and small arteries, associated with high blood pressure (arteriolar nephrosclerosis, essential hypertension).

Renal structure and function

The kidneys are composed of units (nephrons), each consisting of a glomerulus and its associated tubule. A normal human kidney contains about 1.25 million nephrons, sufficient for a considerable reserve. The glomerulus is a collection of capillaries covered by epithelium continuous with that lining the tubule. A thin basement membrane separates the epithelial covering of the glomerular capillaries from the endothelial lining. The basement membrane appears to be a differentiated cytoplasmic product of the endothelial cells. The epithelial cells form a cytoplasmic secretion of mucoprotein or mucopolysaccharide, which is spread over the surface of the basement membrane and which penetrates it at regular intervals. However, some investigators have considered that there are distinct epithelial and endothelial basement membranes, between which there is a connective tissue substance or layer. The total surface of a glomerular tuft is very large, and their aggregate surface is enormous. The glomerulus acts as a filter, and from blood flow-

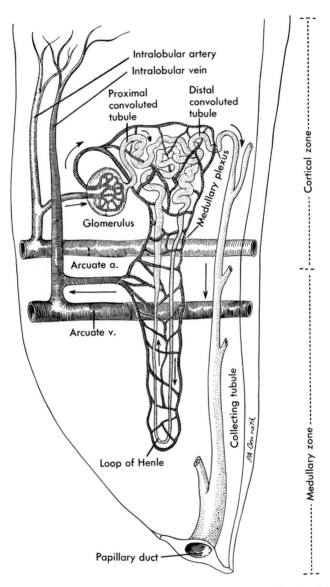

Fig. 13-1. Nephron. Diagrammatic representation of a renal unit, show-ing the circulatory relationships.

ing through its capillaries a protein-free filtrate of the plasma collects in the glomerular space and flows down the tubule. During this tubular passage there is active resorption of water, glucose, chloride, sodium, and other substances. Active secretion by tubules of certain substances, notably creatinine and ammonia, may also occur. For this mechanism to function normally in the nephron there must be (1) a free flow of blood through the capillaries of the tuft; (2) a normal filter; i.e., water, salt, urea, and other waste products must be allowed to filter through, but certain substances such as plasma proteins must be held back; (3) a normal epithelial lining of the tubule and an unblocked lumen. Lesions in the kidney can produce functional disturbance by three corresponding types of qualitative change. Each may occur alone, but combinations of varying degrees of each are the usual occurrence. The large numerical reserve of identical units is such that a fraction of their number can maintain adequate function. Consequently, functional changes in relation to renal lesions must be considered on a quantitative as well as a qualitative basis. When functional deficiency occurs in chronic glomerulonephritis and nephrosclerosis, values for urea and creatinine clearance are closely correlated with the number of functioning glomeruli.

The vessels of the glomerular tuft, after forming the efferent arteriole, again break up into capillaries, which supply the tubule. Hence, obstruction of flow through the glomerulus also interferes with tubular blood supply. Destruction of a glomerulus usually results in atrophy and disappearance of the corresponding tubule, although aglomerular tubules have been demonstrated. Glomeruli do not regenerate. No new glomeruli are formed during adult life, although some compensation may result from hypertrophy of those remaining. Tubular epithelium, on the other hand, regenerates readily. Hence injurious agents that affect the tubular epithelium alone, e.g., mercury bichloride, lead either to death of the person or to complete recovery; i.e., the injury is neither chronic nor progressive. After injury, regenerative tubular epithelial cells may have an atypical flattened form and are most resistant to injury.

Classification of renal diseases

Cardiovascular renal disease includes most conditions accompanying high blood pressure and is a very frequent cause of death in persons past middle age. Renal diseases of different origin and nature may produce similar disturbances of renal function and have much clinical similarity. Also, renal disturbances of different pathogenesis may reach late or end stages that are morphologically similar and difficult to differentiate.

The following classification of the main renal diseases is based on a combined consideration of the portion of the kidney primarily or most prominently affected and the type of involvement. Other parts of the kidney almost always show some secondary or less prominent pathologic change.

Glomerular disease
    Glomerulonephritis
        Diffuse
            Acute
            Subacute
            Chronic
            Membranous
        Focal
Vascular disease
    Nephrosclerosis
        Atherosclerotic
        Arteriolosclerotic
    Polyarteritis nodosa
    Bilateral cortical necrosis
    Diabetic glomerulosclerosis
    Infarcts of the kidney
    Orthostatic albuminuria
Tubular disease
        Toxic and metabolic tubular injury
        Chemical tubular injury
        Genetic or acquired tubular dysfunction
Interstitial disease
    Interstitial nephritis
        Acute diffuse
        Chronic diffuse
        Focal suppurative
        Pyelonephritis
        Syphilis
        Tuberculosis
    Leukemic infiltration
Obstructive disease of the kidney (hydronephrosis)
Metabolic renal disease
    Hyperparathyroid renal disease
    Hypervitaminosis D
    Renal calculi
    Uric acid infarcts
    Renal lesions in gout
Congenital malformations and anomalies
    Agenesis
    Hypoplasia

Fusion
Ectopia
Cysts
Tumors
  Benign
    Hamartoma
    Adenoma
    Fibroma
    Leiomyoma
    Lipoma
  Malignant
    Hypernephroma (carcinoma)
    Wilms' tumor (adenomyosarcoma)
    Carcinoma of the pelvis
    Metastatic

Glomerulonephritis

The classifications and terminologies used in renal disease and particularly in glomerulonephritis have recently entered an era of upheaval. This is partly the result of additional knowledge and understanding obtained by the techniques of percutaneous renal biopsy and electron microscopy. Contributing also has been popularization of usage of terms for clinical syndromes (e.g., the nephrotic syndrome, nephrocalcinosis, etc.), the pathologic basis of which may be one of several distinct renal diseases. Until stability and general agreement is reached, some understanding of different classifications and synonyms is necessary.

The most widely used terms for diffuse glomerulonephritis are those of Volhard and Fahr, whose classification with its later modifications, recognized three main stages or types of the disease—acute, subacute and chronic. The subacute stage was sometimes further divided into two groups, an extracapillary and an intracapillary (or subchronic) type.

Longcope and Ellis each made a classification of diffuse glomerulonephritis into two *clinical* groups, termed types A and B by the former and types 1 and 2 by the latter, but with considerable similarity. The Ellis type 1 has a sudden onset, usually with a preceding history of streptococcal infection (poststreptococcal glomerulonephritis). The Ellis type 2, of insidious onset and lacking a history of preceding streptococcal infection, often showed the clinical picture of the nephrotic syndrome.

The underlying lesion in many of the cases grouped as Ellis type 2 is now termed membranous glomerulonephritis, or lobular glomerulonephritis.

In glomerulonephritis the lesion is primarily an inflammation affecting glomerular tufts. This is manifested by (1) proliferation of glomerular and capsular epithelium, (2) proliferation and swelling of capillary endothelium, (3) thickening of basement membranes, (4) formation of intracapillary fibers, and (5) exudation of leukocytes. Either proliferative activity or exudation may be the predominant change. The glomerular changes result in narrowing or complete closure of the capillaries of the tuft. The condition progresses to hyalinization and disappearance of the glomeruli. Secondary degenerative changes in tubules are constantly present.

The exact cause of glomerulonephritis is unknown, but it appears to be related to infection, particularly with streptococci, and to be an immune or hypersensitivity reaction. Acute glomerulonephritis is frequently preceded by an attack of tonsillitis, scarlet fever, or other streptococcal infection. Infection with certain strains of beta-hemolytic streptococci (e.g., type 12) are followed by acute nephritis with unusual frequency. An allergic reaction of renal tissue to bacteria or their products has been suggested as the exciting cause. Antibodies have been demonstrated to be localized in the glomeruli in experimental glomerulonephritis, and gamma globulins have been shown to be localized in glomerular lesions of nephritis in man. Some investigators believe that the nephrotoxic antibodies are "autoantibodies."

Diffuse glomerulonephritis may be subdivided into acute, subacute, and chronic forms. The acute form is more common in children, lasts only a few weeks, and may entirely clear up or progress to subacute or chronic forms. The subacute type lasts several months and may be a rapidly progressive form with a stormy course, sometimes with severe edema. The chronic form may last many years, often with long periods of latency. The forms leading eventually to failure of renal function present a final stage referred to as uremia.

Acute diffuse glomerulonephritis. In acute glomerulonephritis the kidneys are swollen and pale, with smooth surfaces on which tiny hemorrhages are sometimes visible. Microscopically the glomeruli appear enlarged, cellular, and bloodless. Their apparent increase of nuclei is mainly the result of endothelial hypertrophy and proliferation, but leukocytes are sometimes numerous. Glomerular epithelial cells are little changed except for some cytoplasmic swelling. The endothelial basement membrane occasionally shows slight thickening. Small hyaline intracapillary

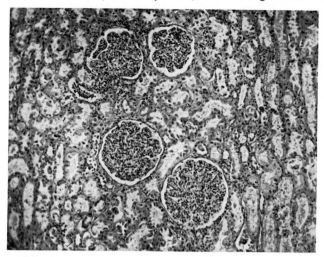

Fig. 13-2. Acute glomerulonephritis. Note the large size and great cellularity of the glomeruli.

fibers are demonstrable by an azocarmine stain. Edema and cellular infiltration of the intercapillary space contributes to narrowing of the capillary lumina. Capillary thrombi may be present. With the electron microscope focal swelling of the basement membrane has been demonstrated. In some studies deposits have been observed on either side of, and within, the basement membrane. Fusion of epithelial foot processes is usually not seen, except occasionally in areas of severely damaged basement membrane.

The effect of all these changes is to impede or entirely obstruct the flow of blood through the glomeruli. This results in diminished urinary output (oliguria), some hypertension, and leakage of albumin and red cells through the glomerular filter into the urine. There is a rough correlation between the degree of glomerular damage and impairment of renal function as measured by inulin clearance. Tubular changes are usually present as dilatation and cloudy swelling, as fatty degeneration, or as a hyaline droplet degeneration when the inflammatory changes are severe. Red cell casts may be found in the tubules. The tubular lesions partly result from a decrease of their blood supply by the glomerular changes and partly result from a direct toxic action. The mortality in treated cases is about 1 or 2%. Severe involvement of a large proportion of glomeruli results in death. Otherwise there is recovery, or if the proliferative glomerular changes are severe, there may be progression to subacute or chronic phases. Circulatory congestion complicating acute glomerulonephritis appears to result from a defect in excretion of sodium and water rather than from any primary myocardial damage or failure.

Goodpasture's syndrome. The association of severe pulmonary hemorrhage and glomerulonephritis has been called Goodpasture's syndrome. Most cases have been in young male adults, hemoptysis is usually the presenting symptom, and the later renal disease usually progresses in a few months to termination with uremia. Gamma globulin has been demonstrated by immunofluorescence in both pulmonary alveolar septa and glomerular basement membranes.

Subacute glomerulonephritis. Rapidly progressive glomerulonephritis, usually terminating in uremia in the course of a few months, is referred to as subacute. The kidneys are enlarged, pale, and soft ("large white kidney"). There may be some slight irregularity of the surface and some adherence of the capsule. Microscopically there is significant proliferative involvement of all glomeruli, with frequent and prominent capsular "crescents" caused by the proliferation of capsular epithelium. Adhesions of tuft to capsule are common. Hyalinized glomeruli are absent or rare. Moderate uniform tubular atrophy is present, and many tubules contain casts. Interstitial connective tissue may appear increased.

Chronic glomerulonephritis. Chronic glomerulonephritis ends by failure of renal function. It may result from an acute diffuse glomerulonephritis that progresses to a chronic phase. In such cases the history may be one of infection, an acute attack of nephritis, progression to a chronic phase, and termination, all in a relatively short period. More frequently there is no history of an acute attack because acute phases were mild and passed unnoticed. The condition may progress over many years, with little clinical evidence except a slowly progressive decrease of renal function. In other cases there are long latent periods of apparent health, punctuated by mild acute flare-ups. The end result in each case is similar, with failure of renal function terminating in uremia.

The failure of renal function is manifested by decreasing

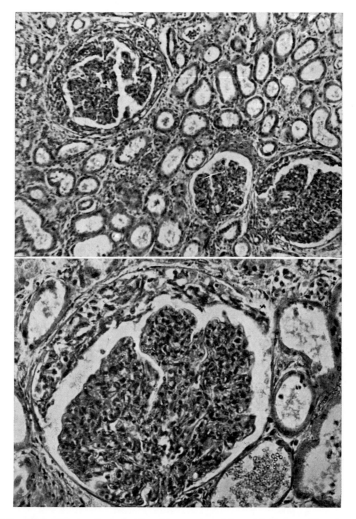

Fig. 13-3. Glomerulonephritis with considerable epithelial proliferation. Note the glomerular crescents resulting from proliferation of the capsular epithelium.

ability to concentrate the urine. Eventually it may have a fixed specific gravity near 1.010, corresponding to that of blood plasma. The dilute urine is excreted in large amounts, resulting in polyuria and nocturia. Albumin and casts are present in the urine but in small or moderate amounts. High blood pressure develops and increases with the progression of renal failure. Failure to excrete nitrogenous waste products is reflected in an increase of nonprotein nitrogen and urea in the blood. Termination occurs with the clinical syndrome known as uremia.

The kidneys are small, contracted, and firm. Their capsules are tightly adherent, and the outer surfaces are roughly and irregularly granular and pitted. The cortices are irregularly narrowed and scarred with loss of normal architectural markings. Microscopically a large proportion of glomeruli are partially or completely changed into hyaline masses. Many tubules are atrophic or have disappeared, and the amount of connective tissue between the tubules and glomeruli shows a great relative increase. Some tubules and glomeruli are permeable and apparently functioning, although none may be completely normal.

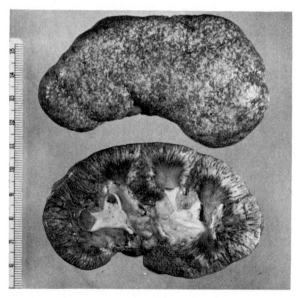

Fig. 13-4. Chronic glomerulonephritis.

Medium-sized and small arteries commonly develop intimal and medial proliferation and thickening. Renal ischemia caused by the glomerular and vascular changes results in the hypertension of chronic nephritis. In some cases the gross and microscopic changes of chronic glomerulonephritis are not readily distinguishable from those of the primarily vascular condition, hypertensive nephrosclerosis.

More severe vascular changes, particularly cellular intimal proliferation and arteriolar necrosis, are associated with accelerated progress of the disease in late stages. Such cases clinically may simulate "malignant hypertension," with very high blood pressures and retinal lesions.

Hereditary nephritis. A hereditary chronic renal disease, usually associated with nerve deafness, has been studied in several families. The lesions have a mixture of features of glomerulonephritis and pyelonephritis, and foam cells in the cortex may be a prominent feature. The foam cells are not pathognomonic, as they occur occasionally in various other renal diseases. In some instances the foam cells can be identified as lipid-filled, degenerated cortical tubular cells.

Membranous glomerulonephritis. Membranous glomerulonephritis is characterized by a thickening of the basement membrane of the glomerular tuft as its predominant feature rather than by a proliferation of cells. However, basement membrane thickening is also in the renal lesions of lupus erythematosus and diabetes mellitus. By electron microscopy there is seen to be a fusion or loss of the foot processes of the epithelial cells (podocytes). This change may be revealed by electron microscopy in early or minimal cases in which the basement membrane thickening is imperceptible in ordinary sections. In certain instances fusion of foot processes is demonstrable without morphologic alterations of the basement membrane, especially in children. Such cases are often referred to as *lipoid nephrosis.* In the advanced forms of the disease the basement membrane is thickened and there are deposits of a dense material between the endothelial cells and the basement membrane. The deposits may extend into the basement membrane in focal areas. At times the electron dense material is deposited on the epithelial side of the membrane, between foot processes. Membranous glomerulonephritis may progress to a sclerosis of glomeruli, sometimes apparently through a stage of lobularity of the tuft (lobular glomerulonephritis).

Membranous glomerulonephritis is usually of insidious onset and does not ordinarily have a preceding history of streptococcal infection. The clinical features are those of the nephrotic syndrome (lipoid nephrosis) with severe proteinuria and edema. It is fairly generally agreed that membranous glomerulonephritis is the underlying lesion of the condition that has long been called lipoid nephrosis. Although the early and mild forms are commonly in childhood, it occurs at any age, and advanced forms are more common in adults. Although the etiology is not established, it is frequently considered a hypersensitivity-immunologic condition.

The kidney in early membranous glomerulonephritis may show few gross changes and has a smooth surface and pale color. Fatty changes into tubular epithelium may be more striking than the basic glomerular lesions. In advanced stages with glomerulosclerosis the appearance may be similar to other types of chronic nephritis with contracted kidneys. It has been observed that the glomerulosclerosis develops first and most prominently in the glomeruli near the corticomedullary junction.

Nephrotic syndrome. The nephrotic syndrome is a clinical entity characterized by massive proteinuria, hypoproteinemia, edema, lipidemia (hypercholesterolemia), and lipiduria. The clinical complex may have underlying it one of a number of distinct diseases, although the condition they have in common is an increased glomerular membrane permeability, which allows the proteinuria and lipiduria.

The condition that most commonly underlies the nephrotic syndrome (including lipoid nephrosis in children) is idiopathic membanous glomerulonephritis. The nephrotic syndrome may be seen in patients with diffuse proliferative glomerulonephritis. In such cases one can demonstrate fusion of epithelial foot processes and thickening of the basement membrane by electronmicroscopy, in addition to proliferation of epithelial and endothelial cells of the glomeruli (membrano-proliferative glomerulonephritis). Other diseases affecting glomeruli that are associated with the syndrome are diabetic glomerulosclerosis (Kimmelstiel-Wilson disease), lupus erythematosus, renal amyloidosis, and renal vein thrombosis. Infrequently the nephrotic syndrome occurs in a wide variety of other conditions, many of which seem to have a hypersensitivity component.

The clinical use of the term *nephrotic syndrome* (or *nephro-*

sis) should not be confused with the older use of the term *nephrosis* in pathology, which referred to an injury or degenerative lesion involving renal tubules.

Uremia. Uremia is the complex clinical condition marking the final stage of renal insufficiency. No particular substance or toxin is known to be causative, but it is probably an autointoxication resulting from the retention of various metabolic products ordinarily eliminated by the urinary mechanism. Azotemia, the retention of nitrogenous metabolites, may also be extrarenal, i.e., caused by diseases other than those of the kidneys.

Failure of function is denoted by an inability of the kidneys to produce a concentrated urine and to adapt to increased work. In final stages of failure the specific gravity of the urine tends to be fixed about 1.010, the urine being almost isotonic with serum. Urea, creatinine, uric acid, sulfate, chloride, ammonia, and phosphate are retained. The hydrogen ion concentration of the urine can no longer be varied to suit the body's need, and there is frequently a retention acidosis, which may be lessened by increased breathing and loss of acid through vomiting. Blood phosphorus increases greatly and calcium falls, resulting in nervous hyperirritability and muscular twitchings. Convulsions may occur when the uremia is associated with hypertension.

Other than the damaged kidneys, there are no constant anatomic changes in uremia. Edema of the brain is common. A mild sterile pericarditis is occasionally present, and degenerative changes have been described in outer portions of the myocardium. In some cases electrocardiographic changes are indicative of hyperpotassemia. Necrotizing colitis is an occasional occurrence in uremia. Pulmonary hemorrhage originating from alveolar septa may be found in some cases of glomerulonephritis, particularly those in which there are necrotizing glomerular or vascular lesions.

Renal edema. Edema in nephritis is influenced by two factors: (1) loss of plasma albumin and (2) salt retention. The albuminuria results from increased permeability of the glomerular tufts, and the protein loss decreases the osmotic pressure exerted by plasma colloids to hold fluid within the vessels. The sodium chloride retention is caused by a lessened ability of the damaged kidney to excrete it. Lowering of plasma albumin is the more important factor. Edema tends to appear when plasma protein is lowered below 5 grams per 100 ml. Loss of albumin

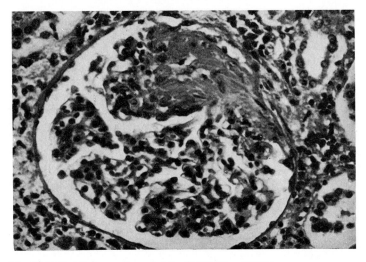

Fig. 13-5. Focal glomerulonephritis. (AFIP No. 80093.)

is particularly important because it exerts four times the osmotic force of globulin. In the so-called "nephrotic" types of renal disease a massive albuminuria and severe edema go hand in hand (p. 370).

The distribution of edema in nephritis is often independent of gravity and may appear first on the face rather than in dependent parts. The edema fluid has a very low protein content and low specific gravity.

Focal glomerulonephritis. Focal glomerular lesions are commonly found in cases of subacute bacterial endocarditis. The kidneys may show scattered reddish dots or tiny petechial areas, which have been described as giving the kidney a "flea-bitten" appearance. Microscopically, occasional glomeruli show a portion of the tuft involved by hyaline necrosis, or so-called "hyaline thrombi." Although often considered to be caused by tiny emboli from the infected cardiac valves, there is much evidence that this is not the correct pathogenesis. The lesion, sometimes referred to as "focal necrotizing glomerulonephritis," probably represents an immunoallergic response to antigenic products of the bacteria. Only a small proportion of glomeruli are altered, and renal function is not usually affected, but hematuria may be manifested.

Vascular disease of the kidney

Sclerosis of renal arteries and intrarenal vessels is extremely important because of the association of these changes with high blood pressure. Ischemic renal tissue releases into the bloodstream a pressor substance, which produces hypertension by constriction of peripheral vessels. Hypertension may be the result of atherosclerosis of a renal artery in those rare instances in which the lumen is constricted sufficiently to cause renal ischemia. In the usual case of hypertension, however, renal ischemia is associated with sclerosis of the smallest arteries or arterioles of the kidney. Sclerosis of the larger arteries within the renal substance is usually irregular and not generalized in its distribution. Hence it rarely results in ischemia of sufficient renal tissue to produce hypertension, nor is there enough destruction to cause renal failure. It produces a few large, gross scars, similar to healed areas of infarction. Because it is a common finding in elderly persons, such a kidney is called a "senile arteriosclerotic kidney."

Senile arteriosclerotic kidney (atherosclerotic nephrosclerosis). The atherosclerotic involvement of larger and medium-sized intrarenal arteries is a patchy change that results in irregular, depressed areas on the kidney surface. The kidney is not much decreased in size unless there is some other pathologic change. Microscopically, fibrous replacement of glomeruli and tubules is present in the scarred subcapsular portions of the cortex. There is some cellular infiltration by lymphocytes and plasma cells. These changes in the kidney rarely are associated with any severe hypertension or renal functional failure.

Hypertension. Cases of high blood pressure commonly are divided into *secondary* and *essential* types. The less common secondary type is the result of renal disease, such as chronic pyelonephritis and glomerulonephritis, of cerebral or cardiovascular disease, or of endocrine lesions, such as an adrenal or pituitary tumor. The common "essential" hypertension was so called because there seemed to be no primary lesion. It has been recognized that renal arteriolar sclerosis is an almost constant postmortem finding in essential hypertension. The arteriolar sclerosis is often a generalized change, particularly common in the spleen, pancreas, adrenals, and brain, but it is only in the kidneys that arteriolar sclerosis and hypertension seem to be closely associated. However, biopsy of the kidneys in hypertensive patients has shown that as many as 28% may have little

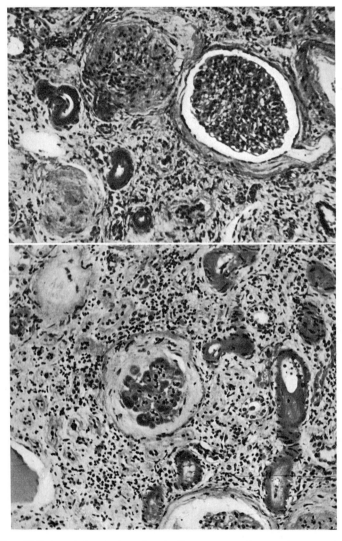

Fig. 13-6. Arteriolar nephrosclerosis. From a case of severe hypertension. Note the extreme hyaline thickening of the arteriolar walls and also the glomerular changes.

or no vascular change. Early in essential hypertension the renal blood flow is reduced by tonic muscular spasm of the renal arterioles. In this stage the glomerular filtration rate and tubular functions are normal. Later the renal ischemia is maintained and increased by structural narrowing or sclerosis of the arterioles and small arteries. Structural change with loss of nephrons is accompanied by reduction of glomerular filtration rate and tubular function.

In a recent series of 2,300 renal biopsies from hypertensive patients, more than 80% had arteriolar nephrosclerosis, about 15% had chronic pyelonephritis, 1.3% had unilateral renovascular lesions, and 1% had chronic glomerulonephritis.

The importance of renal vascular changes in hypertension has been shown by Goldblatt, who produced renal ischemia by means of a clamp on the renal artery. It was demonstrated that the ischemic renal tissue released a pressor substance into the circulation, which resulted in constrictive action on peripheral vessels and produced hypertension.

The substance secreted by the kidney (renin) is not in itself a pressor substance. Renin is an enzyme secreted into the blood, where it acts on a substrate, an alpha-2 globulin (hypertensinogen), to produce a decapeptide called angiotensin I. This in turn is acted upon by a converting enzyme to form angiotensin II, which constricts arterioles and elevates blood pressure. In the sustained elevation of blood pressure in hypertensive patients, other factors, such as hyperaldosteronism, may also be present.

Renin is secreted by specialized cells at the vascular pole of the glomerulus that form a functional structure called the juxtaglomerular complex. This consists of granular juxtaglomerular cells in the media of the afferent arteriole; cells situated in the angle formed by the two arterioles (lacis cells, or "polkissen"); and the macula densa, a specialized adjacent segment of the distal tubule.

The degree of granularity of the juxtaglomerular cells is an indication of their secretory activity. In established arteriolar nephrosclerosis the juxtaglomerular cells are hypertrophied, hyperplastic, and actively functioning. In unilateral renovascular hypertension the juxtaglomerular cell change may be great. In hypertension complicating chronic pyelonephritis, the juxtaglomerular cells do not appear to be hyperplastic and active. Juxtaglomerular cells appear to have a second function in stimulating aldosterone secretion by the adrenal cortex.

Essential hypertension has been divided into "benign" and "malignant" clinical types. They appear to be fundamentally the same in nature. The malignant form more commonly occurs in young adults. Retinal changes are usually severe. It is more rapidly progressive and has severe lesions, but it is of the same general type; death usually results from renal failure. Pathologically the malignant form is characterized by hyperplastic arteriolosclerosis, usually with necrosis in the walls of small arteries and arterioles and small hemorrhages from the severely damaged vessels. These necrotizing vascular changes can be reproduced experimentally by renal ischemia sufficient to cause renal failure.

Common causes of death in hypertension are cerebral hemorrhage, renal failure (uremia), congestive heart failure, and coronary occlusion. Cardiac hypertrophy (left ventricle) is a constant finding in cases of hypertension. Retinal changes are also a constant part of hypertensive disease and consists of sclerosis of small retinal vessels, small hemorrhages, and edema. In the malignant phase retinal changes are severe and may result in blindness.

The cause of essential hypertension is still unknown. Hereditary and racial tendencies are important. Body build and, to a lesser degree, obesity seem to have some association with hypertension. A high dietary intake of sodium chloride appears to predispose to hypertension. Experimental salt hypertension in the rat resembles human hypertensive disease in its evolution and lesions.

The kidney of hypertension (arteriolar nephrosclerosis). In benign hypertension the most constant finding in the kidney is a sclerosis of small arteries and arterioles. Often the smallest preglomerular vessels show the change most severely in the portion just proximal to the tuft. In many cases the kidneys are of normal size and have smooth surfaces. With more severe or prolonged hypertension any degree of atrophy may be found. The capsules are adherent, and the outer surfaces of the kidneys present a finely granular and scarred appearance. Tiny retention cysts are often present in the cortex. With such changes, of vascular origin, the term *primarily contracted kidney* is used to differentiate this from the *secondarily contracted kidney* of glomerulonephritis. In practice it is often impossible to distinguish grossly the contracted kidney of hypertensive nephrosclerosis from that of chronic glomerulonephritis.

Microscopically the essential lesion is a sclerosis of small

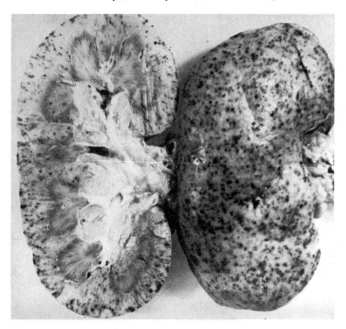

Fig. 13-7. Kidney in malignant hypertension, showing focal hemorrhages from arteriolonecrosis.

arteries and arterioles. Hyaline arteriolar sclerosis, which involves particularly the afferent arterioles, is a hyalinization and decreased cellularity of the wall, with a variable reduction in the size of the lumen. Electron microscopy has indicated this appearance is caused by deposition of a hyaline substance in the arteriolar wall. The vascular hyalin has been described previously (see pp. 33 and 299). Larger vessels, particularly the interlobular arteries, may show a laminated, eosinophilic intimal thickening, often with a prominent, thickened and reduplicated internal elastic lamina (hyperplastic elastic sclerosis). Although the elastic tissue hypertrophy is prominent, the intima particularly is thickened with the production of fibrils and localization of small lipid particles.

The effects of the vascular changes are reflected in the glomeruli, which early show a thickening of the capillary basement membranes and later show varying degrees of hyalinization and atrophy. Hyaline deposits first appear beneath the endothelium,

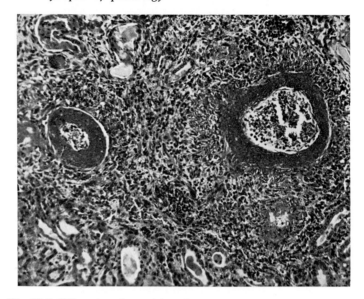

Fig. 13-8. Kidney in polyarteritis nodosa.

but with increase later fill the capillary lumina. Glomerular capsules as well as tufts become thickened and hyalinized. The atrophy of glomeruli and associated tubules produces the renal shrinkage. In end stages with significant renal contraction it is often difficult to distinguish chronic glomerulonephritis and arteriolar nephrosclerosis, even by microscopic examination. Remaining traces of a proliferative inflammatory process, e.g., glomerular crescents, must be searched for as a distinguishing feature.

In malignant hypertension the kidneys often show little atrophy as a result of the rapid progress of the disease. Small hemorrhages on the outer surface of the kidney may cause it to resemble the "flea-bitten" kidney of focal glomerulonephritis. This is caused by acute necrotizing arteriolitis and arteritis. Hyperplastic arteriolar sclerosis of larger arterioles and small arteries may be prominent. The pathologic findings differ somewhat, depending on whether the hypertension was malignant from the beginning or whether it was benign with a superimposed malignant terminal phase. In the latter case varying chronic changes with hyalinization and atrophy of glomeruli are present, but in addition to the usual arteriolar sclerosis, one sees a hyaline necrosis of vessel walls, some inflammatory cellular infiltration, and often hemorrhage about severely injured vessels. The hyaline necrotic changes may extend to involve glomerular capillaries as well as arterioles and small arteries.

While most cases of hypertension are associated with vascular and renal diseases, a few are caused by the involvement of endocrine glands or nervous system. Cushing's syndrome, tumors of the adrenal glands (pheochromocytoma and aldosteronism), and diseases of the brainstem may be associated with high blood pressure.

Infarction of the kidneys. Renal infarcts are quite common as a result of embolism from the heart in cases of bacterial endocarditis, atrial fibrillation, and mural thrombosis after myocardial infarction. In rare cases infarction has been sufficiently extensive to give rise to oliguria or anuria as well as hematuria.

Renal vein thrombosis. Renal vein thrombosis is an uncommon condition that may give rise to hemorrhagic infarction of the kidney, or if the main renal vein is occluded, there may be massive renal necrosis. In adults the renal vein thrombosis is usually secondary extension from the thrombophlebitis of peripheral veins. In childhood a primary renal vein thrombosis may be associated with ileocolitis. Renal vein thrombosis may be associated with the nephrotic syndrome, particularly in adults.

Bilateral cortical necrosis of the kidneys. There is an unusual condition of extensive necrosis of the peripheral layers of renal cortices that is of unknown etiology but is sometimes associated with hemorrhage and toxemias of late pregnancy or acute infections. It has also been described in newborn infants, associated with maternal antepartum hemorrhage. A similar condition results from poisoning by dioxane or diethylene glycol, from injections of staphylococcal toxin, or from choline deficiency in experimental animals. The chief clinical feature is oliguria, and death usually results in a few days. Because of ischemia, irregular areas of necrosis involve the cortical portions of both kidneys. The surface is mottled by patchy opaque areas of reddish yellow color and has a soft consistency. The microscopic appearance is similar to that of infarction, with a zone of congestion and leukocytic infiltration about the margin of the necrotic areas.

The ischemic necrosis of the renal cortices appears to be caused by a widespread organic or functional occlusion of the

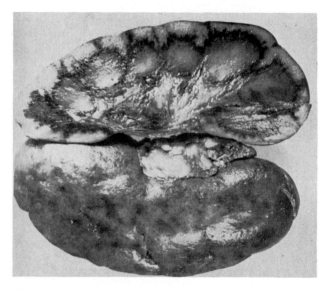

Fig. 13-9. Cortical necrosis of the kidney. A reddened congestive zone outlines the opaque necrotic cortical tissue.

intralobular arteries and their branches, the terminal arteries, and the arterioles of the renal cortices. The actual mechanism of the vascular obstruction, whether by intense vasoconstriction, vasoparalysis, thrombosis, or necrosis of arterial walls, may vary in different cases. The work of Trueta suggests that there may be a vascular mechanism by which the cortex is bypassed, the blood being shunted through the medulla.

Renal lesions in disseminated lupus erythematosus. In disseminated lupus erythematosus glomerular changes are common. There may be proliferation of endothelial cells of glomerular capillaries, fibrinoid deposits, and hyaline thickening of basement membranes, giving a so-called "wire-loop" appearance. With the electron microscope the deposits are seen between the endothelial cells, but sometimes between the epithelial cells, and the basement membrane. Epithelial foot processes occasionally may be fused, especially in areas where the electron dense deposits are extensive. There also occur intracapillary hyaline "thrombi."

Diabetic glomerulosclerosis. Diabetic glomerulosclerosis is a characteristic glomerular lesion that occurs in one third of diabetic individuals over the age of 40 years, has no relationship to the degree or duration of the diabetes, but is a helpful criterion in histologic diagnosis of diabetes mellitus. Glomeruli show focal areas of hyaline sclerosis, which appear to begin as a basement membrane alteration. These hyaline nodules, which characteristically lie in the centers of glomerular lobules, have a vacuolated or laminated structure. Hyalinization of the efferent glomerular arterioles may also be present. In some cases a clinical syndrome is present, which consists of diabetes, hypertension, retinal arteriosclerosis, albuminuria, and edema. There has been described also a nonspecific, diffuse intercapillary sclerosis and a subintimal layer of hyalin in the afferent and efferent arterioles of glomeruli. Electron microscope studies have shown two distinct processes, a thickening of the basement membrane and a precipitation of hyaline masses beneath and between endothelial cells, which correspond to the diffuse and nodular lesions. In the nodular lesions the hyaline deposits increase in size; they isolate the endothelial cells and push them to the periphery and ultimately obliterate the capillary lumen. Some fusion of epithelial foot processes is seen only in severely damaged glomeruli. Other renal lesions often associated with diabetes mellitus include arteriosclerosis, pyelonephritis, and papillary necrosis. In uncontrolled diabetes there may be glycogen accumulation in the cells of the loops of Henle.

Tubular injury and disease

Nephrosis refers to degenerative renal changes, as distinct from inflammation (nephritis) or vascular disease (nephrosclerosis). The degenerative changes are seen in the tubules, particularly in the sensitive convoluted tubules of the cortex. A certain amount of tubular degeneration accompanies glomerulonephritis. Other types are (1) nephrosis of toxic or metabolic origin, (2) nephrosis resulting from chemical poisons, and (3) genetic or acquired tubular dysfunction (e.g., the Fanconi syndrome). Tubular epithelium regenerates readily, so that if a patient survives a severe tubular injury, recovery is usually complete.

Toxic and metabolic tubular disease. Injury of toxic or metabolic origin is the commonest form of tubular change. Most acute infections and toxic conditions cause tubular lesions, which may be cloudy swelling, fatty degeneration, hyaline droplet degeneration, or necrosis of epithelial cells, in increasing order of se-

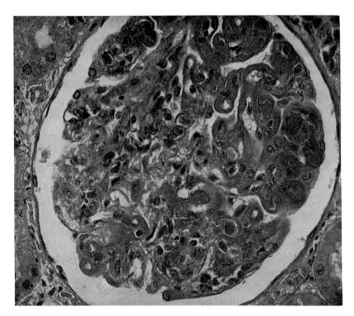

Fig. 13-10. Kidney in disseminated lupus erythematosus, showing "wire-loop" lesions and fibrinoid necrosis of a glomerulus.

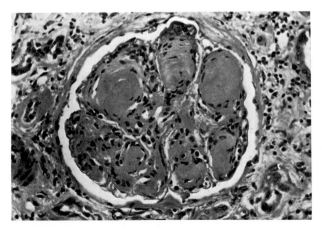

Fig. 13-11. Diabetic glomerulosclerosis. (AFIP.)

verity. Hyaline and lipoid droplets indicate absorption from the tubular lumina and storage in the lining epithelial cells of protein and lipoid material that has passed through damaged abnormally permeable glomeruli. Cholemic nephrosis is a tubular degeneration accompanying severe jaundice. It is uncertain whether it is caused by bile pigments, bile salts, or associated liver damage. Intestinal obstruction, particularly when high in the intestinal tract (e.g., pyloric stenosis), may produce tubular degeneration, sometimes with calcification of the degenerated cells.

A distinctive vacuolar lesion of the proximal convoluted tubules (vacuolar nephropathy) occurs most often with chronic intestinal disease (e.g., ulcerative colitis) accompanied by chronic diarrhea. The reversible lesion appears to be characteristic of acute or severe potassium deficiency, although the cause or mechanism of the potassium depletion is variable. Large clear vacuoles, which fail to react to stains for fat or glycogen, balloon out the tubular cells. Signs of renal dysfunction are inconstant and fail to correlate with the severity of the vacuolation. Chronic potassium deficiency may be followed by the changes of chronic pyelonephritis and interstitial fibrosis.

A vacuolar type of hydropic degeneration also occurs in dioxane and diethylene glycol poisoning, and a more diffuse type

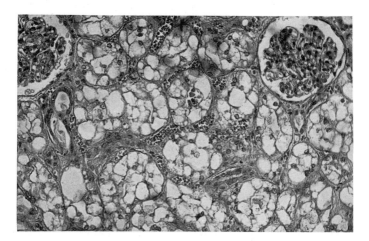

Fig. 13-12. Vacuolar nephropathy of potassium deficiency from a case of regional enteritis. (Courtesy Dr. J. F. Kuzma.)

of hydropic degeneration results from intravenous injection of gelatin or hypertonic solutions of sucrose (osmotic nephrosis). In the latter case it is probable that much of the swelling of the tubular cells seen microscopically is caused by absorption of fluid during preparation of the tissue.

The Fanconi syndrome is characterized by renal glycosuria, aminoaciduria, low serum inorganic phosphorus, and a growth disturbance resembling rickets. A familial form, caused by a recessive gene, is usually evident in childhood. The basic defect appears to be a resorption deficiency of tubules, and micro-dissection shows a thin first part of the proximal convoluted tubules, described as a "swan-neck" appearance, and there is also a fibrosing chronic interstitial nephritis. Some cases have an associated cystinosis.

Adult or acquired Fanconi syndrome (syndrome of proximal tubular dysfunction) may result from an injury by heavy metals or by decomposition products of tetracycline, and it also has been reported with various cancers, including myeloma. Excretion of Bence Jones protein in the urine (in multiple myeloma) produces some tubular degeneration. Precipitation of the protein with blockage of the tubular lumina also occurs.

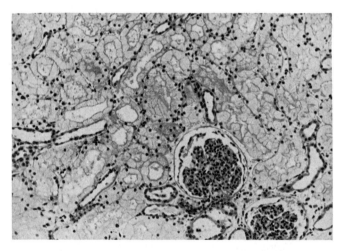

Fig. 13-13. Hydropic degeneration of the kidney, caused by intravenous injection of hypertonic sucrose. (From Anderson, W. A. D.: Southern Med. J. 34:257, 1941.)

Hemoglobinuric nephrosis (acute tubular nephrosis, lower nephron nephrosis). A variety of conditions in which there occur a fairly massive destruction of blood or tissues and shock may be followed by oliguria or anuria and by death from renal failure. The kidneys in such cases are characterized by degenerative changes of the tubules, pigmented casts in the tubular

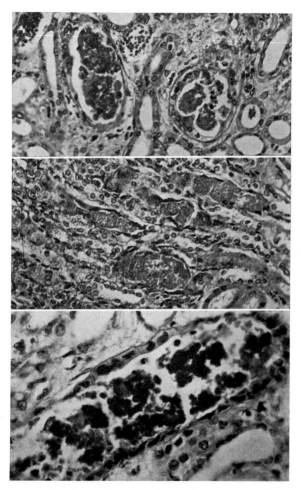

Fig. 13-14. Transfusion reaction in the kidney. The tubules contain pigment casts, and their epithelial lining cells show degenerative changes.

lumina, and edema of renal tissue. While the pathogenesis of the renal lesion has not been completely elucidated, it appears to be on the basis of a disturbance of renal blood flow, in which hemoglobin or myoglobin and derived pigments may play a part in some cases. While the changes are often most prominent in the distal or lower portions of the nephrons, they are not limited to this area, so that the term *lower nephron nephrosis* has been described as "euphonious, but erroneous." Vascular effects on the upper or proximal portions of the nephrons may be of greater importance. Acute tubular nephrosis occurs regularly during secondary shock, resulting from severe reduction of renal blood flow.

Hemoglobinuric nephrosis is characteristically observed in cases of massive hemoglobinemia and hemoglobinuria, such as occur in blackwater fever and after transfusion with incompatible blood. Severe traumatic injuries involving crushing of muscular tissues or prolonged muscular ischemia also produce the condition, and it was a prominent sequel of injuries in World War II (crush syndrome, posttraumatic anuria). Similar renal lesions occur in some cases of severe burns, heat stroke, uteroplacental damage, sulfonamide intoxication, rattlesnake bites, and after certain poisons. Shock and excessive vomiting are often associated with the conditions leading to hemoglobinuric nephrosis. The development of renal functional failure is associated with oliguria, which often progresses to anuria. The urine excreted is highly acid, gives a positive benzidine reaction, and shows pigmented material or pigmented casts on microscopic examination.

The gross appearance of the kidneys is not specific. There is usually some swelling and enlargement, with increase of weight. The outer and cut surfaces of the cortex are pale, but the medulla is dark or dusky and shows accentuated striations.

The microscopic changes are characterized by degeneration and necrosis involving focal portions of the distal part of Henle's loop and distal convoluted tubules. The interstitial tissue around these damaged areas shows edema and cellular infiltration, often with thrombosis of adjacent veins. Reddish or brownish casts of a heme compound are found in the lumina of the distal tubular segments and in the collecting tubules. The glomeruli and proximal convoluted tubules may show relatively slight or no changes. The oliguria or anuria may be mainly caused by a disturbance in renal circulation with inadequate glomerular filtration and may be contributed to by the blockage of tubular lumina with pigment casts and by excessive reabsorption or leakage of glomerular filtrate through the damaged tubular walls.

The pathogenesis of the renal lesion is not completely established, but much evidence suggests that it has a vascular basis, with disturbance of renal blood flow and ischemia. A renal vasomotor mechanism has been demonstrated that, on stimulation, causes renal cortical ischemia and diverts blood flow to the medulla. Hemoglobin and derived pigments may play some part in producing this vascular disturbance, in addition to the effect of tubular blockage.

Nephrotoxins (**chemical nephrosis**). Nephrotoxins are exogenous poisons that injure the kidney, most often by causing degeneration and necrosis of tubular epithelium. Mercury bichloride, a frequent example, causes a pure tubular injury of severe grade and results in oliguria, which usually progresses to anuria and death from uremia. Death occurs most frequently between the fifth and tenth days, at which stage the kidney is swollen and grayish white in color. The epithelium, particularly of the convoluted tubules, is necrotic, broken up, and irregularly desquamated. The interstitial tissue is edematous and often infiltrated by leukocytes. After seven or ten days the kidney appears more red and congested, and calcium is often deposited in the degenerated and necrotic tubular epithelium. Evidence of epithelial regeneration and mitotic nuclei may be found at this time. (See Fig. 10-1.)

Nephrotoxic chemicals and drugs are numerous and are not uncommon as a cause of acute renal failure. The most frequent are carbon tetrachloride, mercury, and ethylene glycol. A few, such as sulfonamides, bee venom, and poison ivy, may cause a hypersensitivity type of injury in the kidney. Excessive phenacetin ingestion has been related to a pyelonephritis-type lesion and papillary necrosis. Degradation products of tetracyclines have been noted to cause severe tubular injury with clinical manifestations similar to those of the Fanconi syndrome.

Interstitial nephritis

Interstitial nephritis, unlike glomerulonephritis, is essentially an exudative rather than a proliferative inflammation. Marked exudates of inflammatory cells may be present focally or diffusely in interstitial tissues.

Focal suppurative interstitial nephritis (pyemic kidney, abscesses of kidney). Lodgment of infected emboli, as part of a generalized pyemia, results in multiple abscesses throughout the kidney substance. The abscesses appear as small, rounded yellowish opaque areas, surrounded by a reddened hyperemic zone. They may be numerous, or a single large abscess (carbuncle) may be found. Staphylococci and *Escherichia coli* are the common organisms.

Pyelonephritis. The term *pyelonephritis* is used when both the parenchyma of the kidney and the renal pelvis are involved by interstitial inflammation. Descending and ascending types are described. In the former, bacteria reach the kidney by the bloodstream, primarily infecting renal tissue and "descending" to infect the pelvis. In the latter case the bladder and pelvis are infected first, and spread occurs by "ascending" to infect

Table 13-1. *Differentiating features of chronic pyelonephritis and chronic glomerulonephritis*

	Chronic pyelonephritis	Chronic glomerulonephritis
Involvement	Unilateral, bilateral, or unequal	Bilateral
Gross	Nodularity of broad coarse scars	Fine granularity
Extent	Patchy	Diffuse
Glomerular changes	Focal or in scarred area	Diffusely involved
Membranous or proliferative glomerular lesions	Rare	Common
Tubular disappearance	In relatively large areas without glomerulosclerosis	Proportionate to sclerosed glomeruli
Dilated tubules with hyaline casts (thyroidlike areas)	Common	Small and uncommon
Hypertrophy of remaining tubules	Slight	Common and marked
Neutrophilic leukocytes	Common	Few
Plasma cells	Common	Infrequent
Vascular changes	Often severe	Usually moderate
Inflammation of pelvis	Usual	Infrequent
Necrosis of papillae	May be present	Absent

renal tissue. This may be upward spread via the lumen or by lymphatics of the ureter. The relative frequency of ascending and hematogenous infection is uncertain and a point of debate. The presence of renal scars appears to predispose to infection of the area by circulating bacteria. The susceptibility of the kidney to infection is also enhanced by urinary tract obstruction. Ascending infection occurs mainly when there is obstruction with consequent stagnation of urine. The so-called pyelitis common in children and pregnant women is really pyelonephritis. Pyelonephritis is the commonest and probably the most important renal disease.

The kidneys show wedge-shaped areas of inflammation extending through the cortex and medulla to the pelvis. Microscopically such areas show interstitial infiltrations of inflammatory cells, often with some tubular destruction and abscess formation. In the acute stages the cells are mainly neutrophilic leukocytes, and in chronic phases they are lymphocytes and plasma cells. The mucosa of the pelvis is roughened, and masses of lymphocytes are found under the epithelium. Continuation of low-grade interstitial inflammation results in gradual atrophy and destruction of tubules and in hyalinization of glomeruli by a process of periglomerular fibrosis and capsular thickening. Hyaline casts are present in enlarged tubules with atrophic epithelium, and some areas may have a thyroidlike appearance. Eventually there results a kidney that is coarsely

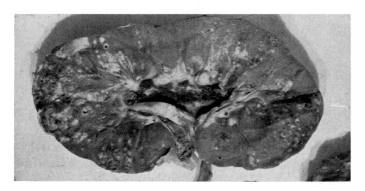

Fig. 13-15. Suppurative pyelonephritis.

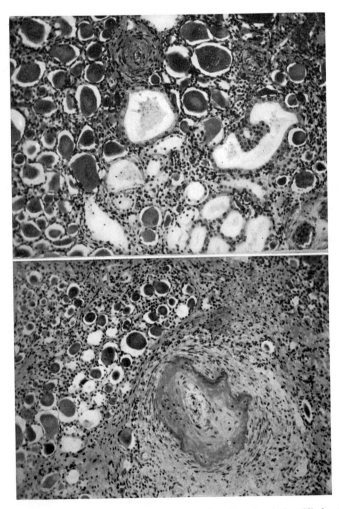

Fig. 13-16. Chronic pyelonephritis. Note the dilated tubules filled with casts and the thickened blood vessels.

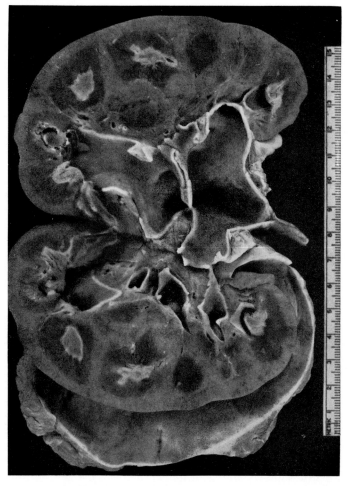

Fig. 13-17. Papillary necrosis of the kidney. From a case of diabetes mellitus with ureteral stenosis and mild hydronephrosis.

pitted by shallow, often broad, U-shaped scars, greatly contracted, and of little functional value. Such a pyelonephritic contracture of the kidney is often unilateral and must be distinguished from unilateral renal hypoplasia. When chronic pyelonephritis is bilateral, its end stages are easily confused clinically with chronic glomerulonephritis. Vascular changes and hypertension are frequently associated with chronic and healed stages of pyelonephritis.

Necrosis of renal papillae (necrotizing renal papillitis). Acute pyelonephritis complicated by necrosis of renal papillae occurs particularly in diabetic patients over 40 years of age, but it may also occur in nondiabetic patients with urinary obstruction. Some cases have been associated with excessive use of acetophenetidin (phenacetin).

Prolonged heavy use of analgesics containing phenacetin may be associated with chronic renal disease characterized by papillary necrosis, without extensive polymorphonuclear leukocytic exudate, and by interstitial fibrosis, with significant atrophy of tubules and peritubular capillaries in the medulla. The cortex may show focal areas of tubular atrophy.

Acute pyelonephritis is a fairly frequent complication of diabetes mellitus, and about 25% of cases show some necrosis of renal papillae. In some the clinical course is fulminating with death in a few days. The necrotic papillae stand out as pale, grayish yellow, infarctlike areas bordered by a reddish zone of inflammatory reaction. Sequestration of the necrotic papillae occurs, and the necrotic material, in late stages, may be sloughed away.

Pyonephrosis. When an obstructive factor is added to pyelonephritis, hydronephrosis and hydronephrotic atrophy are also present in variable degree. When the distended hydronephrotic pelvis is filled with pus, the condition is referred to as pyonephrosis. The end result may be a thin-walled sac filled with pus.

Radiation nephritis. When renal tissue is included in the field of therapeutic deep x-radiation, renal damage may result, sometimes sufficiently severe to lead to hypertension or death from renal functional failure. Symptoms usually begin six to twelve months after the radiotherapy. The kidneys show thickened capsules and pericapsular fibrosis. Tubules are atrophic, with widespread interstitial fibrosis, glomerular damage, and fibrinoid necrotic lesions of arterioles.

Tuberculosis of the kidney

Renal tuberculosis is secondary to an active tuberculous lesion elsewhere, the organisms reaching the kidney by hematogenous spread. The kidneys are usually involved along with other organs in acute miliary tuberculosis, but another form of renal tuberculosis also occurs, in which there is a chronic ulcerative and spreading lesion. This form is usually unilateral, and the primary focus from which spread occurred is often not prominent. Embolic masses of organisms arrested in the kidney produce the first lesion in the cortex. By discharge of this lesion into a tubule, spread occurs to the medulla, where a caseous ulcerative tubercle appears on a renal papilla. From there spread occurs to the mucosa of the pelvis, ureter, and bladder. Reinfection and extension to other portions of the kidney readily follow. Tuberculous strictures of the ureter and individual calices lead to stasis of the urine and hydronephrotic changes. There is a progression of the tuberculous process in the kidney tissue with caseation, loss of tissue through ulceration, and hydronephrosis.

The appearance of the kidney depends upon the state of the process. In an early period a few yellowish opaque tubercles are seen in the cortex and near the tip of papillae. Later, caseous masses of varying size replace the renal tissue, and the ragged hydronephrotic cavities contain a thick creamy pus.

The infected ureter becomes thick walled, rigid, and stenosed. The urinary bladder involvement begins at the ureteral opening and spreads as an irregular area of ulceration.

Hyperparathyroid renal disease

Renal hyperparathyroidism. Deficiency of renal function stimulates hyperplasia and hyperfunction of the parathyroid glands. The actual stimulating factor is probably some disturbance of calcium or phosphorus balance resulting from renal deficiency. Parathyroid hyperplasia and hyperfunction are present in some degree in all cases having severe deficiency of renal function. If the disturbance is severe and long continued, a clinical picture is produced similar to that for osteitis fibrosa cystica or renal rickets (in children).

Renal rickets. Renal rickets (renal dwarfism, renal infantilism) is a condition arising before puberty, in which a prolonged chronic renal insufficiency is associated with stunting of growth, skeletal deformities, and sometimes failure of sexual development. Renal disease develops before bone growth is completed and gives rise to renal insufficiency continuing over a long period. The failure of renal function causes retention of phosphates. A high level of blood phosphorus is characteristic and, in turn, stimulates the parathyroids to hyperplasia and increased function. The bone lesions, particularly in those cases with severe deformities, are those of osteitis fibrosa cystica and are caused by an excess of parathyroid hormone.

The actual lesions in the urinary tract can be divided into two groups. In one there are lesions of a congenital nature, either cystic kidneys or some abnormality of the lower urinary tract resulting in dilatation of the ureters and hydronephrosis. In the other group the renal changes have commonly been called chronic interstitial nephritis. In such cases the picture is that of the end stage of chronic pyelonephritis.

Parathyroid nephritis. Hyperparathyroidism itself may produce renal lesions of a distinctive type and result in a renal failure. The parathyroid hyperfunction may be caused by a localized adenomatous overgrowth of a single parathyroid or by a peculiar diffuse hyperplasia of all the parathyroids. The resulting disturbance in calcium metabolism appears to be the

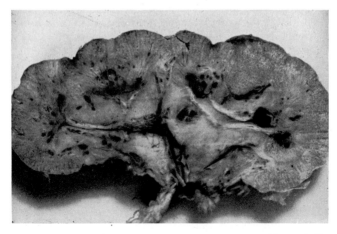

Fig. 13-18. Chronic pyelonephritis and hyperparathyroid renal disease. Black calculous masses are evident in the renal substance and in the pelvis. From a person having hyperparathyroidism caused by a parathyroid adenoma.

main cause of the damage to the kidney. Calcium deposits in the kidney are the characteristic feature. In acute hyperparathyroidism the calcium may be mainly intratubular, but in chronic hyperparathyroidism it is interstitial and peritubular and is accompanied by interstitial fibrosis and cellular infiltration. Renal calculus formation is very frequent and develops on the basis of a parenchymal calcium concretion. Hyperparathyroidism is, however, the underlying cause of only a very small proportion of renal calculi.

Calcification in the kidney (nephrocalcinosis) occurs not only with hyperparathyroidism but also in the disturbance of calcium metabolism of the milk-alkali syndrome, sarcoidosis, and hypervitaminosis D. It also may be the result of skeletal involvement in multiple myeloma and some metastatic cancers, and it occurs in renal tubular acidosis, hypochloremic alkalosis from excessive vomiting, and after tubular injury by nephrotoxins such as mercury bichloride.

Renal calculi

Stones, or calculi, formed in the urinary tract are caused by precipitation of chemical salts in the urine. Calculi are frequently classified as primary and secondary. The primary stones are those formed without apparent causal factors, such as infection, inflammation, or urinary obstruction and stasis. Secondary stones are those that follow evident inflammation or obstruction.

Etiology. The causes of stone formation are of two types: first, those factors that cause increased urinary concentration of the crystalloids that compose stones, and second, changes of a physical or chemical nature in the urine or urinary tract that favor precipitation of crystalloids.

High concentration of crystalline salts in the urine favors precipitation. Colloids in the urine hold the crystalloids in solution in a supersaturated state. The balance is delicate and easily disturbed either by hyperexcretion of crystalloids, such as may occur in hyperparathyroidism, or by decrease of colloids, which may be caused by infection.

Encrustation of solid material with urinary salts is a factor of importance. A nidus for such precipitation may be bacteria, necrotic or degenerated tissue, or other foreign bodies. Encrustation frequently occurs on a small calcified plaque of a renal papilla.

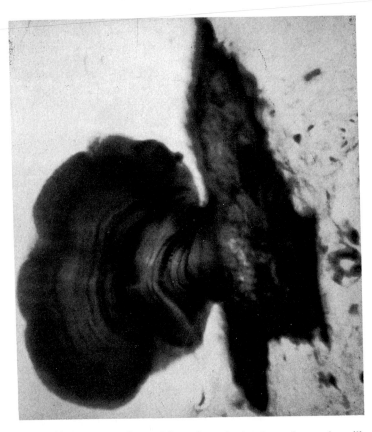

Fig. 13-19. Renal calculus. Calcium plaque in the tissue of a renal papilla with an attached early stone. Note the narrow necklike attachment of the calculus and its laminated structure caused by successive deposits of precipitated material. (From Anderson, W. A. D.: J. Urol. 44:29, 1940.)

Urinary reaction is important in the maintenance of urinary salts in solution and largely determines the composition of the stones. However, reaction alone (e.g., great alkalinity) is probably never the cause of stone formation.

Urinary obstruction acts by promoting stagnation and infection. It is rarely the sole factor.

Hyperparathyroidism has a known direct relationship to renal stone formation but probably accounts for 1% or less of renal calculi. The greatly increased urinary excretion of calcium and phosphorus in the urine and the tendency to deposition of calcium salts in renal tissue result in calculus formation in 30 to 70% of cases of hyperparathyroidism.

Pathogenesis. A mechanism of primary stone formation has been described by Randall. Damage to a renal papilla results in calcium deposit in the injured tissue. When near the surface, this plaque of calcium becomes exposed by ulceration of overlying tissue and becomes a nidus on which any urinary salt may crystallize. Successive depositions produce a laminated stone, often of variable composition. The plaque holds the stone in place until it has time to reach a considerable size before tearing away from its moorings.

Types. While stones are often composed of mixtures of uric acid, calcium oxalate, and phosphates, certain constituents predominate and give the stone distinctive character. *Uric acid stones* are brown, fairly smooth, moderately hard, and on section show concentric laminations. *Calcium oxalate stones* (15 to 30% of renal stones) are very hard, have a rough spiny surface of dark brown color, and are laminated. *Phosphate stones* (20% of renal stones) are soft, smooth, white, and friable. More than 50% of renal stones are composed of a mixture of calcium oxalate and phosphate. Uric acid and oxalates tend to precipitate in an acid urine, while phosphate stones are commonly associated with alkaline urines.

Sulfapyridine administration may be associated with the formation of small stones, caused by the precipitation of acetylated sulfapyridine.

Effects. Renal calculi may obstruct the outflow of urine, promote infection, and cause the pain of renal colic. The point of obstruction may be in the renal pelvis, ureters, or bladder. Partial or intermittent obstruction gives rise to dilatation of the ureter or renal pelvis (hydronephrosis) above the obstructed point. Stasis caused by obstruction promotes infection (pyelonephritis). Passage of a small stone through the ureter produces the severe pain of renal colic.

Oxalosis

Oxalosis is a rare primary disturbance of oxalate metabolism with the deposition of calcium oxalate in the kidneys and other tissues. Hyperoxaluria is accompanied by progressive calcium oxalate urolithiasis and nephrocalcinosis, usually beginning in early childhood. Renal damage occurs with recurrent urinary tract infection, and the cause of eventual death is usually renal failure. Oxalate also may be found in the myocardium, the walls of small arteries, and the rete testis.

Hydronephrosis

Hydronephrosis is a dilatation of the renal pelves and associated atrophy of renal tissue resulting from an obstruction to the outflow of urine. Obstruction may result from a wide variety of causes, e.g., prostatic enlargements, calculi, congenital and inflammatory strictures, pregnancy, and tumors. Obstructions at or below the outlet of the bladder result in bilateral hydronephrosis. With obstruction of one ureter only, the corresponding kidney is hydronephrotic. The degree of hydronephrosis depends upon the degree and duration of the obstruction. Partial and intermittent obstructions result in a greater degree of hydronephrosis than do sudden complete obstructions. The latter tend to produce atrophy with relatively little hydronephrosis. In some cases no mechanical obstruction can be demonstrated (idiopathic

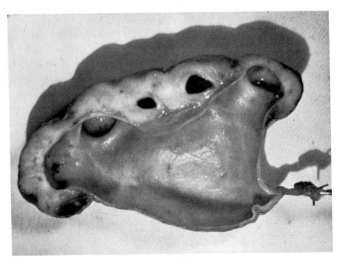

Fig. 13-20. Hydronephrosis caused by obstruction of the upper end of the ureter.

hydronephrosis). Some of such cases result from spinal cord lesions causing paralysis of the bladder. Neuromuscular imbalance has been postulated as a possible explanation for others.

With distention of the renal pelvis the calices flatten, the renal tissue becomes atrophic and thin, and the dilated pelvis assumes a saccular and rounded form. In severe cases the total size of the kidney and pelvis may be increased and the outer surface lobulated. The atrophy and fibrosis of the renal parenchyma affect tubules more rapidly than glomeruli. Hence, except in late stages, the tubular atrophy may seem to be out of proportion to the glomerular changes. Eventually glomeruli become hyalinized. The occurrence of infection converts the condition into pyonephrosis. When hydronephrosis is unilateral, the opposite kidney may undergo a compensatory hypertrophy.

The kidney in toxemias of pregnancy

Renal lesions regularly accompany the toxemias of late pregnancy (eclampsia, preeclampsia, etc.). They are more constant and characteristic than the hepatic lesions (p. 493). The glomeruli are enlarged and bloodless and have narrowed capillaries. Most of the capillary narrowing is accounted for by considerable thickening of the basement membrane of the tufts. Tubular changes are constantly present and often are more

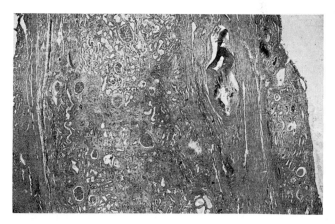

Fig. 13-21. Hydronephrotic atrophy of the kidney. Full thickness of the renal substance, with pelvic mucosa evident at the right.

prominent than glomerular lesions. The convoluted tubules particularly are involved by changes that vary from mild cloudy swelling or fatty degeneration to hyaline droplet degeneration and even necrosis. The tubular changes, although more striking, are probably secondary and of less importance than the glomerular lesions. The lesion characterized by ischemic glomeruli with diffusely and uniformly thickened basement membranes is considered a distinctive variety of membranous glomerulonephritis. An electron dense material may be deposited between endothelial cells and the basement membrane.

In some cases of pregnancy toxemia the renal changes are those of primary glomerulonephritis, pyelonephritis, or hypertensive arteriolar nephrosclerosis. More than half of the women who recover from eclampsia eventually develop hypertensive cardiovascular renal disease. The rare bilateral renal cortical necrosis also may occur in association with pregnancy (p. 379).

Congenital malformations and anomalies of the kidney

Congenital absence. Congenital absence, or aplasia, of both kidneys is rare and incompatible with life. Absence, or aplasia, of one kidney is more common, and the opposite kidney is larger than normal.

Congenital fusion. Congenital fusion of the kidneys, *horseshoe kidneys,* is most commonly a connection of the lower poles, either by a fibrous band or by actual renal tissue. The pelves are separate, and the ureters pass anteriorly across the lower poles of the kidneys.

Duplication of ureters or double pelvis. The duplication of ureters or a double pelvis are common anomalies that usually are of no functional significance. Persistence of some degree of fetal lobulation of the kidneys is also very common and harmless.

Cysts of the kidney

Cysts of the kidney are of three main types: *solitary cysts, retention cysts,* caused by tubular dilatation in vascular or inflammatory disease of the kidney, and the condition of *congenital polycystic kidneys.* A fourth variety, peripelvic lymphatic cyst, is rare.

The solitary cysts are usually serous, but they may be hemorrhagic. They vary from a few millimeters to several centimeters in diameter. Some are congenital in origin, and others result from tubular obstruction. Occasionally they are multilocular.

In advanced renal vascular disease or glomerulonephritis there frequently are multiple small cysts, usually only a few millimeters in diameter, resulting from tubular dilatation.

Peripelvic lymphatic cysts of the kidney are lymphatic distentions associated with obstruction of the lymphatic trunks of the hilus of the kidney. They are usually small and unimportant, but rarely they have caused damage by pressure on renal vessels. They may distort the pelvic outline in roentgenograms.

Congenital polycystic kidneys. Polycystic kidney is a congenital maldevelopment. One or both kidneys may be involved by extremely numerous cysts of varying and often large size. The condition is present at birth, and absence of sufficient functioning renal tissue may result in death at that time or within the next few years. If renal functional tissue is sufficient, life may go on with little or no clinical evidence of the disease until the third, fourth, or fifth decade. At that time renal failure results from the development of vascular disease, other accumu-

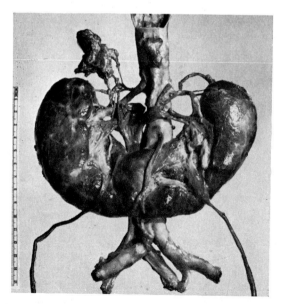

Fig. 13-22. Horseshoe kidney, showing the relations of blood vessels and ureters.

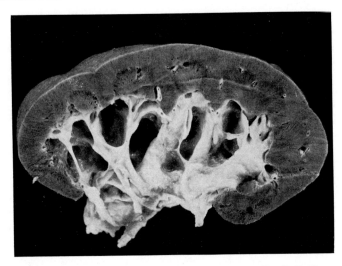

Fig. 13-23. Peripelvic cysts of the kidney. (Courtesy Dr. J. F. Kuzma.)

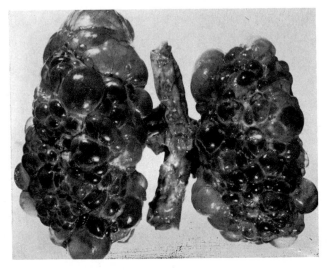

Fig. 13-24. Congenital polycystic kidneys.

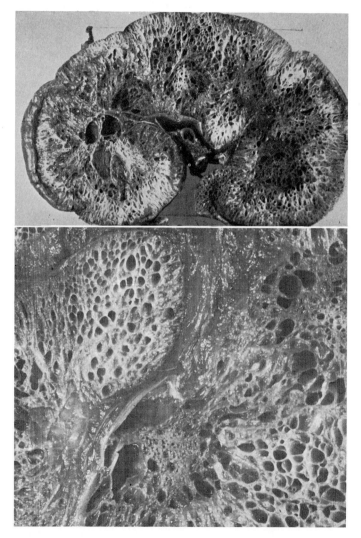

Fig. 13-25. Congenital cystic kidney in a newborn infant. The lower illustration shows a low magnification of the cut surface.

lated injuries of the kidney, or progressive increase in the size of the cysts. The patient may have lumbar pain, palpable mass in the kidney region, and hematuria, a picture simulating renal neoplasm. Other cases simply present acute or chronic renal failure with mild hypertension and cardiac hypertrophy, so that clinical differentiation from other types of renal disease may be very difficult. Attacks of hematuria are a quite distinctive finding and are caused by the rupture of blood vessels into cysts communicating with the pelvis.

The involved kidneys may be moderately or enormously enlarged, which results from an increase in size of individual cysts rather than from an increase in their number. The kidneys have a knobby or irregular outline. The cysts are lined by cuboidal or, more commonly, flattened epithelium. In the newborn group the remaining renal tissue is hypoplastic, the number of nephrons is reduced, and interstitital connective tissue is excessive.

At a later age, in cases without clinical symptoms, the functional renal tissue between cysts is often abundant. The patients dying of renal failure show extreme atrophy of the renal tissue between cysts, which is caused by progressive cystic enlargement and associated development of arterial disease.

Polycystic kidneys can be divided into several distinct types. Type 1, relatively uncommon, is found in newborn infants and is incompatible with continued life. The symmetrically enlarged kidneys have a spongy appearance. The cysts are saccular or

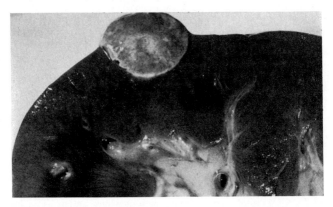

Fig. 13-26. Adenoma of the kidney.

cylindrically enlarged collecting tubules. It appears to result from a hyperplasia of the interstitial portions of the collecting tubules developing from the ureteral buds. Intrahepatic bile ducts are also cystic. The condition is apparently caused by a homozygous recessive gene.

Type 2, seen at any age, may involve a portion of a kidney, one kidney, or both kidneys. Unilateral polycystic kidneys in adults is usually of this type. Bilateral involvement is usually fatal in infancy. The terminal or ampullar portion of collecting tubules is cystic. The condition does not appear to be familial.

Type 3 is the common large bilateral polycystic disease of adults. There is an irregular mixture of normal and abnormal tubules and nephrons. Cysts involve various parts of the nephron. Connective tissue is increased. Cysts of other organs, particularly the liver, may be present. Occasionally, congenital (berry) aneurysms of cerebral arteries also may be present. There is sometimes a familial history.

Type 4 is uncommon. The cysts are small, located mainly in the outer cortex, and are dilated Bowman's spaces. The condition appears to be caused by urethral or ureteral obstruction in early fetal development.

Renal tumors

Benign tumors. Adenoma and fibroma are quite common but remain small and are of little practical importance. Lipoma of the kidney occurs rarely and may grow to a large size or undergo malignant change. Hamartomas of the kidney (angiomyolipomas) are seen mainly in cases of tuberous sclerosis. They are often multiple, bilateral, and composed of an unorganized mixture of fibrous and fatty tissue, blood vessels, and smooth muscle fibers. Angiomyolipomas of the kidney also may occur in the absence of the tuberous sclerosis complex; they are often large and may produce symptoms.

Adenoma. Adenoma of the kidney is commonly seen as a small grayish nodule in the cortex. Microscopically it is composed of dark-staining epithelial cells, forming well-differentiated tubules and sometimes structures resembling glomeruli.

Fibroma. Fibroma is commonly found in the medulla, where it appears as a tiny grayish area. It is composed of irregularly arranged connective tissue fibers. The margin is usually irregular or ill defined, and a few tubules are often enclosed in the tumor. Many of them may be of developmental origin or hamartomas.

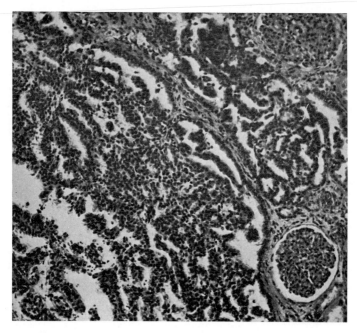

Fig. 13-27. Benign adenoma of the kidney. The edge of the tumor is shown, with glomeruli of the adjacent renal tissue evident on the right.

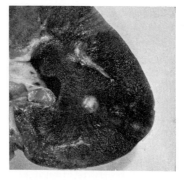

Fig. 13-28. Fibroma in the medulla of the kidney.

Malignant tumors. Malignant renal tumors are of unusual interest. They are of four types: (1) renal carcinoma or hypernephroma (Grawitz's tumor), which occurs particularly in the fifth and sixth decades; (2) embryonal adenosarcoma (Wilms' tumor), occurring in infancy and early childhood; (3) carcinoma of the renal pelvis; and (4) sarcoma.

Hypernephroma (Grawitz's tumor). Hypernephroma or adenocarcinoma is the common malignant renal tumor of adults. It is called hypernephroma because it has been supposed to arise from "rests" of adrenal cells in the kidney. Small areas of adrenal cortical tissue are often found in the outer part of the kidney, just beneath the capsule. Adrenal heterotopia, with all or part of the adrenals within the capsule of the kidneys, is sometimes encountered. Also adrenal tissue is not uncommon on the undersurface of the liver and in internal genitalia. Further evidence of the adrenal nature of these tumors lies in their close microscopic resemblance to the adrenal cortex. They are composed of large clear cells containing abundant, doubly refractive cholesterol esters, and the cells may be arranged in cords as in

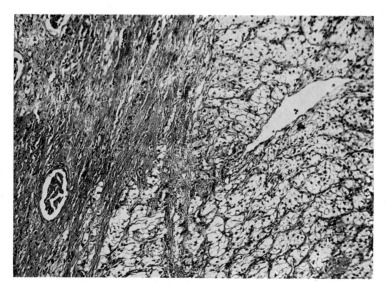

Fig. 13-29. Hypernephroma of the kidney. Compressed atrophic renal substance is seen at the left.

the adrenal cortex. However, this evidence is insufficient proof of their adrenal origin. Hypernephromas never give rise to the endocrine and sexual disturbances that accompany true adrenal cortical tumors. Some areas of the tumor may show a papillary or tubular structure, and all gradations may be found between a close resemblance to adrenal cortex and clear-cut renal carcinoma. Hence hypernephromas are generally considered to be simply renal carcinomas. However, attempts have been made to reconcile the evidences of adrenal and renal origins by suggesting that the tumor arises from cells retaining early embryonic potentialities for differentiation into either type of tissue. Most adenocarcinomas of the kidney occur after the age of 40 years. The frequency in males is more than twice that in females. Occasionally there is an associated polycythemia, which disappears after nephrectomy. Erythropoietic-stimulating activity (erythropoietin) has been demonstrated in the tumor tissue or in the plasma in some instances.

The hypernephroma forms a large rounded tumor in the kidney, at first well encapsulated and separated from the renal tissue. It is microscopically invasive, however, so that it is not easily shelled out or separated from surrounding tissue. The yellowish cut surface shows some connective tissue trabeculae coursing irregularly through the tumor. There is a great tendency to degeneration, necrosis, hemorrhage, and cyst formation. Microscopically the characteristic cells are large, with abundant pale, foamy cytoplasm. In some areas the cells may be smaller, with a denser, slightly granular, and more eosinophilic cytoplasm, more like ordinary renal tubular epithelium. The cells are arranged in solid sheets or as cords and papillary structures with a thin supporting stroma. The well-differentiated tumors of lower grade malignancy form tubular or papillary structures. Tumors of high malignancy have little tubular or papillary formation and show greater variation in size and staining of cells and nuclei and more frequent mitoses.

The growth of the tumor causes atrophy and fibrosis of adjacent tissue. In later stages there is extensive invasion of renal substance. The tumor cells have a tendency to invade veins and grow along the blood vessels. Metastasis occurs by bloodstream, and the lungs, liver, and bones are the common sites for the secondary tumors.

Because of the relatively localized growth of hypernephroma in its early stages, it may attain considerable size with only pain-

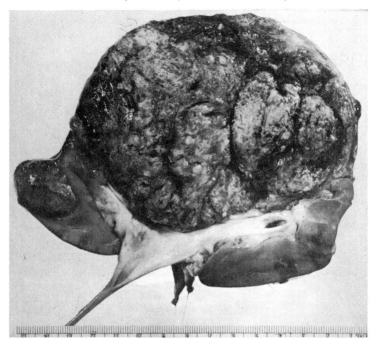

Fig. 13-30. Hypernephroma of the kidney.

less hematuria as clinical evidence of its presence. Metastases in lungs or bones may be the first indication.

Embryonal adenosarcoma (Wilms' tumors). Embryoma is a rare mixed tumor of the kidney, the occurrence of which is almost limited to the first 7 years of life, although a few cases have been reported in adults; the average age is 3 years. These tumors account for about 20% of cancers in childhood. The origin is believed to be from mesodermal cells displaced during development but retaining the ability to grow and differentiate into various types of tissue. Being rapidly growing tumors of embryonic nature, they are highly radiosensitive.

At first the tumor is surrounded by a dense connective tissue capsule and remains separated from the renal parenchyma until quite large. The kidney tissue is pushed into various shapes. Eventually the capsule is ruptured and extension occurs to kidney tissue, omentum, and adjacent viscera. Blood-borne metas-

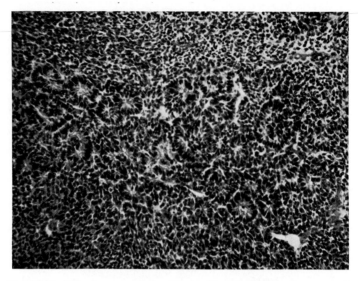

Fig. 13-31. Wilms' tumor of the kidney. Note the tubular or rosettelike structures amid the general sarcomatous appearance.

tases are common in the lungs and brain, but the liver and regional lymph nodes are also frequently involved.

The tumor tissue is uniformly grayish white and moderately firm, but cysts or hemorrhage may be present. Microscopically the predominant tumor elements are an abundant embryonic type of malignant connective tissue surrounding some glandlike tubules of variable size and shape. Epithelial cells may also form solid cords and strands of cells. Occasionally, smooth or striated muscle, cartilage or myxomatous tissue is present.

Sarcoma. Sarcoma may arise from connective tissue of the kidney, but this is uncommon. Examples of fibrosarcoma and liposarcoma have been reported.

Tumors of the renal pelvis. The pelvis of the kidney gives rise to the same types of tumor as are found in the bladder, the common forms being transitional cell papilloma and papillary carcinoma. The papillary carcinomas may give rise to secondary implants lower down in the ureter. Poorly differentiated infiltrating forms, which extend into the renal substance, also occur. An infrequent variety is squamous cell carcinoma.

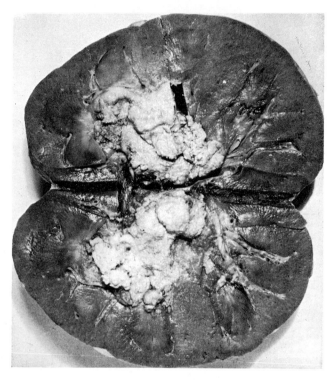

Fig. 13-32. Papillary carcinoma of the renal pelvis.

URETER

The most important pathologic involvement of the ureters is obstruction, which may be by a calculus from the renal pelvis, a fibrous stricture resulting from inflammation, or less frequently caused by tumors, either of the ureter itself or adjacent to and pressing on the ureter. Kinking of the ureter occurs when the kidney is abnormally movable or an aberrant renal artery crossing the ureter causes some cases of partial or intermittent obstruction. Hydronephrosis is the common result unless the obstruction is transitory. Obstruction of the urinary tract below the ureters causes bilateral dilatation of the ureters (hydroureter).

Ureteritis cystica is a fairly frequent condition that may contribute to ureteral obstruction. The cysts develop from the

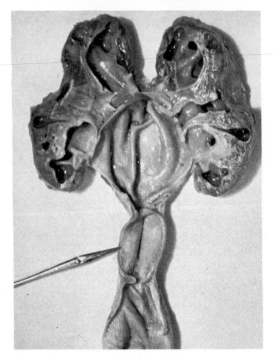

Fig. 13-33. Multiple strictures of the ureter with hydronephrosis.

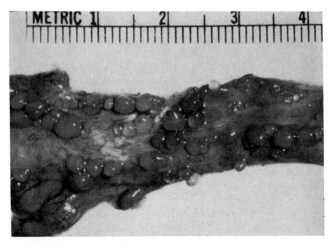

Fig. 13-34. Ureteritis cystica.

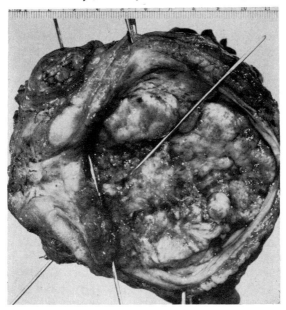

Fig. 13-35. Carcinoma of the urinary bladder. Irregular nodular neoplastic masses project into the lumen, obscuring the ureteral openings.

cell nests of von Brunn, which probably are focal downgrowths of mucosa occurring as a consequence of ureteritis. The upper portion of the ureter is most frequently involved, and there is frequent association with similar cystic lesions of the renal pelvis (pyelitis cystica) and of the urinary bladder (cystitis cystica).

Tumors of the ureter are uncommon and are of the same gross and histologic types as those that arise in the bladder.

URINARY BLADDER

Inflammation, obstruction, and tumors are the important lesions of the bladder; congenital abnormalities and traumatic changes are less common.

Inflammation

Inflammation of the bladder (cystitis) may be acute or chronic. The infection may descend from a pyelonephritis, may reach the bladder by way of the urethra, or may be introduced by catheterization. Obstruction of the bladder outlet, as by a calculus or enlarged prostate, is particularly likely to be associated with chronic inflammation. Important organisms in cystitis are pyogenic cocci and the colon bacillus.

Acute cystitis. In acute cystitis the mucosa is congested, edematous, and may be hemorrhagic or ulcerated. Congestion and inflammatory cells, particularly in submucosa, are evident microscopically.

Chronic cystitis. Chronic cystitis is associated with considerable thickening of the bladder wall by granulation tissue and fibrosis, unless an associated obstruction causes the wall to be dilated. Occasionally the thickened mucosa shows small, fluid-filled cystic cavities, the so-called "cystitis cystica." Other special varieties of cystitis have been given the descriptive names of interstitial cystitis, gangrenous cystitis, follicular cystitis, bullous cystitis, etc.

Malakoplakia. Malakoplakia is an uncommon inflammatory condition characterized by soft, grayish yellow plaques involving the mucosa of the bladder. The etiology is not established, but it is associated with long-standing cystitis. The sessile plaques are formed by accumulations of cells in the mucosa and submucosa. Although there is a mixture of inflammatory cells, large mononuclear or histiocytic cells are most characteristic. Laminated, hematoxylin-staining structures (Michaelis-Gutmann bodies) may be present, and they are similar to the Schaumann bodies of sarcoidosis.

Obstruction

Obstruction to the outlet of the urinary bladder may be caused by prostatic hypertrophy, strictures of the urethra, tumor, calculus, or neurogenic disturbance. The bladder becomes distended and thin walled. Hypertrophy of muscle bundles follows if the obstruction is prolonged, so that the inner surface of the distended bladder is roughened by prominent muscular trabeculae. Distention of weak areas between the trabeculae may produce multiple small (false) diverticula.

Tumors

Tumors of the urinary bladder are more frequent in men and commonly occur in the age group of 50 to 70 years. Etiologic factors are not apparent in most instances. Aniline dye workers excreting the dyes in the urine show a high incidence. The base or trigonal region of the bladder is the favorite site.

The common types are (1) papilloma, (2) papillary carcinoma, and (3) transitional cell carcinoma. Various other varieties, including squamous cell carcinoma, adenocarcinoma, and mucous carcinoma occur only rarely. Some of the mucous adenocarcinomas appear to be of urachal origin and have a poor prognosis.

Papilloma. The papilloma is a delicate pedunculated tumor projecting from the mucosal surface. It has a narrow base and many fine villous processes. Delicate branching villi compose the tumor, each having a thin connective tissue core containing blood vessels, separated by a definite basal membrane from a surface covering of transitional epithelial cells. (See Fig. 11-12.) The epithelial cells are uniform in size, shape, and staining.

Papillomas are frequently multiple and tend to recur. They are always potentially malignant, although they may remain benign for months or years. Evidence of malignancy is most likely to be invasion at the base of the pedicle, so that a section through this area is most important in diagnosis. Other findings suggesting malignancy are a breaking through of the basal membrane separating the stromal core, a growing together of the villi, and atypical staining and morphology of the epithelial cells.

Papillary carcinoma. Papillary carcinomas have a general architecture similar to that of the benign papillomas. They are more frequently single and firmer, have a broader base, and form large, bulky, cauliflower-like growths with a tendency to hemorrhage and necrosis. There is more irregularity of arrangement, size, and shape of the epithelial cells, and mitoses are more numerous than in papillomas. The processes tend to be fused, and there is invasion of the connective tissue stroma or of the wall of the bladder from the base of the tumor.

Transitional cell carcinoma. Transitional cell carcinoma forms a sessile infiltrating type of tumor that spreads widely through the bladder wall and to surrounding structures, although no large tumor may form in the bladder lumen. Necrosis and ulceration tend to occur. A few of these infiltrating tumors are composed of squamous rather than transitional epithelial cells.

Spread of bladder cancer is usually late and not very extensive, particularly in the papillary forms of low malignancy. Invasion of surrounding structures and metastasis to pelvic and prevertebral lymph nodes usually precede spread to the lungs, liver, or bones.

MALE GENITAL ORGANS
Penis

Phimosis. Phimosis is a condition in which the foreskin cannot be retracted.

Paraphimosis. In paraphimosis a retracted foreskin cannot be brought forward. Paraphimosis, as well as phimosis, may be congenital or may be acquired and caused by inflammatory swelling and edema.

Balanitis. Balanitis is an inflammation of the glans. It is predisposed to by phimosis. The gonococcus and the colon bacillus are the common causative organisms.

Peyronie's disease. Peyronie's disease is a plastic induration or fibrosis of the penis; it is of unknown etiology.

Venereal lesions. The venereal lesions that may affect the penis are chancroid syphilis (chancre), lymphopathia venereum, and granuloma inguinale. They have been considered in Chapter 8.

Squamous cell carcinoma. Squamous cell carcinoma is the only important tumor of the penis. It occurs on the glans or prepuce (less commonly), usually in patients past 50 years of age, and often it is preceded by chronic irritation from balanitis, phimosis, or uncleanliness. It begins as a small warty growth, later developing into an ulcerative fungating mass. Metastasis occurs to inguinal and, later, to retroperitoneal nodes.

Urethra

Urethritis. Inflammation (urethritis) is the common lesion of the urethra and is usually of infectious origin. It is accompanied by abundant pus production and much desquamation of epithelium.

Stricture. Stricture of the urethra is a common end result of infection, particularly gonorrhea, but its origin also may be traumatic or caused by a congenital fold of mucosa. The obstruction may cause dilatation of the bladder, ureters, and renal pelves.

Testis and epididymis

Varicocele. Varicocele is a varicose dilatation of the veins of the spermatic cord.

Hydrocele. Hydrocele is the accumulation of clear watery fluid in the tunica vaginalis.

Hematocele. If blood is present, the hydrocele is referred to as a hematocele.

Spermatocele. Spermatocele is a dilatation of the duct of the epididymis.

Epididymitis. Inflammation (epididymitis) is most commonly caused by gonorrhea, the infection usually spreading from the seminal vesicles. One finds suppuration and the formation of small abscesses. Scarring, which follows the inflammation, often prevents the passage of spermatozoa, thus causing sterility, although testicular atrophy and sexual inactivity do not necessarily result. Nongonorrheal epididymitis is less common but may result from staphylococcal or colon bacillus infections.

Acute orchitis. Inflammation of the testicle may result from trauma or complicate certain infectious diseases, particularly mumps, typhoid fever, and smallpox. It is the most serious feature of mumps in young adults. In some cases it is followed by testicular atrophy and sterility.

Tuberculosis. Tuberculosis may involve the epididymis before other parts of the urogenital system. Small conglomerate caseous tubercles are formed, similar in their gross and microscopic appearance to tubercles elsewhere.

Syphilis. Syphilis more commonly involves the testis firstly and the epididymis secondarily. The syphilitic orchitis may be a gumma or a diffuse fibrosis.

Granulomatous orchitis. Granulomatous orchitis of a chronic nature and unknown pathogenesis is not uncommon. Trauma appears to be a factor in some cases.

Hyalinization of seminiferous tubules. Hyalinization of seminiferous tubules has been found associated with hypogonadism and testicular failure. A progressive sclerosis beginning in the basement membranes and tunica propria of the tubules results in hyalinization, with disappearance of germinal and Sertoli cells and an apparent increase and clumping of Leydig cells. Azoospermia and high urinary gonadotropins are associated with this lesion.

Cryptorchism. Cryptorchism is a failure of descent of the testis into the scrotum. The testis is found in the peritoneal cavity or in the inguinal canal. The condition may be unilateral or bilateral. Undescended testicles are usually deficient in spermatogenesis, but they do produce the hormone necessary for secondary sexual characteristics. Malignant tumors are much more frequent in the cryptorchid than in the normally descended testis.

Tumors of the testis. Almost all testicular tumors are malignant and account for about 0.6% of cancer in males. In 11%

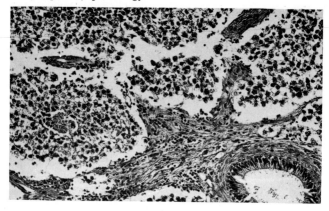

Fig. 13-36. Seminoma of the testis.

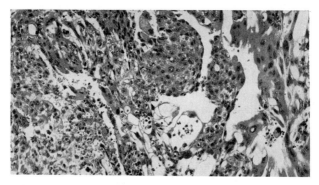

Fig. 13-37. Choriocarcinoma of the testis.

of cases there is an associated cryptorchism or ectopic position of the testis. Most testicular tumors occur between 20 and 45 years of age. The classification and terminology of testicular cancers are variable and confused. Ewing has regarded them all as teratomas, arising from sex cells and capable of reproducing any tissue. Commonly they are divided into two groups only, seminomas and teratomas, but a more detailed classification includes (1) seminoma, (2) teratocarcinoma and teratosarcoma, (3) embryonal carcinoma, (4) adult teratoma, and (5) choriocarcinoma. A benign interstitial cell tumor occurs.

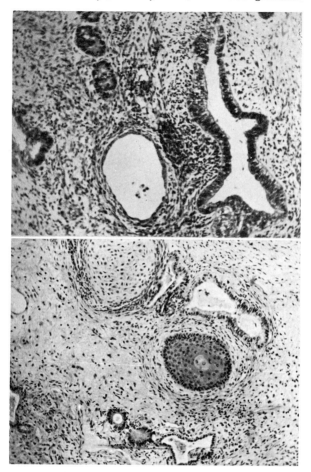

Fig. 13-38. Adult teratoma of the testis. Note the variety of cells and structures.

Seminoma. The seminoma occurs in an older age group and is relatively less malignant than most of the other cancers. It is a firm, homogeneous grayish white mass, circumscribed, and varying up to the size of a grapefruit. Gray or yellowish opaque areas of necrosis may be present. Histologically it is composed of uniform rounded or polygonal cells with prominent round or oval hyperchromatic nuclei, arranged in diffuse sheets or in cordlike or tubular form. A scanty stroma separates groups of cells and is sometimes infiltrated with small lymphocytes. This microscopic appearance is similar to that of dysgerminoma of the ovary (p. 733).

Embryonal carcinoma. The embryonal carcinoma is a more malignant, rapidly growing, and invasive tumor that usually shows more structural variation. Degeneration and necrosis are frequent in areas of the tumor, which tends to be soft, grayish, and opaque. The tumor cells may occur in solid sheets or may have a papillary or glandular structure. The cells tend to be larger and more variable than in the seminoma, with larger pleomorphic nuclei having coarsely clumped chromatin.

Choriocarcinoma. Testicular choriocarcinomas are usually small soft tumors with areas of hemorrhage and necrosis. Two types of cells, the Langhans and syncytial cells, occur, and villuslike structures may be formed. The polyhedral Langhans or cytotrophoblastic cells may form irregular sheets. The syncytial cells are large, multinucleated, with irregular hyperchromatic nuclei. Trophoblastic elements also may be seen in embryonal carcinomas. Rare extragenital choriocarcinomas also occur in the male, and like the testicular tumor, are similar to the choriocarcinoma of the placenta. The choriocarcinomas are all highly malignant.

Teratoma and mixed tumors. Included in the teratomas and mixed tumors are adult or differentiated teratomatous tumors (adult teratomas), containing various types of tissue, and also more highly malignant varieties in which only one type of cell is found (teratocarcinoma and teratosarcoma). The gross appearance is as variable as its microscopic composition. A large size is often attained, and cyst formation is common. Microscopically, undifferentiated and unrecognizable highly malignant tumor cells may be present, or differentiated structures such as cartilage, muscle, fat, glands, and myxomatous tissue may be recognized.

Most malignant testicular tumors are associated with production of pituitary-like hormones. On a quantitative basis hormone tests show some correlation with the histologic type, although not close or very reliable. The adult type of teratoma has a low level of hormones, the seminoma has a higher level, and the choriocarcinoma has a very high level of hormones.

Most of the testicular malignancies are highly radiosensitive. The well-differentiated tumors or adult types of teratoma re-

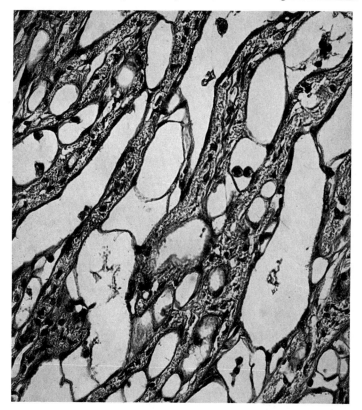

Fig. 13-39. "Adenomatoid tumor" of the epididymis. Flattened cells line thin-walled spaces to give a honeycomb appearance. (From Haukohl, R. S., and Anderson, W. A. D., editors: Pathology seminars, St. Louis, 1955, The C. V. Mosby Co.)

spond least. Metastasis occurs by blood and lymph channels. Lymphatic metastasis is found most frequently in the pelvis and abdominal retroperitoneal nodes. The lungs and liver are the organs most often the site of metastases.

Interstitial cell tumors. The interstitial (Leydig) cells of the testis are numerous in adults and appear increased in atrophic testes, as in elderly persons or in patients with undescended testes. Benign tumors composed of mature interstitial cells are of rare occurrence and have an endocrine function. In children these are a rare cause of hypergenitalism and precocious development of secondary sexual characteristics.

Tumors of the epididymis. Primary tumors of the epididymis are very rare, and most are benign. The most common is the so-called "adenomatoid" tumor. This benign tumor is also found in the female genital tract, most often involving the fallopian tubes, uterus, or ovaries. It shows small glandlike spaces separated by an abundant fibrous and smooth muscle stroma. Its origin is debatable, and it has been variously considered as epithelial, mesothelial, lymphangiomatous, and as a hamartoma of the mesonephros. Leiomyomas of the epididymis also occur.

Prostate

The prostate is a sexual gland. Its secretion is mixed with the sperm in the urethra at the time of ejaculation and functions to activate and prolong the motility of the spermatozoa. The gland has five lobes (median, two lateral, posterior, and anterior) and a group of gland acini in the midline of the urethral floor between the posterior vesical lip and the verumontanum (subcervical urethral glands of Albarran). The median lobe is that part dorsal to the urethra and between the converging ejaculatory ducts. The median lobe, the glands of Albarran, and the lateral lobes are particularly likely to undergo benign enlargement and cause obstruction.

The prostatic glands are lined by cuboidal or cylindric epithelium and often contain concentrically laminated concretions, corpora amylacea. A hormonal secretion of the testis, activated in turn by the pituitary, influences the prostate and causes its rapid maturation at puberty. Involution progresses during and after the fifth decade because of a decrease of hormonal stimulation. Estrogens appear to promote squamous metaplasia in the prostate.

Thrombosis of periprostatic veins is common in elderly bedridden patients. Focal infarctions often occur in enlarged prostates, and around them the glandular epithelium often undergoes squamous metaplasia. Small prostatic calculi are common in patients in older age groups.

The important lesions of the prostate are inflammation, benign enlargement, and carcinoma.

Inflammation. Two common types of inflammation of the prostate are acute prostatitis and tuberculosis.

Acute prostatitis. Acute prostatitis may be caused by gonococci or other pyogenic organisms. The purulent material is confined within acini or extends and forms abscesses. The inflammation may clear up, but it commonly becomes chronic. Septicemias and pyemias also may result in multiple small abscesses of the prostate, the *Staphylococcus aureus* being the most common organism. A rare allergic prostatitis is sometimes seen in asthmatics.

Tuberculosis. Tuberculosis is common in the prostate, usually carried there by the bloodstream, and in less than 20% of cases it is secondary to foci elsewhere in urogenital organs. Typically caseous lesions are formed that are similar to tuberculous lesions elsewhere.

Nodular hyperplasia (benign prostatic hypertrophy). Benign enlargement is the commonest lesion of the prostate, being found in about 30% of men over the age of 60 years. About 17% have symptoms of urinary obstruction as a result, which is its main and important effect. The normal adult prostate weighs about 20 grams. The enlarged prostate is usually two to four times larger, but seldom weighs more than 200 grams. There does not appear to be a transition between nodular hyperplasia and carcinoma.

The *anatomic changes* are the result of hyperplasia in the inner group of prostatic glands. Parts that may be involved include large portions of the lateral lobes, the median lobe, or the subcervical glands of Albarran. The hyperplasia includes a proliferation of periductal, periacinar, and periurethral stroma, including both connective tissue and smooth muscle fibers. Hyperplastic glandular growth also usually occurs, sometimes as a secondary phenomenon. Localized nodules of tumorlike or adenomatous tissue result, in which there are cystic dilatations of acini with papillary infoldings lined by a single layer of high columnar epithelium, and also areas with an increase in number of acini. Occasionally there are nodules composed only of smooth muscle, or there are masses of lymphoid tissue. Prostatic median bar enlargement is predominantly caused by smooth muscle hypertrophy, associated with some interfascicular fibrosis and edema.

The effect of *prostatic enlargement* is to obstruct the outflow of urine. Enlargement of the lateral lobes compresses the urethra into a narrow and irregular slit. Enlargement of the median lobe or of the subcervical glands of Albarran results in a nodular mass, which pushes up the floor of the bladder just inside

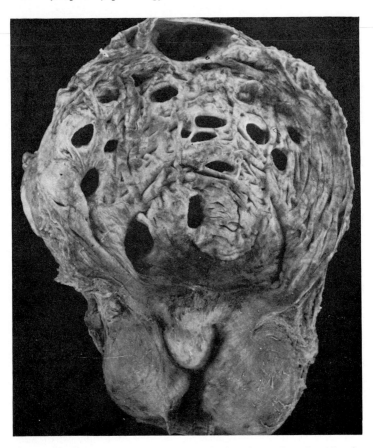

Fig. 13-40. Hyperplasia of prostate gland with obstruction of urethra by large middle lobe; hypertrophied bladder with cellules and diverticula. (From Pessin, S. B., and Anderson, W. A. D.: Lower urinary tract and male genitalia. In Anderson, W. A. D., editor: Pathology, ed. 5, St. Louis, 1966, The C. V. Mosby Co.)

the sphincter or in the proximal part of the urethra. This midline enlargement is particularly effective in obstructing outflow of urine, acting as a plug to close the urethral orifice. A small sac forms behind the prostatic nodule, from which urine cannot be expelled, and contains the so-called residual urine.

Results of the obstruction may be seen in all parts of the

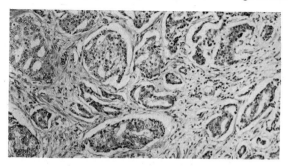

Fig. 13-41. Adenocarcinoma of the prostate.

urinary tract proximal to the prostate. The bladder becomes hypertrophied, with prominent muscular trabeculation evident on its mucosal surface. Diverticula may develop in weak areas between the trabeculae. The ureters and renal pelves undergo dilatation (hydroureter and hydronephrosis).

The etiology has been variously considered to be chronic inflammation, arteriosclerosis, and hormonal imbalance. The concept that the condition is one of true tumor formation has been rejected.

Carcinoma. Carcinoma of the prostate occurs with increasing frequency after the fourth decade, being found in 14 to 29% of males examined at autopsy in the older age groups. In a large proportion of these cases the cancer is occult or latent and has given rise to no clinical manifestations. The incidence of latent carcinoma increases with age. It is morphologically similar to the manifest carcinomas and shows the property of infiltration but lacks the capacity for rapid growth. The occurrence of prostatic carcinoma is associated with senile atrophy of the gland, but it is quite independent of the condition of nodular hyperplasia. Whereas hyperplasia occurs in the inner mass of the prostate, carcinoma arises in the outer mass or near the capsule. Acid phosphatase of the serum is usually increased in patients with carcinoma of the prostate. If there are skeletal metastases, the alkaline phosphatase also may be increased.

The carcinomatous prostate tends to be firm or hard and to lack the elastic consistency of benign enlargement. With invasion through the capsule the prostate becomes fixed to surrounding structures. Microscopically there are numerous acini which tend to be irregular and lined by several layers of epithelium, and also solid cords of epithelial cells irregularly invade adjacent tissue. The latent or inactive carcinomas are not histologically distinguishable from the active and invasive cancers. An epidermoid carcinoma occasionally may be found in the prostate, although adenocarcinoma is the common form. Invasion of the capsular perineural lymphatics occurs early. More distant lymphatic spread to the pelvic nodes is a late occurrence. Hematogenous metastasis to bones, lungs, and liver is common. In bone an osteoplastic reaction is induced by the tumor cells (p. 852). Treatment by castration or with estrogens causes metaplastic, degenerative, and atrophic changes in the tumor cells.

Sarcoma. Sarcoma of the prostate is rare and easily confused with anaplastic carcinoma. Myosarcoma appears to be the most frequent type, but lymphosarcoma, spindle cell sarcoma, and other forms also occur.

Chapter 14

The respiratory tract and lungs

NOSE AND SINUSES

Rhinophyma. The skin of the nose is subject to rhinophyma, a nodular enlargement characterized by hypertrophy of the sebaceous glands. Dilated sebaceous ducts and hypertrophied acini contain epithelial debris and inspissated sebaceous material. The glandular epithelium may at times undergo squamous metaplasia. The surrounding dermis may show some chronic inflammatory reaction and fibrosis.

Rhinitis. Rhinitis, an inflammation of the nasal mucosa, may show characteristics of an allergic inflammation with numerous eosinophils in the mucosa and surface exudate, or it may be nonallergic and infectious in origin. *Atrophic rhinitis (ozena)* is characterized by considerable crusting of the nasal mucosa. Specific types of rhinitis include rhinoscleroma and rhinosporidiosis. *Rhinoscleroma* is characterized by nodular masses in the nose, which are composed of granulation tissue with many lymphocytes and plasma cells, and foamy mononuclear cells (Mikulicz cells), which may contain an organism, *Klebsiella rhinoscleromatis*. *Rhinosporidiosis* is a specific fungous infection.

Polyps. Polyps of the nose and sinuses are predominantly inflammatory masses with edema, marked vascularity, a chronic cellular exudate, and sometimes cysts. Neoplastic polyps (epithelial papillomas) also occur. Other tumors of the nose and sinuses include angiomas, transitional cell carcinomas, squamous cell carcinomas, and adenocarcinomas. Various types of bone tumors may arise in the maxilla and involve the nose or sinuses. Mixed tumors of the salivary gland type, arising in the palate, may invade the nose or maxillary sinus.

LARYNX

Infectious inflammatory lesions of the larynx (laryngitis) are a common component of many respiratory infections, including tuberculosis. Tumors and tumorlike conditions are the most common serious lesions of the larynx.

Carcinomas of the larynx may arise from the epithelium lining the lumen of the larynx or the mucous membranes of the orifice or pharyngeal surface of the larynx. By the clinical and topographic classifications commonly used, they have been divided into two general groups: *Intrinsic* cancers are those arising from the interior of the larynx, and with these are included the subglottic growths, as well as tumors of the vocal cords and ventricles. *Extrinsic* cancers are those of the mucous membranes of the orifice and pharyngeal surface of the larynx. Laryngeal tumors may be classified also as supraglottic and subglottic.

Benign lesions of the larynx that may simulate cancer include cysts, inflammations, keratoses, papillomas, and polyps.

Chronic obstruction of the larynx may be an important aspect of inflammations and neoplasms of the area. Acute obstruction may be allergic or may be caused by a bolus of food. Asphyxiation resulting from the obstruction of the airway by food ("the café coronary") is not uncommon.

Laryngeal cysts. Laryngeal cysts are relatively uncommon. They may be acquired or congenital. The acquired cysts are retention cysts developing in a mucous gland, caused by inflammation or trauma, and may be in the epiglottis, the vocal cords, or the lateral walls of the larynx. The congenital cysts occur in the epiglottis from inclusion of the lymphoepithelium of the entoderm (i.e., a branchial cyst), or they may be in the lateral walls of the pharynx or the aryepiglottic folds from displaced embryonal cells, which normally form the appendix of the ventricle. Laryngeal cysts may be lined by ciliated pseudostratified columnar epithelium or by squamous epithelium.

Keratosis. Keratosis of the larynx, also called hyperkeratosis, leukoplakia, and pachydermia, occurs mainly in adult males as white elevations on the upper surface or edge of the vocal cords. There is hyperplasia of the squamous epithelium with varying degrees of hyperkeratosis and dyskeratosis. The irregularity of the epithelium may be such that distinction from carcinoma is difficult, and some cases appear to undergo transformation to carcinoma.

Papillomas. The papilloma is the most common benign tumor of the larynx. In children papillomas may be of viral origin and usually disappear spontaneously. In adults they are single or multiple and usually involve only the vocal cords. They tend to recur after removal, and about 3% become malignant. They

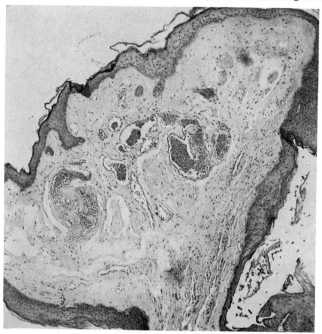

Fig. 14-1. Laryngeal nodule. The polypoid protrusion from the vocal cord is covered by an irregularly thickened and hyperkeratotic squamous epithelium. The central core contains dilated (angiomatoid) vascular spaces and hyalinized connective tissue. (×50.)

are protruding tumors composed of a core of well-vascularized connective tissue, covered by hyperplastic and branched stratified squamous epithelium with variable amounts of keratin.

Laryngeal polyps. A laryngeal polyp (laryngeal nodule or singer's node) is a thickening of the mucosa of the true vocal cord, most commonly found near the anterior commissure but sometimes in subglottic or other areas. Polyps occur in adults, affect men four times as frequently as women, and probably arise as a result of inflammation, trauma, or misuse of the voice. They are usually nodular, but sometimes are polypoid or even pedunculated, and may be seen in any one of four stages. At first there is a fibrous thickening of the stroma of the cord just beneath the squamous epithelium of the edge. In the second stage it becomes polypoid because of edema and dilatation of vessels in the fibrous stroma. In the third stage extreme dilatation of the thin-walled vessels may produce an angiomatous appearance (hemangioma). In the fourth stage the stroma becomes hyalinized and amyloid-like in appearance (the so-called amyloid tumor). In any stage the overlying epithelium may be atrophic, hyperplastic, or dyskeratotic. Only uncommonly does a laryngeal polyp undergo cancerous transformation.

Rarer benign tumors of the larynx include adenoma, chondroma, fibroma, neurofibroma, and myoblastoma.

Carcinomas. Carcinoma of the larynx composes 2 to 4% of all malignant tumors. Among malignancies of the larynx, 98% or more are carcinomas. Men are affected ten to fourteen times as frequently as women. Most cases occur between the ages of 40 and 65 years, the median age being about 60. In 50 to 65% the origin is in a vocal cord. One half to one third are extrinsic. A large majority (96%) are squamous cell carcinomas, and most are fairly well-differentiated, slowly growing tumors. A few are basal cell carcinomas or adenocarcinomas. In the intrinsic group two thirds are Grade I or II squamous cell carcinomas, whereas the extrinsic carcinomas are more likely to be of higher grade or less differentiated.

The tumors vary from a few millimeters up to 6 cm. or more in diameter. They may be papillary or infiltrating and ulcerating. The papillary growths are raised above the surface, rough or granular, grayish white, and friable. Infiltrating growths

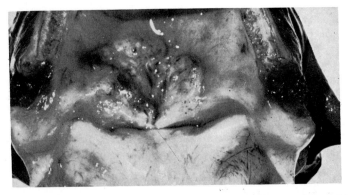

Fig. 14-2. Carcinoma of the larynx. The neoplastic area is roughly nodular and irregularly thickened.

produce a hard, ill-defined thickening, but eventually they tend to become elevated and ulcerated. Histologically they are composed of irregular infiltrating nests and cords of squamous epithelial cells, often with keratin masses. Mitoses vary in number. The stroma also is quite variable in amount. Only a very few are seen in an intraepithelial or carcinoma in situ stage.

Spread of laryngeal cancer may be by direct extension, by lymphatics, and by the bloodstream. Lymphatic spread to lymph nodes of the neck and supraclavicular region is more common and earlier with extrinsic cancers than with the intrinsic growths. Bloodstream spread is relatively uncommon, but when it does occur, metastases are found in the lungs and other organs.

LUNGS
Bronchi

The bronchi are involved in four main types of lesions: inflammation (bronchitis), obstructions (bronchial asthma), dilatations (bronchiectasis), and tumors (bronchogenic carcinoma). These types are frequently mixed; e.g., bronchiectasis and asthma have inflammatory changes as an integral part of the picture, and bronchogenic carcinoma may be associated with obstruction of the bronchial lumen.

Inflammation of bronchi

Acute bronchitis. Acute bronchial inflammations have a varied etiology, and a number of organisms may be found in the associated exudate. In many cases the trachea and larynx are involved as well, so that the condition is a laryngotracheobronchitis. Influenza is primarily a tracheobronchitis. Downward extension of diphtheria produces a fibrinous bronchitis. Pneumonic involvement of the lung has an associated acute bronchitis.

In acute bronchitis the mucosa is thickened, reddened, and eventually covered by exudate, which may be mucoid, fibrinous, or purulent. Microscopically one finds congestion and infiltration of mucosa and often of deeper layers by polymorphonuclear leukocytes. In severe cases necrosis and desquamation of the epithelial surface may be evident, blending with the exudate on the surface. Dilatation (bronchiectasis) may result from the injury to bronchial walls, or abscess formation may follow spread of the infection.

Chronic bronchitis. Chronic bronchial inflammation is a common condition usually associated with one of three conditions: (1) heart disease in which there is a chronic congestion of the lung, (2) infection in the upper respiratory tract, such as chronic sinusitis, and (3) bronchiectasis. It may be caused by prolonged exposure to cigarette smoke, irritating dusts or gases.

The bronchial mucosa is covered with a mucoid or mucopurulent exudate and is reddened and thickened so as to obscure the normal longitudinal markings. Microscopically one finds a widespread infiltration by lymphoid cells and an excess of fibrous connective tissue. The mucosal epithelium may be cubical or flattened and the mucous glands atrophic.

Obstruction of bronchi

Obstruction of a bronchial lumen can be produced by (1) aspirated foreign material, (2) neoplasms, (3) pressure from without, as by enlarged lymph nodes, (4) inflammation or its sequelae, and (5) asthma. A complete obstruction leads to collapse (atelectasis) of the lung tissue supplied by the obstructed bronchus. Incomplete obstruction, or one that allows the entrance of air by active inspiration but blocks its exit on passive expiration, leads to dilatation of the alveoli (emphysema). Aspiration of foreign substances into bronchi often leads to an abscess of the lung.

Bronchial asthma. Asthma is an allergic condition characterized by dyspnea, with particular difficulty in expiration. The sensitivity may be to food, pollens, or bacterial products. However, an allergic basis is not demonstrable in all cases of asthma, and in some persons heredity, emotional stress, or endocrine factors play an influential role. Sputum produced in asthma is often distinctive because of a content of eosinophils, Curschmann's spirals, and Charcot-Leyden crystals. Excessive numbers of eosinophils may be found in the blood. Asthmatic attacks are characterized by spasm of bronchial muscles and overproduction of mucus by bronchial glands. Death during an attack is uncommon.

The lungs in asthmatics are voluminous and distended. Areas of atelectasis also may occur because of persistent bronchial obstruction by mucous plugs.

In the bronchiolar wall there are (1) infiltration of eosinophils, (2) hypertrophy of muscle, (3) a thickened basement membrane and widened submucosal layer, and (4) enlargement and hyperactivity of mucous glands, which may be infiltrated by eosinophils. Excessive mucous secretion is present in the lumen, sometimes in the form of peculiar spiral plugs (Curschmann's spirals).

Bronchiectasis

Bronchiectasis is a dilatation of bronchi, either in a local area or generalized. The dilatation may be cylindrical, fusiform, or saccular if localized to one area. The lower lobes are more commonly involved, and the left is more frequently involved than the right. The condition is frequently associated with (1) chronic bronchitis or (2 multiple abscess formation resulting from the invasion of pyogenic and fusospirochetal organisms.

Etiology. The etiology and pathogenesis have been much debated, but a number of factors are considered causative, their relative importance varying in different cases. These factors are as follows.

Infection of the bronchial wall. Acute respiratory infection

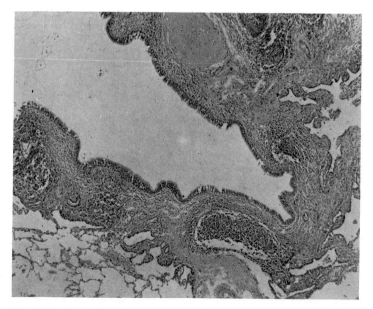

Fig. 14-3. Bronchiectasis, showing bronchial dilatation, chronic inflammatory infiltrate, and fibrosis.

involving the bronchial wall, particularly in children, may injure or destroy muscle and elastic tissue. This most commonly follows bronchopneumonia or bronchitis complicating whooping cough, measles, and influenza. Infection may be associated with tuberculosis, with mucoviscidosis (cystic fibrosis of the pancreas), or with obstructive lesions such as tumors, aspirated foreign bodies, and compression of the bronchi by enlarged hilar lymph nodes (as in the middle lobe syndrome).

Traction on the bronchial wall from without. This may occur either from (1) atelectasis of lung tissue or (2) contraction of scar tissue resulting from inflammation of alveolar and bronchial tissue. Atelectasis brought about by an obstruction of the bronchial lumen exerts elastic pull on the bronchial wall because of the negative pleural pressure and the necessity for spatial adjustment in the thoracic cage. Fibrous contraction of pulmonary tissue, from tuberculosis, fibrosing pneumonia, etc., similarly may exert traction tending to dilate bronchi.

Increased intrabronchial pressure, such as produced by coughing. This may act to dilate bronchi when the wall is already weakened by an inflammatory and destructive process.

Congenital abnormality in bronchial development, particularly of the muscular and elastic components. There is a congenital type of bronchiectasis that includes the lesion referred to as congenital lung cyst. That a developmental factor may be important in the seemingly acquired cases has been suggested by the peculiar distribution of bronchiectasis, its frequent familial occurrence, and its association with other developmental abnormalities.

Lesions. The dilated bronchi are evident on the cut surface of the bronchiectatic lung. In the lower lobes the dilatations are usually cylindric, whereas in the less commonly involved upper lobes they tend to be saccular. When inflammation is severe, particularly with pyogenic and fusospirochetal infections, the bronchiectases appear grossly as multiple abscess cavities.

Microscopically the essential change is absence, damage, or destruction of muscular and elastic elements of the bronchial wall. This may be accompanied by variable degrees of inflammation. In slight and chronic bronchiectasis there may be either atrophy or hypertrophy of mucosa, with infiltration of lymphocytes and plasma cells in the bronchial wall, and eventually fibrosis. Squamous metaplasia of the lining is an occasional occurrence. With severe inflammation there may be necrosis of

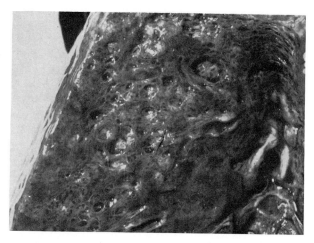

Fig. 14-4. Congenital cystic disease of the lung. The cut surface shows numerous cystic spaces of varying size (honeycomb lung).

tissue, purulent exudate, and abscess formation. A focal necrotizing pulmonary lesion or abscess in the process of healing may become lined by a wall resembling that of a dilated bronchus, so that it is often mistakenly considered as a saccular type of bronchiectasis.

Congenital bronchiectasis and congenital lung cyst. Congenital bronchiectasis is rare and is frequently spoken of as cystic disease of the lung. Anomalous bronchial or pulmonary development results in various-sized cavities, which may or may not have an opening into a bronchus. The cyst is lined by columnar epithelium, and some remnants of muscle and cartilage may be found in the wall. Numerous disseminated cysts, giving the lung a honeycomb structure, may be present. Complications include pneumothorax, and in older patients right-sided heart failure.

A rare type of congenital cystic disease of the lung appears to be a congenital lymphangiectasis. The small, thin-walled cysts are situated in connective tissue close to pulmonary blood vessels and are lined by endothelium.

Tumors of the lung

Tumors of the lung constitute an extremely important group because of a high and increasing incidence of primary bronchogenic carcinomas in males. Tumors of the lung may be classified as follows:

Benign
  Epithelial
    Papilloma of bronchus
    Atypical hyperplasia (tumorlets)
    Peripheral adenoma
  Mesodermal
    Vascular tumors (hemangioma)
    Intrabronchial tumors
      Fibroma
      Chondroma and osteochondroma
      Lipoma
      Granular cell myoblastoma
  Developmental
    Hamartoma
    Teratoma
Malignant
  Epithelial
    Bronchogenic
      Squamous cell (epidermoid) carcinoma
      Small cell undifferentiated (anaplastic) carcinoma
      Large cell undifferentiated (anaplastic) carcinoma
      Adenocarcinoma
      Mixed types
    Bronchiolar carcinoma (pulmonary adenomatosis, alveolar cell carcinoma)
    Bronchial "adenoma"
      Carcinoid type
      Cylindromatous (adenocystic) type
      Uncommon variants
        Oncocytoid
        Mucoepidermoid
        Papillary adenoma
  Mesodermal (sarcoma)
    Undifferentiated sarcoma
    Fibrosarcoma
    Osteochondrosarcoma
    Leiomyosarcoma
    Lymphosarcoma
  Mixed epithelial and mesodermal tumors
    Carcinosarcoma
  Reticuloendothelial tumors (involving lung as part of a generalized process)
    Hodgkin's disease
    Lymphosarcoma
    Letterer-Siwe disease
  Metastatic tumors
  Pleural tumors
    Localized
    Diffuse

Papillomas. Papillomas and papillomatosis of the bronchial tree are uncommon benign lesions similar to those that occur in the larynx. Except as a rarity, they do not undergo malignant change, but they may recur after bronchoscopic removal.

Atypical hyperplasias. Atypical hyperplasias of bronchiolar epithelium with extensions into alveoli are common with chronic pulmonary inflammations. The proliferations may be of a variety of cell types—cuboidal, columnar, syncytial giant cell, or undifferentiated (reserve) cell. A number of infections (e.g., Hecht's giant cell pneumonia), chemical irritations (e.g., cadmium pneumonitis), and other chronic nonspecific inflammations may be accompanied by a proliferation of columnar bronchiolar epithelium extending to line alveolar spaces. Extensive cases may suggest or be confused with pulmonary adenomatosis.

Atypical hyperplasias in which the cells resemble undifferentiated (basal or reserve) cells of bronchial or bronchiolar epithelium occur at the periphery of the lung, frequently in relationship to scars, old infarcts, and bronchiectases. They form tumorlike masses (tumorlets) in bronchiolar walls, in alveolar spaces, or in fibrous areas. They may resemble miniature oat cell (undifferentiated) carcinomas, or they may suggest the appearance of bronchial adenoma. Larger masses of such cells are similar to the tumors reported as "peripheral adenomas." They have sometimes been mistaken for and reported as early or small carcinomas (microcarcinomas). Although benign, their importance as precursors or their relationship, if any, to the numerous examples of "scar cancers," to cancers developing in old pulmonary infarcts, or to other carcinomas of the lung is unknown.

Hemangiomas. Hemangiomas and other primary vascular tumors of the lung are very rare. Microscopic pulmonary "arteriovenous shunts" and arteriovenous fistulas have been described. They may have a relation to circumscribed *sclerosing hemangiomas* (histiocytoma, xanthoma) of the lung, an uncommon lesion showing many of the histologic features of sclerosing hemangiomas elsewhere. They may appear as localized "coin" lesions on roentgenographic examination and must be differentiated from a malignant tumor.

Other tumors. Fibromas, lipomas, chondromas, and myomas are rare benign pulmonary tumors. Primary teratoma of the lung is extremely rare.

Hamartomas. Hamartomas are uncommon benign developmental tumors of the lung. They contain representatives of the histologic components of bronchi or lung tissue, and cartilage is often the predominant tissue. They appear to be new growths of connective tissue with a tendency to metaplasia into cartilage and sometimes adipose tissue. Most are peripheral or subpleural in position, but a few are endobronchial in origin. They are rounded, well-encapsulated masses, which often shell out easily, are firm and grayish white, and have a rough nodular surface. They may be discovered at any age and are more frequent in men. Their chief importance lies in the difficulty of their clinical differentiation from cancer.

Carcinomas. Primary carcinoma of the lung is mainly bronchogenic in origin. It is of frequent and rapidly increasing occurrence and ranks as the leading cause of mortality from cancer in males. It is more common in men (more than 5:1). The highest incidence is between 50 and 60 years of age, but it is also common in the decades before and after. Tracheal carcinoma is rare, accounting for less than 0.1% of deaths from cancer. It is usually of squamous cell type.

Etiology and pathogenesis. The rapid increase in incidence of cancer of the lung during the last few decades appears only partially accounted for by better and newer methods of diagnosis. A real increase, mainly in men and involving the squamous cell and undifferentiated types of bronchogenic carcinoma, appears definitely established. Causation of this increase is a subject of intense interest and hot debate. A mass of evidence, chiefly statistical, indicts cigarette smoking, although the specific carcinogenic factor is unknown. Other suggested etiologic factors with less supporting evidence include carcinogenic agents from atmospheric pollution in cities or tarring of roads and late effects of pneumonitis of viral origin. In certain industries exposure to chromates and arsenicals and the development of asbestosis appear to cause increased incidence of pulmonary cancer. Such industrial exposures are insufficient to account for the large and widespread increase. Occupational pulmonary cancer has been long recognized among certain cobalt miners in central Europe (Schneeberg and Joachimstal), where radioactivity of the ores may be the important factor. Uranium miners in the United States who have had sufficient exposure to irradiation and who are also cigarette smokers have shown an increased incidence of lung cancer of the undifferentiated type.

The relation of squamous metaplasia of bronchial epithelium to the development of carcinoma is still a debatable problem.

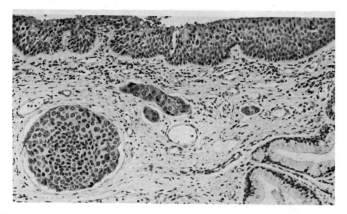

Fig. 14-5. Bronchial mucosa with squamous metaplasia and areas of carcinoma in situ. Underlying vascular spaces contain embolic masses of metastatic squamous cell carcinoma from elsewhere in the lung.

Squamous metaplasia is a frequent occurrence in many chronic pulmonary irritations or in inflammatory lesions such as bronchiectasis. It is evident that it does not regularly proceed to the development of carcinoma. However, much evidence suggests that it may be a frequent precursor or accompaniment of bronchogenic carcinoma. Detailed studies of the whole bronchial tree in cases of bronchogenic carcinoma, and in groups of smokers and nonsmokers, indicate a high frequency of squamous metaplasia and changes of carcinoma in situ in relationship to cancer development.

Natural history. Many lung tumors begin in large bronchi, soon obstructing them or interfering with their function and leading to emphysema, atelectasis, and pneumonitis. Later sequels may be bronchiectasis or abscess, or cavitation in a tumor itself may simulate abscess. Such secondary effects may hinder or obscure clinical and roentgenographic diagnosis. Common initial clinical symptoms are cough, hemoptysis, dyspnea, pneumonia, wheezing, hoarseness, and persistent fever. The course of the disease is variable, depending on the type of tumor and its site. Hyperadrenocorticism with Cushing's syndrome has occasionally been a complication with undifferentiated carcinoma of the lung. Corticotropic substance has been demonstrated in the tumor tissue in at least one instance.

Gross types. While extremely variable in gross appearance, most pulmonary carcinomas fall in one of three groups. The most common is a *hilar infiltrating form*, in which there are large tumor masses about the bronchi at the hilus of the lung, causing stenosis and ulceration of a bronchus and often massively involving mediastinal and peribronchial lymph nodes. In the less common *peripheral* or *nodular form* there may be either a single peripheral tumor or multiple nodular tumor masses scattered through the lung. A *diffuse form,* simulating a pneumonia or organizing consolidation of the lung, may be difficult to recognize grossly. It is often of the terminal bronchiolar or alveolar cell type.

In the apex of the lung and at the thoracic inlet the tumor may result in a distinctive clinical symptom complex, characterized by pain around the shoulder and radiating down the arm, Horner's syndrome (unilateral enophthalmos, miosis, ptosis, and anhidrosis), and atrophy of the muscles of the arm and hand. Pancoast described the lesion in such cases as a *"superior pulmonary sulcus tumor."* These apical tumors are apparently

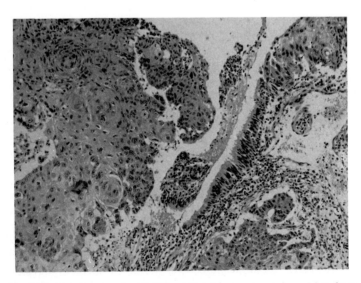

Fig. 14-6. Carcinoma of well-differentiated squamous type arising from the bronchus.

carcinomas of the terminal bronchioles, which extend to involve the inferior cervical ganglion and the brachial plexus.

Microscopic types. Most common is *squamous cell,* or *epidermoid,* carcinoma, constituting 45 to 60% of carcinomas of the lung. Keratinization or intercellular bridges may be seen in the most mature forms, but most examples are less differentiated and may be quite pleomorphic. Variant forms are areas with giant cells, spindle cells, or clear cells may be seen. It most often arises from larger bronchi near the hilus, but it also may be peripheral, where it tends to invade the body wall. Necrosis is frequent, and discharge of the necrotic material may result in cavitation. Compared to other types the well-differentiated squamous cell tumors have a relatively slow course and a good outlook if removed before the involvement of regional lymph nodes.

Undifferentiated, or *anaplastic,* carcinomas constitute about 30% of pulmonary carcinomas. It has been proposed that they arise from "reserve cells" of the mucosa, which are small, dark cells between the basement membrane and the differentiated cells of the mucosal surface. The anaplastic cells sometimes show evidence that they are capable of transformation into glandular or squamous cells, and foci of differentiation may be found in some tumors. Ordinarily the tumors are composed of small round, oat-

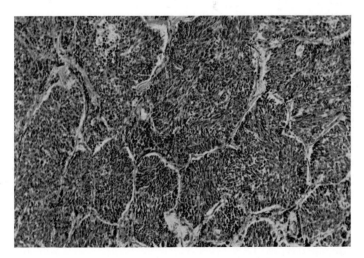

Fig. 14-7. Undifferentiated bronchogenic carcinoma ("oat-cell" type).

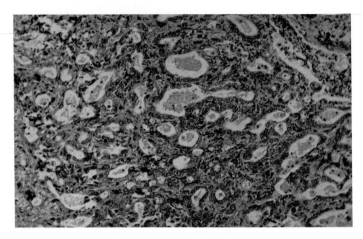

Fig. 14-8. Adenocarcinoma of the lung.

shaped, or spindle-shaped cells without structural formation. Mitoses are numerous. Such tumors are easily mistaken for sarcoma and frequently were so considered until recent years. Rapid growth and a tendency to early spread by lymphatics (intrapulmonary and extrapulmonary) and by hematogenous metastasis are characteristic, with a highly malignant rapid course and a poor prognosis. The anaplastic tumors tend to predominate in the stem bronchi and are uncommonly peripheral. Regional lymph nodes tend to be massively involved, often while the primary tumor is still small and before there is much bronchial obstruction. The tumor tissue is pale, translucent, and with only a slight tendency to necrosis. A large cell type of undifferentiated or anaplastic carcinoma also occurs, and it appears to be a form quite distinct from the small cell type.

Adenocarcinoma, or columnar cell carcinoma, constitutes 9 to 12% of bronchogenic carcinomas. They appear to be as frequent in women as in men. They may arise from surface epithelium or from mucous glands, and mucus is demonstrable in some examples. They are composed of cuboidal or cylindric cells and may be differentiated enough to form glandular or papillary structures. Relatively, more occur peripherally than with other types. They often appear to be associated with lung scars, as many as two thirds in some series of cases. Growth tends

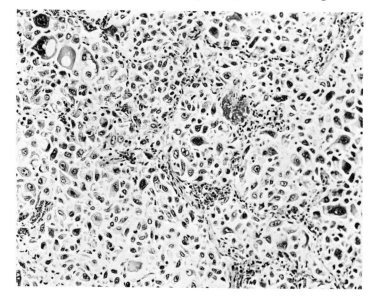

Fig. 14.9. Giant cell carcinoma of the lung. Some of the giant cells contain intracytoplasmic mucin. (×105.)

to be rapid compared to squamous cell tumors, and hematogenous metastasis may be early and widespread.

A *giant cell carcinoma* of the lung, which is characterized by numerous pleomorphic and bizarre cells of giant size, has been noted for a relatively high degree of malignancy and a rapidly fatal course. Most such cases are adenocarcinomas, and intracytoplasmic mucin is often demonstrable. Less frequently there may be areas of recognizable squamous cell differentiation.

Mixed types of pulmonary carcinoma that contain some admixture of squamous, columnar, and undifferentiated cells are not uncommon. Varying methods of classifying such tumors lead to differences in percentage figures given for the common types.

Spread and metastasis. Spread of carcinoma of the lung is by direct extension, by lymphatics, by the bloodstream, and by bronchial "embolism" or aspiration. Although any type of bronchogenic carcinoma may spread by any or all of these methods, squamous cell carcinoma is likely to extend by direct invasion, undifferentiated carcinoma by lymphatics, and adenocarcinoma by the bloodstream. Regional lymph nodes are involved in a high proportion of cases of bronchogenic carcinoma. Other common sites of metastasis are the liver, bones, adrenal glands, kidneys, brain, pericardium, and heart. Hematogenous metastasis is sometimes very widespread, and in some cases metastases produce clinical symptoms before the primary tumor does. Scalene node biopsy is sometimes a useful diagnostic procedure for carcinoma and other intrathoracic lesions, as it reflects the involvement of mediastinal lymph nodes.

Bronchiolar carcinoma. About 3% of carcinomas of the lung are considered to arise from terminal bronchioles or alveolar lining cells *(alveolar cell tumors).* The tumor cells line alveoli, their supporting stroma being the alveolar walls. The area of the tumor is often centered about a bronchiole, and evidence has suggested that bronchioles rather than alveoli are the source of these tumors. However it is probable that most examples are simply variants of adenocarcinoma of the lung which have prominently adopted the alveolar fashion of intrapulmonary spread. What is sometimes considered a benign variant is referred to as *pulmonary adenomatosis,* although there is little evidence that this exists as an entity that can be distinguished from bronchiolar carcinoma.

Nodular and diffuse gross forms occur. The more common nodular form may be multiple and may simulate the appearance of metastatic carcinoma. The diffuse form may involve an entire lobe or occur as a single focus or as multiple foci and simulates the appearance of pneumonia. Whether there sometimes may be a multicentric origin is debatable, as some seeming multicentric tumors are explainable by aspirative or lymphatic spread. The tumor shows little or no necrosis, and the cut surface may be mucoid.

Microscopically the tumor cells are tall, columnar, and usually mucus producing. They may regularly line alveolar spaces or may produce papillary protrusions into the lumen. The cells may be quite uniform, but sometimes hyperchromatic, irregular, and bizarre forms are present. Variations in appearance of the tumor cells do not correlate well with the clinical course. Rare ciliated cells may be found. Mitoses are infrequent. Calcified psammoma bodies are often present. The histologic appearance is similar to an infectious pulmonary adenomatosis of sheep (jagziekte), but an etiologic relationship has not been proved.

Bronchiolar carcinomas occur equally in men and women. There is a wide age distribution, although most cases occur be-

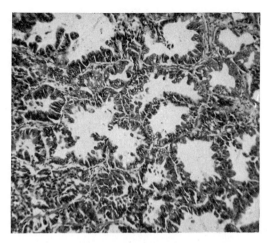

Fig. 14-10. Alveolar cell (terminal bronchiolar) carcinoma of the lung. Alveolar spaces are lined by cancer cells.

tween 40 and 60 years. The condition may be extensive before symptoms develop, which may be mainly dyspnea, cyanosis, and abundant watery or mucoid sputum. Death is most often from respiratory failure caused by progressive replacement of lung tissue, although at the time of termination more than 50% have metastases present, most often to regional lymph nodes, liver, and brain. Both lungs tend ultimately to be involved. Metastatic tumors from other organs (e.g., pancreas) may closely imitate and be mistaken for primary bronchiolar carcinoma.

Bronchial adenoma. Adenomas of a bronchus constitute 2 to 6% of primary tumors of the lung. Although not strictly benign, they are slow in growth and limited in their invasive, destructive, and metastasizing power. Hence their malignant character is of low degree. They are of almost equal sexual incidence, occur mainly under 50 years of age (average 35 to 40 years), and have a slow course and a relatively good prospect of surgical curability.

They grow as polypoid or sessile tumors involving the subepithelial tissues of proximal bronchi, being derived from mucous glands and their ducts. They are more common on the right, involving the lower lobe or main stem bronchus and are least common in the left upper lobe bronchus. Almost all are accessible to the bronchoscope. Although they may project into

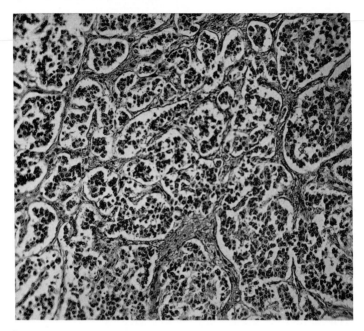

Fig. 14-11. Bronchial adenoma with a characteristic trabecular and alveolar pattern. (From Haukohl, R. S., and Anderson, W. A. D., editors: Pathology seminars, St. Louis, 1955, The C. V. Mosby Co.)

the lumen of a bronchus, causing partial or complete obstruction, most of the tumor is usually beneath the surface. Necrosis and ulceration are uncommon, but vascularity is considerable and hemorrhage may be a complication.

The carcinoid form is most frequent and histologically resembles the carcinoid tumors of the intestine, although argentaffin granules are only rarely demonstrable. Small uniform cells are arranged in strands, sheets, or masses situated about abundant, delicate sinusoidal vessels. Mitoses are infrequent. Invasion and penetration of the capsule quite often occurs, with metastasis to the tracheobronchial lymph nodes in about 9% and metastases to the liver, vertebrae, or kidney occasionally. They are resistant to radiation. Rare examples of carcinoid bronchial adenoma have been reported in which a metastasis in the liver formed serotonin and was accompanied by the clinical functioning carcinoid syndrome.

The cylindromatous type (adenocystic basal cell carcinoma)

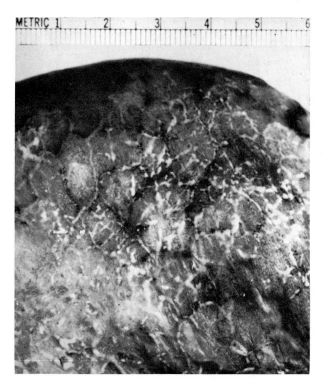

Fig. 14-12. Lymphangitic spread of carcinoma of the lung.

comprises about 15% of bronchial adenomas, tends to be more proximal than the carcinoid form (may involve the trachea), and more often has a sessile or diffuse form. Microscopically cells are arranged in branching cylinders, tubes, or masses and may resemble basal cell tumors of the skin. They may have a secretion that stains with mucicarmine. As compared with the carcinoid form, they have less vascularity and tendency to hemorrhage, they have a greater invasiveness, and they are more radiosensitive. Metastasis may occur in almost one third of the cases, and prognosis for survival is poorer than with the carcinoid type.

The uncommon mucoepidermoid adenoma appears to have recognizable benign and malignant forms. It is composed of a mixture of sheets of squamous-type cells and mucus-secreting cells.

Other infrequent variant forms may be oncocytoid and papillary. The oncocytoid form, a variant of the carcinoid type, is composed of large eosinophilic cells and tends to occur at older ages.

Sarcoma. While examples of hemangiosarcoma, fibrosarcoma, osteochondrosarcoma, and leiomyosarcoma of the lung have been reported, they are all extremely rare. Lymphosarcoma originating in the lung is slightly less rare. It is similar to lymphocytic lymphosarcoma elsewhere. The numerous sarcomas of the lung reported in older literature are now recognized as undifferentiated bronchogenic carcinomas.

Carcinosarcoma of the lung is composed of mixed malignant epithelial and mesodermal elements. Although a few examples have been reported, most cases appear to be anaplastic variants of squamous cell bronchogenic carcinomas.

Reticuloendothelial diseases occasionally involve the lungs as well as other organs. Such involvements may be seen in Hodgkin's disease, nonlipid reticuloendotheliosis (Letterer-Siwe disease) lymphosarcoma, and leukemias. The process in the lung is similar to that in other organs.

International histological classification. Because comparative and statistical studies have been hampered by a wide variation in criteria, classification, and terminology, a standard classification for such purposes has been proposed. Published by the World Health Organization,* it is as follows:

    I. Epidermoid carcinomas
   II. Small cell anaplastic carcinomas
        1. Fusiform cell type
        2. Polygonal cell type
        3. Lymphocyte-like ("oat-cell") type
        4. Others
  III. Adenocarcinomas
        1. Bronchogenic
           a. Acinar } with or without mucin formation
           b. Papillary }
        2. Bronchiolo-alveolar
  IV. Large cell carcinomas
        1. Solid tumors with mucin-like content
        2. Solid tumors without mucin-like content
        3. Giant cell carcinomas
        4. "Clear" cell carcinomas
   V. Combined epidermoid and adenocarcinomas

---

*Kreyberg, Leiv: Histological typing of lung tumours, Geneva, 1967, World Health Organization.

        VI. Carcinoid tumors
       VII. Bronchial gland tumors
              1. Cylindromas
              2. Mucoepidermoid tumors
              3. Others
      VIII. Papillary tumors of the surface epithelium
              1. Epidermoid
              2. Epidermoid with goblet cells
              3. Others
        IX. "Mixed" tumors and carcinosarcomas
              1. "Mixed" tumors
              2. Carcinosarcomas of embryonal type ("blastomas")
              3. Other carcinosarcomas
         X. Sarcomas
        XI. Unclassified
       XII. Mesotheliomas
              1. Localized
              2. Diffuse
      XIII. Melanomas

Metastatic tumors. The lung is a common site for metastatic tumors, spread usually being by the bloodstream. Sarcomas, such as those of skin or bone, frequently produce metastases in the lungs, as do also the renal tumors, hypernephroma and embryonal adenosarcoma. Usually multiple discrete nodular tumor masses are produced. Secondary metastatic spread elsewhere may occur from the metastatic tumors in the lung. Occasionally a lymphatic extension to the lung may occur from cancer of the breast. A peculiar type of tumor metastasis to the lung has been described under the terms *lymphangitis carcinoma* and *diffuse infiltrative carcinoma*. The clinically inconspicuous primary tumor usually is an infiltrative scirrhous carcinoma of the stomach or colon. It should be differentiated from lymphatic spread of primary lung cancer (Fig. 14-12).

Pneumonia

Inflammation of lung tissue is called pneumonia, although sometimes it is quite logically referred to as pneumonitis. Although commonly of bacterial origin, certain types (e.g., lipid pneumonia) are caused by other irritants. The common types are known as lobar pneumonia, lobular pneumonia (bronchopneumonia), and interstitial pneumonia. Lobar pneumonia is almost always caused by pneumococcal infection, whereas bronchopneumonia is caused by a wide variety of organisms. Interstitial pneumonias are mainly nonbacterial (viral) or caused by *mycoplasma, rickettsiae,* or related organisms.

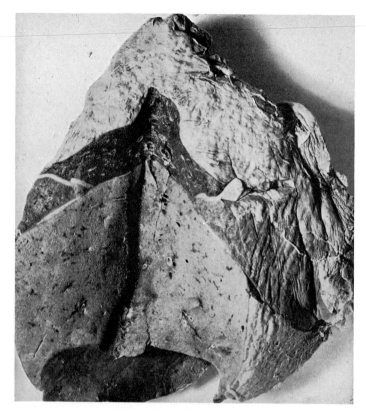

Fig. 14-13. Lobar pneumonia. Gray hepatization of the lower lobe of the lung. The pleural surface has a thick fibrinous exudate.

Viral infections of the lung, including influenza, are considered on p. 166.

Lobar pneumonia. Lobar pneumonia is a diffuse, usually pneumococcal, consolidation affecting one or more lobes of the lungs. It occurs sporadically, at all ages, and in previously healthy persons. The disease has a rapid onset with severe prostration and a serious mortality rate. After a course of one or two weeks, recovery may occur by lysis or crisis, or it may be complicated by organization of the exudate, empyema, abscess formation, pericarditis, endocarditis, or meningitis. In the earliest stage the involved lobe is edematous and congested, followed rapidly by a stage of red hepatization (consolidation), in which a fibrinous exudate is added to the congestion. This in turn is followed by gray hepatization, in which stage congestion is no longer present, and there is degeneration of cells of the exudate. In favorable cases resolution follows, with increase in the proportion of macrophages and finally absorption of the exudate and restitution of the lung tissue to its previous healthy condition.

Etiology. Lobar pneumonia is caused in almost all cases by pneumococci, but it may be caused by Friedländer's pneumobacillus and other bacteria. The pneumococcus is an encapsulated diplococcus, which produces green colonies on blood agar, ferments inulin, and is soluble in bile. Pneumococci are not all alike but have different capsular carbohydrates and form specific immunologic types. The particular type may be determined by noting capsular swelling when the organism is in contact with the type-specific serum (Neufeld reaction) or by agglutination reaction of mouse-cultured organisms with specific sera. Pneumococci may be immunologically classified into about seventy-five serotypes. Although all types are pathogenic for man, the usual ones responsible for lobar pneumonia are types 1, 2, and 3; other significant ones are types 5, 7, and 8. Type 14 causes pneumonia especially in children but rarely in adults.

Accessory etiologic factors believed of importance include acute upper respiratory infection, chilling of the body, and alcoholism. Some evidence suggests that bacterial allergy may have an etiologic role.

Pathogenesis. Organisms reach the lungs by way of the respiratory passages. The bacteremia that often is present is believed to be secondary rather than primary to the pneumonia. Experimental lobar pneumonia has been produced in monkeys by injection of pneumococci into the trachea. This resulted in an interstitial spread of the infection from the hilus to the periphery of the lung with subsequent outpouring of exudate into the alveoli. Further clinical and experimental studies have suggested a different course of events in lobar pneumonia in human beings. There has been produced in the dog a lobar pneumonia closely resembling that which occurs in human beings by implanting pneumococci suspended in a starch-broth paste into the terminal air sacs. A rapid outpouring of edema fluid quickly dispersed the organisms throughout the lobe by way of air passages and through the pores of Cohn in the alveolar walls, followed later by leukocytic exudation.

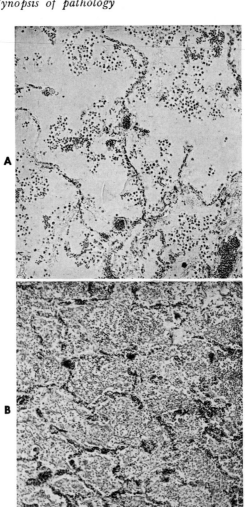

Fig. 14-14. Stages of lobar pneumonia. **A,** Edema and early leukocytic infiltration. **B,** Leukocytic stage: engorgement persists; fibrin is scanty. **C,** Late fibrinous stage: beginning of the contraction of the alveolar exudate; the alveolar walls are ischemic. **D,** Resolution: macrophages predominate; masses of fibrin are free in the alveolar spaces, and the alveolar capillaries are engorged. (From Millard, M.: Lung, pleura, and mediastinum. In Anderson, W. A. D., editor: Pathology, ed. 5, St. Louis, 1966, The C. V. Mosby Co.)

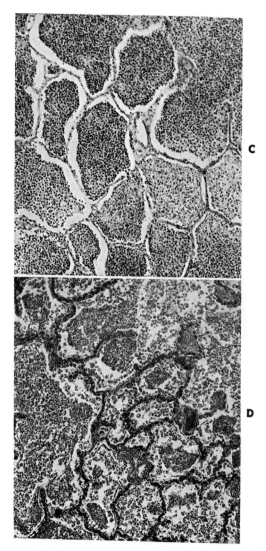

C

D

Fig. 14-14, cont'd. For legend see opposite page.

Morbid anatomy. The pneumonic process goes through a series of stages, which are characteristic and roughly indicate the age of the process. There is no sharp dividing line between these stages, which merge into each other; different stages are often evident in different portions of the involved lung. Acute inflammation in the lung has the characteristics of acute inflammation elsewhere, i.e., vascular congestion and outpouring of a fluid and cellular exudate.

The earliest, the *stage of congestion,* is characterized by engorgement of blood vessels and outpouring of fluid into alveolar spaces. The involved lobe is heavier and less crepitant than normal, is red from the congestion and diapedesis of red cells, and oozes frothy bloody fluid from its cut surface.

The *stage of red hepatization* rapidly follows; the lobe is consolidated by exudate filling the air sacs and has the consistency of liver tissue. The cut surface is dark red in color and distinctly granular. Microscopically the alveoli are filled by fibrin mixed with red cells and neutrophilic leukocytes. These cells are in a good state of preservation, and the vessels in the alveolar walls are congested. Many pneumococci are present in the alveoli. The pleura over the affected lobe is covered by a fibrinous exudate.

In the *stage of gray hepatization* the lobe is still solid and of liverlike consistency, but it is somewhat softer than in the red stage and less granular. The gray color is caused by disappearance of the congestion and of the red cells in the alveoli and by an increased proportion of leukocytes in the alveolar exudate. Microscopically the alveolar exudate contains a large proportion of neutrophilic leukocytes and relatively less fibrin and red cells. In later periods of this stage the cells of the exudate show degeneration and disintegration. Pneumococci are still numerous in the exudate.

In the *stage of resolution* the cut surface of the lung has a somewhat translucent jellylike appearance. At this time many free macrophages are found in the alveoli, arising from transformation of fixed tissue cells. The macrophages engulf and destroy the organisms, which consequently are scarce in this stage. Neutrophilic leukocytes are less numerous and are disintegrating.

During recovery the exudate is removed by being coughed up, by phagocytosis and removal by macrophages, and by liquefaction and absorption. The final result in the uncomplicated case of recovery is restoration of the lung to its previous condition with no residual scars.

The mechanism of recovery is a dual one, consisting (1) of a generalized process of immunization, which localizes the infection and controls bacteremia; and (2) of the local macrophage reaction, which destroys the pneumococci in the involved lobe.

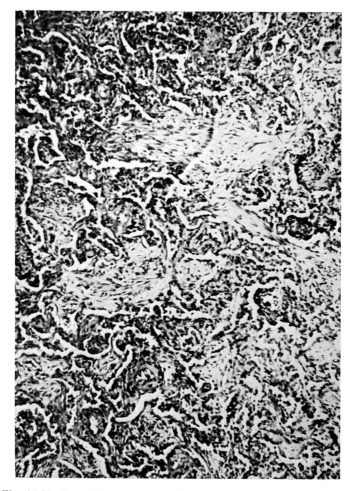

Fig. 14-15. Organizing pneumonia. The strands of connective tissue can be seen passing from one alveolus to another.

Failure of either process results in death. After recovery a local immunity to reinfection persists in the involved lobe as long as macrophages are still present.

Complications. While most cases clear up without persisting lesions, a variety of complications may occur. *Empyema* is a persistent purulent pleurisy that follows the pneumonia. When the purulent effusion is large, the lung tissue collapses proportionately. Spread of pneumonia to cause *pericarditis* occasionally occurs. More rarely there may be metastatic blood spread to cause pneumococcal *meningitis, arthritis,* or *endocarditis.*

In the involved lung tissue several complications may develop. Occasionally there is breakdown of tissue with localized *abscess* formation. Secondary infection of the abscess by fusospirochetal or putrefactive organisms results in *gangrene.* In rare cases resolution of the alveolar exudate fails to occur, and it becomes organized. Such an *organizing pneumonia* is characterized grossly by a dense, solid, fleshy or elastic consistency, to which the term *carnification* of the lung often is applied. Microscopically there are masses of fibrous tissue, which fill the alveoli

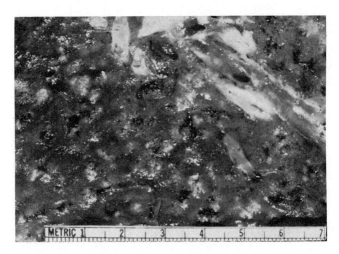

Fig. 14-16. Confluent bronchopneumonia. Some of the opaque grayish areas on the cut surface of the lung appear to be small areas of abscess.

and join by fine strands passing through small openings in the alveolar walls.

Bronchopneumonia (lobular pneumonia). In bronchopneumonia the inflammatory consolidation is patchy and irregular in distribution. It is usually secondary to or a complication of some other disease or infection, and the etiologic agents include a variety of bacteria and other irritants. The most common microorganisms involved are the pneumococcus, streptococcus, influenza bacillus, and staphylococcus. Specific types of bronchopneumonia occur in tuberculosis, tularemia, and plague.

In the pathogenesis of most cases the infection reaches the lung by air passages, with the development of a bronchitis and spread to involve alveoli immediately adjacent to a bronchiole. Direct spread then may involve contiguous lobules. In some cases this spread and confluence may be such that a whole lobe is involved, and distinction from lobar pneumonia is not obvious. Pyemia with numerous septic emboli to the lung setting up many small focal areas of inflammation may produce a condition that is grossly very similar to bronchopneumonia.

Examined grossly, both lungs usually are found to be involved, but unequally, and the lower lobes in their posterior and basal parts are particularly affected. Firm nodular areas of consolidation are palpable, and pus can be squeezed from the cut bronchioles in these areas. There is usually little or no exudate on the pleural surface, but it is likely to be mottled by alternating bluish and red areas. The cut surface of the lung is moist and red with some projecting reddish gray areas of consolidation. These areas can often be felt more easily than they can be seen. Some bluish areas of collapse and lighter areas of emphysema are often present as well. The moist and nongranular character of the cut surface differs from that of lobar pneumonia.

Microscopically the consolidated areas show alveoli containing mononuclear and neutrophilic leukocytes; fibrin and red cells are relatively scarce, although hemorrhagic types may be found, particularly in influenzal and staphylococcal pneumonias. Necrosis of tissue and abscess formation may be present in the cases caused by streptococci and staphylococci. The alveolar walls are congested. Bronchioles in the area contain exudate in their lumina and leukocytic infiltration in their walls that extends interstitially for a variable distance around them.

Types. Types of bonchopneumonia having a particular pathogenesis are often given distinctive names, although they have in common many of the features that have been noted. *Hypostatic,* or *terminal, pneumonia* is that type often found in patients with heart disease or cerebral hemorrhage. The consolidation is found in lower and posterior parts of the lung where passive congestion has been present. *Aspiration pneumonia* is caused by the aspiration of material into the lung; e.g., septic material may be inhaled during an operation, particularly if the operation has involved the mouth, pharynx, or upper respiratory tract. *Postoperative pneumonia* may be of the aspiration type, but often it is related to postoperative atelectasis of areas of lung tissue as a result of plugging of bronchi or bronchioles by secretion or exudate. *Suppurative pneumonia,* is which necrosis and pus formation are distinctive features, may be caused by staphylococci, hemolytic streptococci, or pneumococci. *Chemical pneumonias* are those caused by irritating or poisonous gases, such as may be used in war.

Interstitial pneumonia. An interstitial reaction, particularly with mononuclear cells, occurs in the pneumonias that follow and complicate measles, influenza, adenovirus infections, whooping cough, varicella, psittacosis, and other infectious diseases. This type of response has been regarded as the characteristic pneumonic reaction to a virus or to combined action of a virus and bacteria. Epidemics of viral pneumonia have exhibited interstitial reaction. Viral pneumonias, including the giant cell pneumonia of infancy (Fig. 14-23), are considered on p. 169. Deaths from an Asian influenza epidemic have shown a severe laryngeal, tracheal, and bronchial inflammation associated with a variety of interstitial and secondary bacterial pneumonias and similar to the changes found in the 1918 to 1920 influenza epidemic. Primary atypical pneumonia is caused principally by *Mycoplasma pneumoniae* (Eaton agent). In about 50% of patients with *Mycoplasma* pneumonia, cold agglutinins develop to a titer of 1:40 or more during convalescence.

The gross features of interstitial pneumonia are not characteristic, but microscopically there is an interstitial thickening, particularly around the bronchi and bronchioles and in adjacent alveolar walls. This is caused by an increase in the number of mononuclear cells. Bronchioles and alveoli may contain neutrophilic leukocytes as well, although even in alveoli mononuclear cells and fibrin may predominate.

Farmer's lung is a granulomatous interstitial pneumonitis occurring in agricultural workers and resulting from the inhalation of dust from moldy hay or silage. Exposure may be followed by an acute febrile illness, but the course of the inflammation tends to be prolonged and chronic. The granulomatous pneumonitis is accompanied by varying degrees of focal obliterating bronchiolitis, interstitial fibrosis, and emphysema. The reaction is believed to be the result of hypersensitivity. An allergic interstitial pneumonitis has been described also in pigeon breeders.

Pneumocystis pneumonia. Pneumonia caused by *Pneumocystis carinii* was first noted as occurring in premature and debilitated infants in central Europe. A lymphocytic and plasma cell infiltration of alveolar septa led to use of the term *plasma cellular pneumonitis,* although it is an inconstant and often not a prominent feature.

Recently it has been recognized in more widespread distribution, with cases reported from various areas of North America, and in adults as well as infants. Usually, but not always, it has occurred in persons debilitated by other conditions, including leukemia and malignant lymphomas. It has also occurred in patients with agammaglobulinemia and in patients receiving immunosuppressive therapy, after renal transplantation, appearing related to long-term prednisone therapy. The alveolar lumina contain a peculiar, foamy or vacuolated, lightly eosinophilic material, in which the infective agent, *Pneumocystis carinii,* can be found. Whether it is a protozoon or a yeast is unsettled, but it is generally considered a protozoon. The organisms appear as minute basophilic dots or granules, surrounded by a clear space and a thin homogeneous blue capsule. The tiny cystlike structures are shown best by some silver nitrate stains. Prominent alveolar lining (septal) cells and sometimes hyaline membranes may be present.

Acute diffuse interstitial fibrosis. Hamman and Rich have described an unusual condition of unknown etiology, characterized by a diffuse and progressive fibrosis of alveolar walls. The inflammatory process is marked by edema, hemorrhage, and only a few leukocytes, although eosinophils may be present in the interstitial tissue. There is an absence of stainable bacteria in the lesions. Progressive interstitial fibrosis follows, resulting in deficient aeration of the blood and manifested by dyspnea and cyanosis. Enlargement and failure of the right side of the heart may develop within a few weeks.

Obstruction to the outflow of pulmonary veins may cause

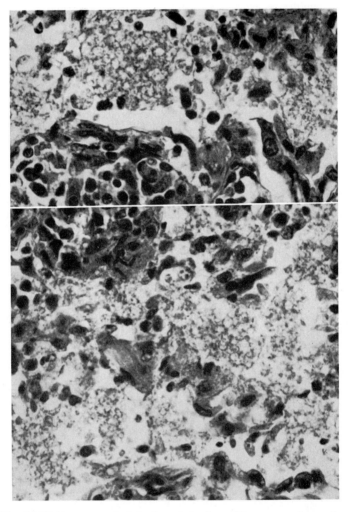

Fig. 14-17. Pneumocystis infection of the lung. The masses of organisms in the alveolar spaces have a foamy appearance. The alveolar walls contain increased numbers of mononuclear cells, plasma cells, and lymphocytes.

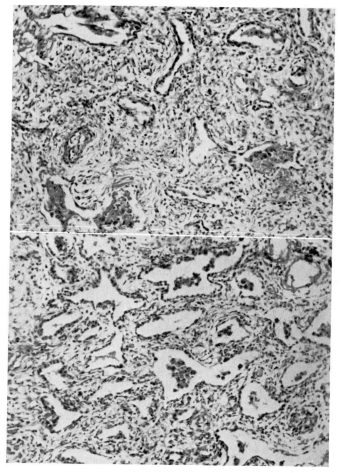

Fig. 14-18. Acute diffuse interstitial fibrosis of the lung. (Courtesy Dr. A. R. Rich.)

pulmonary fibrosis, which in its late stages is similar to that of acute diffuse interstitial fibrosis.

Tularemic pneumonia. Tularemic pneumonia is found in more than half the fatal cases of tularemia. The organisms probably reach the lung by hematogenous spread.

The pulmonary lesion is a nodular or confluent broncho-pneumonia, characterized by focal areas of caseous necrosis. In the exudate around such areas mononuclear cells predomi-nate, although some lymphocytes, plasma cells, red cells, and neutrophilic leukocytes may be present as well. One sees con-gestion of alveolar walls and sometimes a swelling of alveolar lining. Pleurisy with effusion and bronchitis frequently accom-pany the necrotizing pneumonia.

Lipid pneumonia. The reactive lesions in the lung caused by oily and fatty substances introduced by way of the trachea have been termed *lipid pneumonia.* Cod-liver oil and liquid petrolatum are the common causative agents, although olive oil, milk fat, and other substances may produce similar lesions. The fatty or oily materials gain entrance to the lung by way of the trachea because of forced feeding, disturbance of the swallowing mechanism, or excessive use of an oily (liquid petrolatum) base in nasal and laryngeal instillations. The condition is most fre-quent in infants, but an adult type also occurs in which liquid petrolatum is usually the offending agent. The fundamental lesion of lipid pneumonia is an interstitial proliferative inflam-mation, which is essentially a foreign body reaction. Macrophages laden with oil or fat, foreign body giant cells, and increased connective tissue are the essential features. Adult and infantile types have been described. In lipid pneumonia of the infantile type there is pulmonary consolidation resulting from fat-laden macrophages and other inflammatory cells in alveoli and alveolar walls, with little fibrosis. Lipid pneumonia of the adult type (paraffinoma) is a nodular or tumorlike lesion in which fibrous scarring is prominent. The lesions are commonly located around the hilar region of the posterior and dependent portions of the lung. Vascular lesions with weakening of vessel walls may occur, and severe pulmonary hemorrhage has complicated bronchoscopy in some cases. Liquid petrolatum may be identified in tissue sections by its failure to stain black with osmic acid, although stainable by scarlet red. Cod-liver oil in the tissues is charac-terized by shredding of the oil and acid-fat staining by the Ziehl-Neelsen method.

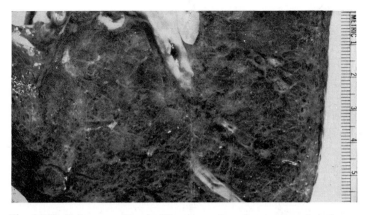

Fig. 14-19. Pulmonary fibrosis. The cut surface shows a prominently trabeculated appearance due to the increased connective tissue.

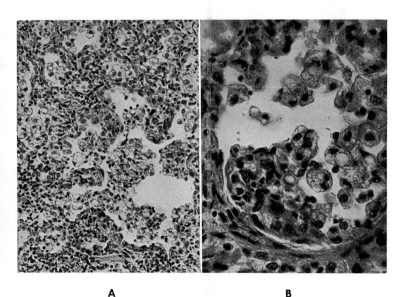

A   **B**

Fig. 14-20. A, Lipid pneumonia in an infant. Low-power photomicrograph. **B,** Foam cells in the alveolus and thickening of the alveolar wall. (From Millard, M.: Lung, pleura, and mediastinum. In Anderson, W. A. D., editor: Pathology, ed. 5, St. Louis, 1966, The C. V. Mosby Co.)

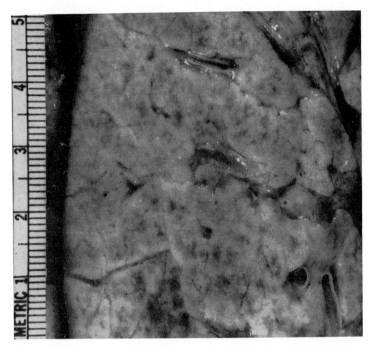

Fig. 14-21. Pulmonary alveolar proteinosis. The cut surface of the lung shows a diffuse grayish consolidation.

Cholesterol pneumonitis. Chronic pneumonitis of the cholesterol type (foam cell pneumonitis) is characterized by alveolar spaces filled with vacuolated macrophages containing cholesterol-rich lipid, associated with necrotizing granulomatous and vascular lesions. Ulceration and obstruction of smaller branches of the bronchial tree, possibly a hypersensitivity phenomenon, has been proposed as the causative mechanism. Endogenous lipid pneumonia is also used as a term for the chronic obstructive lesions of bronchi or bronchioles that are accompanied by lipid, chronic inflammation, and fibrosis. It may simulate the appearance of the aspirative type.

Pulmonary alveolar proteinosis. Pulmonary alveolar proteinosis is a recently recognized chronic disease characterized by the filling of distal air spaces (alveoli and bronchioles) with a granu-

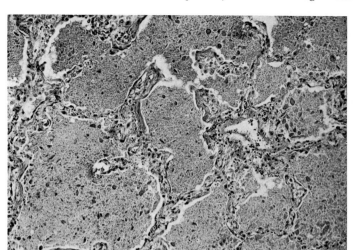

Fig. 14-22. Pulmonary alveolar proteinosis. Alveolar spaces are filled with a granular eosinophilic material, with some darker eosinophilic condensation bodies. Alveolar walls contain little cellular infiltrate.

lar and floccular proteinaceous and lipid-containing material, which stains positively with the PAS technique. This material appears to be derived from proliferating septal cells, which become granular and undergo sloughing and necrosis. Acicular crystals and laminated bodies suggesting early stages of corpora amylacea may be present. The microscopic appearance must be distinguished from that of pulmonary edema, cholesterol pneumonitis, and *Pneumocystis* pneumonitis.

The etiology is unknown. The clinical course is variable. It may or may not begin with a febrile illness and usually has a prolonged course associated with dyspnea and cough.

Various types of pulmonary inflammatory lesions must be distinguished and are given distinctive terminologies. *Desquamative interstitial pneumonia* is characterized by a mass of large cells within alveoli and an apparent proliferation of these cells in the lumina and on alveolar walls. There also may be small lymphoid follicles in the periphery of the lung. *Lymphocytic interstitial pneumonia* is a chronic interstitial pneumonitis with bronchiolitis obliterans and is characterized by massive infiltration and proliferation of lymphocytes in both lungs.

Rheumatic pneumonia. While cardiac lesions are of prime importance in rheumatic fever, pleurisy and pulmonary involvement are common. Mitral stenosis gives rise to a chronic passive congestion of the lung, resulting in brown induration. In addition to such changes, more specific primary rheumatic lesions have been described in the lung. This change is an interstitial pneumonitis, focal or widespread, with a tendency to recurrence. In acute phases congestion and hemorrhage are prominent. Focal areas of inflammation occur, with fibrinoid necrosis, fibrinous exudate in alveoli, proliferation of mononuclear cells and fibroblasts, and eventual fibrosis. The peculiar focal areas of organizing inflammation have been referred to as Masson bodies. The specificity of the lesions is disputed. In subacute and chronic phases the lung is of rubbery consistency, the toughness being caused by interstitial fibrosis and hyperplasia of elastic tissue. Such late changes may be difficult to separate from those resulting from passive congestion. Nodular pulmonary calcifications and ossification may be found in some long-standing cases of mitral stenosis, perhaps by organization of the exudate of rheumatic lesions.

Wegener's granulomatosis. Wegener's granulomatosis, or necrotizing respiratory granulomatosis, appears to be a hypersensitivity disease involving primarily the respiratory tract, but commonly affecting the kidneys and arteries elsewhere. Progressive, severe destructive or ulcerative lesions involve the lungs, with round or oval consolidations around affected bronchi. The lesions show angiitis and an inflammatory exudate in which eosinophils, plasma cells, mononuclear cells, and giant cells may be prominent. In the kidneys focal glomerulitis with necrosis or fibrinoid change is most constant, although there may be some periglomerular granulomatous inflammation. Angiitis, involving medium-sized arteries, may be present elsewhere, e.g., in the spleen. While the severe cases have a short duration of a few months and may terminate in death, there is evidence that milder forms may occur. Possibly Loeffler's eosinophilic granuloma of the lung is a more benign form of a similar condition of hypersensitivity.

Loeffler's syndrome. Loeffler's syndrome is characterized by transitory pulmonary lesions, which are prominent in roentgenograms, an increase of eosinophilic leukocytes in the blood, and a mild clinical course. The lesion has been described as a bronchopneumonia with numerous eosinophilic leukocytes in the

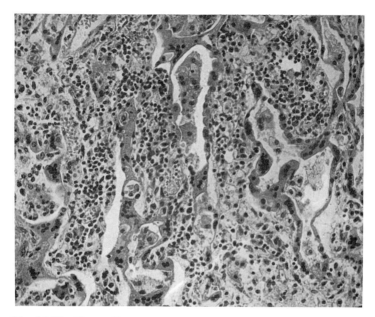

Fig. 14-23. Giant cell pneumonia in a child. Alveolar spaces are lined by cells, some of which are fused to form giant cells.

alveolar exudate, a tendency to organization, granulomatous foci, and necrotizing arteritis and arteriolitis. Bronchial changes may be similar to those in asthma. It has been considered an allergic reaction of pulmonary tissue, although a similarity to eosinophilic granuloma elsewhere and to the reticuloendothelioses has been suggested. Granulomatous pulmonary lesions resulting from the inhalation of cosmetic aerosols have been reported and suggested by some as one cause of Loeffler's syndrome, but the frequency and importance are uncertain and debatable.

Hyperplasia of the pulmonary alveolar lining. Electron microscopic study has suggested that alveoli are lined by a continuous cytoplasm of cells, with infrequent nuclei and few mitochondria. In a variety of pathologic conditions, alveolar lining cells appear in ordinary sections. The hyperplastic cells also may be derived from "septal cells," which are normally found scattered in alveolar walls or in the niches between capillaries or by downgrowth from terminal bronchioles. Such changes have been described in chronic passive congestion, interstitial and lipid pneumonias, around tuberculous foci, in giant cell pneumonias of infancy, and in pneumonia alba of congenital syphilis. Atypical hyperplasias of bronchiolar cells may form minute tumorlike masses (p. 437).

Circulatory disturbances

Congestion. *Active* congestion in the lung accompanies acute inflammations or follows inhalation of irritants. *Passive* congestion is more common, the hypostatic form being found in almost every autopsy. The lower and posterior parts of the lungs are dark red and firmer than normal. More important is the *Chronic passive congestion,* which accompanies pulmonary hypertension and failure in the pulmonary circulation. This generalized pulmonary hyperemia may be present for an extensive period and gives rise to brown pigmentation and increased firmness, a condition called *brown induration of the lung.* The most important cause is mitral stenosis, but aortic stenosis, certain congenital cardiac defects, and other lesions associated with prolonged left ventricular failure occasionally give the same result. The brown color of the lung is caused by hemosiderin pigment, most of which is held in macrophages in alveolar spaces (heart failure cells). The hemosiderin may result from hemorrhages from the bronchopulmonary anastomoses in the mucosa of the terminal bronchioles. Iron pigment in adjacent stroma produces damage and reactive changes. Occasional cases of mitral stenosis may show minute foci of ossification in basal areas. The thickness of alveolar walls, through which oxygen and carbon dioxide must diffuse, may be increased many times. The alveolar walls have increased collagenous interstitial tissue, thickening of capillary basement membranes, dilated capillaries, and edema. Alveolar lining cells tend toward cuboidal shape. Pulmonary vascular changes are common in such cases and consist of intimal thickening and atherosclerosis of arteries, hyperplastic arteriolar sclerosis, and in some severe cases even arteriolar necrosis. These vascular lesions are promoted by the high intravascular pressure, stagnation of blood, and edema.

Edema. Edema fluid in the lung may be (1) of inflammatory origin or (2) a transudate occurring in cases of passive congestion or failure of the pulmonary circulation. Anoxia appears to be an important factor in the pulmonary edema of circulatory failure. Irritant inhaled gases, such as phosgene, produce pulmonary edema by damage to capillaries, making them more permeable to blood plasma. Inflammatory edema is prominent in early stages of pneumonia, and its high protein content causes it to stain well with eosin. The edematous lung is large, pale, and heavy and pits on pressure. Watery, frothy fluid flows or may be squeezed from the cut surface. In sections the edema fluid appears as a faint eosin-staining material in the alveolar spaces. Edema fluid with its protein content provides a medium favorable for bacterial growth and so promotes infection.

High altitude acute pulmonary edema is occasionally found in persons who go to high altitudes for the first time, or it may occur in residents of high altitudes when they return home after some days or weeks at sea level. The edema is severe, with hyaline membranes. Increased capillary permeability, left cardiac insufficiency, and increased pulmonary venous resistance may be important hemodynamic factors.

Pulmonary changes in uremia. A proportion of patients with uremia, hypertension, and left ventricular failure develop a central pulmonary edema, which presents a characteristic roentgenologic appearance. The periphery of the lungs tends to be spared. The combination of a rise in pulmonary capillary pressure resulting from cardiac failure and alteration in capillary permeability resulting from uremia produces a protein-rich or fibrinous type of pulmonary edema. However, the changes may occur in uremia with little or no evidence of heart failure. Improvement in the uremic condition by peritoneal dialysis may be accompanied by improvement in the pulmonary edema. There appears to be some correlation with the degree of acidosis as indicated by depression of the blood carbon dioxide–combining power. Grossly the lungs are rubbery in consistency and yield frothy fluid on firm pressure (solid edema). Microscopically the alveolar walls are thickened and congested, and the alveolar spaces contain an eosinophilic fibrinous fluid with a tendency to hyalinization and formation of eosinophilic (hyaline) membranes lining alveoli. The pathologic changes are similar to those seen in other conditions with cardiac failure and associated vascular damage, such as in rheumatic pneumonitis.

Thrombosis, embolism, and infarction. Blockage to pulmonary arteries by embolism is common, but primary thrombosis is relatively rare. Thrombi that give rise to pulmonary embolism most commonly originate in the iliac veins, femoral veins,

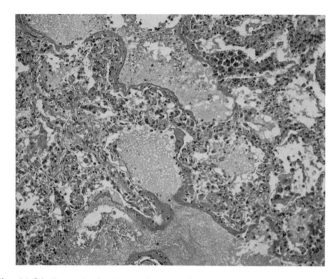

Fig. 14-24. Lung in fatal uremia (uremic pneumonitis). Alveolar spaces contain pale eosinophilic edema fluid with peripheral condensations forming hyaline membranes. Alveolar walls are thick and edematous, and there are some focal accumulations of macrophages containing hemosiderin pigment.

pelvic veins, prostatic venous plexus, vena cava, and right atrium. Pulmonary embolism is common in older age groups and in medical as well as surgical diseases. There is developing evidence that pulmonary embolization in surviving patients may be a precursor of pulmonary arteriosclerosis and pulmonary hypertension. Postoperative pulmonary embolism is most likely to follow abdominal or pelvic surgical procedures. If the embolus blocks the pulmonary artery or one of its large branches, it may cause rapid death and is easily clinically mistaken for coronary occlusion. The actual mechanism of death appears to be a sympathetic-inhibitory reflex or shock. There is insufficient time for development of an infarct of the lung in such rapidly fatal cases. Demonstration of the embolus at autopsy often can be facilitated by opening the pulmonary artery in situ before removal of the heart.

Blockage of smaller pulmonary arteries by emboli results in infarction of lung tissue if there is already some interference with the pulmonary circulation, such as passive congestion or edema. Embolism alone does not result in infarction of the normal lung, probably because blood supplied by bronchial arteries and by anastomoses of pulmonary intralobular arteries is sufficient to maintain nutrition. Pulmonary infarcts are almost always red and hemorrhagic. They form bulging, dark red, firm, conical areas, with their base at the pleural surface. Microscopically the whole area of infarction, including alveolar spaces, walls, and capillaries, is stuffed with blood. In later stages necrosis of alveolar walls may be observed, and there is decolorization of the blood. Extensive pulmonary embolism with subsequent organization may lead to heart failure (cor pulmonale).

An embolus tends to be coiled, twisted, impacted, or riding a bifurcation; its shape may not conform to that of the vessel in which it lies; and it may have freshly broken ends. A thrombus is usually attached to the vessel wall, has a sessile base, and is molded to the shape of the vessel.

Blast injury. Pulmonary hemorrhage associated with thoracic trauma or asphyxia is common in both peace and war injuries. In war experience, "blast injury" or pulmonary concussion caused by a nearby bomb or other high explosive may produce fatal pulmonary hemorrhage without external evidence of trauma. The lungs show bilateral and roughly symmetric hemorrhagic consolidation deep in their substance. There is an associated general pulmonary congestion, and the hemorrhage may be progressive. Microscopically the appearance is similar to that of a recent infarct, but some areas may show fibrin and monocytes as well as red cells in alveolar spaces and so simulate in appearance the red hepatization stage of pneumonia. In compression asphyxia the lesion differs in that the hemorrhages are mainly subpleural and in the lines of the ribs, with emphysema outlining rib markings. In the pulmonary hemorrhage caused by the traumatic impact of a solid, the hemorrhage may be unilateral and related to the site of the blow, and around this point the lung is torn or contused.

Arteriosclerosis. Pulmonary arteriosclerosis of mild degree is common but rarely of clinical importance. In larger arteries it is evident grossly as intimal atherosclerosis. Hypertension and congestion in the pulmonary circulation (e.g., in mitral stenosis) lead to vascular changes. There is a reduction in the pulmonary arterial bed, which is contributed to by thrombosis in larger arteries and peripheral arterial narrowing. The latter may be caused by intimal proliferation (often with thrombosis and organization) or a diffuse arterial contracture with thick walls, narrowed lumina, and indistensibility. Thromboembolic conditions with embolizations of smaller pulmonary vessels may contribute to the development of pulmonary sclerosis and hypertension.

There is also a rare condition of primary sclerosis of pulmonary arteries, associated with hypertrophy of the right side of the heart and usually resulting in death from heart failure. Some of these cases, particularly when associated with severe cyanosis, are designated as *Ayerza's disease*. However, the concept of Ayerza's disease has been variable.

Pulmonary calcification. Calcification in the lung is most commonly a dystrophic calcification occuring in areas of necrosis and inflammation, most often as a result of tuberculosis, histoplasmosis, or other fungous infections. The lung also may be the site of metastatic calcification in severe cases of hyperparathyroidism, the alveolar walls and blood vessels being affected particularly.

Rounded laminated bodies (corpora amylacea) are occasionally seen in alveolar spaces where there has been chronic inflammation. They may be present in association with pulmonary alveolar proteinoses. Rarely they may be present in enormous numbers and may be calcified (microlithiasis alveolaris pulmonum), so that they produce widespread opacity on radiographic plates. The cause is unknown, but probably they result from the calcification of remnants of inflammatory exudate or necrotic material in alveolar spaces.

Atelectasis

Atelectasis is an incomplete dilatation or a collapse of lung tissue. The three main causes are (1) failure of expansion in the newborn infant (congenital), (2) compression of lung tissue, and (3) bronchial obstruction. Atelectasis does not interfere with respiratory function unless areas of considerable size are involved.

In many stillborn children the lungs are completely atelectatic and airless. Infants who live for a few days have lungs with patchy areas of atelectasis or incomplete expansion. Compression atelectasis results from pressure against lung tissue, as by air, transudate, or exudate in the pleural cavity, or by tumors. Bronchial obstruction results in atelectasis because the air is absorbed from the nonaerated portion of the lung.

Atelectatic lung tissue is dark red or blue in color because of congestion, and it is firm, noncrepitant, and depressed below the surrounding surfaces. Microscopically the alveolar walls are pressed together, forming more or less parallel bands separated by narrow elongated alveolar spaces. If atelectasis is present for a considerable period, fibrosis may occur and reexpansion becomes impossible.

Acute massive collapse. Acute massive collapse refers to the rapid atelectasis of the whole or a large part of a lung. The mediastinum is displaced toward the affected side, and there is evidence of respiratory difficulty. It is an occasional complication of abdominal operations, peritonitis, diaphragmatic pleurisy, and paralyses of diphtheria. Bronchial obstruction and interference with the cough reflex are believed to be the important factors in causation. There is some evidence that atelectasis may occur in the absence of obstruction ("contraction atelectasis") because of active contraction of smooth muscle elements in the lung distal to the terminal bronchioles.

Hyaline membrane disease. A condition in newborn infants of failure of pulmonary expansion or pulmonary collapse has as its most prominent microscopic feature hyaline membranes lining the bronchiolar and alveolar ducts.

Clinically the condition is called "respiratory distress syndrome," or "pulmonary syndrome of the newborn." It is particularly common in premature infants, after cesarean section, and in infants from mothers who have diabetes mellitus. The mortality is high.

The lungs are dark red, of liverlike consistency, edematous, poorly aerated, and sink in water. Histologically there is widespread atelectasis and prominent hyaline membranes of eosin-staining homogenous material, lining, particularly, distended bronchioles. The hyaline material may contain some lipid, and a fibrin content has been demonstrated by fluorescein-labeled fibrin antibodies and by electron microscopy. Pulmonary surfactant, a pulmonary surface-active substance capable of lowering alveolar surface tension, has been shown to be deficient. This and the inhibition of a fibrinolytic mechanism may explain the atelectasis and persistence of the hyaline membrane. While the hyaline membrane may contribute to the respiratory diffi-

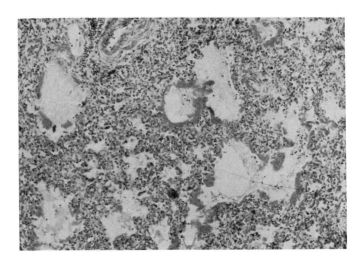

Fig. 14-25. Hyaline membrane disease of the lung in a newborn child.

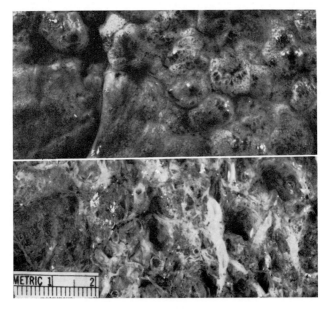

Fig. 14-26. Emphysema of the lung. Small bullae are seen on the pleural surface (above). The cut surface (below) shows increased fibrosis as well as the small cystlike emphysematous spaces.

culty, it is not the primary cause. Pressure ulcers may be found on the larynx.

Hyaline membranes of similar appearance may be found in the lungs of adults in a variety of conditions characterized by pneumonitis and edema, such as uremic pneumonitis, viral interstitial pneumonitis, irritation from inhaled chemicals, and after radiation.

Pulmonary emphysema

Emphysema is the most common chronic disease of the lungs and a major cause of pulmonary disability. Clinical definitions and classifications of emphysema have recently given way to more precise anatomic terms.

Vesicular emphysema is a term used for emphysema of air

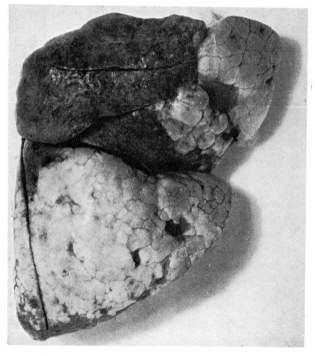

Fig. 14-27. Emphysematous areas in the lung.

spaces of the lung, as distinguished from interstitial emphysema, in which escaped air distends interstitial structures. Vesicular emphysema may be defined as an increase beyond normal size of the air spaces distal to the terminal bronchiole. Some limit the term *emphysema* to those cases in which the enlargement of the air spaces is accompanied by destruction of tissue and use the term *overinflation* if there is dilatation of air spaces without destruction. Emphysema may be grouped into six types, or classes: centrilobular, panlobular, senile (aging lung), localized, secondary, and miscellaneous. The clinical syndrome of emphysema is usually related to sufficiently widespread or severe centrilobular and/or panlobular emphysema.

Centrilobular emphysema is a destructive lesion in which destroyed and enlarged respiratory bronchioles tend to become confluent and form emphysematous spaces situated toward the center of the lobules. The lesions tend to be most frequent and severe in the upper areas of the lungs.

Panlobular emphysema (panacinar emphysema) is characterized by destructive enlargement of all or any part distal to the terminal bronchiole, so that any part or all of the acinus or lobule is affected. Although it occurs in any part of the lung, it tends to become more severe in lower zones. Panlobular and centrilobular emphysema may occur together in lungs in varying degree as well as separately.

In advanced emphysema the lungs are voluminous, pale, dry, and of peculiar pillowlike consistency because of loss of normal elasticity. The lungs fail to collapse when the chest is opened. Large blebs or bullae often occur at the apices and along the margins. Microscopically the alveolar spaces are enlarged, and the walls appear stretched, thin, bloodless, and often ruptured. The constriction of vessels in the alveolar wall causes the pallor and dryness of the lung tissue.

Emphysema is associated with an increase in the residual air content of the lungs and a proportionate decrease in vital capacity. It occurs more frequently in men than in women, and the highest incidence is in persons in their sixth decade. The chest tends to be barrel shaped, with a wide costal angle and a low position of the diaphragm. The decreased pulmonary mobility and elasticity and the obliteration of alveolar capillaries tend to cause stagnation in the pulmonary circulation and throw more work on the right side of the heart. There may be hypertrophy of the right side of the heart (cor pulmonale), and eventually there may be failure and passive congestion. The etiology of these types of emphysema is obscure, but association with chronic bronchitis, smoking, and atmospheric pollution is frequent.

Senile emphysema. Senile emphysema, or aging lung, also associated with a barrel-shaped chest and hyperresonant lungs, is usually seen in persons past middle age. There is an enlargement of alveolar ducts and alveoli, with some loss of elastic tissue and capillaries. The pores of Kohn appear enlarged. Often centrilobular and/or panlobular emphysema are present as well. The lungs follow the change in shape of the chest but are not much enlarged. They collapse on opening the chest, since their elasticity is not greatly impaired. Respiratory function is little impaired except in those cases in which the lung has been overstretched.

Localized emphysema includes bullae in otherwise uninvolved lungs or localized variant forms of centrilobular or panlobular emphysema. **Secondary emphysema** is an overinflation of the intact lung, localized or widespread and usually obstructive in origin. It includes dilated spaces in relation to scars. **Miscellaneous** types of emphysema include types such as emphysema along lobular septa (paraseptal emphysema). The so-called bronchiolar emphysema (muscular cirrhosis of the lungs) is not a true emphysema but a bronchiolectasis with muscular hypertrophy and fibrosis.

Pulmonary interstitial emphysema. Pulmonary interstitial emphysema is a condition in which air is present in interstitial tissues of the lung rather than in alveolar spaces. Air escapes through ruptured alveolar bases into sheaths of pulmonary vessels precipitated by a pressure gradient of air in alveoli to perivascular sheaths in cases where alveoli are overexpanded or blood vessels are not filled to the normal extent. Predisposing conditions are (1) general overinflation of lung tissue, (2) atelectasis of an area of lung with overinflation of adjacent areas, and (3) decreased blood supply to pulmonary vessels with hyperinflation or increased intra-alveolar pressure. The air may travel along vascular sheaths to the mediastinum (pneumomediastinum), work upward to the neck, face, and axillae (subcutaneous emphysema), and work downward along the aorta and esophagus into the retroperitoneum. Cyanosis may result from venous stasis because of collapse of pulmonary vessels and dyspnea because of interference with respiratory movement.

Cardiac disturbance may result from pressure of the distended lungs or pneumomediastinum or from lack of blood because of the venous congestion. Continued accumulation of air in the mediastinum, unless withdrawn, may be fatal from interference with respiration and circulation. Air block in newborn infants may be caused by interstitial emphysema, with pneumothorax resulting from rupture of the pleura.

Pneumoconioses

Pneumoconiosis refers to the pulmonary changes caused by the inhalation of dust. These changes depend on the type and the amount of dust inhaled, the length of time of exposure, and the presence of associated infection, particularly tuberculosis. There are four important types: (1) Anthracosis, caused by the inhalation of carbon pigment, is almost universal in occurrence but is not associated with functional changes and hence is unimportant clinically. (2) Silicosis, caused by the inhalation of free silica, is an important occupational disease among miners and others working in rock. Because of its specific chemical nature it produces a reaction in the lung characterized by the development of nodular areas of hyaline fibrosis. It is often associated with tuberculosis and accelerates this infection. The pulmonary fibrosis predisposes to right-sided heart failure. (3) Asbestosis, caused by the inhalation of asbestos fibers, is relatively uncommon. It produces a diffuse fibrosis of the lung. Characteristic asbestos bodies, which are elongated, club-shaped fibers coated with iron

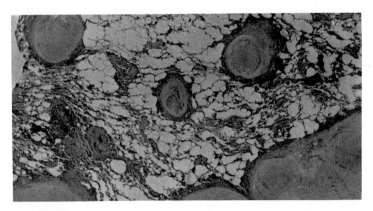

Fig. 14-28. Silicotic nodules in the lung as seen in a low-power photomicrograph.

pigment, are found in the lung tissue and may appear in the sputum. It causes no particular predisposition to tuberculosis. Right-sided heart failure may result from the pulmonary fibrosis. (4) Silicosiderosis occurs among hematite miners and is characterized by lungs of a bright brick-red color.

Anthracosis. A deposit of inhaled carbon pigment is found in some degree in all adult urban dwellers. While the normal color of the lung, as seen in an infant, is grayish pink, the adult lung is flecked by focal and linear deposits of black pigment, evident on both the pleural and cut surfaces. Through function of alveolar phagocytes and lymphocytes the pigment becomes concentrated in the lymphoid tissue of the lungs, peribronchial nodes, and mediastinum. The pigment tends to accumulate particularly in areas where inflammation or fibrosis has blocked lymphatics. The pigment itself does not stimulate fibrosis. Air spaces are visible in the pigmented areas, and respiratory function is undisturbed.

Silicosis. Silicosis is the most important of the pneumoconioses because of its frequency as an occupational disease, the severity of the fibrosis, and its promotion of serious tuberculous infection. Inhaled particles of silica become concentrated in the pulmonary lymphatic system, and here they stimulate connective tissue proliferation. Nodules of hyalinized, collagenous, concentric laminae are formed. Globulins are mixed with the collagen in the nodules. Carbon pigment is usually trapped in the same area, so that some black pigment is evident in the nodules. The particles of silica may be identified by a polarizing microscope. There is evidence that silica can combine with body protein and act as an antigen, so that an antigen-antibody reaction may be a factor in silicosis. Experimentally the reaction of tissues to silica may be modified by the administration of cortisone.

In early stages the silicotic nodules are too small to be identified grossly, but ultimately they develop into nodules, 3 mm. or more in diameter and with sharply defined borders. Islets of this collagenous tissue are scattered through the lung, under the pleural surfaces, and in tracheobronchial lymph nodes. Eventually massive conglomerate areas of fibrosis may result. Most of the fatal cases terminate with tuberculous infection. Other complications that may develop are cardiac hypertrophy and dilatation, particularly of the right side of the heart, emphysema, and carcinoma of the lung. Obliterative vascular changes appear to be important in the pulmonary hypertension and

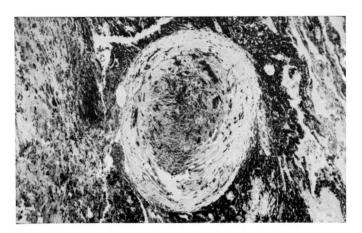

Fig. 14-29. Silicotic nodule of the lung. A large amount of black anthracotic pigment is present also.

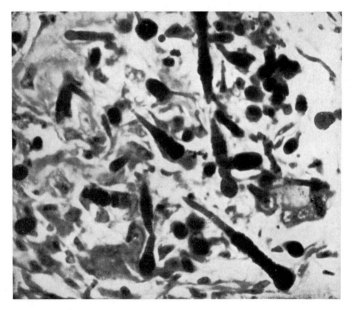

Fig. 14-30. Asbestosis of the lung. Note the bulbous ends and the haustration of the asbestos bodies and also the giant cells.

right-sided cardiac failure. The degree of importance of silicosis in the etiology of pulmonary carcinoma is still undetermined.

Asbestosis. Asbestosis is a mineral fibrous structure, composed essentially of magnesium silicate. Inhalation of the fibers occurs mainly in the factories during the carding process, in which the fiber is separated from the crushed mineral. Inhalation over a period of seven or more years is usually required to produce the disease. The fibers are deposited in the bronchioles and stimulate fibrosis mechanically rather than by specific chemical action. The lower lobes particularly are affected, and the result is a diffuse rather than nodular type of interstitial fibrosis. Emphysema, bronchiectasis, and interference with respiratory function may result. Termination is usually by infection or cardiac failure. Tuberculosis occasionally supervenes, but asbestosis does not particularly predispose to tuberculosis. Bronchogenic carcinoma and pleural mesothelioma occur with increased frequency in association with asbestosis.

Grossly the involved lung shows irregular patches and strands of grayish dense scar tissue. Dilated emphysematous air spaces are evident in the involved tissue.

The characteristic asbestos bodies occur singly or in clumps as elongated fibers of variable size and form (up to 140μ in length). One or both extremities of the fiber are bulbous, and the body is slender and haustrated or segmented. The color is yellowish, greenish yellow, or brown because of the iron pigment deposited on the surface; they stain well with the Prussian blue method for iron. Asbestos bodies may be found in basal lung smears in a considerable proportion of adult urban individuals (20 to 30% in our laboratory) in the absence of the pulmonary lesions of asbestosis.

Silicosiderosis. Silicosiderosis is caused by the inhalation of iron-containing hematite by hematite miners. The lungs have a striking brick-red color. Some silica is usually inhaled as well. A diffuse or nodular pulmonary fibrosis may be produced.

Graphite pneumoconiosis. Inhalation of graphite appears to cause a chronic pneumoconiosis with a predilection for the upper portions of the lung. It is characterized by a granulomatous reaction, with areas of fibrosis, necrosis, cavitation, and obliterative changes in blood vessels and bronchi. The lung tissue is black, and the graphite particles are large and cause a giant cell reaction.

Bauxite fume pneumoconiosis. In the manufacture of alumina abrasive powders, exposure to the white fumes evolved from heating a mixture of bauxite, iron, and coke has resulted in a diffuse pulmonary fibrosis with obliterative endarteritis. Amorphous aluminum and silica dust are the prominent constituents of the fumes.

Beryllium pneumoconiosis. The inhalation of beryllium fumes or dust may cause either an acute pneumonitis or a granulomatous inflammation with diffuse pulmonary fibrosis (p. 243).

Cadmium. Cadmium inhalation may produce a pneumonitis with interstitial fibrosis in addition to some alveolar exudate.

PLEURA

Diseases of the pleura are mainly effusions, inflammations, and tumors. With effusions into the pleural cavity, corresponding collapse of lung tissue occurs. The collapse may be limited to one side by immobility of the mediastinum, or it may be locally limited by adhesions.

Hydrothorax. Hydrothorax is the accumulation of edema fluid or transudate in the pleural cavity. It occurs in conditions of generalized edema, as in renal or cardiac disease, or rarely may be caused by local conditions, such as tumor or aneurysm. The fluid is clear, light yellow, of low specific gravity (below 1.015), and low in protein content. In some cases the fluid is milky because of the fat content (chylous hydrothorax).

Hemothorax. Blood in the pleural cavity may occur in cases of thoracic trauma or from rupture of an aneurysm. A blood-stained pleural fluid is more common than true hemothorax. Its occurrence is usually associated with tuberculosis or with malignant tumor of the lung or pleura.

Pneumothorax. Air in the pleural cavity may be introduced from without by wounds or therapeutic procedures, or it may result from a rupture of the lung into the pleural cavity. The commonest causes of the latter are tuberculosis and rupture of an emphysematous bleb. In many cases air in the pleural cavity is associated with a serous or inflammatory exudate.

Pleurisy. Inflammation of the pleura is usually a spread from the lung. Less commonly it is caused by spread from the abdomen or the mediastinum or is blood borne and appears to be primary in the pleura. Most cases result from infection with tubercle bacilli, pneumococci, staphylococci, or streptococci. The apparently primary forms usually are caused by tuberculosis or rheumatic fever. Major causes of pleural exudate are lobar pneumonia, subpleural tuberculosis, carcinoma, pulmonary infarction, acute mediastinitis, subphrenic abscess, and fractured rib. Pleurisy is classified according to the type of exudate as fibrinous (dry pleurisy), serofibrinous (pleurisy with effusion), and purulent (empyema). The fluid in pleurisy is cloudy or contains flakes of fibrin and has a relatively high specific gravity and high protein content. The exudate containing fibrin and inflammatory cells is evident in sections through the inflamed pleura. Pleurisy may resolve and leave little trace, but often organization results in a thickened scarred area of pleura or fibrous adhesions between visceral and parietal layers.

Empyema most commonly is the result of pneumococcal, staphylococcal, or streptococcal infection of the lung. Organization and formation of adhesions tend to localize the pus in various parts of the pleural cavity. A thick organizing wall of exudate may line the cavity, covering both visceral and parietal surfaces.

Pleural tumors. Most tumors involving pleura are extensions from malignant tumors in the lung, but primary pleural tumors occur also. The primary benign tumors arise from subpleural tissues and include fibromas, lipomas, chondromas, and angiomas.

Mesothelioma is an uncommon primary tumor arising from pleural lining cells. A diffuse malignant form occurs as flattened nodular tumor masses on both visceral and parietal layers or spreads diffusely over pleura, forming a thick layer of tumor tissue. Microscopic characteristics of both epithelial and connective tissue tumors may be present, with a sarcomatous appearance in some areas, but also tending to form glandlike spaces or channels. A papillary pattern or some mucin production may be present. There may be some histologic similarity to synovial tumors (synovioma). Spread may be by invasion of lymphatics and metastasis to mediastinal lymph nodes. Abundant hemorrhagic pleural fluid is a usual accompaniment. A solitary form commonly is fibrous in type but also may contain components of epithelial appearance. It may be benign or malignant.

A frequent association of exposure to asbestos mineral or the finding of asbestos bodies in the lung has been noted in cases of diffuse pleural mesotheliomas. Some association of asbestosis with peritoneal mesothelioma has also been found. Carcinoma of the lung has been noted in about 13% of cases of asbestosis.

MEDIASTINAL TUMORS AND CYSTS

The varied tissue components of the mediastinum may give rise to a great variety of neoplasms, the most frequent being malignant lymphomas, thymomas, teratomas (including dermoid cysts), and neurogenous tumors. Mediastinal teratomas are generally cystic and are located in the anterior mediastinum. Schlumberger has presented evidence that the origin may be from faulty embryogenesis of the thymus. The majority are benign. In malignant mediastinal teratomas, well-differentiated ectodermal derivatives such as skin or nerve tissue and organoid epithelial structures are absent. Their main complications are mechanical effects on the trachea, great vessels, heart, or lungs. The mediastinal neurogenous tumors are almost always in the posterior mediastinum. They are of two main types: (1) ganglioneuromas (benign) and neuroblastomas (malignant) arising from cells of the sympathetic nervous system, which occur mainly in children and young individuals; and (2) nerve sheath tumors, including neurilemomas, neurofibromas, and neurogenous sarcomas, found in adults.

Mediastinal cysts are mainly of developmental origin. Bronchial cysts are considered as developmental reduplication cysts of the respiratory tract. They are lined by ciliated columnar epithelium, and their walls may contain any or all of the tissues normally present in the respiratory tract. They are most common in the posterior part of the superior mediastinum near the bifurcation of the trachea. Esophageal cysts have a muscular wall and a squamous lining. The rare gastroenteric or alimentary cysts have a structure simulating that of stomach or intestine. They are thought to be caused by a pinching off of a diverticulum of the embryonic foregut. Cystic lymphangioma of the mediastinum, a congenital maldevelopment in a group of lymph vessels, is quite rare. It is a nonencapsulated mass of multiple cystic spaces lined by single layers of endothelium, intimately incorporated with surrounding structures. Anterior mediastinal cysts may be of thymic or thymopharyngeal duct origin. Pericardial coelomic cysts (pleuropericardial cysts) are discrete and nonadherent, are situated in the anterior inferior mediastinum, and are composed of a fibrous wall lined by a single layer of flat mesothelial-like cells. A rare mediastinal meningocele, usually associated with von Recklinghausen's neurofibromatosis, may appear as a cystic structure. The wall is composed of dural and arachnoidal components.

Chapter 15

The liver, gallbladder, and pancreas

LIVER
Structure and function

The liver has a double blood supply, portal and hepatic, but the circulation to the right and left sides of the liver is fairly distinct. This circulatory division of the liver does not correspond with the anatomic lobes, but the right and left halves are divided by a line passing through the middle of the gallbladder fossa to the junction of the hepatic veins with the inferior vena cava. The portal stream from the spleen and stomach goes mainly to the left side of the liver and that from the intestines mainly to the right side.

Microscopically the liver appears divided into lobules. At the center of each is a central (efferent) vein, and arranged around the periphery are portal areas, each containing a bile duct, hepatic artery, and portal vein. The cords of liver cells enclose bile canaliculi and blood sinusoids. In the wall of the latter are Kupffer cells, which are highly phagocytic and form a part of the reticuloendothelial system.

The liver is the largest organ in the body, and its functions are many and varied. It is concerned with the excretion of bile, but bile pigment is formed only partly in the liver, the other components of the reticuloendothelial system (spleen and bone marrow) playing a major role. The liver forms bile salts and is important in various other biochemical processes, such as the formation of plasma proteins, heparin, prothrombin, and fibrinogen, fat metabolism and storage, urea and amino acid formation, and glycogen storage. In the fetus the liver is a blood-forming organ. A variety of laboratory tests are useful in determining the efficiency of the various hepatic functions and in clinical study of cases of disease of the liver or jaundice.

An important feature of the liver is a great capacity for regeneration after injury or destruction of its cells, a feature that is important in compensation for effects of injury to liver cells. There is nodular overgrowth of localized regenerating areas (multiple nodular hyperplasia), in which mitoses often can be found, and new bile duct formation is prominent. The compensatory hyperplasia is prevented by deficiency or obstruction in the portal circulation (e.g., in portal cirrhosis) and by confinement and compression caused by fibrosis. Mitotic activity in liver cells may be seen also in patients dying of uremia.

Congenital abnormalities of form are uncommon or unimportant in the liver. *Riedel's lobe* is a downward projection of the right lobe. Acquired changes in form include transverse grooves resulting from tight clothing. Anteroposterior depressions on the upper surface of the liver are caused by the pressure of muscle bundles of the diaphragm.

Congenital biliary atresia is characterized by obstruction of the bile passage, caused by anomalous development of the bile duct. There is severe hepatic fibrosis with distortion of the lobular architecture. Interlobular bile ducts are hypoplastic, with ductular proliferation. The hepatic cells show severe degeneration with giant cell change.

Autolysis

Postmortem autolytic changes develop quite rapidly in liver tissue. Bluish black discoloration may occur in the portion of liver adjacent to the transverse colon. Foamy liver results from postmortem infection of the liver by gas-forming organisms (e.g., *Clostridium welchii*) from the intestinal tract, the bubbles of gas so produced honeycombing the liver tissue.

Retrograde disturbances

Cloudy swelling. Cloudy swelling is common in the liver as a result of acute infections. The liver is enlarged and has a tense capsule, a softer consistency, and a paler, more opaque appearance than normal. Microscopically the liver cells are swollen and have distinct margins and pale granular cytoplasm.

Amyloid infiltration. Amyloid infiltration is common in the liver as well as in the spleen and kidney in cases of tuberculosis and chronic suppuration. The amyloid appears as a hyaline material between the lining cells of the sinusoids and the liver cells. Its continued accumulation causes compression, atrophy, and disappearance of the liver cords.

Hyaline masses. Hyaline masses may be found in the cytoplasm of liver cells in portal cirrhosis. They apparently represent an early and specific type of degenerative change in the liver cells. Intracellular hyaline changes are also noted in yellow fever (Councilman bodies) and in viral hepatitis (acidophilic bodies).

Glycogen. Glycogen is normally abundantly present in the cytoplasm of liver cells but in many diseases is much depleted by the wasting that precedes death. Cytoplasmic glycogen is also reduced in diabetes mellitus, although the amount in the liver cell nuclei may be increased and give the nuclei a clear, glassy appearance. Cytoplasmic glycogen is abnormally increased in *von Gierke's glycogen storage disease.* This is a congenital defect of glycogen mobilization, seen as a rare condition in infants and children. Enlargement because of the accumulation of glycogen may involve the kidneys as well as the liver.

Fatty change. Fatty change in the liver is a common event and may be of very severe degree. Fatty metamorphosis occurs with a variety of infections and intoxications. Prolonged passive congestion tends to cause fatty change in central parts of the lobules. Fatty livers are found in association with obesity, chronic alcoholism, malnutrition and wasting diseases (e.g., tuberculosis and malignant tumors), in some cases of diabetes mellitus, and as a result of certain poisons such as phlorhizin, carbon tetrachloride, chloroform, and ether. In sudden unexpected death in young adults, prominent fatty change in the liver is frequently the only finding. Unexplained death in chronic alcoholism with severe fatty change in the liver has been caused by massive fat embolism in some cases, but this appears to be an infrequent finding. The increase is in neutral fat, the mechanism apparently being some interference with normal carbohydrate-fat metabolism, often by interference with the proper oxidation of fat. Alcohol appears to produce its effect by interference with tissue oxidation.

The fatty liver, such as that seen in chronic alcoholism, is enlarged and has rounded borders, a tense capsule, yellow or yellowish red color, fairly firm consistency, and some greasiness of the cut surface. Microscopically the fat is most prominent around the central part of the lobules, but when the fatty change is great, the distribution is diffuse and the fat is in the form of large globules.

Pigmentation. Pigmentation of the liver is common in a number of conditions. The accumulated pigment may be hemosiderin (in congestion, hemolytic conditions, hemosiderosis, and hemochromatosis), malarial pigment (hematin), bile pigment (in obstructive jaundice), or lipofuscin (in chronic idiopathic jaundice). In obstructive jaundice the bile pigment first appears as small plugs in bile canaliculi, and later it may appear as coarse granules in parenchymal and Kupffer cells.

Chronic idiopathic jaundice. Chronic idiopathic jaundice has been recognized as a distinct condition by Dubin and Johnson, and by Sprinz and Nelson. A benign condition easily mistaken for obstructive jaundice, it is characterized by chronic or intermittent jaundice, with abdominal pain, dark urine, pale stools, a high level of direct-reacting bilirubin in the serum, and nonvisualization of the gallbladder on cholecystography. It appears to be a congenital metabolic deficiency in which the liver can conjugate indirect bilirubin with glucuronic acid but has difficulty in excretion, so that the direct-reacting bilirubin accumulates in the serum and is excreted in the urine. The liver is characterized by a heavy accumulation of a lipofuscin pigment in hepatic cells in the central zones of the lobules. Little or no fibrosis or other morphologic change is evident. The liver may be grossly black or greenish black in color.

Circulatory disturbances

Chronic passive congestion. This disturbance is a common and prominent finding in the liver, an organ highly susceptible to circulatory deficiency. Cardiac insufficiency, e.g., that caused by rheumatic endocarditis, leaves its mark on the liver early and prominently. The effect is particularly in the central parts of the lobules, where stagnation and accumulation of blood dilate the central vein and adjacent portions of the sinusoids. The liver cells, first around the central veins but gradually extending out to the periphery, undergo atrophy resulting from anoxemia and compression. Degenerative changes, particularly of a fatty type, tend to occur. In some severe cases there may be actual necrosis. Grossly the contrasted pattern of red areas (caused by blood-stuffed vessels) and yellowish brown areas (liver cells with fatty degeneration) produces a characteristic "nutmeg" appearance. Long-standing congestion results in the so-called cardiac cirrhosis (p. 505).

Hemorrhage. Hemorrhage in the liver, which occurs in eclampsia and other conditions, is distinguished from congestion by the finding of red cells outside the sinuses, e.g., between the sinusoidal endothelium and the liver cells.

Edema. Edema in the liver is distinguishable by the presence

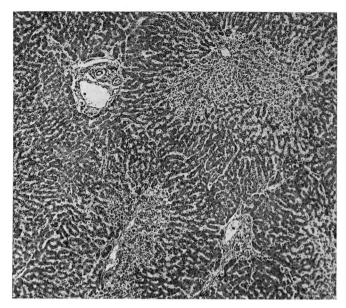

Fig. 15-1. Chronic passive congestion of the liver. The central zones of the lobules show the most severe congestion with centrolobular degeneration and atrophy. (×50.)

of a fine web of granular precipitated protein material between the sinus endothelial lining and the liver cell cords (serous hepatitis).

Infarction. Infarction is rare in the liver, presumably because of the abundant and double blood supply. When it occurs, it is most often caused by blockage of intrahepatic branches of the portal vein, although some infarcts have developed after ligation of the hepatic artery. The so-called Zahn infarct is an area of hyperemia with atrophy of hepatic cells but without actual necrosis.

Thrombosis of hepatic veins. Thrombosis of hepatic veins (Chiari's syndrome) occurs in acute and chronic forms. It may be caused by a primary hepatic endophlebitis or be secondary to various intrahepatic and extrahepatic conditions that favor thrombosis.

Veno-occlusive disease. Veno-occlusive disease of the liver is a peculiar type of obliterating endophlebitis that may progress

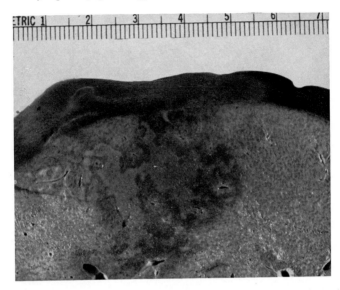

Fig. 15-2. Infarct of the liver. A congested zone outlines the irregular necrotic area.

to nonportal cirrhosis. Described in children and young adults in Jamaica, it appears to be associated with protein undernutrition and possibly with toxic substances in "bush teas."

Peliosis hepatis. Peliosis hepatis is a rare condition in which small focal angiomatoid lesions of hemorrhagic appearance are distributed throughout the liver. It is uncertain whether or not the hemorrhagic lesions are preceded by necrosis. Most instances have been in patients with tuberculosis. It has also been reported in patients treated with the androgenic steroid, norethandrolone. Experimentally peliosis hepatis has resulted after the transplantation of ovarian or testicular tumors in mice or the inoculation of newborn rats with a virus isolated from leukemic rat tissues.

Necrosis

Liver cells undergo necrosis as a result of a variety of poisons of chemical, infectious, and metabolic origin. Adequate stores of glycogen in the liver cells appear to give some protection. The lesions may be classified roughly according to their distribution into the following types: (1) diffuse necrosis, e.g., acute yellow atrophy, (2) "focal" necrosis, i.e., small necrotic foci distributed without any constant relationship to particular areas of the liver lobules, and (3) zonal necrosis, in which the areas of necrosis are in fairly constant relationship to a particular part of the liver lobules. The zonal necroses may be (1) central, i.e., in the central vein region, (2) midzonal, and (3) peripheral, or in portal areas.

Diffuse necrosis. Widespread necrosis of the liver has been called *acute yellow atrophy*. It may be caused by a variety of agents, including infections (viral hepatitis), chemicals (phosphorus, arsenicals, chloroform, carbon tetrachloride, sulfonamides), and metabolic disturbances. It may complicate severe hyperthyroidism ("thyroid storm"). Pregnancy is sometimes complicated by acute yellow atrophy, and also in obstetric practice delayed chloroform poisoning may produce hepatic necrosis. Most cases of diffuse necrosis of the liver, formerly considered idiopathic, now may be accounted for as cases of viral or infectious hepatitis. The hepatic changes are essentially the same as those described in acute and subacute fatal cases of infectious hepatitis. The acute form is fatal after a short duration with fever, gastrointestinal upset, disturbances of hepatic and renal functions, jaundice, crystals of leucine and tyrosine in the urine, and coma.

Except in the most acute cases the liver is shrunken, often to half its normal size. The capsule is wrinkled, soft, opaque, and of mottled, patchy yellowish and red color. In early stages the yellowish color predominates, but later, when the liver cells have extensively disintegrated, a red color is prominent. Microscopically one sees a loss of nuclei, granular and fatty degeneration of cytoplasm, and breaking up, disorganization, or complete disappearance of many cells.

Subacute yellow atrophy refers to those milder cases in which there is recovery or in which progress of the disease is slower, so that death occurs at a later stage or only after repeated attacks. Here there is an opportunity for removal of the necrotic cells, regenerative hyperplasia from the remaining liver tissue, and development of fibrous tissue. Nodules of hyperplastic liver cells are separated by connective tissue, and bile duct proliferation is in evidence. Complete healing may be achieved, but in some cases the changes are progressive and end in hepatic insufficiency, or liver cell carcinoma may develop in the hyperplastic nodules. The healing or healed stage is often referred to as multiple nodular hyperplasia or toxic (postnecrotic) cirrhosis.

Focal and zonal necroses. Multiple small areas of necrosis are more frequent in the liver than are diffuse or massive areas of necrosis. Those that have a fairly constant relationship to some part of the liver lobules are referred to as zonal necroses.

Focal necrosis. Focal necroses, which have no special or constant site in the liver lobules, occur in a variety of severe infections, such as typhoid fever, pneumonia, diphtheria, and tularemia (Fig. 15-3).

Central necrosis. Central necrosis is the commonest type of zonal necrosis. It occurs with severe chronic passive congestion, particularly if there is added infection with streptococci. A variety of poisons, some of industrial importance, such as trinitrotoluene, carbon tetrachloride, and chloroform, produce central necrosis. *Chlorpromazine jaundice* occurs in 0.2 to 5% of patients receiving chlorpromazine. There are central degeneration of liver cells, central bile stasis, and local pigmentation. There is no necrosis, and bile is absent from large ducts, although capillary

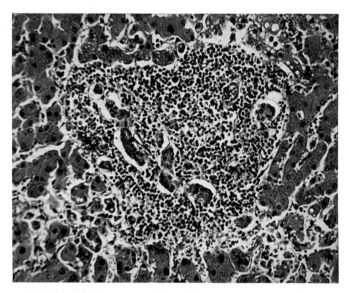

Fig. 15-3. Liver, showing focal necrosis in tularemia.

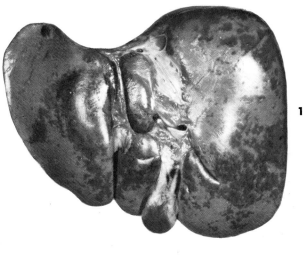

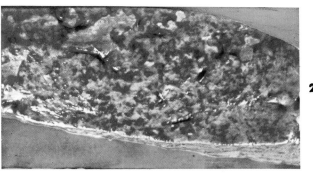

Plate 3. Liver in eclamptic toxemia of pregnancy. **1,** Posterior surface.
2, Cut surface, showing irregular areas of hemorrhage. (From Dieck-
mann, W. J.: The toxemias of pregnancy, St. Louis, 1941, The C. V.
Mosby Co.)

bile thrombi are present in the liver cell cords. Restoration occurs without serious scarring or cirrhosis.

Midzonal necrosis. Midzonal necrosis occurs in certain infective conditions and is particularly characteristic of yellow fever. In this latter condition there are rounded hyaline cytoplasmic masses (Councilman bodies) and also nuclear inclusion bodies in cells of the midzonal region.

Peripheral necrosis. Peripheral necrosis is often seen in phosphorus poisoning and in eclampsia, although in the latter condition the necroses are by no means constant in their position but are often focal in distribution and hemorrhagic in character.

Eclampsia. Eclampsia is a toxic complication of the later months of pregnancy (pp. 399 and 774), in which hypertension, albuminuria, edema, and convulsions are prominent features. The lesions in the liver are the most striking, but they cannot be correlated with the severity of the disease and are probably of less importance than the renal changes. Areas of confluent necrosis and associated hemorrhage may be patchily scattered through the liver substance, and irregular areas of hemorrhage beneath the capsule give the liver a grossly mottled appearance.

Viral hepatitis

Infectious hepatitis is a transient and often mild, icteric condition that occurs sporadically, in epidemic form, and also by inoculation of the infective agent with human blood or serum. There appears to be an asymptomatic carrier state in which the virus may be present in the blood. The sporadic cases often have been referred to as catarrhal jaundice, with the supposition that an inflammatory swelling of the common bile duct caused obstruction. However, there is an actual hepatitis and hepatic necrosis, and in fatal cases the liver lesions are those of acute yellow atrophy. The jaundice appears to be caused by an obstruction of the intralobular bile canaliculi. Associated lesions in fatal cases include cholemic nephrosis, regional lymph node and splenic enlargement caused by cellular proliferation and congestion, and hemorrhagic phenomena in various tissues resulting from disturbances of prothrombin and vitamin K caused by the destruction of liver. In some cases ascites, phlegmonous inflammation of the intestinal tract, and degenerative cerebral lesions may be found. In nonfatal cases there may be complete restoration of the hepatic tissue without significant scarring. This is

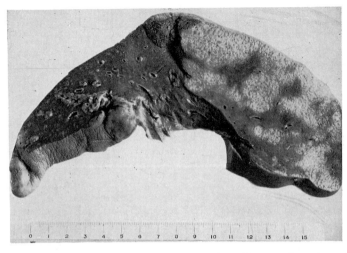

Fig. 15-4. Epidemic hepatitis, nineteenth day. Regenerating tissue is evident on the right. (From Lucké, B.: Amer. J. Path. **20**:471, 1944.)

because of the great regenerative ability of the hepatic cells when the injury is not continued and the hepatic framework and vessels are not destroyed.

The infective agent appears to be a peculiarly resistant filtrable virus. A susceptible experimental animal has not been found. The natural method of spread has not been established with certainty, but it may be by the intestinal route, with the agent waterborne. Hepatitis spread from an infected person by inoculation of serum or blood or by contaminated needles or syringes is termed *homologous serum jaundice*. The mortality in the pandemic of the World War II period was less than 0.4%, but there appears to have been some enhancement of virulence, and the recent mortality, particularly from inoculation hepatitis, seems to have been considerably greater.

Pathologic anatomy. Well-advanced lesions may be present at the time symptoms become manifest. There is degeneration and destruction of hepatic cells, with an associated inflammatory reaction. There may be destruction of scattered hepatic cells or actual focal areas of necrosis. Degeneration of hepatic cells may be a hyalinization similar to that seen in yellow fever. The inflammatory reaction may be perilobular or intralobular, with a

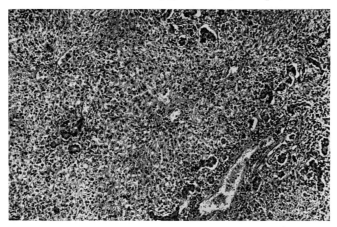

Fig. 15-5. Epidemic hepatitis. Microscopic appearance of the liver shown in Fig. 15-4. (Courtesy Dr. Balduin Lucké.)

predominance of mononuclear cells and some eosinophilic and neutrophilic leukocytes.

In fatal acute cases the liver is usually moderately reduced in size, is very soft in consistency, has a slightly wrinkled capsule, and is dark reddish brown in color. The cut surface may be mottled, purplish red, and congested, but without any distinct pattern. Microscopically there is massive destruction of hepatic cells, but there is preservation of the architectural framework, sinusoids, and bile ducts. Smaller bile ducts may show proliferative changes. Inflammatory cells may be most numerous about peripheral parts of the lobules. Mononuclear cells, lymphocytes, and plasma cells predominate, with fewer neutrophils and eosinophils.

In more prolonged or subacute fatal cases the liver is greatly reduced in size and weight, sometimes to half normal, and severely deformed. The surface is irregular with wrinkling and irregular, projecting coarse nodules. The cut surface has a variegated appearance. Dark red areas of destruction contrast with irregular nodular areas of pale or greenish color caused by regenerative hyperplasia of hepatic cells. The regenerative hyperplastic hepatic cells are often arranged in atypical fashion with poor lobular architecture.

The severity of the jaundice observed clinically does not correlate with the degree of hepatic destruction. The jaundice appears to be partly caused by the obstruction of small intralobular bile canaliculi, in which plugs of bile often may be evident.

While in most recovered cases there is complete restoration of the liver without significant scarring, there is evidence that prolonged, recurrent, or chronic hepatitis may occur and that cirrhosis may be an occasional sequela of hepatitis.

Cirrhosis of the liver

Cirrhosis refers to a fibrosis or scarring of the liver, which is progressive and is not simply the stationary healed end stage of an injury. It is a chronic disease, often accompanied by some degree of liver cell failure and portal hypertension. All parts (although not necessarily each lobule) of the liver are involved, with fibrosis. In some cases there are connective tissue bands disorganizing the lobular architecture and uniting centrolobular zones with portal tracts, accompanied by nodular parenchymal regeneration. Necrosis of hepatic cells is usually present at some stage of the disease.

There are several varieties of cirrhosis, differing in etiology, nature, form, and effects. Numerous classifications are extant, and even more numerous terminologies. Generally agreed to are the three morphologic varieties of portal (Laennec's) cirrhosis, postnecrotic cirrhosis, and biliary cirrhosis. Differentiated among the cases of portal cirrhosis are the fatty cirrhosis of malnutrition or alcoholism, and the pigmentary cirrhosis associated with hemochromatosis. Table 15-1 outlines some of the morphologic features that aid in differentiating some of the varieties. Usually distinctive are the forms of cardiac or congestive cirrhosis (the result of a passive congestion of long standing), parasitic cirrhosis (caused by schistosomiasis or clonorchiasis), and syphilitic cirrhosis. The type known as posthepatitic cirrhosis is characterized by fine scarring and fine, uniform nodularity and is believed to be the result of a smoldering form of inflammation, not necessarily viral. This is in contrast to the postnecrotic cirrhosis that results from massive necrosis, which is sometimes caused by viral hepatitis. Posthepatitic cirrhosis bears some resemblance to nutritional cirrhosis in its gross features.

The effects and complications of cirrhosis are mainly obstruction of the portal circulation, gastrointestinal hemorrhage, disturbance of liver function, and development of carcinoma of the liver. The incidence of primary carcinoma of the liver in cirrhosis is usually reported as 4 to 8%.

Portal cirrhosis. Portal cirrhosis (Laennec's cirrhosis, fatty nutritional cirrhosis, alcoholic cirrhosis, septal cirrhosis, hobnail liver) occurs at any age but most commonly in middle life, and it is more frequent in males. A history of chronic alcoholism is present in 50 to 80% or more of cases, but it also develops in total abstainers. Bouts of jaundice or other evidences of hepatitis occur in some cases. Major clinical signs are ascites, edema, jaundice, enlargement of the liver and spleen, telangiectasis, hematemesis, dermatitis, and disorientation. Ascites is the most constant and striking result. There is obstruction of the portal circulation, and collateral channels of venous return develop. Death may be sudden from the rupture of varices of the esophagus.

The causes of death in portal cirrhosis are mainly acute and chronic infections, hemorrhage from esophageal varices or gastric erosions, hepatic insufficiency, carcinoma of the liver, and cardiac failure. Death may occur from acute hepatic insufficiency in chronic alcoholics before a late stage of hepatic fibrosis and atrophy has developed.

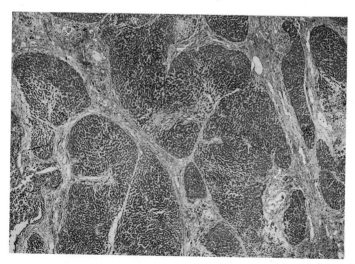

Fig. 15-6. Portal cirrhosis of the liver.

Gross appearance. The disease goes through stages in which both morphologic appearances and associated clinical effects are distinctive. The early stage is an enlarged liver with severe fatty change. In this period there may be few symptoms, but at any time an acute necrosis may develop with sudden hepatic insufficiency. With the progression and development of fibrosis, a fibrofatty stage follows, in which hepatic insufficiency and portal hypertension are clinical manifestations. In the final, late stage of fibrosis and atrophy, portal hypertension and its

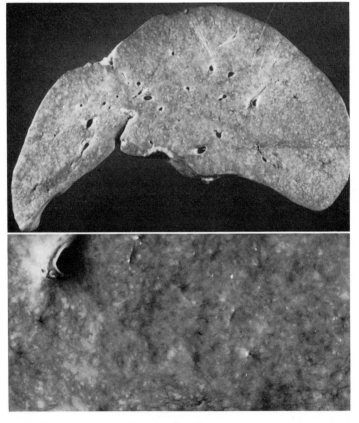

Fig. 15-7. Cirrhosis of the liver, fibrofatty stage.

complications may be dominant clinically. When seen in late stages the liver is atrophic and smaller than normal (hobnail liver). The general shape is normal, and the color is reddish brown, or is yellowish if there is associated fatty change. The whole outer surface is nodular because of rounded, projecting masses of liver cells, 2 to 5 mm. in diameter, separated by retracted grayish connective tissue. Consistency of the tissue is much increased. On the cut surface an interlacing network of gray translucent connective tissue separates prominent nodules of liver cells.

Microscopic appearance. Microscopically the normal architecture of the liver is completely upset by bands of connective tissue, which redivide the liver into irregular nodules having no constant relationship to central veins or portal regions. Most of the connective tissue is fairly young, only slightly hyalinized, and infiltrated by mononuclear chronic inflammatory cells, mainly lymphocytes and plasma cells. Bile canalicular and pericanalicular changes may be associated with cholestasis and jaundice. Small bile ducts are numerous and prominent in the connective tissue areas. In all stages of the process degenerative changes and necrosis may be evident in the liver cells; most

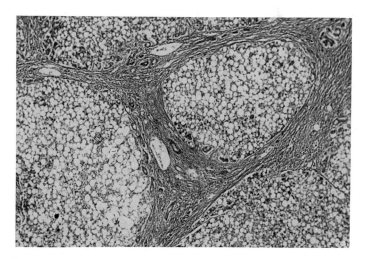

Fig. 15-8. Cirrhosis of the liver, microscopic appearance of fibrofatty stage.

characteristically there is a hyaline accumulation in their cytoplasm, as described by Mallory. The hyaline Mallory bodies are differentially stained by chromotrope aniline blue. Electron microscopic studies suggest that the Mallory bodies are related to mitochondrial changes of clumping, enlargement, and bizarre forms. In early stages fatty change is a prominent feature, preceding or associated with the development of fibrosis. Fatty cysts tend to persist in the fibrous trabeculae even in late stages. Regenerative nodules of liver cells form the bulk of the tissue in advanced cirrhosis and contribute to the distortion of architecture and vascular relationships and to the development of portal hypertension.

Etiology. The etiology is still unsettled and much debated. Cirrhosis has been produced experimentally in animals by repeated doses of certain poisons, such as carbon tetrachloride, tars, and combinations of phosphorus and alcohol, manganese chloride and phenylhydrazine, and chloroform with infection. Mallory also found that lead would induce cirrhosis. Alcohol alone has quite regularly failed to produce cirrhosis in experimental animals, although it has done so when combined with a high fat diet in a prolonged experiment. Dietary deficiency also has resulted in cirrhosis. Nutritional cirrhosis in experimental animals has been produced in rats by a diet low in casein, but is preventable when methionine or cystine plus choline is added to the diet. The cirrhosis is similar to portal cirrhosis of man except for the presence of a golden brown fluorescent pigment, ceroid. Ceroid is believed to be of lipoidal nature and is developed from liver cells containing fat during the development of cirrhosis.

Clinical experience indicates that alcoholism is a factor in many cases of cirrhosis, although the relationship is not necessarily a direct one. It appears that it is dietary insufficiency in combination with alcoholism that results in the liver damage, although there may be a direct metabolic effect of alcohol. The fatty liver so characteristic of chronic alcoholism proceeds gradually to the development of portal cirrhosis if the individual survives and the insults to the liver continue. Obstruction of lymphatics and sinusoidal blood vessels in the liver by cells swollen from fat or injury may be part of the pathogenetic mechanism. Alcoholism and malnutrition may be associated with a florid type of cirrhosis or chronic toxic hepatitis, which is characterized by severe hepatocellular damage and inflammation and which rapidly progresses from a fatty liver to cirrhosis.

No doubt other types of recurrent or continuing hepatic injury can proceed to cirrhosis as the terminal stage. In some cases the acute exacerbations of hepatitis are clinically evident. The possible role of methionine or cystine and choline deficiency in the production of cirrhosis in man has not yet been made clear by sufficient investigation.

Effects. The effects of portal cirrhosis in disturbing the portal circulation are usually more prominent than failure of liver function. Ascites is an outstanding feature and is partly the result of congestion and increased pressure in the portal veins, causing extravasation of fluid along the peritoneal serosa, but reduction of plasma proteins is an important factor contributing to the accumulation of fluid. Additional causative factors are considered to be renal retention of sodium and water (resulting from hyperaldosteronemia and increased secretion of antidiuretic hormone) and increased production of hepatic lymph because of intrahepatic congestion with exudation of lymph through Glisson's capsule. Perfusion experiments have indicated that in some cases portal hypertension may be contributed to by an increased hepatic arterial inflow transmitted to the portal side by abnormal arterioportal anastomoses.

The gradually developing obstruction in the portal circulation permits the development of a collateral venous circulation. The cutaneous vessels over the abdomen and back become dis-

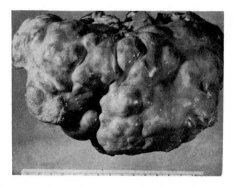

Fig. 15-9. Coarse nodular cirrhosis of the liver. (From Anderson, W. A. D., editor: Pathology, St. Louis, 1957, The C. V. Mosby Co.)

tended and prominent. Varices of esophageal veins commonly develop, and the anastomoses with these from the portal circulation are composed of vessels from the coronary veins and from the left gastroepiploic veins and vasa brevia. In the lower third of the esophagus the rich anastomoses of submucosal veins are poorly supported by connective tissue. Hence, this is a frequent site for varices and venous rupture. Severe hemorrhage complicating cirrhosis also may be from erosive gastritis or peptic ulcers. Varices of hemorrhoidal veins are much less common in association with cirrhosis.

Testicular atrophy is a common accompaniment of cirrhosis, particularly in patients under 50 years of age. The extensively damaged liver apparently fails to inactivate estrogens, particularly in the absence of sufficient intake of the vitamin B complex. A similar explanation is possible for the occasional occurrence of gynecomastia, palmar erythema, and arterial spider nevi of the skin.

The spleen is enlarged and congested in cases of portal cirrhosis as a result of the obstruction to the portal circulation. *Banti's syndrome* (p. 540) frequently includes portal cirrhosis.

Postnecrotic cirrhosis. Postnecrotic cirrhosis (coarse nodular cirrhosis, toxic cirrhosis) is characterized by irregular involvement of the liver, often with areas of preserved architecture. There may be broad bands of fibrous tissue that follow collapse of the parenchyma. The nodules represent persisting parenchyma. It may result from a variety of causes, which produce a massive necrosis of hepatic tissue, insufficient to cause death but too great to allow structural recovery. The causes include viral hepatitis and hepatotoxic chemicals and drugs. It may follow directly an acute hepatitis or appear after months or years.

The liver is smaller than normal and is characterized by large nodules (1 cm. or more in diameter) irregularly distributed in the liver. Thick dense grayish septa of fibrous tissue, of varying width, separate the nodules. The nodules are composed of groups of hepatic cells, in which the arrangement may vary from normal to great distortion. Bizarre liver cells may be seen, but fatty change is not usually present.

In *Wilson's disease* (hepatolenticular degeneration) cirrhosis is associated with degenerative changes in basal ganglia of the brain. It appears to be an inherited disturbance of copper metabolism. There is a defective synthesis of serum ceruloplasmin, a low serum copper, but an increase of albumin-bound copper in

Table 15-1. *Differential diagnosis of cirrhosis**

Diagnostic features	Post-necrotic	Nutritional	Post-hepatitic
Macroscopic			
Size	Normal or reduced	Enlarged	Normal or reduced
Color	Gray-brown	Yellow	Reddish brown
Texture	Tough ++	Tough ++ Greasy	Tough ++
Scarring			
Type	Coarse	Fine	Trabecular
Distribution	Irregular	Uniform	Uniform
Breadth	0.1-5.0 cm.	0.01-0.1 cm.	0.1-0.3 cm.
Nodule			
Size	Fleck-7 cm.	0.2-0.3 cm.	0.5-1.5 cm.
Uniformity	Irregular	Uniform	Uniform
Microscopic			
Intact lobule	±	0	+++
Pseudolobulation	++	+++	±
Fat	±	+++	±
Pseudoductule	+++	+	+
Hemosiderin	±	+	0
Bile stasis	+	+	0
Central veins	+	0	+++

*From Gall, E. A.: Amer. J. Path. **36**:244, 1960.

the serum. Increased accumulation of copper is found in the liver, brain, kidneys, cornea, and other tissues. Clinical symptoms usually arise during adolescence. Symptoms and lesions either of hepatic cirrhosis or of the nervous system may be predominant. Kayser-Fleischer corneal rings, a pigmentation of Descemet's membrane, is characteristic. The cirrhosis is usually the coarse nodular type.

Biliary cirrhosis. Much less common than the portal type, biliary cirrhosis is caused by an obstruction in some part of the bile duct system. There may or may not be an associated infection (cholangitis). The obstruction may be intrahepatic or the result of stricture, gallstone, or pancreatic carcinoma interfering with the common bile duct. The liver is a deep green color (bile stained) and is usually increased in size and weight. Its surface is smooth or only finely granular, and during the early phase the lobular pattern is preserved. The portal areas are

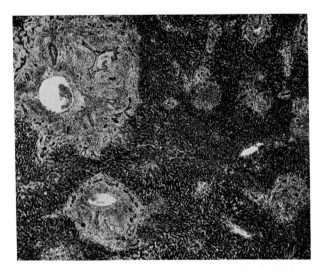

Fig. 15-10. Biliary cirrhosis of the liver. (From Edmondson, H. A., and Anderson, W. A. D.: Liver. In Anderson, W. A. D., editor: Pathology, ed. 5, St. Louis, 1966, The C. V. Mosby Co.)

lengthened, widened, and appear prominent. Hepatic cell degeneration is associated with bile stasis. Intrahepatic bile ducts are dilated and often contain neutrophilic leukocytes. Inspissated masses of bile distend the bile canaliculi, and there is increased connective tissue in portal areas and around the periphery of the lobules. Chronic inflammatory cells, mainly lymphocytes and plasma cells, infiltrate this fibrous tissue.

Cholangitic or cholangiolitic biliary cirrhosis is associated with viral hepatitis. There is a prominent inflammatory exudate in portal areas, with active proliferation of cholangioles. Xanthomatous (pericholangiolitic) biliary cirrhosis is characterized by chronic inflammation about the smallest bile ducts in portal areas, with duct blockage and intralobular bile stasis. Observed mainly in females, it is associated with high cholesterol and lecithin values of the serum and xanthomas of the skin.

Pigment cirrhosis. The liver changes in hemochromatosis may be referred to as pigment cirrhosis. The gross and microscopic features of the liver are those of a mild portal cirrhosis with the addition of large amounts of hemosiderin pigment

(p. 50). Marked pigmentation of the liver (hemosiderosis) with cirrhosis is common in natives of some areas of South Africa.

Syphilitic cirrhosis. The liver is commonly involved in congenital syphilis, and many spirochetes may be demonstrable in that organ. In some cases there is a diffuse fibrosis within the lobules. In acquired syphilis the liver is not so regularly affected, but gummas may occur, which heal by fibrous scars and leave a severe distortion of the organ (hepar lobatum).

Cardiac or congestive cirrhosis. Long-continued chronic passive congestion of the liver leads to atrophy of liver cells around the central vein areas, with a relative increase in the connective tissue. There may also be a diffuse fibrosis and alteration of architecture. It is most commonly associated with constrictive pericarditis and rheumatic heart disease.

Parasitic cirrhosis. As a result of the lodgement of ova in the liver, cirrhosis may be produced by infection with *Schistosoma mansoni* and less frequently with *S. japonicum* and *S. haematobium*. Dense whitish zones of fibrosis develop about intra-

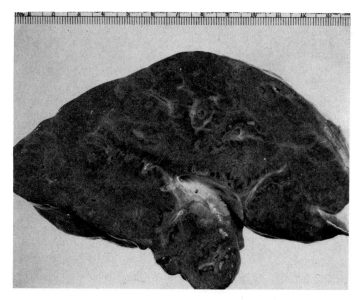

Fig. 15-11. Cirrhosis of the liver caused by *Schistosoma mansoni* infection.

hepatic portal branches. The external surface may be nodular and similar in gross appearance to Laennec's cirrhosis. Small fibrous nodules, 1 or 2 mm. in diameter, may be scattered through the liver. Microscopically the ova or remains of their shells may be found in the fibrous areas. Brownish pigment granules are held in Kupffer's cells. Splenomegaly, ascites, and esophageal varices develop in late stages (p. 231).

The liver fluke, *Clonorchis sinensis,* may produce a biliary type of cirrhosis caused by lodgment in biliary channels. There is fibrous thickening with dilatation of bile ducts, and fibrosis and cellular infiltration develop in the portal spaces. Flukes or their remnants may be found in involved areas. Severe visceral leishmaniasis (kala-azar) also may be complicated by cirrhosis.

Weil's disease

Weil's disease, or spirochetal jaundice, is caused by infection with *Leptospira icterohaemorrhagiae* and affects particularly the kidneys, liver, capillaries, and skeletal muscles (p. 197). The liver is usually enlarged and bile stained. Microscopically one sees degeneration and inflammation of liver structure. Areas of necrosis may be slight and focal, or they may be so extensive as to simulate acute yellow atrophy. Biliary stasis is evident in the central part of the lobules. There may be some evidence of regeneration of hepatic cells.

Granulomatous hepatitis

Granulomatous lesions in the liver may be produced by numerous infections, by hypersensitivity, and by various generalized granulomatous diseases. Among the more frequent are tuberculosis, sarcoidosis, and fungal infections.

Abscesses

Abscesses of the liver may be (1) pyogenic, (2) amebic, or (3) actinomycotic.

Pyogenic abscesses. Pyogenic abscesses may result from (1) spread of organisms to the liver by way of the portal vein (pylephlebitis) from the appendix, rectum, or other parts of the bowel; (2) extension of organisms to the liver by way of the bile ducts (cholangitis) from the gallbladder; (3) spread to the liver from contiguous infected tissue, e.g., a subphrenic abscess; (4) infection carried to the liver by hepatic arteries in septicemia; and (5) penetrating traumatic injuries. The bac-

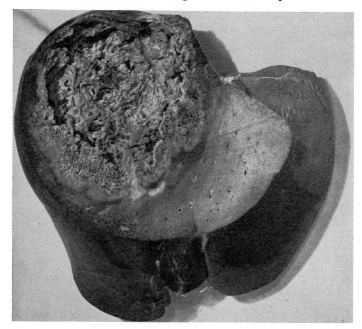

Fig. 15-12. Amebic abscess of the liver.

teria most commonly found are *Escherichia coli,* staphylococci, and streptococci.

Pylephlebitis with multiple liver abscesses most frequently is an extension from an acute suppurative appendicitis. The abscesses are more abundant in the right lobe. The areas of necrosis vary from microscopic size to a diameter of several centimeters and by coalescence can form large cavities. Necrosis, cellular disintegration, and leukocyte accumulation are found in the areas of abscess. Occasionally there is the complication of rupture or spread of the infection to adjacent tissues. *Pyogenic hepatic abscesses* resulting from the spread of organisms to the liver by the hepatic arteries are usually only a part of a general septicemia, and abscesses are present in other organs as well.

Amebic abscesses. The amebic abscess (tropical abscess) is caused by the spread of *Entamoeba histolytica* from intestinal lesions by way of the portal vein. The lesion begins in the portal areas, with lysis of tissue and only a little accompanying inflammatory reaction. As noted previously, although the lytic lesion is called an abscess, it is not a true abscess. Adjacent abscesses coalesce to produce lesions of considerable size. The larger abscesses tend to become walled off by connective tissue (p. 219).

Actinomycotic abscesses. Actinomycotic abscesses of the liver are the result of spread from intestinal lesions by way of the portal blood. Multiple small ragged abscess cavities in which the actinomycotic colonies can be found are produced (p. 204).

Cysts

Cysts in the liver are commonly of the following types: (1) hydatid (echinococcus) cysts, (2) cystic distentions of ducts (hydrohepatosis), and (3) congenital cysts.

Hydatid cysts. Hydatid cysts are caused by the lodging in the liver of the larval form of the dog tapeworm *Echinococcus granulosus* (p. 233). The liver is a commonly involved organ. The cyst wall is composed of concentric hyaline laminae, lined by germinal cells from which grow "daughter" cysts. Scolices and hooklets of the worm may be identified in the cyst wall or its contents by microscopic examination. Old cysts, in which the parasites are dead, contain a yellowish gray, puttylike material. Alveolar hydatid disease is caused by *E. multilocularis* (p. 235).

Cystic distention of bile ducts. Cystic distention of the bile ducts, known as hydrohepatosis, is the result of obstruction to bile passages, particularly if such obstruction is intermittent, incomplete, or slow in development.

Congenital cysts. Congenital cysts are uncommon but are sometimes found associated with a congenital cystic condition of the kidneys. They are usually small and cause no disturbance.

Tumors

Hemangioma. The commonest tumor of the liver is a cavernous hemangioma similar to those occurring elsewhere. At autopsy it is often encountered as an incidental finding. It grows very slowly or remains stationary in size.

Adenoma. Benign hepatoma is relatively infrequent. It is a circumscribed mass of well-formed liver cells that grows expansively, compressing the surrounding liver substance. Bile duct adenoma also occurs and tends to be cystic.

Hamartoma. Hamartoma of the liver is a benign tumorlike malformation of a portion of the liver. It consists of both proliferating hepatic cells and bile ducts (mixed adenoma of the

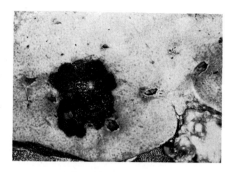

Fig. 15-13. Hemangioma of the liver.

liver). Most cases occur in infants and children. The lesions are frequently multiple and cystic.

Carcinoma. The liver is a very common site for metastatic tumors, whereas *primary carcinoma* is less frequent in the United States. In the Orient and Africa primary carcinoma of the liver is much more common. It is a frequent malignant tumor among Japanese males and is very common among Negro males in some parts of Africa. The high incidence in certain regions appears to result from environmental rather than racial reasons and is associated particularly with nutritional disturbance and cirrhosis or with prevalence of *Clonorchis sinensis* infestation. Cancer of the liver occurs at all ages, even in young infants, but the highest incidence is between 50 and 60 years. A considerable proportion (more than 50% in some series of cases) are associated with cirrhosis in a chronic or late stage. Postnecrotic cirrhosis appears to have a particularly high incidence of liver cell carcinoma as a late complication. Pigment cirrhosis also is a significant precursor. The incidence of carcinoma is much higher in males than in females.

There are three gross forms: (1) nodular, in which various circumscribed tumor nodules are present throughout the liver; (2) massive, in which a single large tumor occupies one of the lobes; and (3) diffuse, in which the tumor cells are found extensively invading every part of the liver.

Histologically there are two types, hepatocarcinoma (liver cell carcinoma) and cholangiocarcinoma (bile duct carcinoma), but some highly undifferentiated tumors are difficult to classify. *Hepatocarcinoma* (hepatocellular carcinoma) is more frequent

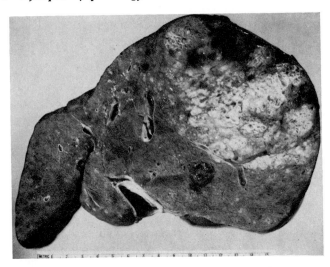

Fig. 15-14. Primary carcinoma of the liver (liver cell type).

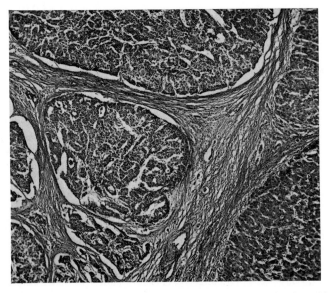

Fig. 15-15. Hepatocarcinoma associated with cirrhosis of the liver. Non-cancerous liver tissue is shown at the lower right.

and is composed of cells arranged in columns resembling normal liver cords. These cells are often hyperchromatic and multinucleated, or they are of giant size. Atypical lobules may be formed, and there is often some bile in or near the tumor cells. A delicate network of capillaries is found in the stroma. *Cholangiocarcinoma* is a glandular carcinoma arising from bile ducts. The columnar or cuboidal cells may be in solid clusters or attempt to form tubules. The connective tissue stroma is dense and shows only a few capillaries. Cholangiocarcinoma has a more rapid course than hepatocarcinoma. Combined liver cell and bile duct carcinomas also occur.

Intrahepatic spread is more common, but extrahepatic metastases are not unusual, particularly in regional lymph nodes and lungs. The symptoms are variable, multiple, and often ap-

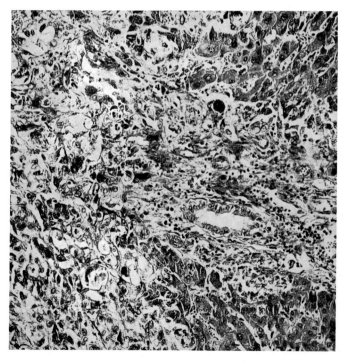

Fig. 15-16. Cholangiocarcinoma of the liver.

pear unrelated, so that antemortem diagnosis is rarely accomplished.

Primary carcinomas of the liver in infancy and childhood (hepatoblastomas) are among the most frequent cancers of this age group. They are of the liver cell type, although the cells tend to be smaller, more anaplastic, and more embryonal in appearance than in adults. The condition is to be distinguished from the giant cell transformation of the neonatal liver, which appears to be the response of an immature liver to various injuries or disease processes.

Hemangioendothelial sarcoma (Kupffer cell sarcoma) is a rare tumor of the liver of adult man. It occurs as multiple hemorrhagic nodules, which are composed of blood-filled spaces lined by cells resembling Kupffer cells, or as solid masses of similar cells.

GALLBLADDER

The gallbladder is a thin-walled sac, in which bile is concentrated by active mucosal absorption of water. The function of the gallbladder is as a reservior for bile. The chief lesions are inflammation, stone formation, and carcinoma. Inflammation (cholecystitis) interferes with reabsorptive concentrating activity of the organ. Gallstones (cholelithiasis) result from the precipitation of constituents of bile. They may produce obstruction in the gallbladder, cystic duct, or common duct. Carcinoma is the only common type of tumor of the gallbladder.

Jaundice

Jaundice, or icterus, is the condition of hyperbilirubinemia and deposition of bile pigment in the tissues. Bile pigment is formed from the breakdown of hemoglobin by reticuloendothelial cells, particularly in the spleen, liver, bone marrow, etc. Prehepatic bilirubin so formed has a protein linkage and gives an indirect van den Bergh reaction. The polygonal cells of the liver divest the indirect-reacting bilirubin of its protein, conjugate the bilirubin, and pass the pigment into the bile canaliculi. This form of bilirubin gives an immediate direct reaction with van den Bergh's reagent and is readily soluble in water and so may be excreted in the urine. Bilirubin excreted with the bile is changed within the bowel to urobilinogen and then to the brown pigment of the stool, urobilin. Urobilinogen may be reabsorbed from the bowel and reexcreted by the liver and kidney.

Table 15-2. *Differences between the types of jaundice*

	Retention jaundice	*Regurgitation jaundice*
Van den Bergh reaction	Indirect	Direct
Stool	Increased urobilinogen and urobilin	Decreased or absent bilirubin, hence decreased urobilinogen and urobilin
Urine	Increased urobilinogen and urobilin No bilirubin or bile salts	No urobilinogen or urobilin Bilirubin and bile salts present

Jaundice may be classified (Table 15-2) into two main types: retention jaundice and regurgitation jaundice. In retention jaundice the liver cells are unable to remove all the pigment from the bloodstream. The increased bilirubin thus is indirect reacting and is not excreted by the kidneys (acholuric jaundice). The amounts of urobilinogen and urobilin in the stool and urine are usually increased. In regurgitation jaundice there is leakage back into the bloodstream of bilirubin that has been acted upon by liver cells. The van den Bergh reaction is usually direct, and bilirubin is present in the urine. The color of the stool will depend on the amount of bilirubin reaching the intestinal tract. The causes of jaundice may be classified as follows:

Retention jaundice, caused by
  Anoxemia, resulting from
    Anemia
      Hemolytic anemias—familial or acquired hemolytic jaundice, sickle cell and pernicious anemia, erythroblastosis fetalis
      Hemoglobinemias—mismatched transfusions, paroxysmal hemoglobinuria
      Certain hemolytic drugs
     Chronic passive congestion
    Febrile disease, associated with anoxemia, resulting from
      Anemia—hemolytic septicemias, malaria, and blackwater fever
      Pulmonary consolidation—pneumonia
    Immaturity of liver cells in newborn—icterus neonatorum
    Constitutional hepatic dysfunction
Regurgitation jaundice, caused by
  Necrosis of liver cells, resulting from
    Severe grades of hepatic cell anoxemia

Toxic agents
  Poisons—chloroform, phosphorus, mushroom poisoning, etc.
  Organisms—viral hepatitis, yellow fever, Weil's disease, congenital syphilis, etc.
  Undetermined—"idiopathic" acute yellow atrophy
Obstruction of biliary tree, resulting from
  Plugging—calculi, parasites, neoplasms, etc.
  Stricture—congenital scarring, neoplasms, etc.
  External pressure—inflammatory, neoplastic, or parasitic masses
Chronic idiopathic jaundice (Dubin-Johnson syndrome)

The effects of jaundice other than pigmentation of tissues may be slight in the pure retention type. In regurgitation jaundice they are probably largely the result of retention of bile salts and their absence from the intestinal tract. Such effects include pruritus and the interference with absorption of fats and fat-soluble vitamins (including vitamin K). The latter may give rise to a bleeding tendency caused by prothrombin deficiency. Other effects are on the central nervous system and kidney (cholemic nephrosis).

Cholecystitis

Inflammation of the gallbladder may be acute or chronic. Chemical damage to the gallbladder wall because of the action of concentrated bile, promoted by an obstruction of the cystic duct, usually by a stone, is probably the commonest cause of cholecystitis. In some cases, bacterial infection supervenes. The presence of stones within the gallbladder also may promote an inflammatory process. In nonobstructive or noncalculus cholecystitis, primary bacterial infection may be responsible, usually caused by streptococci, colon bacilli, and staphylococci. Infection may reach the gallbladder wall from the bloodstream, by direct spread from adjacent organs, from the liver, from the intestine through lymphatics, or by ascending bile ducts from the duodenum.

Acute cholecystitis. In acute cholecystitis the gallbladder is enlarged, gray or reddish in color, and has a thick edematous wall. The mucosa shows areas of necrosis and ulceration, and leukocytes are present in the wall. Purulent exudate may fill the cavity (empyema of the gallbladder). Calculi are often associated with the inflammation and may obstruct the neck of the gallbladder, or they may erode through the softened and necrotic wall.

Chronic cholecystitis. Chronic cholecystitis may be catarrhal, with merely slight thickening, lymphocyte infiltration, and congestion of mucosal folds. In other cases the changes are greater, with areas of destruction of the mucosa, fibrous thickening of the wall, and a more diffuse infiltration of lymphocytes. Gallstones or duct obstruction often complicates a chronic cholecystitis.

Cholecystitis glandularis. Cholecystitis glandularis is a term sometimes applied when there are epithelium-lined sinuses in the wall of the gallbadder. Epithelium-lined spaces seen in the wall of the gallbladder may be of three types. The commonest type is formed by outpouchings of the mucosa or sinuses, which

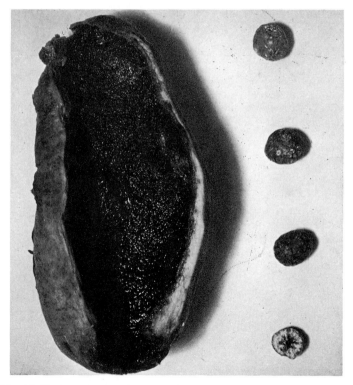

Fig. 15-17. Chronic cholecystitis and cholelithiasis. Note the thickness of the wall of the gallbladder. The lowest stone is cut to show its radiating structure.

communicate with the lumen of the gallbladder (Aschoff-Rokitansky sinuses). They may become dilated to form diverticula or cysts, and sometimes calculi are formed within them. The lining epithelium is similar to that of the mucosa of the gallbladder or bowel. A second type of epithelium-lined space in the gallbladder is formed by aberrant bile ducts, which communicate with intrahepatic ducts but not with the gallbladder (Luschka ducts). Their lining epithelium is similar to that of intrahepatic bile ducts. The third type is composed of subperitoneal gland-like spaces lined by flattened or cuboidal cells, which are apparently of mesothelial origin.

Cholesterolosis

In cholesterolosis (strawberry gallbladder) multiple, tiny, yellowish deposits of cholesterol are present in mucosal folds. These yellow areas on the reddish background of a congested mucosa suggest the appearance of a ripe strawberry. There is usually an associated increase of cholesterol in bile and blood. Cholesterolosis is often of little significance, but it may be associated with chronic inflammation in the gallbladder wall. Pedunculated mucosal folds containing cholesterol sometimes are pinched off and form the nuclei of stones.

Cholelithiasis

Important factors in the formation of gallstones are disturbances of cholesterol metabolism, infection, and stasis. The incidence increases with age, is greater in women than in men, and is greater in the white race than in Negroes. They may be in any part of the biliary tract, but they are commonest in the gallbladder.

Types of gallstones. Three normal constituents of bile, cholesterol, calcium bilirubinate, and calcium carbonate, are the main substances composing gallstones. *Pure gallstones,* which constitute about 10%, are composed almost entirely of one of these substances. *Mixed gallstones,* which are the most frequent type and account for about 80%, contain a mixture of the three substances in varying proportions. *Combined gallstones* are those in which one type of gallstone forms a nucleus, and another type forms the outer shell (Table 15-3).

Pure gallstones form when the bile contains an excess of the stone-forming substance, which is usually caused by disturbances of metabolism or of liver function rather than by a local inflam-

Table 15.3. *Classification of gallstones**

Type	Composition	Appearance	Factors in origin	Changes in gallbladder
Pure gall-stones, 10%	Cholesterol (crystalline)	Solitary, crystalline surface	Hypercholesterolemia	Cholesterolosis
	Calcium bilirubinate	Multiple, jet black, crystalline or amorphous	Hyperbilirubinemia	No change
	Calcium carbonate	Gray-white, amorphous	Unknown	No change
Mixed gall-stones, 80%	Cholesterol and calcium bilirubinate	Multiple, faceted, or lobulated, laminated and crystalline on cut surfaces: hue depends on content: cholesterol—yellow, calcium bilirubinate—black, calcium carbonate—white	Chronic cholecystitis plus increased content in bile of cholesterol, calcium bilirubinate, or calcium carbonate	Chronic cholecystitis
	Cholesterol and calcium carbonate			
	Calcium bilirubinate and calcium carbonate			
	Cholesterol, calcium bilirubinate, and calcium carbonate			
Combined gall-stones, 10%	Pure gallstone nucleus with mixed gallstone shell	Largest of gallstones, when single; hue depends on composition of shell	As in pure gallstones, followed by chronic cholecystitis	Chronic cholecystitis
	Mixed gallstone nuclei with pure gallstone shells		As in mixed gallstones, followed by increased content in bile of cholesterol, calcium bilirubinate, or calcium carbonate	Chronic cholecystitis

*From Halpert, B.: Gallbladder and biliary ducts. In Anderson, W. A. D., editor: Pathology, ed. 5, St. Louis, 1966, The C. V. Mosby Co.

matory reaction. Cholesterol stones are the most frequent, and calcium bilirubinate (pigment) stones are second in frequency. Calcium carbonate stones are the rarest of the pure gallstones.

The *cholesterol stone* is usually single. It is a crystalline calculus, light in weight, and soft and has a radiate structure evident on its cut surface. It occurs in the absence of infection and is probably of metabolic origin. The gallbladder may show cholesterolosis. The formation of a cholesterol stone appears to be influenced by hypercholesterolemia, dietary disturbances, diabetes, pregnancy, etc. Low bile salt concentration in gallbladder bile decreases the ability of cholesterol to remain in solution and thus favors precipitation. Inflammation of the gallbladder may influence this by causing abnormal absorption of bile salts. Disturbances in absorptive and secretory functions of the gallbladder, promoted by neurogenic and hormonal factors, have been thought to favor calculus formation. The solitary large cholesterol stone may give rise to few or no symptoms and is usually too large to enter and obstruct ducts. It is nonopaque to roentgen rays.

Calcium bilirubinate (pigment) stones are multiple, small, dark brown or black, hard, and brittle. Formed by precipitation of bile pigment in an uninfected gallbladder, they are associated with conditions having increased bilirubin concentration of the bile, such as hemolytic jaundice or pernicious anema. Stasis favors their formation.

Calcium carbonate stones are rare, soft, white stones, usually formed only when there is complete obstruction of the cystic duct. Stasis may be a factor in deposition of bile pigment and calcium. The more complete the obstruction the greater the proportion of calcium, which is deposited from the gallbladder wall.

Mixed gallstones are the commonest variety (accounting for about 80%). They are composed of varying mixtures of cholesterol, calcium bilirubinate, calcium carbonate, and some organic material. They form in gallbladders in which function is altered, so that the solvents, bile acids, are resorbed faster than the stone-forming substances they hold in solution. The exact mechanism of their formation is uncertain. Chronic cholecystitis is usually associated, although how much this may be the cause or the effect often cannot be determined. The association with cholecystitis has led to the term *infective stones* for this type, although association with a specific bacterial infection is not usually evident. Mixed stones are usually multiple and some-times are present in huge numbers. They vary from 0.1 to 2 cm. in diameter, are often hard, rough-surfaced stones, and are of varying color and structure according to their composition. Adjacent surfaces may be faceted. They often seem to be composed of concentric laminae laid down over a small nucleus. Some have a lobulated surface with the contour of a mulberry. The mulberry stones appear to form around polypoid projections of the mucosa that contain lipoidal material, and when small, may remain attached to the mucosa.

Combined gallstones constitute about 10% of gallstones. They occur most often as a solitary stone with a cholesterol nucleus and an outer shell similar to a mixed gallstone. Less often the nucleus is a mixed stone, and the outer shell is of cholesterol or calcium bilirubinate. The gallbladder containing combined gall-stones usually shows chronic cholecystitis.

Effects of gallstones. Biliary calculi do not of themselves produce symptoms, but they may produce injury in three ways: (1) their presence causes continuation of a chronic inflammatory process; (2) the chronic irritation of calculi may be a factor in the development of carcinoma of the gallbladder; and (3) stones may cause obstruction at the neck of the gallbladder or in the bile ducts.

The effects of obstruction of bile passages depend on the site and completeness of the obstruction. Large stones such as the solitary cholesterol calculus are often too large to get into bile ducts, although they may obstruct the neck of the gallbladder. Passage of a small calculus, distending biliary ducts, elicits the severe pain of biliary colic.

Complete obstruction of the neck of the gallbladder or cystic duct leads to hydrops or mucocele of the gallbladder, in which condition the pigmented bile has been absorbed and replaced by a mucoid secretion from the lining of the gallbladder. In some instances, empyema of the gallbladder may develop. Obstruction by a stone in the common duct results in only a little distention of the gallbladder if the wall has been thickened by inflammation, although bile passages themselves are usually visibly dilated above the obstruction. *Courvoisier's law* states that obstruction of the common bile duct by pressure from the outside, as by a carcinoma of the pancreas, produces a distended gallbladder, whereas obstruction by a stone produces little or no distention of the gallbladder. The usual explanation is that in

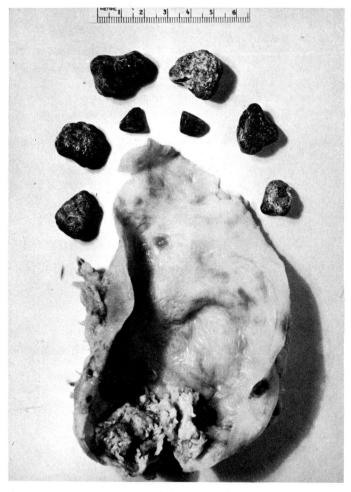

Fig. 15-18. Carcinoma of the gallbladder. Papillary adenocarcinoma of the fundus and cholelithiasis.

the latter instance the gallbladder wall is thickened and contracted as a result of inflammation.

If biliary obstruction is present for a considerable time, the bilirubin excretory function of the liver may become suppressed, and a watery or mucoid fluid, the so-called "white bile," is found in bile ducts. Other complications include ascending cholangitis and biliary cirrhosis of the liver.

The pancreas may be affected when a stone is impacted in an ampulla of Vater, which acts as a common opening of pancreatic and bile ducts. In such a case, reflux of irritating bile into the pancreatic duct may give rise to acute pancreatitis (p. 523).

In rare cases, perforation of a gallbladder into a viscus may release a gallstone, which produces intestinal obstruction. Inflammatory reaction and adhesions after perforation of the gallbladder also may result in obstruction of the bowel.

Carcinoma

The only important tumor of the gallbladder is carcinoma. About 75% of cases occur in women, commonly between 50 and 70 years of age. About 75% of carcinomas of the gallbladder are associated with calculi, which are often thought to have some causative role, probably by mechanical irritation. Among patients in whom gallstones are present at necropsy, about 3% have a carcinoma of the gallbladder. Papillomas and adenomas of the gallbladder occur, but it is uncertain how frequently these precede development of carcinoma. Many so-called papillomas appear to be nonneoplastic cholesterol polyps, and most lesions appearing as polyps by cholecystography are not true adenomas.

Cancer of the gallbladder is an adenocarcinoma in more than 90% of cases but occasionally is of squamous or mixed cell type. Adenocarcinoma may be subdivided into (1) an infiltrating scirrhous type, (2) a papillary type, and (3) a mucous type. The *infiltrating scirrhous type* is most common (65%). It forms a firm tumor, which spreads widely through the gallbladder wall, causing it to be greatly thickened. The lumen is narrowed and eventually obliterated. Microscopically it is an infiltrating adenocarcinoma, often with abundant dense fibrous stroma. The *papillary adenocarcinoma* (22%) forms a friable fungating tumor, which grows into the lumen of the gallbladder. Microscopically it presents stalks of connective tissue stroma covered by atypical columnar epithelium and infiltrated by glandular acini. The papillary type is less malignant and slower in its growth and spread than is the infiltrating adenocarcinomatous variety. The *mucoid adenocarcinoma* (7%) forms a bulky gelatinous mass, in which the tumor cells are distended with mucoid material and may have a signet-ring form. *Squamous cell carcinoma* (4%) of the gallbladder is a variety assumed to arise on the basis of metaplasia of the epithelial lining.

Spread of cancer of the gallbladder is by direct extension to the liver and metastasis to regional lymph nodes. Further spread may occur by lymphatic and bloodstream metastasis, but widespread extension is not the usual occurrence.

PANCREAS
Heterotopia and malformations

Heterotopic pancreatic tissue is found in about 14% of autopsies. Such misplaced tissue occurs in the duodenum (80%), stomach, jejunum, or Meckel's diverticulum. It is most commonly asymptomatic, but it may give rise to digestive disturbance

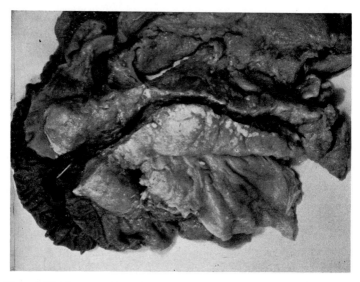

Fig. 15-19. Fat necrosis and acute pancreatitis. The white opaque areas represent fat necrosis. A small white rod is in the duct opening into the duodenum.

or be the site of tumor growth. *Annular pancreas* is a rare maldevelopment in which a band of pancreatic tissue encircles and may narrow or obstruct the second part of the duodenum. The pancreatic tissue often intermingles with the muscularis of the duodenum, so that simple resection or division of the ring of pancreatic tissue may be insufficient.

Fatty infiltration

Fatty infiltration of the pancreas is quite common in obesity and may be of severe degree (lipomatous pseudohypertrophy). A minor amount of fatty replacement of atrophic pancreatic tissue is common.

Acute pancreatitis

Acute pancreatitis is characterized by edema, necrosis, hemorrhage, and suppuration in varying degrees of predominance. The effects are caused by the escape of active lytic pancreatic enzymes, which act on the parenchyma of the gland, blood vessels, and fatty tissue. The condition appears to be brought about by increased pancreatic secretion with partial or complete obstruction of outflow and raised intraductal pressure. It may occur suddenly with severe abdominal pain, if extensive it may

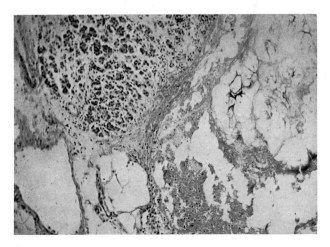

Fig. 15-20. Fat necrosis of the pancreas.

be accompanied by peripheral vascular collapse or shock, and it is frequently fatal. Occurring almost entirely in adult life, it is more common after 40 years of age, and 60% of the cases are in women. Cholelithiasis or alcoholism is frequently associated. Pancreatitis may complicate hyperparathyroidism, occurring in about 7% of cases.

Pathogenesis. Although the characteristic destructive damage and reaction in acute pancreatitis are brought about by release of pancreatic enzymes, the mechanism has been a matter of theory and debate. A variety of factors may be responsible and have variable relative importance in different cases. The *common channel theory,* derived from a case described by Opie, involves obstruction of a common opening into the duodenum of the biliary and pancreatic ducts, so that the reflux of bile into the pancreatic duct activated or released enzymes. Although such an obstruction may be by an impacted stone, spasm of the sphincter of Oddi, edema, mucus, etc., it is evident that such a mechanism can account for only a few cases. However, duct obstruction, partial or complete, may be an important factor, particularly when combined with a stimulus to increased secretion such as may be brought about by a heavy meal or by alcohol intake. The obstruction may be in the smaller ducts, as well, and in some cases appears to be caused by squamous metaplasia of the duct lining. The important factor appears to be increased intraductal pressure, with rupture and release of enzymes. Proteolytic enzymes increase the permeability of blood vessels in the pancreas, with extravasation of fluid into interstitial spaces. Venous obstruction augments the fluid extravasation and prevents enzyme absorption. Retained enzymes act upon blood vessels and parenchyma, producing hemorrhage and necrosis.

Infection, when it occurs, appears to be a later or secondary complication rather than a primary cause of the pancreatic necrosis. However, various bacterial and viral infections may cause pancreatitis of a different nature, as in the case of scarlet fever, typhoid fever, mumps, and Coxsackie virus infection. Vascular disease also may cause focal areas of pancreatitis with necrosis. Pancreatic vessels are occasionally involved in the severe arteriolar degeneration and necrosis of malignant hypertension, but a resulting pancreatic necrosis is usually small and overshadowed by the severe renal involvement. Terminal acute pancreatitis is an occasional incidental finding at autopsy in a variety of conditions, but especially with circulatory failure.

More rarely, acute pancreatic necrosis is found as a cause of sudden death, particularly in alcoholics. Trauma rarely appears to be a cause of acute pancreatitis.

Acute pancreatitis is accompanied by leukocytosis, increased serum amylase in early stages (although it may later return to normal), increased serum lipase, and increased amylase in the urine. The increase of serum amylase does not correlate with the severity of the pancreatitis. Hypocalcemia may be present in severe cases, and glycosuria is found in a small proportion of cases.

Pathologic appearance. The pancreas is enlarged and firm with softer friable areas of necrosis. Various degrees of hemorrhagic and gangrenous changes may involve portions of the pancreas or the whole organ. The gangrenous changes progress rapidly post mortem. Areas of fat necrosis affect the fat of the pancreas, mesentery, and omentum. These appear as firm, dry, opaque yellow or gray nodules. The necrotic areas of fatty tissue are surrounded by a zone of hyperemia and leukocytes. The pancreatic tissue is edematous but is infiltrated by relatively few leukocytes. Blood vessels may have necrosis of their walls and thrombi in their lumina. Inspissated secretion may be found in pancreatic ducts, and metaplasia of duct epithelium with associated acinar dilatation is present in about 50% of the cases. Complications include the development of multiple suppurative abscesses or sinus tracts and of pseudocysts. The peritoneal cavity may contain a turbid yellowish or brownish fluid, in which globules of fat may be evident and which has an increased concentration of amylase.

Chronic pancreatitis

Chronic pancreatitis is manifested by perilobular and interacinar fibrosis, often with increased firmness of the organ. A variable degree of acinar and islet atrophy may be present. The latter type may be associated with diabetes. Dilatation of acini with appearance of a central space or channel suggests some duct obstruction, as does also the presence of inspissated material in the lumina of ducts. Dilatation of ducts, hyperplasia of duct epithelium, and lymphocytic infiltration also may be present. Precipitation of calcium salts, mainly calcium carbonate, in pancreatic ducts may form single or multiple calculi. As with acute pancreatitis, there is frequent association with alcoholism or biliary tract disease.

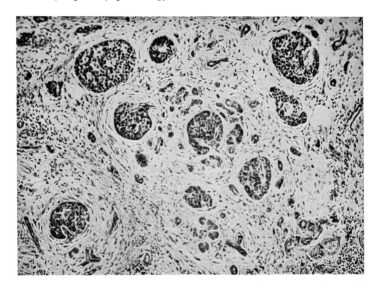

Fig. 15-21. Pancreas; acinar atrophy following duct obstruction. The islet tissue is left relatively intact.

There appears to be a definite relationship of pancreatic fibrosis and insufficiency to the development of fatty change in the liver and cirrhosis, and both are commonly associated with chronic alcoholism.

Pancreatic cysts

True cysts in the pancreas may be congenital or caused by duct obstruction. Pseudocysts, which do not have an epithelial lining, result from pancreatitis with degeneration and softening of tissue or from hematomas. Some pancreatic tumors are cystic.

Dilatation of pancreatic acini with inspissation of secretion is quite commonly seen in adults in association with uremia, gastric cancer, small intestinal obstruction, and ulcerative colitis. The genesis and significance of the lesion are unknown.

Cystic fibrosis of the pancreas

Cystic fibrosis of the pancreas (mucoviscidosis) is a familial, mendelian recessive genetic disease of children, adolescents, and young adults, in which there is abnormality of secretion by exocrine glands. Because many of the glands affected produce a thick viscid mucus, the term *mucoviscidosis* has been used, although an abnormality of sweat is most consistently present. The incidence is variously estimated at about one case in 600 or one in 3,700 live births, and it is rare in Negroes. Mild or incomplete forms that are difficult to recognize probably exist. Characteristic sweat electrolyte patterns may be present in asymptomatic relatives of known patients.

The pancreas and lungs are most seriously involved and, less commonly, the liver and salivary glands. In the pancreas, amorphous inspissated eosinophilic material obstructs ducts, with dilation of ducts and acini. There is progressive atrophy of the parenchyma and gradual replacement by fibrosis, with infiltration by some lymphocytes and mononuclear cells. Fatty replacement of atrophic parenchyma as well as fibrosis may occur. The islets of Langerhans remain intact, although there are some reports of an increased incidence of diabetes mellitus. The pancreas may show little gross change except to be firmer and thinner than normal.

In about 10% of cases there is "meconium ileus" at birth, an intestinal obstruction caused by abnormal inspissated meconium, which possibly results from deficiency of pancreatic secretion before birth. The obstruction is usually in the distal part of the small intestine, and proximally the dilated ileum is filled with a large amount of tenacious viscid meconium.

With pancreatic involvement and deficiency of the pancreatic enzymes trypsin, amylase, and lipase, food is poorly digested and absorbed. Fatty foods particularly are poorly digested, and steatorrhea is commonly present. Malnutrition, including deficiency of vitamins A, D, and K, may be a prominent feature.

Pulmonary involvement is present in almost all cases at some time during the course of the disease and is the important factor in most deaths. The paranasal sinuses also are consistently involved, and nasal polyposis is sometimes present. A respiratory infection with increased mucus production may initiate pulmonary disturbance. Inspissated abnormal bronchial secretions cause obstruction, leading to secondary infection, emphysema or atelectasis, bronchial damage, and bronchiectasis. Squamous metaplasia of bronchial linings, in which vitamin A deficiency may be a factor, complicates the problem of the removal of secretions. Mucous glands of the trachea, bronchi, and bronchioles become distended with inspissated material similar to that in pancreatic acini and ducts. Recurrent resistant bronchopneumonia and lung abscesses are common results and often appear to be caused by *Staphylococcus aureus* infection. Pulmonary hypertension and cor pulmonale develop in some cases.

The liver may show a focal fibrosis in portal areas, with amorphous eosinophilic material plugging bile ductules. There is usually some bile duct proliferation and inflammatory reaction in the areas of fibrosis. The hepatic changes vary greatly in their severity and extensiveness. A few cases may progress to widespread and severe biliary cirrhosis with portal hypertension and enlargement of the spleen.

Salivary glands have increased secretion and show a similar mucinous obstruction. Submaxillary glands are consistently enlarged by the age of 6 years. Sweat glands show a consistent abnormality of sweat electrolytes, and sodium and chloride are increased two to four times above normal. The sweat also contains unusual types of mucoproteins containing large amounts of a sugar (fucose). Various sweat tests (e.g., pilocarpine iontophoresis sweat tests) have been devised that are important diagnostically and as simplified screening procedures. Hand prints on filter paper or agar plates impregnated with silver chromate have been used as a simplified screening test. Abnormally high losses of sodium chloride in the sweat during hot weather may lead to massive salt depletion in these patients, which may be followed by peripheral vascular collapse, hyperpyrexia, coma, and death.

Diabetes mellitus

Diabetes mellitus is a disease caused by an absolute or relative deficiency of the hormone insulin, which is produced by the islets of Langerhans of the pancreas. This, in turn, gives rise to a disturbance of carbohydrate metabolism, with the inability to store glycogen in the liver, excessive accumulation of glucose in the blood (hyperglycemia), and excretion of the excessive sugar in the urine (glycosuria). Fat metabolism also is upset. The fats cannot be completely oxidized, ketone bodies accumulate, and acidosis results. Clinical features are excessive appetite, thirst, and urination. In older persons, obesity and severe arteriosclerosis are common accompaniments. There often appears to be a hereditary factor in the disease. Death in diabetic patients is most commonly caused by cardiovascular complications, diabetic coma, infection, or uremia.

The relation of the pancreatic islets to diabetes has been

proved by extirpation of the organ, which results in diabetes, and by the isolation of the hormone insulin from the islets after selective atrophy of the acinar tissue. Injection of insulin will control most cases of diabetes.

The exact causation of diabetes mellitus in many cases is unknown, and in various cases different factors may have some role. Heredity appears to be a most important basic factor, and the tendency to diabetes appears to be inherited as a modified recessive mendelian factor. Two distinct clinical types are juvenile diabetes, which has a relatively acute onset, usually before the age of 15 years, and maturity-onset diabetes, which develops gradually and usually after 40 years of age. Latent tendencies to diabetes may be present in individuals before development of the clinical disease. Demonstrable pathologic changes in the pancreatic islets are present in many cases and apparently are related to the failure of sufficient insulin secretion. In some cases functional abnormalities of the pituitary or adrenal glands appear to be important factors; e.g., diabetes is often associated with acro-

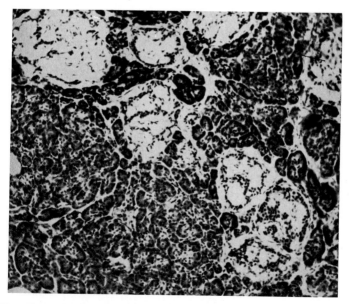

Fig. 15-22. Hyalinization of the islets of Langerhans of the pancreas. From a case of diabetes mellitus.

megaly. Hypophysectomy or the rare destruction of the pituitary, as by metastatic cancer, may ameliorate clinical diabetes (Houssay phenomenon). Similarly, Addison's disease with adrenal cortical destruction may improve a diabetic state, whereas some adrenal cortical hyperplasias or tumors may be associated with the development of diabetes. Obesity often appears to be a factor precipitating diabetes in older susceptible individuals.

Alloxan, the ureide of mesoxalic acid, has been found to produce a specific necrosis of the islets of Langerhans in experimental animals and to result in diabetes mellitus.

The anatomic changes in diabetes mellitus to be considered are (1) the lesions in the pancreas and (2) the lesions in other organs resulting from the disturbed metabolism.

Lesions in the pancreas. Pathologic changes in the pancreas in diabetes mellitus are concerned with the islets of Langerhans. In about 20% of cases no anatomic pancreatic change is demonstrable by the usual histologic methods. Frequently the changes in the islets are slight and cannot be closely correlated with the clinical severity of the disease.

Gross changes in the pancreas in diabetes are uncommon. Occasionally the pancreas may be small, under 35 grams. Gross fibrosis may be related, but lipomatosis is not significant. Pancreatic lithiasis may or may not be associated with diabetes. In hemochromatosis associated with diabetes the pancreas is a rusty brown color because of the deposition of hemosiderin. If more than five sixths of the pancreas has been destroyed by other disease processes, such as carcinoma or pancreatitis, diabetes may be produced. However, the bulk of the islets of Langerhans are situated in the tail of the pancreas, and consequently extensive destruction of other portions of gland will do relatively little harm to them. Since the islets have a structure and blood supply independent of the acini, there is frequently little disturbance of the islets even in advanced involvement of the pancreas by carcinoma or other destructive processes.

The islets comprise 1 to 3% of the weight of the pancreas. There is a wide range of normal variation in the numbers of islets, estimates ranging from 750,000 to 3,750,000. Sometimes there is a distinct quantitative reduction. It is possible that this quantitative variation may be a factor in hereditary aspects of diabetes.

Histologically, three different types of cells can be identified within the islets: alpha cells, beta cells, and D cells or undifferentiated cells. The beta cells, which are the insulin-producing cells, comprise 60 to 70% of islet cells. They can be specifically stained with aldehyde fuchsin, which gives a purple color to the secretory granules. The alpha cells, comprising 20 to 30% of islet cells, and the D cells, 2 to 8%, also can be differentially stained. With fluorescent antibody techniques it has been demonstrated that beta cells contain insulin and alpha cells contain glucagon. The secretory product of the D cell is unknown.

By electron microscopy the alpha, beta, and D cells can be differentiated on the basis of their ultrastructure. The secretory granules of the *beta* cells appear as round, dense irregular structures enclosed within smooth membranous sacs. The secretory granules of *alpha* cells, by contrast, show great variation in ultrastructure within a single cell and may appear round, irregularly shaped, or as crystalline bars. In the D cell the secretory granules appear smudged and indistinct.

Electron microscopic studies on beta cell granules show their formation in the ergastoplasm, appearing first as an amorphous substance between the two membranous components of the lamellar ergastoplasm, and subsequently within sacs that pinch off from the ergastoplasm. Ribonucleoprotein granules attached to the outer surface of the ergastoplasmic sacs disappear, and the beta granule condenses into a dense structure surrounded by a smooth membranous sac. When the beta cell is stimulated to secrete insulin, the granules within their encasing sacs move to the surface of the cell, where the membranous sac fuses with the plasma membrane. It then ruptures, and the granule is liberated into the extracellular space, where it undergoes dissolution. This mechanism of secretion is called emiocytosis. Before the insulin of the liberated granules can enter the bloodstream it must traverse a basement membrane associated with the beta cell, a space, and finally the capillary endothelium. Theoretically blockage or impairment of the rate of transfer through any one of these steps in insulin secretion could result in production of a diabetic state.

Pathology of the islets. Distinct differences occur in the pathologic changes in a patient with classic juvenile diabetes and one with maturity-onset diabetes. In the juvenile diabetic the number of islets is usually reduced. Degranulation of beta cells and fibrosis of the islets may be present, and in occasional instances lymphocytic infiltration is observed. In the maturity-onset diabetic patient the number of islets is usually normal, the degree of beta granulation may be normal or moderately reduced, and hyaline deposition may be observed within the islets. In approximately 20% of patients with maturity-onset diabetes, no distinct pathologic changes can be found in the islets.

Hyalinization is the commonest change observed in the islets in the maturity-onset diabetic patients. The hyalin appears as an eosinophilic amorphous material deposited around the capillaries of the islets, compressing and displacing the islet cells. By electron microscopy the hyaline material appears as a fibrillar protein interposed between the basement membrane of the capillary and the basement membrane of the islet cells. The hyalin is apparently amyloid, since it has the same ultrastructural and staining properties as experimental and human amyloidosis. The hyalin encases the sinusoids, rarely occluding them, but it ultimately replaces nearly all the epithelial cells of the islets. Sometimes the peripheral cells of the islets attempt to proliferate and the hyaline masses continue to encroach upon the new cells, so that masses of hyaline material much larger than the original islet may be produced. In 97% of cases with hyalinization of the islets, the patients are over 40 years of age. Hyalinization of the islets is also seen to a minor degree in about 2% of nondiabetic persons over the age of 40 years.

"Hydropic degeneration" of beta cells is occasionally seen in untreated, inadequately treated or comatose diabetic patients. In cases adequately treated with insulin it is almost never seen. The cytoplasm of the beta cells first becomes vacuolated and later disappears, leaving nuclei and cell membrane alone visible. Histochemical studies show that the vacuoles contain glycogen. Electron microscopic studies show that the glycogen accumulates first as small focal masses within the cytoplasm of the beta cell, and as the hyperglycemic state becomes more severe, the masses increase in size and displace the normal intracellular organelles. Since insulin is formed within the ergastoplasm, obviously the accumulations of glycogen would interfere with insulin synthesis, thus resulting in a further increase in the severity of the diabetic state. Glycogen accumulation in the beta cell is a reversible change and is removed after treatment with insulin and return of the blood sugar level to normal.

Lymphocytic infiltration of the islets is rare but may be observed in juvenile diabetic patients. It is particularly evident in those patients who come to autopsy within days or weeks after the onset of diabetes. Its significance is unknown. In involved islets there may be complete or extensive disappearance of epithelial cells, with scattered lymphocytes replacing them. Some investigators have considered that lymphocytic infiltration may be a transient lesion in the interval between necrosis in the islets and the development of fibrosis.

Fibrosis of islets may develop after "hydropic degeneration" or necrosis of the insular epithelium as well as after lymphocytic infiltration. It varies from a slight change to an almost complete replacement of the islet by dense collagen. Even in advanced examples there is little extension of fibrosis into adjacent acinar tissue. Fibrosis may occur either alone or combined with other types of pancreatic lesions, such as chronic pancreatitis.

Eosinophilic infiltration may sometimes be observed in and around the islets in the children of diabetic mothers, and invariably associated with islet hypertrophy and hyperplasia. These changes are diagnostic of diabetes mellitus in the mother.

Hemochromatosis. Hemosiderin may accumulate within beta cells of the islets as well as within acinar cells in hemochromatosis. Alpha cells do not contain hemosiderin but tend to be reduced in number. Atrophy of acinar cells and interstitial fibrosis are usually present.

Infants born of diabetic mothers are large and often stillborn and may show severe hypertrophy of their pancreatic islets. It appears that infants born of women with a latent diabetic tendency but without clinical diabetes may sometimes show similar effects.

Lesions in other organs. Pathologic changes in organs other than the pancreas depend on the disturbed metabolism and include changes in the distribution and amount of glycogen in certain tissues. Such changes will not be present in cases in which the metabolic disturbance is controlled by insulin administration. Glycogen may be demonstrated in tissues by prompt fixation in alcohol followed by staining with Best's carmine. The glycogen appears as a bright red intracellular material.

The kidney contains excessive glycogen in the epithelium of Henle's loops and occasionally in convoluted tubules so that the cells have a water-clear cytoplasm or hydropic appearance (Armanni-Ebstein lesion). This change may be associated with glycosuria from any cause. Diabetic glomerulosclerosis (Kimmelstiel-Wilson lesion) is a specific renal lesion frequently associated with diabetes mellitus (p. 380). Chronic pyelonephritis is also common in diabetes and may be complicated by papillary necrosis (p. 392).

The liver has decreased glycogen storage within the cytoplasm of the liver cells, although the nuclei of the liver cells may have increased glycogen content and appear clear and glassy. The skin, voluntary muscle, and heart may also show some changes in glycogen content.

Vascular lesions involving small blood vessels (diabetic microangiopathy) are widespread in diabetes mellitus. The changes include thickening of basement membranes and accumulation of material resembling basement membrane in the walls of capillaries and arterioles. The lesions appear soon after disturbances in carbohydrate metabolism become apparent, although their pathogenesis is not fully known.

Arteriosclerotic lesions of medium-sized and larger arteries also are likely to develop in diabetic patients at an earlier age and with enhanced severity.

Proliferative retinopathy appears to be a specific diabetic lesion and is found particularly in severe diabetes of long duration (average about 17 years). Retinal neovascularization and microaneurysms of capillaries are the characteristic changes. There is frequent association of diabetic retinopathy and diabetic renal lesions. Blindness results in about 25% of cases.

Tumors

Primary tumors of the pancreas may be carcinoma arising from ductal or acinar tissue, cystadenoma, or adenoma arising from cells of the islets of Langerhans.

Cystadenomas of the pancreas are uncommon. They occur mainly in women, in middle age periods, and most often in the tail of the pancreas. They are rounded, coarsely lobulated cystic tumors, which grow slowly and by expansion. The cystic spaces are lined by flattened or cuboidal epithelium, occasionally with papillary infolding. A malignant counterpart, cystadenocarcinoma, also occurs.

Carcinoma. The majority of carcinomas of the pancreas arise in the head of the organ, where early in their course they cause obstruction of the common bile duct. The obstruction produces dilatation of bile ducts and the gallbladder and clinically gives rise to a painless, ever-deepening jaundice. Spread to neighboring tissue and by metastasis is a late feature. In the less common tumors arising in the body or tail, earlier and more widespread extension and metastasis result in a greater variety of clinical symptoms, and multiple and sometimes widespread venous thrombosis is a frequent complication. A large proportion metastasize to lung and thoracic lymph nodes and often lead to mistaken diagnosis of primary lung cancer.

The tumor forms a hard nodular mass within the pancreatic tissue, often fibrous or scirrhous in character, and it is difficult to distinguish grossly from chronic pancreatitis. Microscopically it may be a cylindric cell adenocarcinoma originating from the pancreatic duct system or, less frequently, an acinar cell type resembling the parenchyma of the pancreas.

Adenomas, papillomas, and carcinomas of the ampulla and papilla of Vater, of biliary tract origin, compose the largest proportion of tumors of the duodenum.

Islet cell tumor. Tumors composed of islet cell tissue occasionally occur in the pancreas, most frequently in the head or tail of the organ. They are usually small, less than 2 cm. in diameter, and only rare examples have measured up to 6 cm. in diameter. They usually appear well circumscribed, and some have a fibrous capsule. Their increased consistency may make them palpable, and their homogeneous color in contrast with the surrounding lobulated yellowish pancreatic tissue may make them visible. About 80% are single, about 90% are benign, and about 60% produce excessive insulin and clinical symptoms.

The benign islet cell adenomas are usually circumscribed or encapsulated. In some cases there seems to be microscopic evidence of invasion, but no metastases are present, and there is a clinically benign course. The carcinomas of islet tissue tend to be larger and more infiltrative, but metastasis is often the only good evidence of malignancy. Carcinomas tend to produce more severe evidence of hyperinsulinism. Some metastasizing islet cell carcinomas are well differentiated microscopically.

Microscopically the islet cell tumors are usually composed of well-differentiated tissue, often with the characteristics and architecture of normal islet tissue, and appearing simply as a gigantic islet. The cells, which often seem comparable to beta cells of normal islets, tend to occur in ribbons or cords, with only occasional solid masses or glandular structures. Degenerative changes such as fibrosis, hyalinization, or calcification may be present. The appearance may simulate that of carcinoid tumors or some bronchial adenomas. It is probable that these tumors may arise from ductal tissue, as well as from preexisting islet tissue.

Functioning islet cell tumors may give rise to episodes of severe hypoglycemia, often precipitated by fasting or exercise.

Nervous system manifestations and even loss of consciousness may occur. The attacks are relieved by administration of glucose. Multiple petechial hemorrhages and acute degeneration of nerve cells and astrocytes have been described in the central nervous system. The severity of the clinical episodes does not correlate with the size of the islet cell tumor.

Noninsulin-producing islet cell tumors are sometimes associated with gastric hypersecretion and the development of severe and intractable or recurrent peptic ulcers (Zollinger-Ellison syndrome). The ulcers may be atypically located, characteristically resist therapy, and frequently are fatal. Electron microscope studies indicate that the cells of the ulcerogenic adenomas are of alpha cell origin. The ulcerogenic tumors are sometimes multiple and often malignant. A gastrinlike hormone has been demonstrated in these tumors. Multiple adenomas involving the pituitary, adrenal, and parathyroid glands, as well as the pancreatic islets, are sometimes found in this syndrome.

Pancreatic adenomas have also been associated with a syndrome characterized by profuse watery diarrhea, hypokalemia, and hypercalcemia. Gastric hypersecretion and ulcer are not part of the syndrome. Pancreatic adenomas producing this syndrome may be part of a multiple endocrine adenopathy and have a genetic basis.

Chapter 16

The reticuloendothelial system, spleen, and lymph nodes

T RETICULOENDOTHELIAL SYSTEM

he reticuloendothelial system is composed of widespread cells having the essential and common ability to phagocytose particulate foreign material, such as injected vital dyes or India ink. Some of these phagocytic cells are endothelial cells lining the blood sinuses of the spleen, liver, and bone marrow and the lymph sinuses of lymph nodes. Also, all connective tissues contain elements (undifferentiated mesenchymal cells) that are capable of assuming mobility and phagocytic function. These cells are called histiocytes, clasmatocytes, polyblasts, resting wandering cells, adventitial cells, etc. Both the endothelial cells and the undifferentiated mesenchymal cells are capable of becoming macrophages.

The concept of the reticuloendothelial system has been furthered by Maximow, who pointed out that in the spleen, bone marrow, and lymphatic tissue generally there exists an undifferentiated mesenchyme, called reticulum, in the form of a nucleated syncytium with an abundant meshwork of fibrils. These fibrils (reticulin) are not seen well in ordinary sections stained by hematoxylin and eosin. However, reticulin fibers are argyrophilic and are stained black by silver salts, which are converted to the black oxide. This syncytium or reticulum is not in itself phagocytic, but under the stimulus of an injury or inflammation there differentiates from it the mobile phagocytic macrophage. Since the undifferentiated mesenchyme is widespread throughout the body, macrophages likewise have diverse origin. Microglial cells are the corresponding phagocytic cells in the nervous system.

The monocyte of the circulating blood is also phagocytic and is commonly believed to be of reticuloendothelial origin. The other two main views regarding its origin are that it may arise from the lymphocyte or from the myeloblast. The ordinary lining endothelium of blood vessels and lymphatics, other than in the spleen, lymph nodes, liver, bone marrow, adrenal cortex, and hypophysis, is not actively phagocytic.

Reticuloendothelial cells are important in the normal breakdown of hemoglobin and formation of bile pigment, in fat metabolism, and in defense of the body. The blood is cleared of particulate matter, foreign material, and bacteria in its filtration through the liver, spleen, and bone marrow. The phagocytic cells ingest and remove dead tissue fragments, pigments, bacteria, fungi, and protozoa. For larger masses of particulate matter they fuse and form foreign body giant cells. The osteoclast of bone is a particular type of such a giant cell. The reticuloendothelial system plays a role in immunity, and it has a function in antibody formation.

Diseases of the reticuloendothelial system fall into three main groups: (1) infections and inflammations, in which proliferation and phagocytosis by reticuloendothelial cells are prominent, of which histoplasmosis and malaria are excellent examples; (2) lipidoses, or lipid storage diseases, in which, because of disturbed metabolism, fatty substances accumulate in reticuloendothelial cells; the fatty material may be kerasin (Gaucher's disease), sphingomyelin (Niemann-Pick disease), or cholesterol (Schüller-Christian disease, xanthomas); and (3) tumors and tumorlike conditions, which form a large and confusing group of conditions and include the leukemias, Hodgkin's disease, reticulum cell sarcoma, lymphosarcoma, and reticuloendotheliosis.

Since the large storehouse of reticuloendothelial cells is in the spleen, lymph nodes, bone marrow, and liver, the reticuloendothelial involvement is considered in conjunction with diseases affecting these organs.

SPLEEN

The average normal adult spleen weighs 150 to 170 grams, but the size and weight vary widely. Many of the diseases of the spleen bring about an enormous increase in its size and weight, sometimes to 2,000 grams or more. The adult spleen is usually not clinically palpable unless it weighs more than 300 grams. The cut surface of the normal spleen is moderately firm and light red; the malpighian corpuscles are just visible as small grayish white areas. Small accessory spleens are not uncommon. Microscopically the discernible structures are (1) the malpighian bodies (lymph follicles), which are cylindrical masses of lymphoid tissue surrounding small arteries; (2) the pulp, consisting of sinusoids separated by reticular tissue; and (3) trabeculae or fibromuscular bands, which connect with the splenic capsule. An accessory spleen is present in about 10% of persons. The tail of the pancreas is a frequent site.

The spleen is not essential to life, but it has important functions, particularly as the main component of the reticuloendothelial system. Thus it is important (1) in the breakdown of hemoglobin and formation of bile pigment, (2) in the filtration of organisms or other foreign material from the bloodstream, (3) probably in the formation of antibodies and immunity, (4) as the reservior for blood, and (5) for blood formation in the fetus or when there is severe anemia.

Functioning of the spleen in the storage and breakdown of blood elements may get out of balance or equilibrium because of primary (idiopathic or hereditary) factors, or this may be secondarily caused by various disease processes, mainly of the reticuloendothelial system. The resulting hypersplenism may destroy excessive numbers of circulating red blood cells (congenital hemolytic icterus), platelets (thrombocytopenic purpura), or neutrophilic leukocytes (splenic neutropenia). All three elements may be excessively destroyed (panhematopenia). Surgical removal of the spleen and accessory splenic tissue is effective in such cases when clinical study has established that bone marrow function is normal and is not a contributing factor. In primary hypersplenism there is a diffuse or nodular hyperplasia of the reticulum cells of the spleen proportional to the severity of the disease. In acute stages of hemocytopenia there is also sequestration in the red pulp and splenic sinusoids of the decreased formed elements of the blood. In secondary hypersplenism small hemolytic or cytolytic foci may be found in the spleen.

Splenectomy may be beneficial in rupture of the spleen, familial hemolytic jaundice, thrombocytopenic purpura, hypersplenism or primary splenic neutropenia, thrombosis or anomalous obstruction of the splenic vein, and early stages of splenic anemia or Banti's syndrome.

Retrograde conditions of the spleen

Atrophy. Reduction in size of the spleen may occur in old age, usually in association with severe arteriosclerosis of splenic vessels. Extreme atrophy may be present in late stages of sickle cell anemia.

Arteriosclerosis. Hyaline sclerosis of small arteries and arterioles in the spleen is very common, its frequency and severity increasing with age. While more pronounced when there is hypertension and when arteriosclerosis is present elsewhere, the vascular change may be present in the spleen alone. When severe, it may cause multiple small infarcts or necroses in the spleen.

Amyloid. The spleen is a common site for amyloid deposit (p. 35).

Pigmentation. Pigment deposits in the spleen follow excessive breakdown of hemoglobin caused by hemolytic anemias (pernicious anemia, sickle cell anemia), malaria, or chronic congestion (e.g., in Banti's syndrome). Some brownish hemosiderin pigment in the spleen is a normal finding. In malaria the pigmentation is excessive, so that the enlarged organ grossly exhibits a slate gray color (p. 221). In sickle cell anemia and Banti's syndrome curious areas of fibrosis and pigmentation occur in the spleen (siderofibrotic nodules, Gandy-Gamna bodies, pp. 49 and 568).

Multiple necroses of the spleen (Fleckmilz). Speckling of the spleen may be caused by widespread and irregular areas of necrosis as the result of confluence of many minute infarcts. The splenic arterioles commonly show marked degenerative changes with frequent thromboses. Most cases are associated with renal disease and uremia.

Circulatory disturbances

Infarction. Infarction in the spleen is common and is usually the result of arterial embolism (p. 101).

Congestion. Chronic passive congestion in the spleen may be present in conditions of circulatory failure. The spleen is moderately enlarged and firm. Microscopically the sinusoids appear dilated. Fibrosis occurs if the process continues for a long period.

Chronic congestion is also associated with obstruction of the portal circulation, e.g., from cirrhosis of the liver and with the Banti syndrome. Severe congestion of the spleen is a feature of sickle cell anemia in its earlier phases and of congenital hemolytic jaundice. In the long-standing, chronic congestion related to portal hypertension (including Banti's syndrome) and in the late stage of sickle cell anemia, foci of fibrosis with deposits of iron and calcium may be seen (Gandy-Gamna bodies).

Banti's syndrome. Banti's syndrome is a symptom complex

dominated by splenic enlargement, nonhemolytic anemia, and leukopenia. The splenomegaly is characterized by congestion and fibrosis. It is accompanied by portal hypertension and often is complicated in later stages by ascites, hematemesis, portal cirrhosis of the liver, and thrombosis of splenic and portal veins.

Rupture of the spleen. Rupture of the spleen is usually the result of direct trauma over the splenic area. Occasionally there is delayed splenic rupture, with a latent period following the traumatic injury. Splenic rupture also may complicate malaria, infectious mononucleosis, primary splenic tumors, and other conditions on rare occasions. Unless there is prompt operation, fatal intra-abdominal hemorrhage usually results. Implants of splenic tissue on peritoneal surfaces (splenosis) may complicate nonfatal splenic rupture. The splenic implants contain characteristic splenic pulp, but they differ from accessory spleens in that the supporting framework is not complete.

Inflammations

Acute splenitis (acute splenic tumor). Splenic reaction with moderate enlargement accompanies acute systemic infections, particularly bacteremias or septicemias. In such cases the causative organisms are usually obtainable in cultures from the spleen. Acute splenic tumor appears to be a reaction to the presence of foreign protein, whether bacterial or nonbacterial.

Two forms occur, a gray or septic type and a red or typhoid type. In the gray type of acute splenitis the spleen is moderately enlarged and very soft. On the cut surface the soft swollen pulp has a grayish color with a purplish tinge. The tissue is so soft as to be almost fluid, and it is easily scraped away with a knife. The red type occurs with bacillary infections such as typhoid fever. The enlarged soft spleen is very red from intense congestion.

Microscopically the changes in acute splenitis are congestion and cellular accumulation in the pulp. In some cases many of the cells are neutrophilic leukocytes, but commonly they are large basophilic mononuclear cells that are lymphoid in character. Eosinophilia has been noted in the spleen in cases of sudden death.

Tuberculosis. The spleen is usually involved in generalized miliary tuberculosis. In rare cases a large localized tuberculous lesion develops in the spleen, while the original focus remains quiescent or heals. Small, rounded, hyalinized fibrous nodules,

1 to 3 mm. in diameter, are a frequent finding in the spleen and in most cases represent healed tubercules.

Malaria. The spleen is enlarged and heavily pigmented in malaria (p. 221).

Histoplasmosis. The spleen is often greatly enlarged in histoplasmosis because of marked proliferation of reticuloendothelial cells. The small organism can be seen in the cytoplasm of these phagocytic cells (p. 208). Similar splenic lesions occur in kala-azar.

Cysts and tumors

Cystic cavities in the spleen are rare. Most are pseudocysts resulting from encapsulation of an area of hemorrhage or degeneration in the pulp. Epidermoid cysts and parasitic (hydatid) cysts are rare occurrences.

Tumors of the spleen, either primary or metastatic, are rather uncommon. Hemangioma, although rare, is the most frequent primary benign tumor. Hamartomas and sarcomas, including the malignant lymphomas, also occur. The reason for the relative infrequency of metastatic tumors in the spleen is not known,

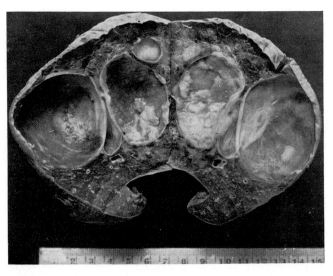

Fig. 16-1. Multiple cysts of the spleen.

but it may result from the inequality of exposure to metastasizing tumor cells or from lesser susceptibility than other tissues.

LYMPH NODES

The lymph nodes are focal collections of lymphoid and reticuloendothelial cells. Lymphoid tissue is widely distributed in other tissues as well, such as the alimentary canal and spleen. The main elements in lymph nodes are (1) lymph follicles (germinal centers), which appear to be related to immunologic function and particularly to secondary immune response; (2) lymph sinuses, lined by endothelium; and (3) the medulla or pulp, consisting of lymphocytes and reticulum cells in a delicate meshwork of reticulin fibers.

The lymph nodes are an integral part of the reticuloendothelial system and participate in its diseases. In agammaglobulinemia the lymph nodes may show an absence of germinal centers and of plasma cells, even after injection of an antigen. Lymphoid aggregations in the spleen and elsewhere may be similarly nonreactive. The main lesions of lymph nodes are inflammations (lymphadenitis) and tumors (primary and metastatic).

Lymphadenitis. Acute lymphadenitis occurs in lymph nodes draining an area of acute inflammation, e.g., in cervical lymph nodes in acute infections of the throat, or in axillary lymph nodes in infections of the hand or arm. The lymph nodes are swollen and tender, and in pyogenic infections suppuration may occur. Microscopically the sinuses of the lymph nodes are found filled by neutrophilic leukocytes or mononuclear cells. In certain infections the lesions in lymph nodes are of a characteristic nature, e.g., in tularemia, lymphogranuloma venereum, and tuberculosis. In disseminated lupus erythematosus the lymph nodes are enlarged in 66% of cases, showing edema, engorgement, and sometimes necrosis.

Chronic lymphadenitis, which may be found in nodes draining an area of low-grade inflammation, shows proliferation of mononuclear cells, which fill the sinuses. Fibrosis usually does not occur.

Chronic dermatitis with pruritus may have an associated enlargement of lymph nodes. The nodes show reticular hyperplasia, melanin pigment, intracellular fat, and a few eosinophils (lipomelanotic reticular hyperplasia, dermatopathic lymphadenitis).

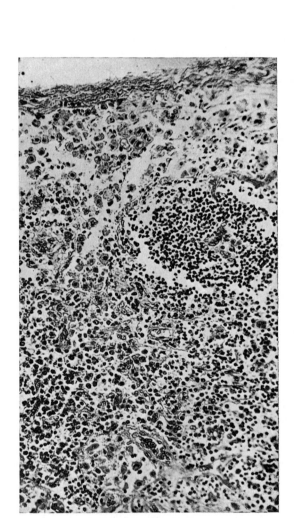

Fig. 16-2. Chronic lymphadenitis. Many large mononuclear cells seen in dilated peripheral lymph sinus. (From Richter, M. N.: Spleen, lymph nodes, and reticuloendothelial system, In Anderson, W. A. D., editor: Pathology, ed. 5, St. Louis, 1966, The C. V. Mosby Co.)

Infectious mononucleosis (glandular fever). Infectious mononucleosis occurs most frequently in children and young adults. It is characterized by slight enlargement of superficial lymph nodes, splenomegaly, sore throat, and an increase of mononuclear cells (atypical lymphoid cells) in the blood. Actually a great variety of tissues may be involved, so that the clinical manifestations are protean. The mortality is almost nil, but fatality has occurred as a result of rupture of the spleen, central respiratory paralysis, and myocarditis.

The large abnormal lymphocyte found in the blood is characterized by a large, eccentric, indented nucleus with a sievelike, coarse network of chromatin. The cytoplasm is basophilic and vacuolated. Occasionally more immature types may be present. The cell is not pathognomonic, and similar cells may be seen in various viral infections and allergic states. However, the presence of such cells accounting for more than 10% of white blood cells is very suggestive of infectious mononucleosis. Absence of anemia in uncomplicated cases assists in differentiation from leukemia.

Of diagnostic importance is the Paul-Bunnell test showing heterophil antibodies in the serum, which agglutinate sheep red cells in high dilutions (a titer of 1:160 or more). The highest titers are usually found in the second or third week, and the reaction sometimes persists for several months. However, several other conditions, including viral hepatitis, viral pneumonitis, undulant fever, and serum sickness, may be associated with heterophil antibodies in the serum. The Davidsohn exclusion test is useful in the presence of relatively low titers. It is based on the fact that the heterophil antibodies of infectious mononucleosis are not absorbed by guinea pig kidney tissue as are the heterophil antibodies of serum sickness and of normal serum. Beef erythrocytes will absorb the heterophil antibodies of both infectious mononucleosis and serum sickness but not of normal serum.

The lymph nodes show a maintenance of architecture (albeit distorted) with distinguishable lymph sinuses and germinal centers. Throughout the pulp, in the sinuses, and on the edges of the germinal centers are large numbers of the specific large mononuclear cells, identical with those characteristic in the blood. Much proliferative activity is evident in the pulp.

The spleen, other lymphoid tissues, and bone marrow show similar changes with an accumulation of the characteristic cells.

Focal areas of mononuclear infiltration, and necrosis occur in the liver, kidneys, nervous system, heart, and lungs. Involvement of the nervous system may give variable clinical manifestations, and fatalities have resulted from acute polyradiculitis with respiratory paralysis (Guillain-Barré syndrome). Hepatitis similar to that of nonfatal viral or epidemic hepatitis is common, and evidence of hepatic dysfunction or jaundice may be present. The liver shows lymphoid accumulations about portal areas, degeneration and regeneration of hepatic cells, and activity of the Kupffer cells. In rare cases the hepatic damage is severe, and viral hepatitis may be simulated clinically.

Acute infectious lymphocytosis. Under the term *acute infectious lymphocytosis* there has been described an infectious condition in children characterized by a relative and absolute lymphocytosis of small lymphocytes of normal appearance. Biopsied lymph nodes show a great proliferation of the reticuloendothelium of the sinuses and hyaline degenerative changes in the lymph follicles. Acute infectious lymphocytosis is differentiated from leukemia and infectious mononucleosis by the normal appearance of the predominating small lymphocytes and the negative heterophil agglutination reaction.

Metastatic tumors. Carcinomas particularly tend to metastasize to regional lymph nodes. The tumor cells are first seen in the sinuses of the periphery or pulp, but lymphoid tissue eventually is replaced by tumor, and invasion occurs through the capsule.

TUMORS OF THE RETICULOENDOTHELIAL AND LYMPHOID TISSUES

Apart from the infections, in which proliferation of reticuloendothelial cells is a distinctive feature (malaria, histoplasmosis, kala-azar), and the lipid storage diseases (Gaucher's disease, etc.), there occurs a variety of tumors and tumorlike conditions involving lymphoid and reticuloendothelial structures (reticuloses). Since they are of obscure causation, etiologic classification fails. The following simplified morphologic classification should be viewed with the realization that gradations and overlappings preclude sharp lines of distinction. The cellular structure of the lymphatic tumors is very labile, and, as they are all derived from the same mesenchymal stem cells, transitions are sometimes observed from one type to another.

Reticuloendotheliosis
Malignant lymphoma
  Lymphocytic type (lymphosarcoma)
  Reticulum cell type (reticulum cell sarcoma)
  Hodgkin's disease
  Mycosis fungoides
Leukemia (p. 572)
  Lymphocytic
  Myelocytic or granulocytic
  Monocytic

Reticuloendotheliosis. Nonlipid reticuloendotheliosis (Letterer-Siwe disease, malignant reticuloblastomatosis, aleukemic reticulosis) is a rare condition in which there is diffuse hyperplasia of the reticuloendothelial system to the point of replacement of normal structures. It may occur at any age but is more frequent in infants and young children. The characteristics include splenomegaly, hepatomegaly, anemia, purpura, and bony changes such as areas of rarefaction and cyst formation. A fatal ending is reached in two weeks to two years, usually from acute infection. The nonfamilial infantile form has been termed nonlipid reticuloendotheliosis to distinguish it from the lipid storage diseases, and it is also called Letterer-Siwe disease, after Letterer and Siwe, who described cases in 1924 and 1933.

The greatest changes are found in the spleen, lymph nodes, liver, and bone marrow. The enlarged spleen shows scattered, indefinite grayish yellow nodules on the cut surface, and similar nodules may be seen in the liver. In addition there may be diffuse or nodular lesions of the lungs and involvement of the intestinal lymphoid tissue. Microscopically there is a great proliferation of large mononuclear cells in organs of the reticuloendothelial system, with distortion of normal structure. These cells are rounded or polyhedral, and some may be very large (up to 50μ). Multinucleated giant cells may be seen. Occasional mitoses are present. Silver staining shows a proliferation of reticulin fibers in contact with the atypical cells. In some cases there may be a few neutrophilic or eosinophilic leukocytes.

Reticuloendotheliosis is closely related to monocytic leukemia and Hodgkin's disease. By some observers it is considered simply an aleukemic form of monocytic leukemia. However, the rarefaction of bone and formation of bone cysts appear characteristic of reticuloendotheliosis; in monocytic leukemia the cell type is more uniform and the process is more widespread, with the

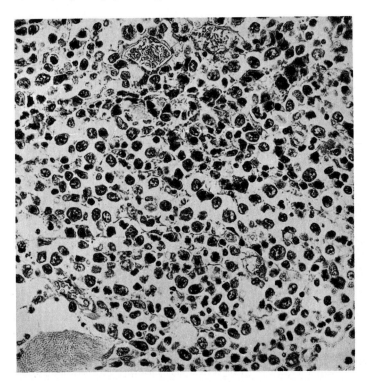

Fig. 16-3. Reticulum cell sarcoma. The highly pleomorphic cellular neoplasm is without organized arrangement. (From Haukohl, R. S., and Anderson, W. A. D., editors: Pathology seminars, St. Louis, 1955, The C. V. Mosby Co.)

appearance of infiltration rather than of hyperplasia in situ. Leukemic reticuloendotheliosis denotes a proliferation of reticular cells in the blood. By some this is divided into a primitive cell type, a monocytic type, and a lymphocytic type.

In monocytic leukemia there is hyperplasia of the reticuloendothelial tissues, with enlargement of the spleen, liver, and often lymph nodes. The bone marrow is almost always involved. A tendency to hemorrhage, ulceration, and necrosis is prominent, the oral cavity being the commonest site of such involvement. Infiltration with monocytes and a general reticuloendothelial hyperplasia is the main microscopic finding, evident particularly in the spleen, liver, lymph nodes, bone marrow, and skin. Areas of necrosis and hemorrhage are also common in these tissues. In chronic cases the microscopic appearance may simulate that of Hodgkin's disease, with eosinophils and Reed-Sternberg cells.

Chronic forms of reticuloendotheliosis may be associated with erythroderma. The Sézary form of erythrodermic reticulemia is associated with a specific cell in the peripheral blood. The Sézary cell is a large, monocytoid mononuclear cell with abundant clear cytoplasm.

Waldenström in 1944 described a syndrome characterized by serum macroglobulinemia. In addition to the hyperglobulinemia the patients have fatigue, mucosal hemorrhages, moderate lymphadenopathy, bone marrow lymphocytosis, anemia, and a greatly elevated erythrocyte sedimentation rate. The condition is fatal. A clinical variant of macroglobulinemia, with central nervous system involvement, is known as the Bing-Neel syndrome. Infiltrations that are pleomorphic or of variable cell types are found in the lymph nodes, bone marrow, and spleen and often in a variety of other organs, including the brain. Lymphoid plasma cells containing intranuclear PAS-positive material have characterized some cases. It has been suggested that Waldenström's macroglobulinemia is a neoplastic reticuloendotheliosis that may be a variant of multiple myeloma or a type of lymphoma.

Myeloid metaplasia (aleukemic myelosis) of the spleen is considered on p. 576.

Malignant lymphoma. Malignant lymphoma is a malignant tumor that can arise from any aggregate of lymphoid tissue. It is more frequent in males. It may occur at any period of life, but the peak frequency is in the decade of the fifties. Constitutional symptoms and blood changes are lacking in early stages. External lymph node enlargement is the most frequent beginning, and the cervical nodes are most often affected. The gastrointestinal tract, nasopharynx, spleen, skin, liver, and other tissues are frequently involved. Direct invasion and extension to contiguous lymph nodes occur early. Later widespread extension, probably by the bloodstream, often results in involvement of many tissues. The tumor tissue is generally radiosensitive.

In a central zone of Africa through the equatorial region, lymphoma occurs with high incidence in children between 2 and 14 years of age, with a peak incidence at 5 years of age (Burkitt's lymphoma). Most of the cases involve the jaw or

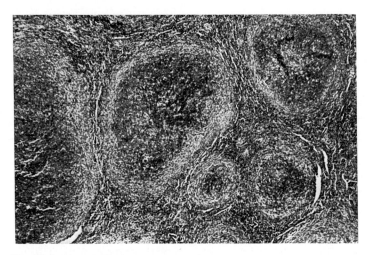

Fig. 16-4. Giant follicular lymphoma of the spleen.

abdomen. The distribution is geographic rather than racial, suggesting an infective spread by an insect vector. This and additional immunologic evidence suggest that a viral agent contributes to the pathogenesis of this lymphoma.

A commonly used classification of malignant lymphomas is (1) lymphocytic lymphosarcoma, (2) reticulum cell sarcoma, (3) follicular lymphoma, and (4) Hodgkin's disease. Mixed types also occur. Mycosis fungoides is a type of malignant lymphoma of the skin. Classification of malignant lymphomas is of value, since there appears to be a varying degree of malignancy as evidenced by survival time.

The essential microscopic feature of malignant lymphoma is disruption and obliteration of the architecture of the lymphoid tissue by the cellular overgrowth. In diffuse *lymphocytic lymphosarcoma* or *reticulum cell sarcoma,* dominance of one cell type (e.g., lymphocytes or reticulum cells) and obliteration of the sinuses of lymph nodes are other criteria important in signifying a malignant lymphoid neoplasm. Pleomorphism is not a feature; most of the cells are similar in appearance, although some giant cell forms (as in reticulum cell sarcoma) may occur. Mitoses are present but not necessarily abundant. In lymph nodes the capsule eventually is penetrated, and there is invasion of surrounding tissue. In the intestinal tract, invasion occurs throughout the walls of the bowel. Fibrosis or granulomatous changes are lacking. Silver stains show a variable number of fine reticulin fibers in the reticulum cell sarcoma.

Follicular lymphoma. Lymphoma of follicular or nodular type (giant follicular lymphoblastoma, Brill-Symmers disease) is a neoplastic condition of lymph nodes, spleen, and other lymphoid tissues and is characterized by a prominent follicular architectural pattern. As in the diffuse forms of lymphoma, there may be classification according to the predominant cell types, with corresponding prognostic significance. However, the presence of a follicular rather than a diffuse architectural pattern is in itself a differentiation that appears to indicate a lesser degree of inherent malignancy. Some cases in later stages become transformed into a corresponding diffuse type of lymphoma, but other cases retain some degree of follicular differentiation to the end. The tumor tissue is very radiosensitive. About half the patients survive for more than five years, and a few survive for ten years or more. The blood picture is normal, and constitutional symptoms are mild. It occurs in adults, the average age being above 40 years.

The lymph nodes are enlarged, firm, and discrete (until late). The spleen is usually greatly enlarged (average 1,600 grams). The cut surface is studded by grayish areas, 1 to 3 mm. in diameter.

Microscopically the essential change is loss of lymph node architecture and the presence throughout the node of numerous, neoplastic, follicle-like nodules consisting of lymphocytic or reticulum cells or both types of cells. The large nodules may fuse and assume irregular shapes. Invasion of the capsule and pericapsular tissues occurs.

The condition is easily distinguished microscopically from the other types of malignant lymphoma by the maintenance and exaggeration of the follicular architecture. It is most easily confused with the lymphadenitis of secondary syphilis (p. 185), rheumatoid arthritis, and other inflammatory hyperplasias. There is no evidence that follicular lymphoma arises from or is preceded by inflammatory follicular hyperplasia. The latter benign reaction of lymphatic tissue to infections or irritative processes is most severe in children, whereas follicular lymphoma occurs in late adult life. The histologic differences between follicular lymphoma and inflammatory hyperplasia are outlined in Table

Table 16-1. *Histologic differences between follicular lymphoma and reactive hyperplasia*

	Follicular lymphoma	Follicular hyperplasia of inflammatory or toxic origin
Follicles	Loss of normal architecture of node	Preservation of nodal architecture
	Closely packed	Scattered
	Diffuse throughout node	More prominent in cortical portion of node
	Slight variation in size and shape of follicles	Great variation in size and shape of follicles
	Fade into surrounding tissue without sharp demarcation	Sharply demarcated reaction centers
	Neoplastic cells of follicles show pleomorphism with nuclear irregularities	Centers composed of reticulum cells and derivatives with little cellular or nuclear irregularity
	Lack of phagocytosis	Active phagocytosis in reaction centers
	Few mitoses, with no significant difference in number inside and outside the follicles	Typical mitoses often frequent in reaction centers, with few outside the follicles
Interfollicular tissue	Cells densely packed	Cells scattered
	Condensation of reticulum fibers at periphery of follicles	Little alteration of reticulum framework
	Similarity of cell type inside and outside follicles	Lymphocytes at margin of reaction centers small, mature, and uniform
	Extensive infiltration of capsule and pericapsular fat, sometimes with follicles outside capsule	No or slight infiltration of capsule and pericapsular fat

16-1. Toxoplasmic lymphadenitis (p. 225) may be confused with malignant lymphomas, including Hodgkin's disease. It is distinguished from malignant lymphoma by the facts that the lymph node architecture is not completely destroyed, only normal mitoses are present, the characteristic Reed-Sternberg cells of Hodgkin's disease are lacking, the sinuses are crowded with macrophages, and the cellular infiltrate is characteristically inflammatory.

Hodgkin's disease. Hodgkin's disease involves lymph nodes or lymphoid tissue elsewhere, as in the alimentary tract, spleen, and often, bone marrow. It is sometimes called a lymphogranulomatous type of malignant lymphoma. The etiology is unknown and its nature is a matter of debate. The most popular concepts are that it is (1) a chronic infective granuloma, (2) a viral infection, or (3) a true neoplasm of lymphoid or reticuloendothelial origin. At least one form or stage, often termed Hodgkin's sarcoma, has the characteristics of a malignant tumor. The belief that it is an atypical form of tuberculosis has been almost abandoned. Organisms of the *Brucella* group have been considered, but an etiologic relationship has not been established. There is an immunologic defect in Hodgkin's disease, with an inability to develop delayed hypersensitivity and delayed homograft rejection. The most widely held opinion is that Hodgkin's disease is a form of malignant lymphoma.

A fatal ending occurs after an average duration of two years, but length of life varies from a few months to ten years or more. Males are affected more than twice as frequently as females. It may occur at any age, but the highest incidence is in young adults.

The beginning is usually a painless enlargement of a group of lymph nodes, most frequently in the neck. Itching is often an accompaniment. Blood changes are inconstant, but there may be a moderate neutrophilic leukocytosis with lymphopenia, and eosinophilia is occasionally present. Anemia develops in later stages. The disease progresses by further involvement of lymphoid tissue, as in other groups of nodes, spleen, etc. In late stages various viscera become involved. Almost any tissue eventually may be affected, although the nervous system is seldom involved except by Hodgkin's sarcoma. Radiation, to which the tissue is moderately sensitive, is the usual method of therapy.

The enlarged involved lymph nodes are at first discrete, but in late stages they become matted together. The cut surface of the Hodgkin's tissue has a grayish, translucent, "fish-flesh" appearance. Diagnosis is usually made by biopsy of a lymph node. The whole of an enlarged node should be resected for such purpose.

The histologic picture in Hodgkin's disease is that of a diffuse progressive neoplastic process. beginning with lymphoid hyperplasia. With progression of the lesion there is a gradual loss of

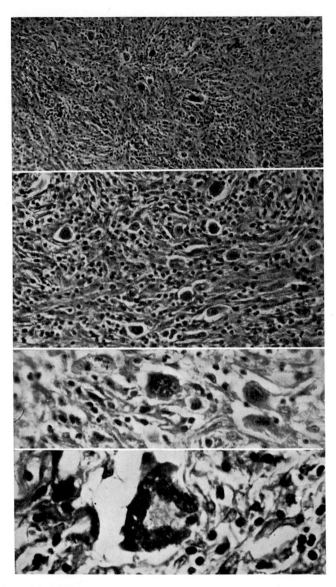

Fig. 16-5. Hodgkin's disease. Note the characteristic large hyperchromatic cells, which stand out prominently. Some fibrosis is evident in the upper figures.

normal architecture because of replacement by a pleomorphic cellular tissue in which large hyperchromatic characteristic cells (Reed-Sternberg cells) are an essential constituent. Eosinophils are often numerous, but they are not invariably present. In certain cases there is invasion, and the tissue has a sarcomatous aspect. Areas of necrosis may occur. Fibrosis with hyalinization is a late development. A follicular or nodular form of Hodgkin's disease is sometimes seen.

The important histologic features are (1) the Reed-Sternberg cells, (2) the pleomorphism of the cellular tissue, (3) the presence of eosinophils, and (4) fibrosis. The Reed-Sternberg cells are large (12 to 40μ), often irregular in shape, and with lobulated or multilobed nuclei. Multinucleated and binucleated forms also occur. The nuclear chromatin is abundant and dark staining and usually is condensed at the periphery, so that the nuclear membrane appears thickened and a clear zone may be evident around the prominent, usually eosinophilic, nucleolus. Their hyperchromatism may cause them to stand out prominently in the first glance at a microscopic field. The cytoplasm is abundant and may be either eosinophilic or basophilic. The appearance of Reed-Sternberg cells is often similar to that of megakaryocytes, from which they can be distinguished by their failure to react strongly with the periodic acid–Schiff method. With this method the mucoprotein or glycoprotein in the cytoplasm of the megakaryocyte stains a red-purple color. Identification of Reed-Sternberg cells is essential in the diagnosis of Hodgkin's disease.

Pleomorphism is prominent in the usual case of Hodgkin's disease in that there is a mixture of the specific cells, giant cells of Hodgkin's disease, plasma cells, lymphocytes, neutrophils, and eosinophils. The occurrence of eosinophils is important. While not invariably present in Hodgkin's disease, they rarely occur in large numbers in lymph nodes in any other condition. Fibrosis is important in distinguishing Hodgkin's disease from other lymphoblastomatous conditions such as lymphosarcoma and lymphatic leukemia.

Attempts have been made to divide Hodgkin's disease into histologic types, from which an estimate of the course and prognosis sometimes can be made. Clinical staging, based on the extent of the disease, also has been used as a basis for prognosis. Histologic types in common use have been those defined by Jackson and Parker. In this classification the most benign form, Hodgkin's lymphoma or paragranuloma, is essentially a disease of lymph nodes, most frequently of the cervical group. There is a proliferation of lymphocytes, the predominant cell, with disturbance of the architecture of the lymph nodes varying from slight to severe. Variable numbers of Reed-Sternberg cells are present, on which the diagnosis is based. Pleomorphism, necrosis, and fibrosis are absent. In time this type may become transformed into Hodgkin's granuloma. Hodgkin's granuloma, the most frequent variety, is characterized by pleomorphism. Reed-Sternberg cells, eosinophils, necrosis, and fibrosis. Widespread involvement ensues. Hodgkin's sarcoma or lymphoreticuloma has a neoplastic character and is characterized by anaplastic cells, often with frequent mitoses, lymphocytic and reticulum cell hyperplasia, and scattered typical Reed-Sternberg cells. Pleomorphism and fibrosis are not prominent features. The behavior is that of a highly malignant and invasive tumor. This type has a higher proportionate incidence in older age groups.

In the histologic types of Jackson and Parker, classification into the paragranuloma or sarcoma groups appears to have prognostic usefulness. However, only about 10 to 20% of cases of Hodgkin's disease fall into these groups.

Based on studies by Lukes and Butler, a histologic classification into four groups, which appears to have prognostic significance, has been proposed: (1) lymphocytic predominance type, which may have a variable histiocytic component and may be nodular or diffuse; (2) nodular sclerosis type, characterized by orderly bands of connective tissue subdividing abnormal lymphoid tissue into nodules; (3) mixed cellularity type, having a variety of cellular components, which include eosinophils, plasma cells, and neutrophils as well as lymphocytes, histiocytes, and Reed-Sternberg cells, with a variable degree of irregular fibrosis; and (4) lymphocytic depletion type, which may have variable amounts of fibrosis or reticular proliferation or be similar to the Hodgkin's sarcoma type.

LIPIDOSES

The lipidoses (lipid storage diseases) are a group of conditions in which an abnormal accumulation of fatty substance occurs within reticulum cells or tissue histiocytes. Often congenital or familial, they are the result of an abnormality of fat metabolism. It has been debated whether the large fat-holding cells are active participants in the disturbed metabolism or if they simply passively accumulate the lipids in abnormal amount.

Table 16-2. *Lipidoses*

Disease	Lipid substance	Organs and tissues involved
Gaucher's disease	Cerebroside (kerasin)	Spleen, liver, bone marrow, skin, brain (infantile or acute neurologic form)
Niemann-Pick disease	Phospholipid (sphingomyelin principally)	Generalized—reticuloendothelial, epithelial, and connective tissue cells
Amaurotic family idiocy (Tay-Sachs disease)	Ganglioside	Central nervous system —glial and ganglion cells
Xanthomatoses Hand-Schüller-Christian disease	Cholesterol ester	Multiple involvement of skeletal system—bone marrow of skull and femur particularly; lung sometimes involved
Xanthoma palpebrum	Cholesterol	Skin, particularly of upper eyelids
Xanthoma tuberosum multiplex	Cholesterol	Skin, tendons and tendon sheaths, and periarticular tissues

The main types of lipidoses and the fatty materials involved are outlined in Table 16-2.

Gaucher's disease. Gaucher's disease (cerebroside lipidosis) is a chronic familial disease in which a cerebroside (kerasin) accumulates in reticulum cells of the spleen, liver, lymph nodes, and bone marrow. Rare cases in infancy may have an acute course with early death. Beginning in childhood, it extends into adult life, and the course of the disease may extend twenty years or more. The spleen increases progressively in size to reach a weight of 2,000 to 3,000 grams. The liver and lymph nodes are enlarged to lesser degrees. Hemosiderosis, pigmentation of skin and conjunctiva, mild anemia, and leukopenia are usually present. An acute infantile form of the disease in which neurologic manifestations are prominent also occurs.

The hypertrophied spleen is firm, reddish brown in color, and studded with grayish white translucent masses. The liver

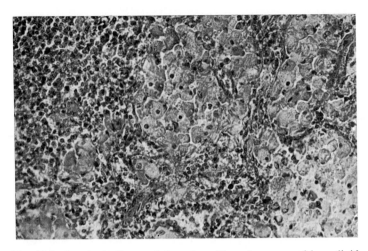

Fig. 16-6. Gaucher's disease of the spleen. Note the masses of large lipid-filled cells.

also is pigmented and shows discrete whitish nodules, and similar masses involve lymph nodes and bone marrow. Microscopically the distinctive feature consists of the large pale Gaucher cells, which compose the grayish translucent areas. These cells measure 20 to 40μ or more in diameter and have a small eccentric nucleus and abundant pale cytoplasm containing fine striations or threads. Multinucleated forms occur. The intracytoplasmic lipid does not stain with the ordinary fat stains. Electron microscopic examination has disclosed that the cellular striations correspond to round, ovoid, or irregular cytoplasmic bodies, which appear related to mitochondria. It has been suggested that the mitochondria are pathogenetically important in the intracellular defect.

Niemann-Pick disease. In Niemann-Pick disease (phosphatide lipidosis, lipid histiocytosis), a phosphatide, sphingomyelin, accumulates in cells of the reticuloendothelial system and in histiocytes in many organs and tissues. Young infants are affected, and death usually occurs before the age of 2 years. The neutral fat, fatty acid, and cholesterol of the blood are increased.

The spleen, liver, lymph nodes, lungs, and bone marrow are most involved, but the lipid-containing cells may be found in any organ. The characteristic cells are smaller than Gaucher cells and have a foamy appearance, caused by many fine vacuoles of lipid in the cytoplasm. There is no hemosiderosis. The disease resembles in some respects the infantile form of amaurotic family idiocy (Tay-Sachs disease), in which a ganglioside is present in the glial and ganglion cells of the nervous system.

Xanthomatosis. Xanthomas are localized accumulations of cells containing lipid (mainly cholesterol). The lesions have a yellow color in the gross appearance and microscopically are made up of large cells filled with doubly refracting lipids. In some cases they are primary or idiopathic, and in other instances they are secondary to disturbances of fat metabolism, as in diabetes mellitus. The commonest sites are in the skin or about tendons. The xanthoma cells are large, rounded, and have a vacuolated cytoplasm. Unlike the other lipidoses, the cells of a xanthoma tend to break down and release their fat, so that a granulomatous reaction and fibrosis may be elements in the lesion.

The *Hand-Schüller-Christian syndrome* is an osseous type of xanthomatosis, the skull particularly being affected. It may occur in childhood or adult life. There is often a characteristic triad of symptoms: defects of membranous bones, exophthalmos, and diabetes insipidus. Blood cholesterol is not increased. The defects in bones are filled by yellow granulomatous material, with many xanthoma cells containing cholesterol. Similar deposits in the pituitary region cause diabetes insipidus and in the orbit lead to exophthalmos. The lung may be involved and become diffusely fibrosed. There is not much generalized storage in the reticuloendothelial system. It is probable that Letterer-Siwe disease and eosinophilic granuloma are variants of this disease or related conditions. Because the pathologic lesions caused by Hand-Schüller-Christian disease, eosinophilic granuloma, and Letterer-Siwe disease have certain common features, the generic term *histiocytosis X* is sometimes used for this group of disorders.

Chapter 17

The blood and blood-forming organs

The conditions in which alteration in the constituents of the blood is the prominent feature are primarily diseases of blood-forming tissue, especially of bone marrow. The changes in the blood, which are most easily studied clinically, are reflections of the basic defect in hematopoietic structure and function. The following is a simplified classification:

Diseases involving red cells
   Deficiency of red cells and hemoglobin—anemia
   Excess of red cells—polycythemia
Diseases involving white cells
   Deficiency of white cells—leukopenia and agranulocytosis
   Excess of white cells—leukocytosis and leukemia
Hemorrhagic diseases

DISEASES INVOLVING RED BLOOD CELLS
Anemia

In anemia there is a quantitative deficiency of hemoglobin, and usually it is accompanied by a corresponding decrease in number of red blood cells. About 14.5 grams of hemoglobin per 100 ml. of blood is the normal for an adult. Different types of anemia show varying degrees of dissociation between the reduction of hemoglobin and of red cells.

General features of anemia. Although anemias of particular types have certain pathologic changes that are more or less characteristic, there are also features common to all severe anemias. These include pallor of skin, mucous membranes, fat, and muscle and fatty change in the heart and liver. In severe anemias fatty degeneration of the myocardium is often of extreme degree and is especially prominent on the endocardial surface where thrush-breast markings may be seen (p. 26). Atrophic changes frequently affect the mucosa of the alimentary canal. Small hemorrhages of the skin and of the mucosal and serous surfaces are common terminally. Red blood cells show variations in size (anisocytosis), shape (poikilocytosis), and staining properties (polychromasia).

Classification of the anemias. An etiologic classification of the anemias is, in many cases, readily correlated with morphologic and other changes in the red cells that can be determined by laboratory tests. It is also helpful as a guide to rational therapy. It is recognized, however, that not all anemias are as yet readily classifiable on this basis.

Anemias resulting from defective erythrocyte formation caused by
    Deficiency
        Deficiency of iron (microcytic and hypochromic anemia)
            Inadequate iron intake or absorption
            Excessive iron loss—as in chronic bleeding
            Chlorosis
            Idiopathic hypochromic anemia
        Deficiency of a specific hematopoietic principle (macrocytic and
            hyperchromic anemia)
            Pernicious anemia
            Sprue
            Megalocytic anemias of pregnancy, etc.
        Other factors
            Aplastic anemia
            Anemia of nephritis
            Anemias resulting from carcinomatosis of bone and osteosclerosis
              (myelophthisic anemia)
            Anemias of thyroid deficiency (myxedema) and scurvy
Anemias resulting from decreased erythrocyte survival (hemolytic dis-
        eases)
    The hemoglobinopathies (e.g., sickle cell anemia)
    Hemolytic disease of newborn (erythroblastosis fetalis)
    Other hemolytic anemias—congenital and acquired
Anemias resulting from loss of blood
    Acute posthemorrhagic anemia
    Chronic posthemorrhagic anemia (leads to iron deficiency)

Iron-deficiency anemias. When there is deficiency of iron supply, hemoglobin cannot be formed in sufficient quantity. Hence the red cells are hypochromic, or have a low concentration of hemoglobin, and tend to be of smaller size (microcytosis). Insufficient dietary intake of iron may be responsible for this type of anemia, but other factors such as failure of absorption or faulty metabolism of the iron may be at fault. Blood loss, particularly chronic bleeding, is a significant cause of iron-deficiency anemia.

Chlorosis is an anemia characterized by a faintly greenish pallor of the skin, and it responds remarkably to iron therapy.

Rarely encountered now, it is said formerly to have been very common among young women.

Idiopathic hypochromic anemia is frequent among middle-aged women. There may be soreness and atrophy of the mucosa of the tongue, and achlorhydria is often present. Dysphagia is a peculiar complication of some cases (Plummer-Vinson syndrome). Iron therapy is effective.

Pernicious anemia. Pernicious anemia (Addison's anemia) was formerly referred to as a primary anemia. It is caused by a deficiency, chiefly of vitamin B_{12}, which occurs predominantly because of a lack of gastric secretion. The gastric deficiency may be related to hereditary predisposition and advancing age, but it also may be brought about by local disease of the stomach or surgical removal of the stomach. In the absence of this substance the normal maturation of erythroblasts to normoblasts is interfered with, and large primitive red cells (megaloblasts) are formed, some of which are passed into the bloodstream along with other immature forms of red cells. The average size of the circulatory red cells is large (i.e., the anemia is macrocytic), and the cells are usually well filled with hemoglobin

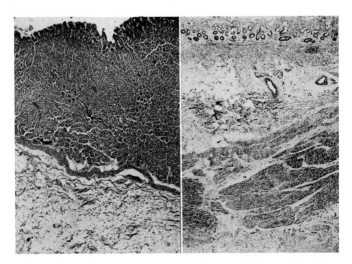

Fig. 17-1. Atrophic gastric mucosa (right) of pernicious anemia contrasted with normal gastric mucosa (left). (×23.)

(hyperchromic). Excessive hemolytic activity (increased destruction of the defective red cells) also is present, as is evident from an abundant hemosiderin deposit in the liver and spleen.

The highest incidence occurs in middle-aged persons. Severe degrees of anemia develop, but temporary remissions are common. Soreness of the tongue, achlorhydria, and gastrointestinal disturbances are usually present. Remarkable results follow liver therapy, which supplies the missing substance necessary for normal blood formation. A few cases are complicated by degenerative lesions in the dorsal and lateral columns of the spinal cord (subacute combined degeneration, p. 891).

In fatal cases the skin and fat may be noted to have a lemon yellow tinge. Fatty degeneration is often prominent in the heart and may be evident also in the liver and kidneys. There is excessive hemosiderin deposit in the liver and spleen. The mucosa of the stomach is atrophic, particularly in the proximal two thirds, with disappearance of oxyntic and peptic cells and replacement of the fundic type of glands by less differentiated abnormal glands. The pyloric portion may be altered only slightly (p. 602). Atrophic changes also affect the epithelium of the tongue.

The hematopoietic tissue of the bones is hyperplastic, and a deep red marrow is found in the long bones, which normally harbor a yellow fatty marrow. The hyperactive marrow is composed almost entirely of erythroblastic tissue.

Sprue and celiac disease. In sprue and celiac disease (steatorrhea) there is intestinal dysfunction or malabsorption syndrome. Macrocytic anemia is often present in these and other intestinal dysfunctions and nutritional deficiencies. The significant deficiency here may be of pteroylglutamic (folic) acid or citrovorum factor (folinic acid). Involvement of the gastrointestinal tract in other ways is followed at times by macrocytic anemia, e.g., in carcinoma of the stomach and *Diphyllobothrium latum* infection.

Aplastic anemia. In aplastic anemia there is a failure of maturation of blood-forming cells at an early undifferentiated stage. An extreme degree of anemia results, in which evidence of regenerative activity of the blood is lacking and the red cells present are of approximately normal size, shape, and staining (normocytic, normochromic). Leukocytes are also depressed. The condition is rapidly progressive and fatal, with hemorrhagic and purpuric phenomena prominent in late stages. The causation is usually unknown, but in some cases chemical poisons such as benzol and trinitrotoluene act as the specific marrow depressant. The greatest incidence is in women during adolescence or early adult life.

The postmortem findings are those of a severe anemia, such as fatty change of the heart and petechial hemorrhages of serous surfaces. The changes actually found in the bone marrow are variable. The normally red marrow may be aplastic, appearing yellow and fatty. In other cases, however, the marrow is active or even hyperplastic, but it exhibits failure of maturation of the hematopoietic cells at an early stage.

Anemia of nephritis. A hypochromic anemia is a common accompaniment of nephritis, sepsis, and other infective conditions. It apparently results from some toxic effect on the bone marrow and responds poorly to treatment unless the causative factor is removed.

Myelophthisic anemia. Myelophthisic anemia is caused by the replacement of the blood-forming tissue of the bone marrow. Widespread tumor growth replacing marrow tissue may act in this way as a result of multiple myeloma (p. 849) or metastatic carcinoma from the breast, thyroid, prostate, kidney, etc. A similar effect is observed in osteosclerotic bone disease in which overgrowth of dense bone encroaches on the marrow (p. 830). Some cases of aleukemic myelosis (myeloid metaplasia) may be associated with marrow fibrosis (p. 576).

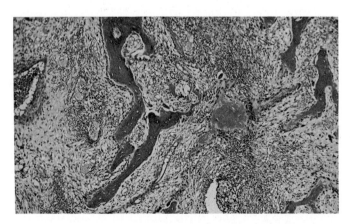

Fig. 17-2. Myelofibrosis associated with metastatic carcinoma.

Anemias of myxedema and scurvy. The anemias of myxedema and scurvy are usually hypochromic. There is evidence that adequate thyroxin and vitamin C are necessary for normal blood formation.

Sickle cell anemia. A mendelian-dominant hereditary peculiarity of red cells is found in about 8% of Negroes. This peculiarity, referred to as sicklemia or the sickle cell trait, is the tendency to assume bizarre shapes when exposed to low oxygen tension, many of the cells becoming elongated, pointed,

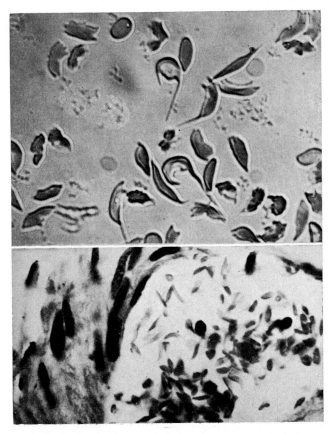

Fig. 17-3. Sickled red blood cells in a moist preparation, above, and in the lumen of a blood vessel, below.

and sickle shaped. The sickling can be observed in blood preserved in sealed moist slide preparations or in tissues fixed in formalin or Zenker's solution. Sickled cells are found in high percentages in the venous circulation in sickle cell anemia but not in the peripheral circulation of persons who have only the sickle cell trait. The anemia is at least partially hemolytic in type, as the sickled red cells have greater mechanical fragility, and there are signs of red cell destruction, as well as of increased regenerative activity on the part of the bone marrow.

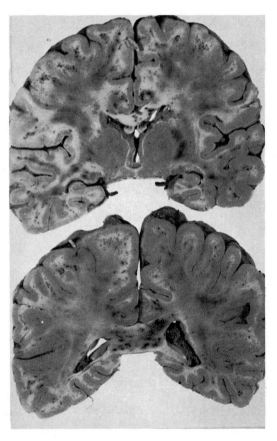

Fig. 17-4. Cerebral lesions in sickle cell disease.

Studies have demonstrated chemical differences in hemo-globins, and several varieties are distinguishable by elec-trophoresis. Sickling or distortion of red blood cells is caused by the presence of hemoglobin S, which in the absence of oxygen is no longer soluble and forms crystals and "tactoids." Hemo-globin S is inherited, wholly or in part. A heterozygous person with a mixture of normal adult hemoglobin and hemoglobin S has the sickle cell trait, and sickling may not occur in the bloodstream, although it may be produced in vitro by depriva-tion of oxygen. A homozygous person with only hemoglobin S may have a sickle cell anemia, as many of the red cells undergo sickling in the peripheral circulation at venous oxygen tensions.

The broader term, *sickle cell disease,* has been used to include all the hereditary and hematologic conditions in which the sickle cell hemoglobin (HbS) is present, including sickle cell trait (Hb A-S), sickle cell anemia (Hb S-S), and various combina-tions of hemoglobin S with other abnormal hemoglobins (e.g. C, D, and E) and with other hereditary diseases such as thalas-semia and spherocytosis.

A milder form of sickle cell anemia has been found in per-sons with a mixture of hemoglobin S and hemoglobin C (sickle cell-Hb-C disease). Thrombotic and hemolytic phenomena similar to those of other sickle cell anemias may be present, sickling occurs in the peripheral blood, and stained smears of the blood show a prominent proportion of target cells.

Pathologic features of sickle cell anemia include the sickled erythrocytes and the thrombi in small vessels, with the develop-

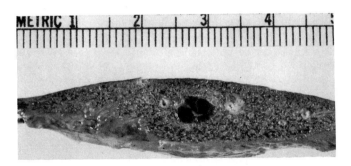

Fig. 17-5. Atrophic and fibrotic spleen of sickle cell anemia.

ment of areas of infarction and fibrosis. Thrombi in cerebral vessels may lead to infarction of the brain. Hemosiderin deposits are found in the spleen, liver, bone marrow, lymph nodes, and kidney. The bone marrow is hyperplastic, and its activity is evident from the regenerative blood picture. The splenic changes in sickle cell anemia are particularly noteworthy. In early stages the spleen is enlarged, and extreme congestion or hemorrhage is noted around the malpighian corpuscles. Later fibrosis develops with noticeable pigment deposits and the formation of siderofibrotic nodules (Gandy-Gamna bodies, p. 540). Fibrotic atrophy of the spleen may progress to an extreme degree.

Sickle cell crises may occur at intervals in individuals with sickle cell disease. The crises may be caused by vascular occlusions in various areas or may be hematologic crises of aplastic or hemolytic type. Persons with sickle cell disease have developed symptoms and lesions when exposed to low oxygen tensions during airplane flights and at high altitudes in mountains. Necrosis in the spleen is particularly common, but infarcts also have been observed in kidneys, brain, and adrenal glands.

Erythroblastosis fetalis. Erythroblastosis (hemolytic disease of the newborn) is a congenital disturbance in which immature red cells are present in the circulation in excessive number. There is an accompanying excessive hemolysis, and extramedullary hematopoiesis (particularly in spleen and liver) is often present. Some cases have severe edema and ascites (hydrops fetalis), while intense and persistent jaundice is prominent in others (icterus gravis neonatorum). The basal ganglia of the brain may show bile pigmentation (kernicterus). Fatty change or even more severe degeneration is sometimes present in the liver. In cases of severe edema of the infant, the placenta is usually enlarged and thick, with an increase in size of the villi.

The Rh factor is important in the pathogenesis of erythroblastosis. About 15% of persons are said to lack the Rh factor in their blood. The child of an Rh-negative mother and an Rh-positive father tends to inherit the dominant Rh factor. In this case the fetus may cause the production of anti-Rh agglutinins in the maternal blood, which in turn penetrate the placental barrier and cause destruction of fetal red cells.

For a similar reason, Rh-negative mothers are likely to suffer serious hemolytic reactions if transfused with Rh-positive blood.

Cooley's anemia is another type of erythroblastic anemia, which has a familial occurrence among Mediterranean races. The bone marrow is hyperplastic, and in the thickened skull trabeculations are prominent on x-ray examination.

Other hemolytic anemias. In addition to sickle cell and erythroblastic anemias there are other forms of hemolytic anemia, congenital and acquired. Among these is hereditary spherocytosis (congenital hemolytic icterus). It is a familial disorder that may become manifest at any age but usually is first detected in childhood. The red cells are rounded, forming biconvex discs (spherocytes), and are excessively fragile. Their fragility is demonstrated by their decreased resistance to hypotonic saline solutions. In such solutions laking begins at a concentration of about 0.7% and is complete at 0.46% (corresponding normal figures are 0.44% and 0.35%). The spherocytosis is regarded as a congenital abnormality in the form of the red cells, which renders them less resistant. It is to be noted, however, that spherocytosis (and increased fragility) may be present in acquired hemolytic anemias also, the changed form resulting from the action of a lytic agent on mature red cells. Hemolysins may be demonstrable in the acquired form. Jaundice results from the excessive bilirubin production, and when the hemolytic action is violent, there may be hemoglobinuria also. Pigment stones often form in the gallbladder. Extreme normoblastic hyperplasia of the bone marrow occurs in an attempt to replace the destroyed red cells, and numerous reticulocytes in the circulating blood reflect this regenerative activity.

The spleen shows the changes of greatest interest, being very much enlarged, with distention and congestion of the pulp sinuses. Excess pigment deposit and even siderofibrotic nodules may be present. Histiocytic proliferation, with phagocytosis of red cells and giant cell formation, is observed in certain cases. Multiple areas of thrombosis and infarction also may be present. Splenectomy is usually followed by prompt clinical recovery. This is apparently caused by removal of the major mechanism of destruction of the fragile red cells, although the fragility of the red cells is not corrected.

Hemolytic anemias of acquired nature may be caused by a variety of infectious, physical, and chemical agents. It also may be the result of immunologic mechanisms, seen in association with known diseases (e.g., collagen diseases), or may be idiopathic. Pernicious anemia also is associated with excessive red cell destruction.

Anemias caused by hemorrhage. Loss of blood is one of the commonest causes of anemia. The loss may be acute and severe, or there may be repeated mild hemorrhages. The anemia is hypochromic in type and may be of severe grade.

Polycythemia

Polycythemia is an increase in number of red blood cells. Counts of 7,000,000 to 10,000,000 red cells per cubic millimeter of blood may occur. The cases can be divided into two groups: (1) *erythrocytosis,* which is a mild type secondary to or compensatory for various conditions in which there is poor oxygenation, such as in congenital heart disease of certain types, pulmonary arteriosclerosis (Ayerza's disease), high altitudes, etc., and (2) *erythremia (polycythemia rubra, Vaquez-Osler disease),* in which the polycythemia is more pronounced and of unknown etiology or not obviously secondary to a condition of poor oxygenation.

Polycythemia rubra usually appears in middle life. It is frequently considered a neoplastic change of erythropoietic cells,

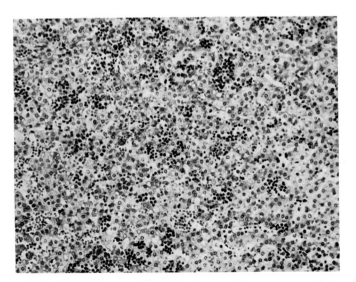

Fig. 17-6. Extramedullary hematopoiesis in the liver.

comparable to a leukemia. Some evidence suggests that it may be caused by local anoxemia in the bone marrow itself as a result of arteriosclerotic or inflammatory changes in skeletal vessels, with excessive erythrogenesis as misdirected overcompensation. The increase of red cells is caused by overproduction rather than by any greater longevity or decreased destruction of the cells. Leukopoietic overactivity also develops in some cases, and there may be termination with leukemia or a myelofibrotic syndrome.

The main pathologic finding is engorgement and hyperplasia of bone marrow. The liver and spleen are enlarged and hyperemic. Engorgement of vessels is widespread; hemorrhages and thromboses are common.

DISEASES INVOLVING WHITE BLOOD CELLS
Agranulocytosis

Agranulocytosis is a depression of leukocyte formation with an extreme decrease in the number of white cells in the blood. It is frequently associated with severe infection and with necrosing ulceration of the mucosa of the mouth and pharynx (agranulocytic angina). The absence of severe anemia distinguishes agranulocytosis from aplastic anemia, and the absence of thrombocytopenia distinguishes it from aleukemia. Most cases are caused by hypersensitivity to the toxic effects of certain drugs, aminopyrine being the most frequent and serious offender. Other cases are caused by dinitrophenol, arsphenamine, thiouracil, and the sulfonamides. The findings in the bone marrow are variable. While usually aplastic, in some cases the marrow appears normal or even hyperplastic.

Primary splenic panhematopenia. A condition in which there appears to be excessive destruction of neutrophilic leukocytes and other blood elements by the spleen has been termed primary splenic panhematopenia, or hypersplenism. In addition to the decrease of granular leukocytes, platelets, and red cells in the peripheral blood, there are splenomegaly and hyperplasia of the bone marrow. Splenectomy is curative, but unremoved accessory spleens may cause recurrence. Examination of the spleen shows enlargement and increase of reticuloendothelial cells throughout the pulp with stagnation or sequestration of blood elements in pulp and sinusoids. It is uncertain whether the mechanism is simply a phagocytic destruction of blood elements or the operation of humoral factors (p. 539).

Leukemia

Leukemia is a condition of lawless overgrowth of white blood cells and proceeds to a fatal ending. It is probably best regarded as a neoplastic change in blood-forming tissue, in most cases accompanied by flooding of the blood and tissues with the excess of white cells, many of which are immature or abnormal forms. Those unusual cases in which excessive or abnormal white cells are not found in the blood are referred to as aleukemic leukemia. The aleukemic condition may be only a transient phase in the course of the disease, but in rare cases it is present from beginning to end.

The etiology of human leukemia is not known, although much effort has been directed in the search for a specific agent. Ionizing radiation as a cause of human leukemia has been long suspected and has been confirmed by studies on atomic bomb victims in Hiroshima and Nagasaki. Acute leukemias and chronic granulocytic leukemia was increased in the irradiated population. Exposure to ionizing radiation during fetal life and childhood appears to have more dangerous leukemogenic effect than in adult life.

Among chemical poisons, benzol appears to have a best established leukemogenic activity.

A possible viral etiology of leukemia has had much recent study. Although viral agents have been accepted as a cause of leukemia in mice, the evidence in human leukemia for a viral etiology is still incomplete. Outbreaks of leukemia cases in "clusters" have suggested an infective agent. Electron microscopy has provided suggestive evidence of the association of virus-like particles and mycoplasma (PPLO) in cells of human leukemia, although a viral agent has not been isolated and propagated.

Most patients with chronic myelocytic leukemia have shown an abnormal chromosome, the ph^1, or Philadelphia, chromosome, and other chromosomal abnormalities have been observed with less regularity in various leukemias. Genetic damage and somatic mutation may be the mechanism of neoplastic transformation in leukemogenesis.

The bone marrow, considered as a blood-forming organ, is large and labile in activity. In the adult it comprises about 1,400 ml., almost the size of the liver. Only a small proportion of this organ, represented by red marrow, normally is active in blood production. The remaining latent yellow or fatty marrow is replaced by active red marrow when there is greater demand for blood cells. In leukemias the entire marrow may be activated into grayish red, densely cellular, leukocyte-forming tissue. Crowding out of erythroblastic tissue results in anemia.

According to the type of white cell involved, the leukemias are classed as myeloid, lymphatic, and monocytic. Each of these may be acute or chronic, but the acute types are difficult to distinguish from each other. In the lymphogenous leukemias, the lymphatics of the spleen are involved with leukemic cells, but they are not appreciably affected in myelogenous leukemia. In the liver, portal space lymphatic spaces are similarly affected in lymphatic leukemia. whereas in myeloid leukemia the hemic vascular system of the liver and spleen are involved. There is a different age incidence for the various types. Acute leukemia has its maximum incidence in the first decade; chronic myeloid leukemia occurs between 25 and 45 years and chronic lymphoid leukemia, between 45 and 60 years. The monocytic type tends to occur more frequently in middle or older age periods. There is evidence that the occurrence of leukemia is persons over 50 years of age is increasing.

Acute leukemia. Acute leukemia may begin suddenly and it runs a rapid course of a few weeks or months. Early stages may be aleukemic, but later the white blood count becomes very high although less than the extreme figures of chronic leukemia. Anemia and thrombocytopenia are often severe. The majority of white cells in the blood are myeloblasts or lymphoblasts, the distinction between these primitive cells being difficult and unreliable. At autopsy the bone marrow is everywhere hyperplastic and packed with the same primitive white cells. The spleen, lymph nodes, and tonsils are usually moderately enlarged, and their sinuses are filled by the leukemic cells. These cells may also be found infiltrating the liver, heart, kidneys, and other viscera.

Chronic myeloid leukemia. In the myelogenous type of leukemia there is a great increase in granular leukocytes in the blood, and many immature cells (myelocytes and myeloblasts) are recognizable in blood smears. The total white count may become very high, reaching 500,000 or more per cubic millimeter in some cases. Platelets also may be increased, but red cells progressively diminish in number. The course of the disease may extend over several years before the inevitably fatal end.

The essential lesion is a myeloid hyperplasia throughout the

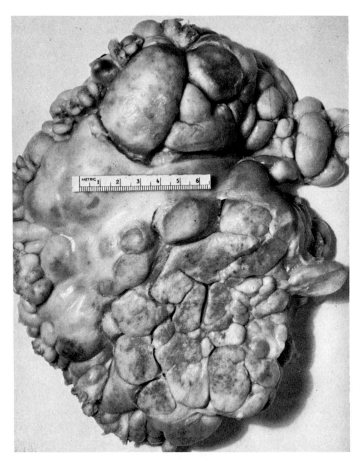

Fig. 17-7. Mesenteric lymph nodes in chronic lymphatic leukemia.

bone marrow, including the marrow of long bones, which normally is yellow and fatty. The marrow tissue is grayish brown and fairly firm. Myelocytes are predominant microscopically, but granular leukocytes in all stages of development are present. The spleen becomes enormously enlarged, dark red, and firm. Masses of myeloid cells replace the tissues and obscure the usual splenic architecture. The liver is also considerably enlarged and is infiltrated by myeloid cells. Similar but milder

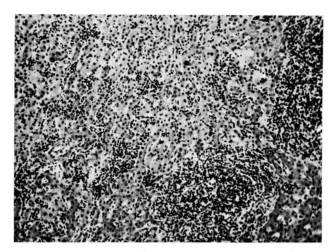

Fig. 17-8. Leukemic infiltration of the liver.

myeloid infiltration is found in the kidneys, heart, and other viscera. The unusual number of leukocytes in the lumina of blood vessels may be noted in any organ or tissue. Lymph nodes are only slightly enlarged. Infarcts occur commonly in the spleen, more so than in chronic lymphatic leukemia.

Chronic lymphatic leukemia. The white count is lower in lymphatic leukemia than in the myeloid type. It is usually below 100,000, and often 90% or more are lymphoid cells. Red cell reduction and anemia occur in late stages but to a lesser degree than in myeloid leukemia.

The lymph nodes all over the body are enlarged, and their normal microscopic architecture is replaced by a diffuse mass of lymphoid cells. Other lymphoid tissue, as in the tonsils, thymus, intestine, etc., is similarly affected. The spleen is moderately enlarged by lymphoid hyperplasia, but not to the extreme degree characteristic of myeloid leukemia. Lymphoid accumulation is found also in the liver, kidneys, skin, etc. The bone marrow is hyperplastic throughout, firm, grayish red, and similar grossly to the marrow of myeloid leukemia. Except in early stages, the hyperplastic marrow is composed largely of lymphoid cells.

Monocytic leukemia. The leukemia in which mature and

immature monocytes are prominent in the blood are referred to as monocytic. Two varieties are often included. The *Naegeli type* is characterized by immature cells intermediate between myeloblasts and monocytes and is probably a variety of myeloid leukemia. In the *Schilling type* the immature cells resemble monocytes and reticuloendothelial cells. In this latter variety there is hyperplasia throughout the reticuloendothelial system, and to such cases the term *leukemic reticuloendotheliosis* has been applied (p. 548). The histologic appearance may resemble that of Hodgkin's disease.

Monocytic leukemia tends to run a rather acute course, often with swelling and hemorrhages of the oral mucosa. Skin lesions are more frequent than in the other types of leukemia.

Leukosarcoma. A localized tumor composed of either lymphocytic or myelogenous cells, with the development of a leukemic blood picture, is referred to as a leukosarcoma.

Chloroma. Rare cases of myeloid leukemia of rather acute type and in children or young adults, have associated tumor masses of a pale greenish color, referred to as chloroma. The greenish color fades rapidly on exposure to air. The tumor masses are found in close relationship to the periosteum of the bones of the face, ribs, sternum, or vertebrae and, less commonly, in viscera. Microscopically chloroma is composed of myeloblastic cells.

Myelofibrosis. A condition variously termed primary myelofibrosis, myelosclerosis with myeloid metaplasia, aleukemic myelosis, agnogenic myeloid metaplasia, and leukoerythroblastic anemia is considered by some a variant form of myeloid leukemia and by others a nonspecific response of potential hematopoietic cells of the spleen and liver to a wide variety of stimuli, and of a fundamentally different nature from leukemia. It is characterized by a slowly progressive splenomegaly, with diffuse myeloid metaplasia in a person of middle age or beyond, sometimes with some enlargement of the liver. The liver, and sometimes lymph nodes, also show foci of proliferating myeloid cells and of giant cells of megakaryocytic type. Usually there is no significant peripheral lymph node enlargement. Occasionally tumorlike masses of extramedullary myeloid tissue are found. The peripheral blood picture is variable, but there may be anemia with the presence of immature red blood cells and leukocytosis with or without leukemoid features. Sometimes there is an antecedent history of polycythemia ruba vera. The bone marrow is variable. It may be fibrotic, normocellular, or even hyperplastic. The clinical course is often prolonged but slowly progressive and irreversible. Splenectomy is contraindicated. Radiotherapy appears to be of little benefit. Myelofibrosis, sometimes associated with metastatic cancer, may produce a similar picture.

HEMORRHAGIC DISEASES

The oversimplified classic theory of blood coagulation has been expressed as two equations:

Prothrombin + thromboplastin + calcium = thrombin
Fibrinogen + thrombin = fibrin

It has been shown that the chemistry of blood coagulation is much more involved and complicated than depicted in the foregoing equations and that numerous factors which have been given various names play some role in the process. The more common hemorrhagic disorders may be classified in this fashion.

Diminished prothrombin caused by
    Lack of vitamin K
        Dietary origin
            Hemorrhagic disease of the newborn
        Faulty absorption
            Lack of bile salts
            Obstructive jaundice
            Biliary fistula
            Sprue
    Liver damage
        Faulty utilization of vitamin K
            Acute yellow atrophy
            Chloroform poisoning
Deficiency of platelets or thromboplastin generation
    Diminished number of platelets
        Thrombocytopenic purpura
    Deficiency of antihemophilic globulin
        Hemophilia
Decreased fibrinogen
    Acquired
        Nutritional deficiencies
        Diseases of blood-forming organs
        Severe liver damage
        Amniotic fluid embolism
        Visceral carcinomas
        Severe burns
    Congenital

Anticoagulants in the blood
  Circulating anticoagulants
      During or following pregnancy
      In leukemia and other neoplasias
      In systemic lupus erythematosus
  Excessive anticoagulant therapy
Primary vascular defects
  Hereditary
      Hereditary hemorrhagic telangiectasia
  Acquired
      Vitamin C deficiency
      Allergic purpura

Purpura

Purpura is the condition of petechial and ecchymotic hemorrhages in the skin and mucous membranes. Symptomatic purpura occurs in various conditions, such as leukemia, severe
anemia, and severe infections such as smallpox, streptococcal
septicemia, etc. One type of purpura, however, appears to be a
disease entity. It is associated with a decrease in the number of
blood platelets (thrombocytopenia).

Thrombocytopenic purpura. Thrombocytopenic purpura
(purpura hemorrhagica, Werlhof's disease) not only has a deficiency of platelets but also has some weakness or dysfunction of
the walls of small blood vessels. Spontaneous hemorrhages occur
into the skin, mucous membranes, joints, and intestinal tract.
It occurs chiefly in children and young adults.

The bone marrow is of normal appearance and contains a
normal proportion of megakaryocytes. It has been suggested
that the platelet deficiency is caused by thrombocytolysis rather
than by deficient formation. Megakaryocytes may be found in
the sinuses of the spleen and liver. The spleen also shows enlarged and hyperactive germinal centers. The finding of anti-
platelet antibody in patients with this disease suggests that an
autoimmune mechanism may play a role in the pathogenesis.

**Thrombotic thrombocytopenic purpura (diffuse platelet
thrombosis, thrombocytopenic verrucal angionecrosis).** Thrombotic thrombocytopenic purpura appears to be a disseminated
disease of capillaries and arterioles, characterized by diffuse
hyaline or platelet thromboses. The arterioles and capillaries are
partially or completely occluded by a hyaline or finely granular
eosinophilic material that may be covered by an endothelial
lining. A degenerative process in the vascular walls may be
the primary process. The myocardium, renal cortex, capsular

zone of the adrenal gland, and brain are mainly involved, but other organs also may show the lesions. The clinical syndrome is characterized by acute onset with fever, hemolytic anemia, thrombocytopenic purpura, and sometimes bizarre neurologic manifestations (the *Moschcowitz syndrome*). The disease is fatal within a few weeks. The etiology is unknown, but some evidence suggests that hypersensitivity may be concerned, and there may be similarities to some of the so-called collagen diseases (p. 805).

Hemophilia

Hemophilia is an inherited abnormality of the blood, transmitted as a sex-linked recessive mendelian factor and appearing only in males. The coagulation time of the blood is prolonged, but the bleeding time, clot retraction, prothrombin time, platelet count, and tourniquet test are normal. Severe and prolonged hemorrhages follow trivial injuries. The classical hemophilia (or hemophilia A), which is referred to here, is caused by a deficiency of factor VIII (antihemophilic globulin). Certain hemophilia-like disorders exist in which other factors are deficient (e.g., factor IX [Christmas factor], factor X, etc.).

Chapter 18

The mouth, throat, and neck

T he skin of the face and neck is subject to most of the diseases that involve skin elsewhere (see Chapter 23). The face is a common site for carcinoma. Carcinomas of the upper half of the face are usually of the basal cell type, whereas squamous carcinoma is more likely to be found on the lower part of the face. The face and neck are common sites for malignant melanoma, sometimes as a transformation of a benign nevus.

MOUTH
Congenital malformations

The most important developmental abnormalities are cleft lip (harelip) and cleft palate. Clefts occur at places where embryonic processes that should join have failed to unite during embryonic development. In harelip there is a failure of fusion of the processus globularis and the maxillary process on one or both sides, the cleft being slightly to one side of the midline. Cleft palate may be present with or without associated harelip. Hereditary influence is important.

Inflammations

Inflammation in the mouth (stomatitis) may be a local condition or part of a generalized disease.

Scarlet fever. In scarlet fever one sees hyperemia and reddening of the mucosa of the mouth and tongue.

Aphthous stomatitis. Aphthous stomatitis is characterized by painful, recurrent, erosive oral ulcerations, covered by a gray membrane and surrounded by a thin erythematous ring. The primary cause is unknown but possibly is a complex of infection, probably streptococcal, and hypersensitivity.

Measles. In measles Koplik's spots are an early sign. They are small yellowish spots on a red background, seen on the mucosal surface of the cheeks in the upper molar region.

Mercurial or arsenical compounds. Mercurial or arsenical compounds may cause ulcerative stomatitis.

Vincent's organisms. Vincent's organisms, a spirochete and fusiform bacillus, cause ulcerative and membranous inflammations of the gums as well as in the tonsillar and pharyngeal regions.

Agranulocytosis. Severe ulcerative inflammations of the mouth or pharynx often complicate agranulocytosis.

Leukemias. In leukemias, infiltration of the gingiva is common, with hemorrhage and ulceration.

Thrush. Debilitated infants and children particularly are subject to thrush, a local membranous lesion of the mouth caused by *Candida albicans.*

Noma. Noma is a progressive gangrenous ulcerative condition, which may lead to perforation of the cheeks.

Syphilis. Syphilis may be represented by lesions of the lips or mouth in either primary or secondary stages (p. 185).

Tuberculosis. Tuberculous lesions of the mouth are uncommon.

Tumors

Cancer of the mouth is in most cases squamous carcinoma. It may arise from the lip or any area of the oral mucosa, but in more than half of the intraoral cases it involves the tongue.

Leukoplakia. In leukoplakia of the mouth there are irregular whitish areas on the mucosa of the lips, cheeks, tongue, or elsewhere. Oral cancer is frequently preceded by leukoplakia and begins as carcinoma in situ, so that leukoplakia probably corresponds to the precancerous keratoses of the skin. The squamous epithelium is thickened, with acanthosis or thickening of the prickle cell layer and chronic inflammatory cells in the subepithelial layers. As transformation occurs, the rete pegs become more irregular and prolonged, and there is intraepithelial development of cells of malignant appearance. Later, infiltration or invasion may occur.

The in situ cancer frequently extends beyond the apparent gross margin of the tumor. Oral carcinomas tend to have a greater extension laterally than in depth. Leukoplakia appears to be associated with about 20% of oral cancers. Oral carcinoma is frequently multiple or appears to arise in a multicentric or multifocal manner.

A verrucose, well-differentiated squamous carcinoma, of a low degree of malignancy, sometimes develops in the gingivobuccal groove in "snuff dippers," who leave tobacco snuff in this location for extended periods of time.

Carcinoma of the lip. Cancer of the lip is common, particularly in males. About 95% occur on the lower lip at the mucocutaneous junction, and almost all are of the squamous cell type. The infrequent carcinomas of the upper lip are more often of the basal cell type and show little difference in sexual incidence. Trauma and chronic irritation resulting from jagged or carious teeth, pipe smoking, etc. are believed to be contributing causes. Lesions such as keratoses, leukoplakia, and chronic fissures may precede the development of actual cancer. The greatest incidence is in the fifth and sixth decades of life.

The early cancer may be a small nodule, warty excrescence, or chronic fissure. It develops into a painless ulcer, which grows slowly. It is to be distinguished from a syphilitic chancre of the lip, which is less well defined and shows evidence of inflammation. Biopsy and microscopic diagnosis are essential in most cases.

Metastasis occurs to lymph nodes of the submental and submaxillary groups and from there to the jugular chain of lymph nodes. More distant metastasis is rare. Extension to lymph nodes occurs earlier in the forms with microscopic evidence of high malignancy.

Carcinoma of the tongue. Cancer of the tongue is more common in men and has its greatest incidence in the sixth through eighth decades. Its most frequent sites are the lateral borders and undersurfaces of the anterior two thirds of the tongue. Chronic irritations and leukoplakia may be contributing etiologic factors, as in other cancers of the mouth. The most usual form is a small ulcer or fissure, but papillary or fungating lesions also occur. The tumors are squamous carcinomas of varying grades of differentiation. Metastasis occurs most frequently to upper deep cervical lymph nodes adjacent to the bifurcation of the common carotid artery. Extension to other groups of nodes and metastasis to other tissues tend to be more widespread than in carcinoma of the lip. Cure rates are higher for cancer of the dorsum and the anterior one third of the tongue than for the posterior one third.

Epulis. The term *epulis* is rather loosely used to indicate any benign connective tissue tumor of the gums. There are two main histologic forms: (1) giant cell epulis, in which giant cells and blood vessels are prominent, and (2) fibromatous epulis, in which connective tissue is predominant. The giant cell form is similar histologically to the benign giant cell tumors found elsewhere (p. 847). The variable histologic form may simply represent stages in the development of an epulis. Epulis is often preceded by local mechanical injury to the place of origin, or it may grow in the socket of an extracted tooth. The tumors are benign and do not metastasize, but they may recur if incompletely removed. The rare congenital epulis occurs mainly in the incisor region of the maxilla in females. It is histologically distinct and probably is a hamartoma of a tooth bud. The focal form of gingivitis gradivarum, or "pregnancy tumor," may simulate an epulis. Developing during the first two or three months of pregnancy, it appears to be on a hormonal basis.

The so-called congenital pigmented epulis of infancy also has been called melanotic adamantinoma, retinal anlage tumor, etc. It is a rare benign lesion of the maxilla of infants, probably of neural crest origin. The tumor has an abundant connective tissue stroma, with tubular or gland spaces lined by cuboidal cells with abundant pigment granules.

JAWS
Tumors

The various tumors that occur in other bones may also be found in the bones of the jaws (p. 842). In addition a group

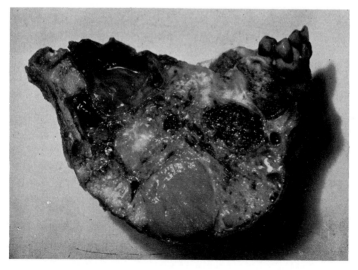

Fig. 18-1. Adamantinoma of the jaw.

of tumors arise from epithelial or mesoblastic tissues of developing teeth. A simple classification of these includes (1) odontogenic cysts and (2) odontogenic tumors (epithelial and mesodermal).

Odontogenic cysts. *Dentigerous cysts* are benign cystic structures in the jaws, are lined by epithelium, and contain one or more imperfectly developed teeth. Trauma may be important in the development of a cyst about an unerupted tooth. *Radicular cysts,* formed by chronic inflammation at the opening of the pulp canal, are lined by a squamous epithelium derived from epithelial rests of Malassez in the periodontal membrane.

Odontogenic tumors. Tumors of odontogenic origin are infrequent but of considerable variety and complexity. They may be grouped into epithelial and mesodermal types. The epithelial odontogenic tumors include a variety of ameloblastic tumors, dentinomas, and various odontomas.

Odontomas are the result of disturbances of tooth development that may lead to an atypical growth of enamel, dentine, cementum, or all three hard substances. Odontomas grow slowly and are surrounded by a capsule. The rare soft odontoma is formed either from the dentinal papilla or periodontal membrane.

Ameloblastomas (adamantinomas) are epithelial tumors arising from cells with a potentiality for forming the enamel organ. Their histologic structure resembles certain developmental stages of the enamel organ, but origin as a downgrowth from oral epithelium has also been considered. They are composed of irregular masses of epithelial cells divided by a connective tissue stroma. The epithelial masses are outlined by a palisade of dark-staining columnar epithelial cells. In rare instances some keratinization occurs. Cyst formation is common within the epithelial masses, so that solid, cystic, and combined forms occur.

The tumor is most common in the mandible and usually appears in persons before the age of 35 years. While ordinarily it does not metastasize, irregular local extension occurs, and the tumor will recur unless removal is complete. A few malignant forms with metastasis have been reported.

Tumors histologically similar to those of the mandible arise in the pituitary region (craniopharyngioma, p. 671) and in the tibia (p. 849).

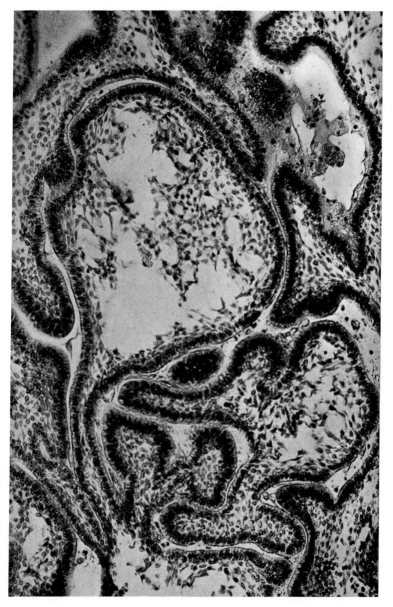

Fig. 18-2. Adamantinoma of the jaw (microscopic section of the tumor shown in Fig. 18-1).

Mesodermal odontogenic tumors include odontogenic fibro-myxomas and cementifying fibromas.

PHARYNX
Inflammations

Pharynigitis is commonly caused by streptococcal infection, although diphtheria, viruses, and Vincent's organisms also cause characteristic pharyngeal inflammations. The tonsils are most frequently involved and are swollen and reddened with exudate on the surface and in tonsillar crypts. When the crypts are prominently distended with pus, it is often termed follicular tonsillitis. Epidemic tonsillitis is sometimes a milk-borne streptococcal infection. *Quinsy* is a peritonsillar abscess that may complicate acute tonsillitis. *Ludwig's angina* is a diffuse cellulitis or spread of the infection to involve structures of the neck.

Tumors

Highly malignant tumors occur in the pharynx, arising most commonly from the posterior wall of the nasopharynx or from the tonsil. They are characterized by an earlier age incidence than that of cancers in general, by predominance in the male, and by a tendency to early metastasis to the lymph nodes of the neck, to the orbit, or to the cranial cavity. Metastasis may appear before the primary growth is noted. As a group they are highly radiosensitive tumors. This factor, plus their surgical inaccessibility, makes radiation the usual form of treatment.

Most of these tumors can be classified as (1) squamous cell carcinoma, (2) transitional cell carcinoma, (3) lymphoepithelioma, and (4) lymphosarcoma. Teratomas of the pharynx and solitary myelomas (plasmacytomas) also occur.

Squamous cell carcinoma. Squamous cell carcinoma forms a coarsely granular elevated tumor with an indurated border and ulcerated surface. Its histologic appearance is similar to that of squamous carcinoma elsewhere, with evidence of keratinization.

Transitional cell carcinoma. Transitional cell carcinoma is an epidermoid cancer in which keratinization is absent. It forms a smaller, flatter lesion than does the squamous type, with a finely granular surface. Histologically the tumor is composed of small uniform cells having large hyperchromatic nuclei and scanty cytoplasm. The cells are more undifferentiated than those of the squamous variety.

Lymphoepithelioma. This tumor, described by Regaud and Schmincke, is one in which wide sheets and cords of undifferentiated malignant epithelial cells are intimately associated with lymphoid tissue or infiltrated with lymphocytes. Many believe that this is not a distinct type of tumor but that its representatives are more properly classified as transitional cell carcinomas, although electron microscopic studies suggest that many of the undifferentiated tumors are squamous cell carcinomas.

Lymphosarcoma. Lymphosarcoma may occur in a localized form or as part of a generalized lymphomatosis.

Nasopharyngeal fibroma. Nasopharyngeal fibroma is an uncommon tumor developing mainly in boys at or near the age of puberty and tending to undergo spontaneous regression by about 25 years of age. It has been considered to arise from periosteum of bone of the vault or posterior wall of the nasopharynx, but a vascular or angiomatous origin with sex-endocrine relationships also has been proposed. The hard tumor is composed of dense but highly vascular connective tissue. It is essentially benign but may be serious because of its progressive growth before sexual maturity and its tendency to profuse hemorrhage.

Laryngeal tumors are considered on p. 428.

SALIVARY GLANDS

Disturbances of the salivary glands include inflammations, duct obstruction (usually caused by calculi), and tumors.

Inflammations

Acute parotitis. Acute parotitis occurs in the epidemic virus disease *mumps* (p. 176) and, as a result of staphylococcal infection, is an occasional complication after surgical operations.

Mikulicz's syndrome. This condition is a bilateral enlargement of the parotid glands, sometimes with involvement of the other salivary glands and lacrimal glands. It may be of inflammatory origin (tuberculosis, sarcoid, etc.) or be caused by leukemic infiltration or Hodgkin's disease.

Mikulicz's disease. Also known as *benign lymphoepithelial lesion,* Mikulicz's disease is of unknown cause and is characterized by enlargement, usually bilateral, of the parotid and sometimes the submaxillary glands. Microscopically, atrophied acini are replaced by considerable lymphocytic infiltration, and there are islands of epithelium resulting from ductal proliferation.

Sjögren's syndrome. Sjögren's syndrome occurs mainly in

women over the age of 30 years. It is characterized by dryness of the conjunctiva, mouth, nose, pharynx, and larynx, with intermittent swelling of the lacrimal glands and in many cases rheumatoid arthritis. The etiology and the relationship to arthritis is obscure. Autoimmunity has been suggested as an etiologic factor. The conjunctival, lacrimal, and salivary glands and the submucous glands of the respiratory and upper alimentary tract show atrophic changes, which account for the impaired function. The involved glands are enlarged, and there is parenchymal atrophy with replacement by lymphocytic infiltration and epithelial islands of ductal proliferation as in Mikulicz's disease.

Ranula. Ranula is a cyst in the floor of the mouth, such as may result from a sublingual gland, a mucous gland, or the submaxillary duct.

Uveoparotid fever. Uveoparotid fever (Heerfordt's syndrome) is a granulomatous involvement of the parotid glands and uveal tract (iris, ciliary body). It appears to be a form of sarcoidosis (p. 799).

Tumors

A variety of tumors occur in the salivary glands, including both the major salivary glands and the minor foci of salivary gland tissue of the palate and other areas of oral mucosa. However, a very large proportion of salivary gland tumors occur in the parotid gland, are benign, and are "mixed tumors." The submaxillary glands are involved with some frequency; the sublingual gland is involved only rarely.

Benign mixed tumor. Benign mixed tumors of salivary gland tissue show varying proportions of epithelial and connective tissues. They may develop at any age, but the highest incidence is in early or middle adult life. About 90% occur in the parotid gland, and about 60% occur in females. Although there are various theories of origin, most evidence suggests that origin is from salivary gland or intercalated duct epithelium and that the components of the connective tissue type arise by metaplasia. Theories of origin from embryonal rests or branchial cleft tissue have little supporting evidence.

Benign mixed tumors are solitary, round or oval, and usually 2 to 5 cm. in diameter, occasional examples being much larger. Although circumscribed and encapsulated, irregular local extensions through the capsule are common. Complete removal is often difficult, and recurrence is a common event (20 to 30%).

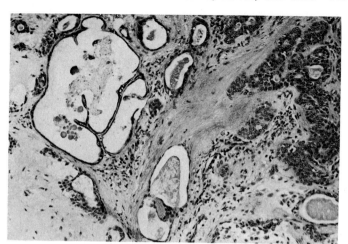

Fig. 18-3. Mixed tumor of the parotid gland.

Recurrent tumor masses are commonly multiple separate nodules. One of the serious complications of the removal of a parotid tumor is injury to the facial nerve.

The histologic picture is complex and variable. The neoplastic cells in these tumors may be secreting epithelial cells, myoepithelial ("basket") cells, or both. These are types of cells normally found in salivary glands. There are usually irregular masses or anastomosing strands of stellate or epithelial cells surrounded by connective tissue. The connective tissue portion is often myxomatous in appearance but may be fibrous or cellular. Myxomatous transformation of epithelial elements has been described. Areas of true cartilage or bone may be formed by metaplasia. More common is pseudocartilage, a chondroid myxomatous degeneration of the stroma resulting from the secretion of myoepithelial mucin of the "connective tissue" type. Glandular areas and occasionally metaplastic squamous epithelium may be present.

Mixed tumors often grow very slowly and may be present for years with few symptoms. Rapid enlargement in a tumor that has been present for years and is stationary or only slowly growing suggests a malignant change in the tumor. Also a mixed tumor that has become malignant is more likely to produce local severe pain.

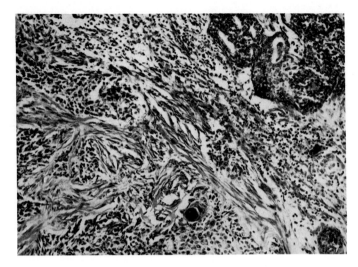

Fig. 18-4. Malignant mixed tumor of the parotid gland.

Malignant mixed tumor. Malignant mixed tumors of salivary gland tissue probably arise most often as a malignant change in a previously existent benign tumor and at an average age of about 10 years more than with benign mixed tumors. They are usually larger than benign tumors and tend to be fixed to underlying tissues or to the skin, which may be ulcerated. Regional lymph nodes may be enlarged by metastasis. Although the gross appearance may be similar to that of the benign mixed tumors, there is a greater tendency to areas of softening, necrosis, hemorrhage, or cyst formation. The histologic appearance may be predominantly that of glandular or solid carcinoma, but occasionally it is that of squamous carcinoma.

Mucoepidermoid carcinoma. Mucoepidermoid carcinomas of salivary tissue are of ductal origin and contain both mucus-secreting and epidermoid cells. They vary greatly in degree of malignancy. About 90% occur in the parotid gland and the remainder occur in the submaxillary glands. Rare examples have been reported within the mandible. They are more common in females and occur most often in the fourth and fifth decades. Those of higher grade malignancy tend to be larger, occur with equal frequency in males, occur at a slightly later average age,

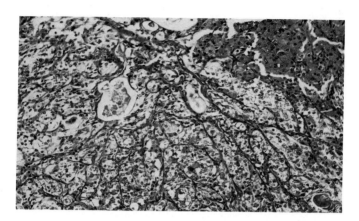

Fig. 18-5. Mucoepidermoid tumor of the parotid gland.

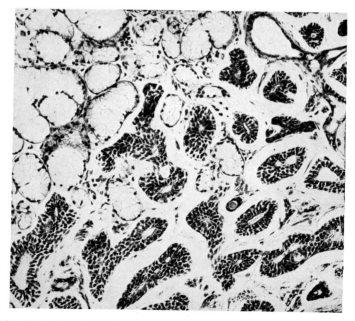

Fig. 18-6. Adenoid cystic tumor of a salivary gland.

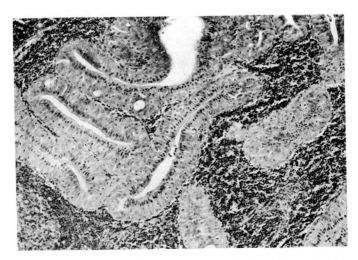

Fig. 18-7. Adenolymphoma (Warthin's tumor) of a salivary gland.

and are more likely to produce pain or to be associated with facial nerve paralysis. Encapsulation of the tumor is usually incomplete or lacking, and a cystic structure is common. Rare squamous cell carcinomas without a mucus-secreting element also occur.

Adenocarcinoma. Adenocarcinoma (adenoid cystic carcinoma, cylindroma) is a relatively infrequent salivary gland tumor arising with about equal frequency in parotid and submaxillary glands. These tend to be of relatively slow growth and low grade of malignancy. The tumor cells are small and dark staining, with relatively abundant cytoplasm, and they grow in solid masses, in anastomosing cords, or with an adenoid cystic pattern. Acellular areas between strands of tumor cells contain mucoid material and tend to undergo hyalinization. Perineural lymphatic extension of the tumor is common. Adenocarcinomas of various other patterns or of anaplastic appearance also occur but are infrequent.

Acinic cell adenocarcinoma. Acinic cell adenocarcinoma is an uncommon parotid tumor of low-grade malignancy; it is composed of cells with abundant clear or slightly granular cytoplasm and small dark eccentric nuclei. The tumor cells resemble the serous cells of the salivary gland acini.

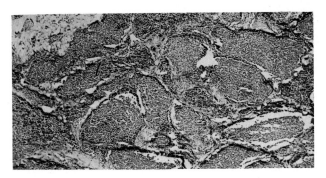

Fig. 18-8. Carotid body tumor. The tendency to rounded masses of tumor cells is evident.

Oncocytoma (oxyphil cell adenoma). Oncocytoma is a rare, benign, encapsulated salivary gland tumor composed of cells with eosinophilic granular cytoplasm and small dark nuclei.

Papillary cystadenoma lymphomatosum (adenolymphoma, Warthin's tumor). Papillary cystadenoma lymphomatosum is a benign, encapsulated cystic tumor occurring in or attached to the parotid gland. It is rounded, soft, and 2 to 6 cm. in diameter. Microscopically it is composed of papillary, tubular, or cystic epithelial structures having a double layer of deeply eosinophilic cells and set in a lymphoid tissue. It occurs predominantly in males. Although the origin is debatable, most evidence suggests that it is from salivary gland or duct tissue inclusions in lymph nodal tissue either in the parotid gland or adjacent to it.

NECK
Carotid body tumors

The rare tumors of the carotid body are found at the upper end of the common carotid artery in close relationship to the point of bifurcation. They are slowly growing tumors that remain encapsulated until a late stage but are potentially malignant. A few reported cases have metastasized. Microscopically they are composed of rounded groups of large polyhedral epithelial cells with small uniform nuclei and poorly defined boundaries. The cells have a tendency to an alveolar arrangement and are closely associated with a vascular fibrous stroma. Some of the tumors are more sarcomatous in appearance. An abundant innervation has been demonstrated as well as cells containing argentaffin granules. Rare tumors of the middle ear arise from the glomus jugularis of the temporal bone and have a similar character and histologic appearance (glomus jugularis tumors). Similar tumors also may arise from other so-called paraganglionic glomera in relation to various vessels and nerves in the neck and upper mediastinum. Tumors composed of such chemoreceptor cells associated with parasympathetic nerves have been called chemodectomas.

Cysts of the neck

Cysts of the neck, arising from vestigial rests, may be of thyroglossal duct origin (midline) or branchiogenic origin (lateral). Lymphatic vessels may also give rise to cysts.

Thyroglossal cysts. A thyroglossal cyst may occur anywhere between the base of the tongue and the thyroid. They are smooth-walled cysts lined by columnar or flattened epithelium.

Branchial cleft cyst. The branchial cleft cyst most frequently appears near the angle of the jaw. The cyst lining is squamous epithelium, and lymphoid tissue is abundant in the wall.

Cystic hygroma. The cystic hygroma is a lymphangiomatous cyst of the neck, usually of congenital origin (p. 316 and Fig. 12-14).

Chapter 19

The alimentary tract

Although divided into the anatomic regions of esophagus, stomach, duodenum, small and large bowel, etc., all portions of the alimentary canal consist of a hollow tube, lined by secretory mucosa and having a muscular wall with peristaltic or sphincteric actions controlled by nervous influences. The same types of disease processes occur in each and follow the same general rules but vary in their relative frequency and importance in the different portions. These types are (1) congenital malformations, (2) diverticula, (3) inflammations and ulcerations, (4) obstructions of the lumen, acute and chronic, and (5) tumors. Table 19-1 outlines the main lesions of the alimentary canal.

ESOPHAGUS

Congenital atresia. Congenital atresia of the esophagus is the only developmental abnormality that is common. In most cases there is an associated tracheoesophageal fistula.

Diverticula. Diverticula may be of the *pulsion* type, with pressure within the esophagus forcing the wall outward at a weak point, or it may be the result of *traction* caused by inflammatory adhesions to surrounding structures. The pulsion type is more common and usually involves the posterior wall at the upper end of the esophagus. The traction type is usually anterior and at about the level of the tracheal bifurcation. Adhesions to tuberculous mediastinal lymph nodes are the usual initiating factor.

Esophagitis. Esophagitis resulting from infection is not a common lesion, although thrush (monilial) esophagitis may occur in malnourished infants. Acute and subacute erosive esophagitis occur near the lower end of the esophagus, especially as a terminal event in elderly or debilitated patients. In subacute erosive esophagitis there are erosion, hyperemia, and an exudate composed largely of desquamated epithelial cells. The inflammatory process appears to begin or to localize largely in

Table 19-1. *Lesions of the gastrointestinal tract*

	Esophagus	*Stomach*	*Duodenum*
Congenital malformations	Atresia	Pyloric stenosis caused by hypertrophy and spasm of muscle of pylorus	Rare
Diverticula	Pulsion type—pressure from within, bulging at weak point; at upper end Traction type—caused by pull of inflammatory adhesions; usually at level of tracheal bifurcation	Uncommon	Fairly common
Inflammations and ulcerations	Relatively unimportant; follows swallowing of corrosive chemicals Varices at lower end in obstructions of portal circulation (cirrhosis of liver) sometimes associated with overlying inflammation and/or ulceration	Gastritis results from various poisons and irritants Chronic peptic ulcer is very frequent and important	Chronic ulcer (peptic) very common in first portion Acute ulceration may accompany severe burns
Obstructions	Congenital Fibrosis following ingestion of corrosives Tumors Cardiospasm and functional strictures of lower end Pressure from without	Usually at pylorus May be Congenital (infancy) Scar of healed ulcer Carcinoma Bezoars or concretions (masses of indigestible material)	Uncommon, except at pylorus

Small intestine	Appendix	Colon	Rectum and anus
ncommon, except for abnormalities of mesenteric attachment and rotation and for Meckel's diverticulum	Rare	Congenital dilatation (megacolon—Hirschsprung's disease)	Atresia
Meckel's—persistence of omphalomesenteric duct; 1 to 3 feet proximal to ileocecal junction; other types uncommon	In rare cases may follow appendicitis	Common in descending and sigmoid regions—often become inflamed (diverticulitis)	Uncommon
yphoid—ulcerations of lymphoid areas of ileum regional ileitis—a chronic inflammation of terminal ileum tuberculosis—chronic ulcerations of lower ileum chemical poisons and uremia—may cause ulcerations of ileum lesions of jejunum are rare	Acute appendicitis is common; complicated by perforation, abscess formation, peritonitis, pylephlebitis	Dysentery—bacillary Dysentery—amebic Chronic ulcerative colitis Cholera Tuberculosis—may involve cecal region Actinomycosis—in cecal region Uremia Mercury	Nonspecific chronic inflammation with sinus or fistula formation is common Involvement in lymphogranuloma venereum
aralytic—e.g., in mesenteric thrombosis mechanical—blockage of lumen strangulation—obstruction and interference with blood supply biochemical disturbance, with dehydration and electrolyte loss resulting	Commonly caused by a fecalith or by fibrosis Important in pathogenesis of appendicitis	Acute obstruction as in small bowel Chronic obstructions from tumors and inflammatory fibrosis	Acute obstruction is uncommon Chronic obstruction from tumors, impacted feces, and in lymphogranuloma venereum

Table 19-1. *Lesions of the gastrointestinal tract*—cont'd

	Esophagus	*Stomach*	*Duodenum*
Tumors	Benign—uncommon Carcinoma—prognosis almost hopeless Squamous cell type—common Adenocarcinoma—rare; occurs at lower end	Benign—uncommon Malignant—carcinoma is very common and important Types Polypoid Ulcerating Scirrhous or infiltrating Sarcoma—uncommon	Rare

the lamina propria of the mucosa, and the erosive action of regurgitated gastric juice appears to have a secondary role. However, acid peptic erosion (peptic esophagitis) appears to be a relatively common condition.

Gastroesophageal lacerations at the cardiac orifice of the stomach (Mallory-Weiss syndrome) are an infrequent cause of gastric hemorrhage. The longitudinal lacerations through the cardioesophageal junction have occurred in a variety of conditions associated with vomiting, and atrophic gastritis is present in some cases. Complete rupture of the esophagus (Boerhaave syndrome) is a more serious surgical emergency, with a high mortality from chemical mediastinitis.

Stenosis. Stenosis of the esophagus may be caused by the swallowing of corrosive chemicals such as lye. The resulting dense fibrous tissue repair causes such stricture of the lumen as to make impossible the swallowing of solids, and eventually even liquids. Tumors of the esophagus also obstruct the lumen and give rise to dysphagia. Pressure on the esophagus from without, as by a mediastinal or pulmonary tumor, enlarged lymph nodes, or aortic aneurysm, produces variable degrees of esophageal obstruction.

Cardiospasm. Cardiospasm or functional stricture of the lower end of the esophagus is caused by spasm of the cardiac sphincter. It appears to result from neurogenic imbalance of sphincteric action. Degenerative changes have been found in afferent vagal fibers. As in other types of obstruction, the esophagus above the stricture becomes dilated. Idiopathic muscular hypertrophy of

Small intestine	*Appendix*	*Colon*	*Rectum and anus*
are Carcinoids similar to those of the appendix occur but more rarely; may metastasize to liver and produce carcinoid syndrome (serotonin production)	Carcinoid—a benign, yellow argentaffin tumor, which histologically may resemble carcinoma True carcinoma is rare	Benign—polyps and adenomas are common Carcinoma—common, particularly in distal portions of colon and rectum: gross types are (1) annular constricting and ulcerating and (2) papillary; histologic varieties are (1) adenocarcinoma, (2) mucoid, (3) scirrhous	

the lower esophagus is a rare condition sometimes associated with spasm.

Varices. Varices at the lower end of the esophagus occur in cirrhosis of the liver because of obstruction of the portal circulation. Hemorrhage from the varices is influenced both by the increased hydrostatic pressure and by mucosal ulceration.

Benign tumors. Benign tumors are uncommon. Fibrous polyps, polypoid lipomas, and leiomyomas may project into the lumen and occur mainly at the level of the cricoid cartilage. Intramural leiomyomas may be found at any level.

Congenital cysts. Cysts containing derivatives of the primitive foregut occur in the middle and lower thirds of the esophagus.

Carcinoma. Carcinoma is the only type of tumor common in the esophagus. It occurs more frequently in persons after the age of 50 years, and more than 80% occur in men. The three common sites are (1) in the middle third of the esophagus, at the level of the tracheal bifurcation (50%); (2) in the lower third, about the level of the diaphragm (25%); and (3) in the upper third, about the level of the cricoid cartilage. Some investigators have found the highest incidence in the lower end of the esophagus.

The *gross types* are (1) an infiltrating or scirrhous form, which grows around the esophagus and soon produces stenosis and obstruction of the lumen; (2) a medullary type of soft, bulky ulcerating tumor; and (3) a polypoid form, which is least common.

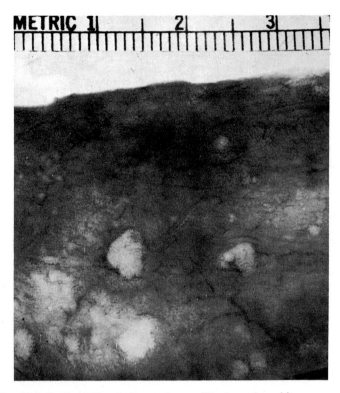

Fig. 19-1. Leukoplakia of the esophagus. The irregular white areas are prominent on the mucosal surface.

These tumors are *squamous cell carcinomas* of varying degree of differentiation. In rare instances an *adenocarcinoma* may be present at the lower end of the esophagus. It may arise from ectopic gastric mucosa or may be an upward extension of an adenocarcinoma of the cardiac end of the stomach. Carcinoma with both squamous and glandular patterns (adenoacanthoma) also occurs in the cardioesophageal region.

Metastasis is more widespread in the highly undifferentiated tumors, the liver, lungs, and lymph nodes draining the area being most frequently involved. The outlook in carcinoma of the esophagus is usually hopeless because of surgical inaccessibility, although radiologic treatment may result in palliation.

STOMACH AND DUODENUM
Congenital pyloric stenosis

Great hypertrophy of the circular muscle fibers of the pylorus is characteristic of this condition. Usually accompanied by spasm, it produces stenosis and obstruction of the pyloric orifice. Symptoms begin shortly after the first week of life, with vomiting, visible gastric peristalsis, and often a palpable hardened pylorus. Symptoms may subside in a few weeks or continue for months. Recovery results after surgical splitting of the circular muscle fibers of the pylorus. Although the condition is congenital, its pathogenesis is unknown, and the relative importance of spasm and muscular hypertrophy in the production of symptoms is a debatable point. Myenteric ganglion cells and nerve fiber tracts have been shown to be fewer in number in the hypertrophied pyloric region, and the ganglion cells show degenerative changes. The condition occurs predominantly in males. Duodenal obstruction in infancy also may be caused by an *annular pancreas,* a malformation in which a band of pancreatic tissue is wrapped around the duodenum.

Poisons

Various ingested corrosives leave their mark on the stomach as well as on the mouth, pharynx, and esophagus. The effects vary with the type and strength of the poison. Certain powerful poisons such as phenol and mercuric chloride cause immediate death and fixation of the gastric mucosa. The fixed tissue is firm and grayish white or brownish; microscopically the cells appear well preserved. Little or no inflammatory reaction is evident because of the rapidity with which death occurs.

Strong acids, such as hydrochloric and sulfuric, burn the tissues, which then appear of yellowish or brown color, necrotic, and hemorrhagic. Action on the blood in contact with the acid results in dark brown pigmentation because of hematin formation. Microscopically the tissue appears massively necrotic and disintegrated. The degree of inflammatory reaction depends on the period of survival after ingestion of the poison.

Strong alkalies, such as lye and lysol, also produce necrosis with softening and discoloration, although the pigmentation may be less distinct.

Various weaker corrosive poisons result in lesser degrees of the same type of change, with more opportunity for the development of severe inflammatory reaction.

Gastritis

Acute gastritis. An acute gastritis may be caused by various irritant foods, alcoholic drinks, and poisons.

Chronic gastritis. Chronic gastritis occurs in hypertrophic and atrophic forms.

Chronic hypertrophic gastritis. Chronic hypertrophic gastritis is characterized by thickening of the mucosa and submucosa. The lining of the stomach is excessively rugose or even polypoid. There is a hyperplasia of the mucosal epithelium, and in the submucosa there is a connective tissue increase with infiltration of chronic inflammatory cells. Multiple polyps may develop. The condition is rather rare but clinically may be difficult to differentiate from a cancer. Chronic gastritis with hypertrophy of the rugae is sometimes associated with loss of protein into the lumen (Menétrier's disease).

Chronic atrophic gastritis. Chronic atrophic gastritis is a nonspecific change that becomes more frequent with advancing age. In may be particularly prominent in persons with chronic alcoholism, chronic pellagra, and pernicious anemia. The normal rugae of the stomach are less prominent. Hypochlorhydria or achlorhydria is a common accompaniment. Microscopically the mucosa is atrophic, with a scarcity of mucosal glands, and there is an increase of leukocytic infiltration and lymphoid aggregation in the mucosa and submucosa. The mucosa of the pylorus and fundus may be metaplastic and transformed to an intestinal type, and there may be a change of parts of the mucosa of the fundus to a pyloric type (pyloric gland heterotopia). There is an increase of mucus-producing gland cells at the expense of the chief and parietal cells. Small cysts may be present in deeper parts of the mucosa. The interglandular connective tissue and the muscularis mucosa are thickened. The importance of chronic gastritis with metaplasia in predisposing to carcinoma of the stomach is debatable, but the two conditions are commonly associated.

In pernicious anemia there is an extreme atrophy involving all coats of the stomach wall. This change is localized in the upper two thirds of the stomach and does not affect the pyloric antrum or duodenum. In the involved area the stomach wall is extremely thin, but there is an abrupt transition to normal thickness at the junction with the pyloric mucosa. In the involved area only a few scattered glands remain, the specialized oxyntic and peptic cells having entirely disappeared. (See Fig. 17-1.) Absence of inflammatory changes suggests that a purely atrophic process has occurred. These changes appear to be the morphologic basis of the achylia gastrica present in pernicious anemia. The atrophic change is not reversed by treatment with liver or vitamin B. Carcinoma of the stomach is at least three times more common in persons with pernicious anemia.

Specific gastritis. Rarely in syphilis, tuberculosis, and mycoses, local granulomatous or ulcerative lesions may occur. In some instances, as in syphilis, a diffusely infiltrative lesion occurs that may be of the leather-bottle (linitis plastica) type and is grossly indistinguishable from scirrhous carcinoma.

Sarcoidosis, eosinophilic granuloma, and xanthomatosis on occasion produce lesions in the stomach.

Bezoars

Bezoar is a term applied to an accumulation of foreign material in the stomach and intestine. There are four varieties: (1) trichobezoar, or hair ball; (2) phytobezoar, or food ball; (3) trichophytobezoar, a combined hair and food ball; and (4) shellac bezoar, or concretion.

Pyloric obstruction

In adults, stenosis and obstruction at the pylorus may result from the contracting scar of an ulcer or from carcinoma. The stomach becomes greatly dilated and filled by stagnant food and fluid. Persistent vomiting results in loss of chlorides and acid and the production of so-called gastric tetany; i.e., alkalosis and a chloride insufficiency occur. An increase in nonprotein nitrogen of the blood and evidence of renal insufficiency may be present. The kidneys show significant tubular degeneration and often calcium deposits in the degenerated tissue. Other obstructions high in the intestinal tract produce a similar result.

Peptic ulcer

The term *peptic ulcer* refers to ulceration in areas that may be acted upon by acid gastric juice, i.e., the stomach, the first portion of the duodenum, and after gastrojejunostomy, the jejunum. Acute ulcerations or erosions are superficial and often hemorrhagic areas of mucosal loss. These common acute ulcers heal easily and give rise to little trouble. It is believed, however, that they may form the starting point for chronic peptic ulcers. Chronic peptic ulcers are more important than the acute forms because of their persistence, annoying symptoms, and the complications of hemorrhage, perforation, and malignant change. The term *peptic ulcer,* when unqualified, usually refers to this serious chronic type.

Acute ulcer. Acute ulcers or erosions are quite common and may be produced by a variety of injuries, such as coarse or excessively hot foods, septicemias, and burns of the skin. The variety complicating extensive superficial burns is known as a Curling ulcer. Found in only a small proportion of fatal burns, it is most common in the duodenum but also occurs in the stomach or intestine. Acute hemorrhagic ulcerations of the stomach or intestine occasionally occur in patients with acute central nervous system lesions, especially of the hypothalamus (Cushing ulcer), with other types of stress, with shock, or who have been treated by adrenal steroid hormones. Acute ulcers are usually small, involve only the mucosa and superficial layers of submucosa, and are often hemorrhagic. They usually heal readily but in certain areas and circumstances may become chronic. Acute ulcers are more frequent in the stomach than in the duodenum. The gastric ulcers apparently tend to heal more readily, while duodenal ulcers tend to be chronic.

Chronic peptic ulcer.

Etiology. The etiology of chronic peptic ulcer is not thoroughly understood. The one factor of established importance is the *action of acid-pepsin gastric content.* Chronic peptic ulcers develop only in areas exposed to acid-pepsin secretion: the duodenum, stomach, lower part of the esophagus, jejunum at the site of a gastrojejunostomy, and Meckel's diverticulum containing gastric mucosa. In the rare Zollinger-Ellison syndrome (hypersecretion of gastric acid secretion associated with pancreatic adenoma) peptic ulceration occurs in the jejunum as well as in the duodenum. Ulceration does not occur in acid-pepsin secreting mucosa but in adjacent areas. When there is achlorhydria, as in pernicious anemia, peptic ulcer does not occur.

Although chronic ulcers in the duodenum and stomach, the two common sites, have certain features in common, there are obvious differences that have led some investigators to consider them different disease entities. Duodenal ulcers are much more common and occur most often in males, usually be-

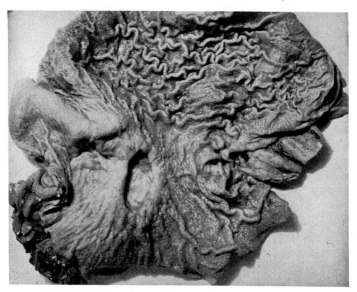

Fig. 19-2. Chronic ulcer of the stomach.

tween 20 and 50 years of age. Individuals with Group O blood and those unable to secrete AB substances in the saliva and gastric secretions are more susceptible to duodenal ulceration. It is the duodenal ulcer that tends to occur in the professional or executive person who is hard driving and under mental stress. Most patients with duodenal ulcers secrete a greater than normal amount of gastric acid and have a greater than normal number of parietal (acid-secreting) cells in the stomach. On the other hand, chronic gastric ulcers are not characterized by the great preponderance in males as are the duodenal ulcers, tend to occur in an older age group, and are associated with a normal or low amount of gastric secretion with no increase in the number of parietal cells. Despite these differences, it can be said that the peptic ulcers in both sites are caused by too much gastric acid secretion with respect to the degree of protection provided for the mucosa.

The factors that normally protect the gastroduodenal mucosa against digestion by gastric secretions include (1) a layer of mucus, (2) dilution or buffering of gastric juices by swallowed food and saliva and by the alkaline small intestinal juices, and

(3) an adequate blood supply. Although it has been suggested that decreased resistance of the mucosa plays a role in the development of peptic ulcers, there is no general agreement on this point. Significant changes of the aforementioned protective factors have not been demonstrated conclusively in ulcer subjects. Impaired tissue resistance is considered by some to be more important in the pathogenesis of gastric ulcers than duodenal ulcers. Chronic gastritis is frequently but not always associated with chronic gastric ulcers. The possible relationship of these ulcers to local trauma such as that caused by the passage of coarse, indigestible foods has been noted. Localized mucosal damage caused by changes in vascular supply (e.g., vasospasm, thrombosis, embolism) or by bacterial infection has been thought by some to be responsible for ulcer formation, but such a mechanism is not regarded by many writers today to be of major significance. Smoking may favor ulcer production or interfere with healing of one already present.

The influence of the nervous system has long been considered a factor in the cause of peptic ulcers. A hypersecretion of gastric acid may be mediated through the vagus nerve and possibly through adrenal cortical steroids as a result of hypothalamic-anterior pituitary stimulus brought about by anxiety, other emotional states, or other types of stress.

A familial history is present in many patients with peptic ulcers, suggesting an hereditary predisposition in certain instances. It is of interest to note that there is an increased incidence of peptic ulcers in patients with chronic lung diseases such as pulmonary emphysema, with hyperparathyroidism, with rheumatoid arthritis, or with polycythemia vera. Most frequently the ulcers are of the duodenal type.

Various factors have been thought to prevent healing once the ulcer is established. These include hyperacidity and stasis, the traumatic effects of food, tobacco smoking, and the pull of muscle about the ulcer. The rather constant location of gastric ulcers on the lesser curvature has caused emphasis on functional and anatomic factors. Contraction of oblique muscle fibers forms a groove (magenstrasse) along the distal part of the lesser curvature, along which food or liquid may be forced without mixing with the rest of the gastric content. Usually gastric ulcers are located in or near the magenstrasse. This region, in comparison with other parts of the gastric mucosa, is exposed to more trauma, lacks protective mucin production, and is subjected to greater muscle traction.

Gross appearance. Peptic ulcers are highly constant in location, being found in the pyloric portion of the stomach, most commonly on the posterior wall near the lesser curvature, and in the first portion of the duodenum proximal to the ampulla. The gastric ulcers are usually situated a few centimeters proximal to the pyloric ring. Ulcers right at the pylorus are more commonly carcinomatous. Duodenal ulcers occur in the first portion (duodenal bulb) on the anterior or posterior wall. Peptic ulcers are usually single but may be multiple.

The ulcers vary in size from a few millimeters to 3 cm. in diameter. They usually do not extend and become very large. Large ulcers of the stomach are usually carcinomas rather than chronic peptic ulcers. An ulcer in the duodenum is almost never a carcinoma.

The chronic ulcers appear as indurated, deep punched-out or funnel-shaped areas. The proximal or cardiac side of the gastric ulcer is usually steep with overhanging edges, while the distal or pyloric side tends to be sloping or terraced. The base of the ulcer is covered by roughened, grayish, necrotic material or may contain granular or blood-tinged exudate. Hyperemia or some fibrous thickening may be present around the edge of the ulcer. Variable degrees of fibrosis and distortion of the organ develop. When marked fibrosis spreads around the stomach, contraction tends to produce an hourglass deformity. Fibrous adhesion to adjacent organs, such as the pancreas or liver, may be present. Fibrosis about a duodenal ulcer shortens the distance between the pyloric ring and the opening of the ampulla.

Microscopic appearance. At the edge of the ulcer the mucosal and muscular layers end rather abruptly, although there may be some overhanging of the epithelium. Occasionally there is some downward proliferation of the marginal epithelium, producing an appearance that should not be confused with malignancy.

The whole thickness of the base of the ulcer is composed of fibrous scar tissue, the muscle layers usually being completely gone. Over this fibrous base are successive layers of granulation tissue, necrotic and hyalinized material, and exudate. Inflammatory cells may be found not only in this layer of exudate on the surface but also in the granulation tissue and about the edges. Blood vessels in the base often show inflammation in early ulcers and later show intimal thickening with narrowing or even obliteration of the lumen.

When healing occurs, it is by organization and fibrosis, the mucosa from the edges growing inward to cover the area. Contraction of the scar tissue sometimes produces an hourglass deformity of the stomach or pyloric stenosis.

Complications. The complications and sequelae of peptic ulcer include hemorrhage, perforation, malignant change, and scar contraction with pyloric stenosis or deformity of the stomach.

Small hemorrhages commonly accompany peptic ulcers. Repeated small hemorrhages produce secondary anemia. A severe or even fatal hemorrhage may follow erosion of a larger vessel. Endarterial changes in the vessels of the base protect against this to some extent. On the other hand, the vessel walls, being held in rigid scar tissue, may be unable to retract after erosion. Alimentary azotemia may occur after massive hemorrhage from a peptic ulcer, apparently because of absorption of digestive products of the erythrocyte fraction of the blood.

Perforation results when the ulcer continues to penetrate deeply. Perforation into the peritoneal cavity produces shock and soon results in peritonitis. In other older ulcers, adherent to some surrounding structure, perforation may occur into the adherent organ.

Relationship to carcinoma. Malignant change may develop in a chronic gastric ulcer, but this is extremely rare in duodenal ulcers. While the frequency of this occurrence in gastric ulcer is debated, the consensus is that 5 to 10% of benign gastric ulcers undergo malignant change. In some areas, such as Japan, the frequency of malignant change appears to be greater.

In an ulcerating gastric cancer, evidence that it arose from a previously benign chronic ulcer is given by (1) complete destruction of the muscle layers of the stomach in the base of the ulcer, (2) fusion of the muscularis mucosa and muscle wall at the margin of the ulcer, (3) intimal thickening of blood vessels, and (4) the presence of carcinoma in only one part of the wall and its absence in the base of the ulcer and in other portions of the wall.

Distinguishing points of benign and malignant gastric ulcers are given in Table 19-2. A malignant ulcer tends to be bowl shaped, with an edge that is raised and nodular but does not overhang the crater and with a smoothing out of the mucosal folds around the margin. Benign ulcers are less frequent than

Table 19-2. *Comparison of benign and malignant gastric ulcers*

	Ulcerating carcinoma	Chronic ulcer
Duration	History less than two years	History often more than two years
Age	More frequently past 40 years of age	Frequently begins under 40 years of age
Size of ulcer	Usually over 2.5 cm. in diameter	Diameter usually less than 4 cm.
Position	Usually at or very near pylorus	Commonly 2 to 3 inches from pylorus
Edge of ulcer	Raised, rounded	Sharp, punched-out, terraced on pyloric side

malignant ulcers on the greater curvature and in the region of the cardia. If hypochlorhydria or achlorhydria is present in a patient, a gastric ulcer is more likely to be malignant rather than a simple peptic ulcer. The reverse is true if there is severe hyperchlorhydria. None of the criteria for distinction of benign and malignant gastric ulcers is uniformly reliable. Sometimes the distinction is impossible without microscopic examination and application of the usual histologic criteria of malignancy.

Tumors of the stomach

Benign. Benign tumors of the stomach are uncommon compared to carcinoma and are of little clinical significance unless they obstruct the pylorus. Leiomyoma and adenoma are the most frequent types. The mucosa may be involved by a polypoid adenoma or by multiple polyps. Regenerative polyps, usually less than 2 cm. in diameter, are more common than neoplastic true adenomatous polyps and have not been shown to become malignant. Adenomatous polyps may undergo malignant change, but as they are uncommon, they account for few gastric cancers. Some of the fibroid polyps appear to be of inflammatory origin. Fibroma and lipoma also occur.

Carcinoma of the stomach. Malignant tumors of the stomach are a major factor in the cancer problem, causing about 10% of all cancer deaths (25,000 per year) in the United States. However. the death rate from cancer of the stomach appears to be steadily declining, the reason for which is unknown. Carcinoma of the stomach is more common in males (in proportion of almost 2:1). More than 90% occur in persons after 50 years

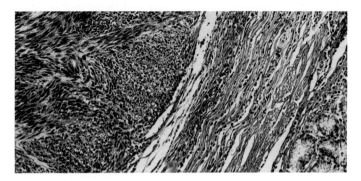

Fig. 19-3. Leiomyoma of the stomach. The margin of the tumor is shown (center), with a few mucosal glands at the right.

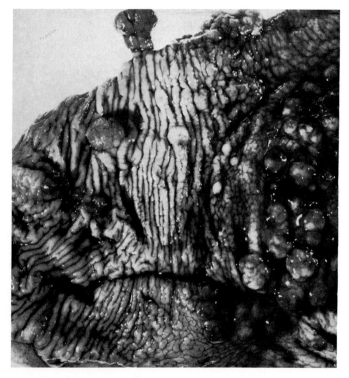

Fig. 19-4. Benign polyps of the stomach.

of age. Differences in racial or geographic incidence are striking, carcinoma being particularly common among Icelanders and Japanese and relatively less frequent among Indonesians and African Negroes. The high incidence in Iceland may be related to dietary intake of carcinogens, particularly in smoked meat and fish. Hereditary susceptibility appears to be of some importance, and numerous studies have indicated a relatively high incidence in certain families or among relatives. The high incidence in the Napoleon Bonaparte family is of historic interest. Studies on correlation of the incidence of certain blood group factors and gastric cancer have confirmed the importance of a genetic basis of susceptibility. Blood group A appears to be significantly associated with prepyloric and cardiac gastric carcinomas, and blood group O is associated with fundus lesions.

Conditions that may be associated with, and sometimes precede or predispose to, carcinoma of the stomach are chronic gastritis, chronic gastric ulcer, and adenomatous polyps. The proved frequency of these conditions progressing to carcinoma is not sufficient to account for more than a small proportion of gastric cancers.

Carcinoma may occur anywhere in the stomach, but the majority develop from mucus-secreting cells of the antrum and pylorus and more particularly along the lesser curvature. A few are found on the greater curvature and about 5% in the fundus

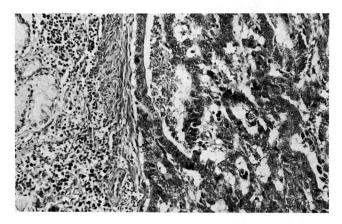

Fig. 19-5. Adenocarcinoma of the stomach. A few normal mucosal glands are at the left.

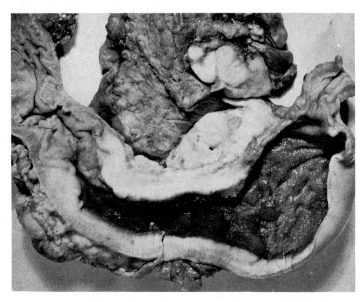

Fig. 19-6. Diffuse scirrhous carcinoma of the stomach (linitis plastica). Note the considerable diffuse thickening and contraction of the wall.

or region of the cardia. Although the relative proportions vary in the different sites, as compared with benign ulcers, there is much overlapping.

Types. Gross pathologic classification of carcinoma of the stomach appears of greater practical usefulness than does microscopic classification. A classification proposed by Borrmann,* or some modification of it, has been very commonly used. In order of increasing malignancy, cases may be arranged as follows:

Group I. Polypoid carcinoma: an exophytic, circumscribed, solitary tumor, without important ulceration

Group II. Ulcerated carcinoma: an endophytic, penetrating growth, with wall-like marginal elevation and sharply defined borders

Group III. Ulcerated carcinoma: an endophytic penetrating growth, but in part with diffuse spread

---

*Borrmann, R.: Geschwülste des Magens und Duodenums. In Henke, F., and Lubarsch, O., editors: Handbuch der speziellen pathologischen Anatomie und Histologie, Berlin, 1926, Julius Springer, vol. IV, part 1, pp. 812-1054.

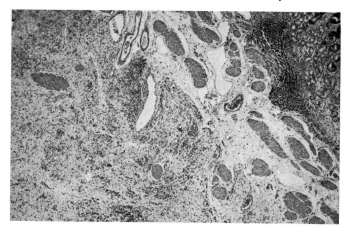

Fig. 19-7. Linitis plastica (sclerosing carcinoma) of the stomach. The mucosa is at the right.

> Group IV. Diffuse carcinoma: an infiltrating growth, without bulky localized tumor or severe ulceration, and often with a dense fibrous stroma

The *polypoid* or *fungating* carcinoma is a soft, bulky tumor that projects into the cavity of the stomach. The size of the tumor may be large before many symptoms are produced. The surface tends to become ulcerated and infected, and it bleeds easily. Eventually the tumor infiltrates and penetrates the muscular wall, but the course may be relatively slow. This fungating form constitutes up to 25% of gastric cancers and is a relatively favorable form for surgical removal.

The *ulcerative* or *penetrating* carcinoma is the most frequent form of gastric cancer, constituting up to 30%. The growth is primarily away from the lumen, and ulceration is early and prominent. The ulcer tends to be shallow and bowl shaped, with an edge that is raised and nodular but does not overhang the crater. The mucosal folds around the ulcer's margin tend to be smoothed out. Despite the described differences, a gross distinction from a benign ulcer is sometimes difficult. If the diameter of the ulcer is more than 4 cm., it is usually an indication of malignancy, but size alone is not a reliable criterion.

The *diffuse, spreading,* or *infiltrating scirrhous* carcinoma is the least common of the distinctive types. The growth extends in the wall of the stomach without producing either a localized tumor mass or a prominent ulcer. Abundant fibrous stroma forms, so that the involved portion of the stomach becomes contracted, thick walled, and firm. It may begin at the pylorus, encircling this region and producing obstruction. The proximal extension may be only a short distance, or the whole stomach may be involved. The diffuse infiltrating type *(linitis plastica)* results in a small, very thick-walled stomach (leather-bottle stomach). Histologically, malignant cells are sometimes quite scarce in the midst of the abundant connective tissue stroma and may be difficult to find. The outlook is poor and cure is rare. Extensive intramural (tubal) spread along the alimentary tract sometimes occurs.

Superficial spreading carcinoma extends in the mucosa and submucosa, only later penetrating deeply and metastasizing. It may begin as a carcinoma in situ. It is found mainly in the antrum and pylorus. The mucosa and submucosa may be thickened by the tumor, but abundant fibrous stroma is lacking.

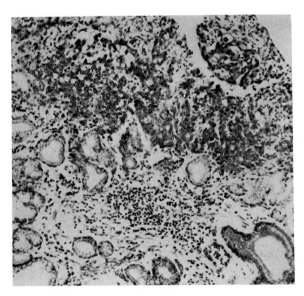

Fig. 19-8. Superficial spreading carcinoma of the stomach. The gastric mucosa only is shown, and the neoplastic cells are in the upper half of the photomicrograph.

A considerable number of late extensive cancers of the stomach cannot be classed into the gross types because their distinctive features have been lost.

Microscopic classification is relatively unimportant from a practical standpoint. Carcinomas of the stomach are adenocarcinomas, derived from mucus-secreting and glandular cells, with varying degrees of differentiation. Mucus production may occur in any of the varieties of gastric carcinoma, either in small localized areas or involving the whole tumor. Large mucoid areas grossly appear translucent and gelatinous. Accumulation of mucus in the cytoplasm of the tumor cells displaces and flattens the nucleus at one side of the cell, giving it a signet-ring appearance. Also there may be areas of extracellular mucus. Other microscopic varieties may show a predominance of gland formation or papillary structure, infiltrating spheroidal cells, or highly anaplastic undifferentiated cells. A metaplastic squamous cell component (adenoacanthoma) or squamous cell carcinoma rarely occurs in the pyloric area.

Grading of gastric carcinomas has been done on a histologic basis (Broder's system), according to the degree of spread (Duke's system), and by combinations of the two. Although grading is not widely used or standardized, it appears to be one of the features having significance in prognosis. Lymphocytic reaction in the stroma of the tumor and sinus histiocytosis in regional lymph nodes have been considered to indicate a

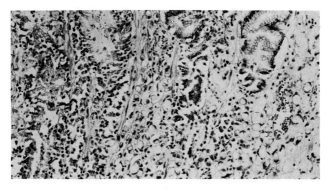

Fig. 19-9. Adenocarcinoma of the stomach. Mucin-containing tumor cells of the signet-ring type are infiltrating the gastric mucosa.

better prognosis, although the degree of importance of this feature is somewhat uncertain.

Spread and metastases. Carcinoma of the stomach spreads by direct growth and invasion, by lymphatics, through the peritoneal cavity, and by the bloodstream.

Direct spread in the stomach wall is very important in prognosis. Diffusely infiltrative tumors of the linitis plastica type have the poorest outlook, but also in other types the degree of intramural spread is important. Intramural extension that is rapid or extensive, or spread beyond the limits of visibility or palpability, is associated with poor chances of survival, whereas sharp circumscription of the tumor is an important feature suggesting a good prognosis. Direct spread may also extend intramurally into the esophagus, the first portion of the duodenum, the gastrohepatic and gastrocolic omenta, and adjacent areas of the pancreas, spleen, transverse colon, liver, and diaphragm. When the peritoneal surface is reached, peritoneal dissemination may occur, with numerous peritoneal deposits or ovarian metastases. The ovaries may be involved by bilateral (Krukenberg) tumors.

Metastasis to perigastric regional lymph nodes is one of the main factors affecting prognosis in resectable tumors. From tumors in the distal portions of the stomach, metastases are found in the inferior gastric, subpyloric, and superior gastric nodes. From cancers in the proximal portion of the stomach the pancreaticolineal group of nodes is most often involved. Further spread by lymphatics occurs to the celiac, lumbar, mesenteric, pelvic, and mediastinal nodes and to the thoracic duct. From thoracic duct involvement miliary carcinomas of the lungs may develop.

Bloodstream metastasis of gastric carcinoma most frequently involves the liver, lungs, and bones.

Cytologic diagnosis. Cytologic study for diagnosis has not been readily applied to gastric cancer because of the difficulty of getting exfoliated malignant cells for study, the hazard of cellular digestion by gastric enzymes that destroys cytologic features, and difficulties in interpretation of morphology of some types of gastric tumor cells. Tumor cells have been more readily obtained by use of an abrasive gastric balloon and by lavage with mucolytic agents such as chymotrypsin or papain. Proper preparation by first controlling food intake and gastric lavage keeps digestive effects on the exfoliated tumor cells to a

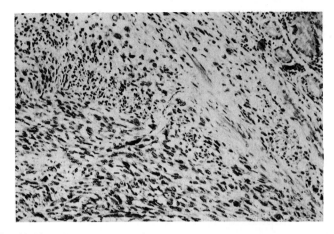

Fig. 19-10. Leiomyosarcoma of the stomach. Mucosal glands are at the upper right.

minimum. By proper technique and careful interpretation of the nuclear characteristics of enlargement, variation in size, increase in chromatin, irregular borders, large nucleoli, and mitoses, gastric cancer cells can be recognized with dependable frequency.

Sarcoma of the stomach. Sarcoma constitutes about 2% of cancers of the stomach. The varieties include leiomyosarcoma, fibrosarcoma, and malignant lymphoma. Some of the so-called round cell sarcomas probably are highly anaplastic carcinomas. Malignant lymphoma is the commonest variety. It forms an intramural tumor, is similar to malignant lymphoma elsewhere, and is highly radiosensitive. It may be primary in the stomach or be only part of a more generalized involvement. The mucosa may be greatly thickened, with giant rugae, multiple nodules, or a single bulky polypoid growth. Ulceration occurs in late stages. The pylorus is not often involved, and obstruction is unusual. Histologic varieties include a giant follicle form (rare), a small lymphocyte type, and a reticulum cell type (most frequent). The last variety may be difficult to differentiate from anaplastic carcinoma.

Carcinoma of the duodenum

The duodenum is a rare site for cancer, even as a malignant change in a chronic duodenal ulcer. Most carcinomas of the

Table 19-3. *Inflammations and ulcerations of the intestinal tract*

	Etiology and pathogenesis	*Region of bowel involved predominantly*	*Nature of lesion*
Chemical poisons	Corrosive action of ingested salts of mercury and other heavy metals	Ileum and colon	Hemorrhagic and diphtheritic
Uremia	Localized blood vessel changes (?) Ammonia poisoning	Lower ileum, cecum, and ascending colon	Hemorrhagic, diphtheritic and ulcertive lesions
Burns	In 1 to 6% of fatal burns; possible relation to adrenal damage	First part of duodenum, stomach, and small intestine—in order of frequency	Acute, ulcerative
Typhoid and paratyphoid	Organisms ingested in contaminated water and food; generalized infection	Ileum—Peyer's patches and solitary lymph follicles	Hyperplastic and necrotic; involvement of lymphoid tissue
Bacillary dysentery	Ingested dysentery bacilli produce localized infection of intestine	Large intestine, especially distal portion	Diphtheritic inflammation, with widespread necrosis abundant exudate
Amebic dysentery	Ingested *Entamoeba histolytica* locally affect intestine	Large intestine	Local invasion and tissue lysis by parasite
Chronic ulcerative colitis	Etiology uncertain	Large intestine, especially distal portion	Chronic ulcerative inflammation
Cholera	Ingested cholera vibrios of Koch produce infection of intestine	Whole intestinal tract, but particularly colon	Acute catarrhal inflammation, reddening of mucosa sometimes hemorrhages
Regional enteritis	Etiology uncertain	Ileocecal region	Great thickening of a segment of ileum

Character of ulcers	Microscopic appearance	Complications
gged, small, superficial; ay be coalescing and ex- nsive		
specific form, hemor- agic, multiple, some- mes extensive	Hyaline thickening, inflam- mation, and necrosis of small arteries in affected area	
ute, usually single, may long and narrow		Hemorrhage, per- foration
ers involve Peyer's tches, oval, in long is of bowel	Proliferation of large mon- onuclear phagocytic cells	Perforation, hemor- rhage
llow, ragged, very nu- erous and coalescent, t undermined	Superficial fibrinopurulent exudate	Dehydration, steno- sis may follow healing
dermined edges; flask- aped on section	Amebae in tissues; leuko- cytic infiltration when secondarily infected	Perforation, liver abscess
ensive, ragged, chronic, alescing ulcerations sur- unding islands of hy- rtrophic mucosa		Stricture of bowel wall; sometimes malignant change in polypoid mu- cosal islands
ulcers but superficial squamation of surface ithelium	Loss of epithelium from mucosa	Extreme dehydration
specific	Extreme thickening of sub- mucosa; sarcoidlike ag- gregates of epithelioid and giant cells	Obstruction of bowel, mesenteric lymph nodes af- fected; perfora- tion rare

Table 19-3. *Inflammations and ulcerations of the intestinal tract*

	Etiology and pathogenesis	Region of bowel involved predominantly	Nature of lesion
Tubercu-losis	Usually secondary to pulmonary lesion, caused by swallow-ing sputum; occasionally primary from infected milk or food	Ileocecal region—starts in lymphoid tissue	Tubercle formation in lymphoid tissue of bowel; sometimes hyperplastic with thickening of bowel wall
Actinomy-cosis	Ingested ray fungus	Ileocecal region and appendix	Suppurative and ulcerative, with thickening of bow wall
Lympho-granulo-ma vene-reum	Agent of psittaco-sis—LGV group; Frei reaction positive	Usually large intes-tine	Chronic suppurativ and granulomatou

duodenum arise at or about the ampulla of Vater and hence usually obstruct the bile and pancreatic ducts, with the early appearance of jaundice. Some probably originate from bile duct epithelium rather than from duodenal mucosa, and others originate from aberrant pancreatic tissue. Cysts of the duodenum are rare. They may be cysts of Brunner's glands or enterogenous cysts.

INTESTINAL TRACT

The main types of diseases of the small and large bowel are (1) inflammatory and infective conditions, including inflammations of diverticula and of the peritoneum, (2) obstructions, and (3) tumors.

Inflammations

Inflammations may involve large portions of the tract, but often one region is affected exclusively or more prominently, so that the terms *enteritis* (small intestine), *ileitis, appendicitis, colitis, sigmoiditis,* and *proctitis* (rectum) may be used to indicate inflammation of the particular region. The causes are of two main groups: (1) poisons, either endogenous (e.g., in nt'd

Character of ulcers	Microscopic appearance	Complications
fect lymphoid tissue but end to encircle bowel	Caseous necrosis, epithelioid cells, giant cells, lymphoid cells	Stenosis of gut, perforation and peritonitis
t specific	Suppuration; characteristic ray fungus in lesions	Pylephlebitis; chronic draining sinus or fistula
t specific	Often not characteristic; focal abscesses	Obstruction of lumen

uremia) or exogenous (mercury poisoning, botulinum food poisoning); and (2) infections (typhoid, dysentery, cholera, tuberculosis, etc.).

The inflammation may be (1) catarrhal, i.e., a superficial inflammation involving the mucosa of the bowel; (2) follicular, in which in addition to catarrhal inflammation there is a severe hyperplasia of the lymph follicles; (3) diphtheritic, characterized by the formation of a false membrane composed of necrotic mucosa and a fibrinous exudate; and (4) ulcerative, in which sloughing of necrotic areas and ulceration are often of distinctive nature. Some types of infection of the bowel may be catarrhal, diphtheritic, or ulcerative, etc., depending on their stage or degree of severity.

Intestinal inflammations caused by poisons

Endogenous. *Uremia* is accompanied by intestinal lesions in about 20% of the cases. The earliest changes in the mucosa are areas of hyperemia and edema, followed by hemorrhage, necrosis, diphtheritic change, sloughing, and ulceration. Uremic ulcers are commonest in the lower ileum, cecum, and ascending colon, but they also occur in other parts. The change is probably caused by localized interference with circulation to the involved area of bowel, and sclerotic or necrotic changes in blood vessels are often evident in the affected region. Irritation from excessive ammonia in the intestinal content, because of excretion of excess urea, also has been suggested as a causative factor.

Exogenous. Poisoning by heavy metals, such as mercury bichloride and other corrosives, may produce an intense hemorrhagic and diphtheritic inflammation of the bowel. The ileum and colon are most greatly involved (Chapter 10).

Enteric-coated tablets containing potassium chloride appear to have been responsible for ulcerative lesions of the small intestine. Administered to relieve potassium deficiency in patients receiving thiazide diuretics, a small proportion of users have developed serious circumferential lesions, which appear to be hemorrhagic infarcts. Rapid release and absorption of the potassium chloride in a short segment of intestine appears to initiate the vascular stasis leading to infarction and ulceration.

Intestinal inflammations caused by infection

Among the most important intestinal infections are those caused by the coli-typhoid-dysentery group of organisms. This group consists of aerobic gram-negative bacilli. One division of the group, distinguished by the inability to ferment lactose, consists of highly pathogenic organisms, such as those of typhoid, paratyphoid, and dysentery. A second division, composed of lactose fermentors, includes the colon bacillus and closely related organisms. They are of very low pathogenicity.

Typhoid fever. Infection with the typhoid bacillus is characterized by involvement of lymphoid and reticuloendothelial tissues, with hyperplasia of large mononuclear phagocytic cells. It is in all cases a generalized infection, but involvement of the lymphoid tissue of the intestine (Peyer's patches and solitary lymph follicles) is usually the most prominent feature, and ulceration there gives rise to the most dangerous complications of perforation and hemorrhage.

The organisms are ingested with water, milk, or food that has been contaminated, usually by chronic carriers. The febrile illness often has severe mental clouding and toxic symptoms in addition to intestinal disturbances, and it lasts for about four weeks. The blood culture is usually positive during the first week but is less regularly so later. The stool culture is more frequently positive during the second and third weeks. Urine culture is positive in about 20% of cases in the third and fourth weeks. The Widal reaction, which is the demonstration of specific agglutinins in the patient's serum, is usually positive after the first week. This test may be invalidated as a diagnostic procedure if the patient has had a recent inoculation with typhoid vaccine, which may produce a positive reaction. At autopsy the organisms are most easily isolated from the spleen or gallbladder. The leukopenia that occurs, with a decrease in the number of granulocytes and relative increase in nongranular white blood cells, is in accordance with the body's reaction to the organism, i.e., proliferation of mononuclear cells rather than exudation of polymorphonuclear leukocytes.

Intestinal lesions. The lower ileum and cecum, where lymphoid tissue is most abundant, is involved earliest and most severely. The more proximal parts of the small intestine and the more distal parts of the large intestine show a later and less severe reaction. Goodpasture has demonstrated in early cases the growth of a small gram-negative form of the organism in young plasma cells of the lymphoid follicles. The early changes in Peyer's patches and lymphoid follicles are congestion and edema, followed soon by a great proliferation of mononuclear leukocytes, the characteristic cells of typhoid. These involved lymphoid regions stand out as irregular projecting prominent areas on the mucosal surface. The large mononuclear cells in the lesions are actively phagocytic and in their cytoplasm can be seen remnants of ingested lymphocytes, plasma cells, and sometimes the large gram-negative typhoid bacilli.

At about the seventh to tenth day necrosis begins in the affected patches. Tiny necrotic areas slough off, leaving small ulcers, which by their coalescence form rounded or oval areas of ulceration having the size, shape, and situation of Peyer's patches. The long axis of these ulcers is in the direction of the long axis of the bowel, in contradistinction to tuberculous ulcers, which tend to encircle the gut.

This process of ulceration, particularly if rapid, may result in hemorrhage. The ulcers usually involve only the mucosa and submucosa, but deeper extension and perforation may occur, particularly as the result of secondary infection. Perforation is most likely to occur in the lower ileum, where the lesions are earliest and most severe. Generalized peritonitis follows, except in cases of slower perforating processes, which allow a walling off and localization of the peritonitis.

On recovery, surface epithelium grows over the ulcerated area, but there is little regeneration of the glandular epithelium or lymphoid tissue. There is no scar formation or contraction of the bowel.

Lesions in other organs. While intestinal lesions are usually primary and predominant in typhoid fever, the infection is a generalized one, and various other organs, such as the lymph nodes, spleen, liver, bone marrow, and gallbladder, are rather constantly involved. The reaction tends to be similar everywhere, with proliferation of large mononuclear cells and foci of necrosis. The necroses are mainly caused by the endotoxins of *Salmonella typhosa,* but vascular blockage by accumulated mononuclear cells is a contributing factor.

The *spleen* is enlarged up to 400 or 500 grams. It is red, soft, and exceedingly engorged with blood. In addition to this extreme congestion, collections of large mononuclear cells are seen microscopically. Small focal areas of necrosis may be present.

The *liver* likewise shows small focal necroses, irregularly distributed in the lobules.

Mesenteric *lymph nodes* also have microscopic necroses and great accumulation of large mononuclears. Similar changes may be found in *bone marrow,* where the formation of granulocytes is in abeyance.

The *gallbladder* is usually infected, and the organisms can be cultivated from the bile. Morphologic change in the gallbladder usually is slight, but acute cholecystitis may accompany or follow typhoid. A focus of infection may remain here, however, and excretion of organisms by way of the bile and intestinal tract results in a chronic carrier of the disease.

Cloudy swelling and even fatty degeneration affect the heart, liver, and kidneys in typhoid fever as in other acute infections. Zenker's degeneration of voluntary muscle is not uncommon. Rarer complications of typhoid fever include meningitis, suppurative periostitis or osteomyelitis, hemorrhagic pneumonia, and thrombosis of the veins of the legs.

Paratyphoid fever. The illness of paratyphoid infection is similar to that of typhoid, although it is of shorter duration, is less severe, and has a lower mortality. The lesions produced are essentially similar but of less severe degree. There is a somewhat greater tendency to pus production and abscess formation.

The *Salmonella* group of organisms are causative agents in certain types of food poisoning.

Bacillary dysentery. *Dysentery* is a term loosely used to indicate diarrhea with pus, blood, or mucus in the stools. Several unrelated conditions may thus be included under this term. The important types of dysentery are caused by the *Shigella dysenteriae* and by *Entamoeba histolytica*.

There are several varieties of dysentery bacilli, which may be distinguished by fermentative and antigenic reactions. They produce an endotoxin that has a local effect on the intestinal mucosa, and some also produce an exotoxin that may affect the nervous system.

The dysentery organisms reach the intestinal tract with contaminated food and drink. Dysentery is endemic but also tends to break out in epidemics, particularly in hot weather and when many persons live together under crowded and unhygienic conditions. An acute febrile illness lasting six to eight weeks results, but the infection is localized in the bowel, and positive cultures cannot be obtained from the blood. Repeated flare-ups or even a chronic condition may occur.

The large intestine is involved almost exclusively, specific lesions being rare in other organs. The distal parts of the colon are more severely affected. Occasionally the terminal ileum becomes involved. The lesion is of a diphtheritic or even membranous type, with necrosis and desquamation of surface layers and abundant fibrinopurulent exudate. In some very acute cases, death occurs from toxemia before any severe lesions have developed in the bowel. In most cases, however, there are widespread necroses of the mucosa of the large intestine and abundant exudate. Sloughing of necrotic areas leaves an extremely ragged ulceration of the colon. The ulcers are usually shallow, not undermined, and vary a great deal in size and shape. Their coalescence denudes large areas, leaving only occasional islands of intact mucosa. Severe diarrhea, excessive fluid loss, dehydration, and exhaustion accompany this condition of the bowel. Severe hemorrhage is uncommon. Perforation also is unusual and usually results in localized rather than generalized peritonitis.

Microscopic study shows the necrosis or ulceration of the mucosa with exudate on the surface. All layers of the bowel wall are edematous and infiltrated by neutrophilic leukocytes, but the submucosa is most greatly involved. Recovery is ac-

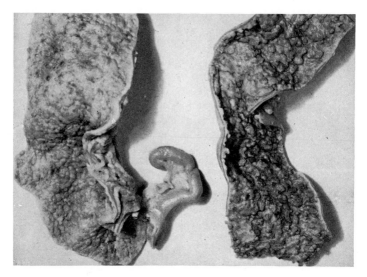

Fig. 19-11. Bacillary dysentery in the large intestine.

companied by healing of the ulcers and sometimes by scar formation and stenosis of the bowel. In healing, small mucosa-lined cysts may be formed, which continue to harbor the organisms.

Amebic dysentery. *Entamoeba histolytica* infection of the large intestine produces large, undermined, and flask-shaped ulcerations. The amebae can be identified microscopically in the adjacent tissues. Leukocytes are present when there is secondary infection. Occasionally a localized amebic granuloma may clinically simulate other inflammations or tumors of the colon. For detailed consideration see p. 217.

Balantidial dysentery. A rare ulcerative dysentery is caused by the ciliated protozoan parasite, *Balantidium coli,* the natural host of which is the pig. The parasites invade the mucosa of the large intestine and may produce chronic ulcers, sometimes deep and undermined. Lymphocytes, eosinophils, and neutrophils may form a mild inflammatory exudate. The parasites are easily recognized in the lesions by their large size (50 to 100μ) and the large, dark elongate nucleus (Fig. 19-12).

Cholera. Cholera is an Asiatic and tropical disease caused by

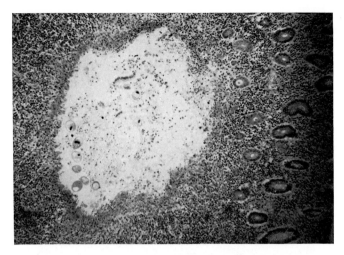

Fig. 19-12. *Balantidium coli* infection of the bowel. (Courtesy AFIP.)

the cholera vibrio or comma bacillus. It spreads in epidemic fashion, particularly by contamination of water and food. The infection is almost limited to the intestinal tract, where there is an acute catarrhal inflammation and distinct reddening of the mucosa. Profuse diarrhea, with flakes of whitish material in the watery stools (rice water stools), is characteristic and results in profound dehydration.

Pseudomembranous enterocolitis. Pseudomembranous enterocolitis is an occasional postoperative complication of surgical procedures on the intestinal tract. There is extensive denudation of the intestinal mucosa with variable degrees of pseudomembrane formation and great exudation of fluid into the lumen of the bowel. The clinical features are profuse diarrhea, dehydration, shock, and a fulminant course to a usually fatal outcome. A *Micrococcus pyogenes* resistant to most antibiotics has been found in some cases and in some cases appears to have followed the disturbance of the normal balance of intestinal flora by the use of antibiotics.

Chronic ulcerative colitis. Chronic ulcerative colitis is of debatable etiology but is usually considered as a specific entity. Among suggested causes are infection, allergy, lack of protective enzymes in the bowel wall, neurogenic and psychogenic disturbances, mucolytic and proteolytic enzymes acting on the

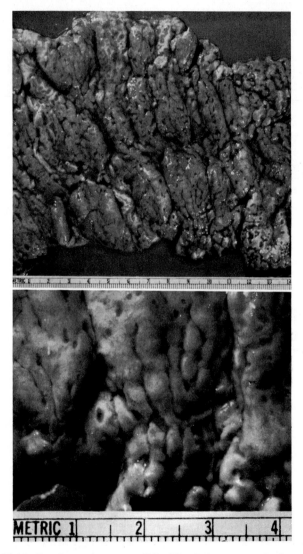

Fig. 19-13. Pseudomembranous colitis. The lesion occurred after a surgical procedure and antibiotic therapy.

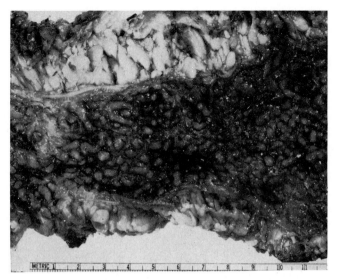

Fig. 19-14. Chronic ulcerative colitis with polypoid regeneration of mucosa.

mucosa, and alterations in the ground substance of the connective tissue. The disease has not been produced in experimental animals. Most cases occur in early or middle adult life. The course frequently extends over years, with remissions and relapses.

The large intestine is involved, the rectum and sigmoid being affected earliest and most severely, but in one third or less of cases the ileum also may be affected. Hyperemia and edema of the mucosa are followed by the appearance of small areas of necrosis and ulceration. Their coalescence produces large irregular and ragged ulcerations. Strips and tags of mucosa surrounded by the ulcerations become edematous and hyperplastic, projecting as inflamed polypoid masses. Myenteric ganglion cells appear to be increased in number. Eventually the bowel wall undergoes a considerable fibrotic thickening, and the ulcers heal by scar tissue. Stricture or stenosis of the bowel is thus a complication. Severe hemorrhage sometimes occurs. About 40% of deaths result from perforation of the colon with peritonitis. Malignant change not infrequently occurs in the polypoid mucosa and may be highly malignant with early metastasis. Patients with ulcerative colitis have eight times the frequency of death from cancer of the colon than others of the same age and sex. The cancer appears at an earlier average age, may arise from multiple sites, and tends to be less well circumscribed and to have a very fibrous stroma. Cancers occurring with ulcerative colitis are more evenly distributed through the colon. Other complications may include renal tubular degeneration, particularly of a hydropic or vacuolar type (p. 383), fatty change or cirrhosis of the liver, interstitial pancreatitis, fluid and electrolyte disturbances, protein loss, arthritis, venous thromboses, and amyloidosis.

Regional ileitis. Regional ileitis (Crohn's disease) is a hyperplastic granulomatous condition affecting distal portions of the ileum. It is characterized grossly by considerable regional thickening of the bowel wall with corresponding stenosis of the lumen, mucosal ulceration, and enlargement of regional mesenteric lymph nodes. Histologically its unique feature consists of focal masses of epithelioid and giant cells in the involved submucosa and in mesenteric lymph nodes. These lesions may occur in small numbers or even be entirely absent. Important clinical features are a palpable mass in the abdomen, signs of chronic obstruction, abdominal pain, and loss of weight.

The etiology is unknown, although it has been ascribed to a wide variety of infective, toxic, and vascular factors. Histologic similarity has suggested a possible relationship to Boeck's sarcoid, and there appears to be a disturbed lipid absorption metabolism. It is to be distinguished from the granulomatous lesions of tuberculosis and actinomycosis, which also commonly involve the ileocecal region, by the different histologic picture and demonstration of the specific causative organisms of the latter conditions. Lymphogranuloma inguinale may involve the bowel and is differentiated by the presence of a positive Frei reaction, its microscopic appearance (p. 200), and its usual involvement of colon rather than ileum.

Regional ileitis appears grossly as a garden-hose thickening of a segment of ileum, either at or within a few feet of its termination. In its acute stage the involved area is red and edematous. Later it tends to be rigid, firm, fibrous, and ulcerative. The bowel is dilated proximal to the constricted lumen of the involved segment. The adjacent mesentery contains enlarged lymph nodes. Perforation may occur, but the effects are usually limited by peritoneal adhesions.

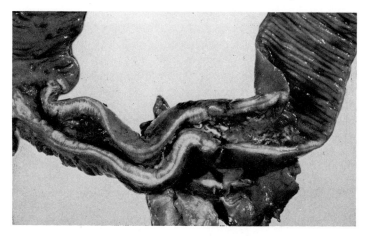

Fig. 19-15. Regional ileitis.

Microscopically the main feature is extreme thickening of the submucosa. There is a progressive granulomatous lymphangitis with focal lymphatic obliteration that produces elephantiasis of the intestinal wall, mesentery, and regional lymph nodes. There is also a severe hyperplasia of lymphoid tissue and the development of noncaseating aggregates of epithelioid cells and multinucleated giant cells. Tubercle bacilli cannot be demonstrated in these lesions. Similar sarcoidlike lesions are often present in the enlarged mesenteric nodes. Obstructive lymphedema is constantly present in the thick submucosa. Ulcerations of various depths develop, floored by granulation tissue. Eventually a diffuse cellular infiltration involves the bowel wall, with thickening of the muscular coat and adhesions of the serosa.

Complications of regional ileitis include intestinal obstruction, perforation, fistula formation, malabsorption syndrome, fluid and electrolyte disturbances, protein loss, arthritis, and amyloidosis.

Tuberculosis. Tuberculous infection of the intestine may be primary, the organisms being ingested with milk or other food. More commonly it is secondary to a pulmonary lesion because of the swallowing of infected sputum. A considerable proportion of fatal cases of pulmonary tuberculosis show intestinal lesions.

The lesions begin and are most common in the lower ileum

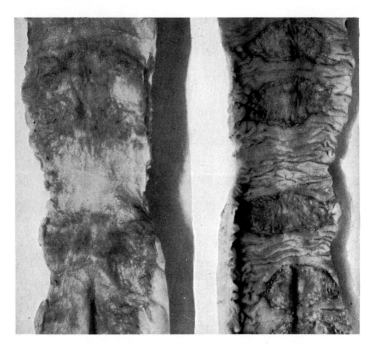

Fig. 19-16. Tuberculous enteritis. Note the oval ulcers tending to encircle the bowel. The change in the serosal surface is seen on the left.

but from there extend upward and downward to involve the small intestine and colon. The lymphoid tissue of the bowel is affected, and yellowish areas of caseous necrosis develop in the mucosa and submucosa. Ragged ulcers result from sloughing of this necrotic material. The lesions extend by lymphatics, which run laterally, encircling the gut. Hence the ulcerative lesions tend to be of elliptical shape, extending laterally and partially encircling the bowel. When such an ulcer is deep and extensive, its healing may produce significant contraction and stenosis of the bowel. The microscopic appearance is similar to that of tuberculosis elsewhere, with caseous necrosis and lymphoid, epithelioid, and giant cells. Perforation of a tuberculous ulcer is uncommon and usually results only in a localized peritonitis or abscess formation, as peritoneal reaction has walled off the area. Severe hemorrhage rarely occurs because blood vessels in the lesions are involved by periarteritic and endarteritic changes as they are in tuberculous pulmonary cavities. Occasionally a hyperplastic form of tuberculosis occurs around the ileocecal region, with great thickening of the bowel wall. Such lesions may be difficult to distinguish grossly from regional enteritis and tumors.

Actinomycosis. The ileocecal region or appendix is one of the common sites for actinomycosis. Characteristic features are thickening of the bowel wall, ulceration, and suppurative areas containing the ray fungus. Pylephlebitic spread to the liver is a frequent complication. Appendectomy is likely to be followed by a chronic sinus or fistula if the appendiceal infection was actinomycotic.

Appendicitis

Inflammation in the appendix has the same features and follows the same course as inflammation elsewhere. Its importance is caused by its frequency as a serious surgical condition with significant complications. Obstruction of the appendiceal lumen by fecaliths and interference with vascular supply are important features in its pathogenesis. Spread of the infection beyond the appendix rather than the lesion in the appendix itself is the factor that causes mortality.

Acute appendicitis.

Etiology. The full story of the cause of acute appendicitis is not yet known. The nervous strains and dietary habits of modern life have been vaguely suggested as predisposing factors. The essential thing in causing the wall of the appendix to react with inflammation is invasion by bacteria. The common organisms in the inflamed appendix are colon bacilli and varieties of streptococci, organisms commonly found in the intestinal lumen. Obstruction and vascular occlusion are factors of tested importance in the etiology of appendicitis. They probably act by breaking down the appendiceal wall's resistance to invasion by the potential pathogens in the lumen.

The importance of luminal obstruction has been emphasized. An obstructed appendix having a normal mucosa may develop a secretory pressure approaching systolic blood pressure, thus presumably interfering with the blood supply of the tissue. Such obstruction may act as the exciting cause of typical acute appendicitis.

Morbid anatomy. Acute appendicitis is often classified as (1) catarrhal, (2) diffuse, and (3) gangrenous. Catarrhal appen-

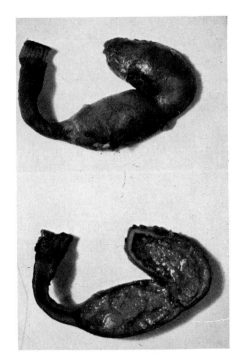

Fig. 19-17. Acute appendicitis. The lumen is distended and filled with pus.

dicitis is one in which the inflammation is limited to the mucosal and submucosal layers. It is usually a mild type or an early stage of the diffuse type. In diffuse appendicitis the muscular and serosal layers are involved as well. In gangrenous appendicitis there is the added condition of necrosis.

The beginning of acute appendicitis is usually a superficial ulceration of the mucosa. Spread occurs from the mucosa to the serosa in a wedge-shaped area and then travels rapidly lengthwise in the muscular and serous coats. Grossly the appendix appears swollen, the serosal vessels are congested, and the surface of the serosa has lost its normal shininess or may be covered by discernible fibrinous exudate. The muscular walls are thick and edematous. The mucosa may show areas of hemorrhage and ulcerations. The causes of luminal obstruction may be

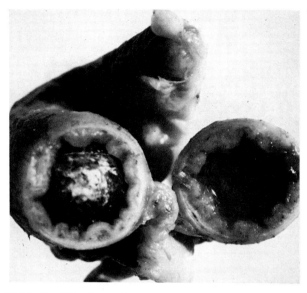

Fig. 19-18. Fecalith obstructing the lumen of the appendix and acute appendicitis.

swelling of lymphoid tissue, the formation of a calculus or a fecalith (a firm, dried, fecal concretion), or marked fibrous thickening of a portion of the appendiceal wall. Over a large fecalith the wall is likely to be thin and gangrenous. Gangrenous areas show a grayish green or black discoloration, have a thick flaky layer of fibrin on the surface, and often have a small perforation.

Microscopically the early stage of acute appendicitis is often difficult to discern, particularly if the section is not through exactly the right area. The normal lymphoid cellularity of the mucosa and submucosa may be confusing. Ulceration of the mucosa or a purulent exudate in the lumen may be seen if the section is through the proper area. In most cases of acute appendicitis the diagnosis is obvious from the infiltration of leukocytes in the muscular and serous layers.

Complications. Many milder cases of acute appendicitis subside without surgical interference, but in other cases spread of the infection may occur with serious or fatal results. Such spread is usually to the peritoneum as a result of gangrene or perforation. If there has been opportunity for the walling off and limitation of the infection to the region around the appendix, a localized abscess may result. This localized peritonitis is much less dangerous than the generalized peritoneal spread that quite commonly occurs. In some cases spread from the appendix is by infection of portal veins draining the inflamed organ (pylephlebitis) and leads to the production of multiple abscesses in the liver. A false diverticulum of the appendix may follow appendicitis.

Chronic appendicitis. Chronic appendicitis has been a subject of controversy because it is often difficult to correlate the clinical symptoms attributed to the appendix with the anatomic findings. In some cases there is evidence of obstruction from a fecalith or other cause, but without any active inflammatory process discernible in the wall of the appendix. Very often the anatomic finding is a fibrous thickening of the submucosa and mucosa, with atrophy of the mucosal glandular elements and with or without a hyperplasia of the submucosal lymphoid tissue. In its extreme degree such fibrosis may completely obliterate the lumen. This fibrosis is believed, in many cases, to be the end result or healed stage of previous, recurring attacks of acute inflammation. An appendix with complete obliteration of the lumen is unlikely to become inflamed again, but partial obliteration may predispose to recurrent inflammation.

Masson's studies have indicated that in some cases the thickening of the submucosa and obliteration of the lumen are largely caused by proliferation of smooth muscle bundles and nervous elements associated with Meissner's plexus, the so-called musculonervous complex of the appendix.

A lymphoid type of chronic appendicitis has been described. Lymphoid tissue is a normal constituent of the submucosa of the appendix, and in young persons it may be very abundant, but in older people it gradually atrophies. There may be, however, a severe chronic hyperplasia of this lymphoid tissue associated with atrophy of the glandular elements of the mucosa and gradual submucosal fibrosis. The condition may progress to fibrous obliteration of the lumen.

Tuberculous appendicitis is secondary to tuberculosis elsewhere. The lesions show little tendency to heal, and they predispose to secondary infection with the occurrence of acute symptoms.

Lesions of the appendix in measles. In measles the lymphoid

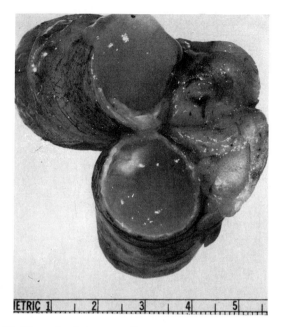

Fig. 19-19. Mucocele of the appendix.

tissue of the appendix, as well as in the throat, spleen, and remainder of the intestinal tract, is distinctly hyperplastic. In early stages there are characteristic giant cells in the mucosa and lymph follicles. (See Fig. 7-9.)

Oxyuris vermicularis infection of the appendix. In children, pinworms commonly infect the appendix, where they may obstruct the lumen. In most instances they cause little damage, but in some cases they may be associated with the clinical picture of acute appendicitis (p. 226).

Mucocele of the appendix. Complete obstruction of the proximal portion of the appendix sometimes results in a cyst-like dilatation (mucocele) of the distal part. The contents of the dilated sac are a thick mucoid material. Malignant mucoceles are lined by a thick papillary layer of mucus-secreting cells. In some instances rupture of the mucocele may cause pseudomyxoma peritonei. This latter condition is more commonly a complication of ovarian mucinous cystadenoma.

Diverticula of the intestine

A diverticulum of the intestine may be true or false. A true diverticulum has all layers of the bowel in its wall; the common example is the congenital Meckel's diverticulum. False diverticula are acquired herniations of the mucosa through a weak place in the muscularis of the bowel. Their walls contain only mucosal and serosal layers. They occur in both small and large intestine and are particularly common in the latter.

Meckel's diverticulum. Meckel's diverticulum is caused by the persistence of the proximal portion of the omphalomesenteric duct, which normally atrophies during early fetal life. It is found in 1 to 2% of persons. It varies up to 30 cm. in length but is usually about the size of a small finger. It is situated 1 to 3 feet proximal to the ileocecal junction (averaging 80 cm.). Its structure is similar to that of the bowel wall, but heterotopic tissue, such as gastric or duodenal mucosa, or pancreatic tissue

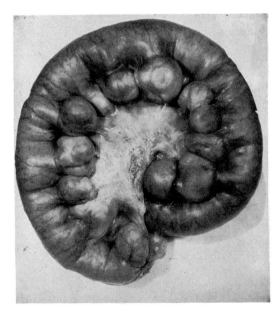

Fig. 19-20. Diverticulosis of the small intestine. The diverticula are located at the mesenteric border and have large stomas. (Courtesy Dr. J. R. Schenken.)

may be found in it. Peptic ulcer, subject to the complications of hemorrhage and perforation, has been reported in such tissue.

The commonest lesion of a Meckel's diverticulum is inflammation. Pathologically this is similar to appendicitis, which it may mimic clinically. More rarely it may promote intestinal obstruction by intussusception or adhesions, or it may be the seat of a tumor. Hemorrhage from the bowel is an important complication of the diverticula containing gastric mucosa.

Patent omphalomesenteric (vitelline) duct is comparatively rare. A communication is demonstrable between the umbilicus and the ileum. The intestine may prolapse out through the umbilical fistula.

Acquired diverticula. The common sites for diverticula are the esophagus, duodenum, and colon, but they also occur in the small intestine. These are commonly false diverticula, although some may have muscle fibers in their walls. In the small intestine they occur along the mesenteric attachment, whereas in the colon they are situated away from the mesenteric attachment between the taeniae or longitudinal muscular bands of the colon. The descending and sigmoid portions of colon have the highest incidence. The protrusion often is into appendices epiploicae, so that the diverticula are readily overlooked. They

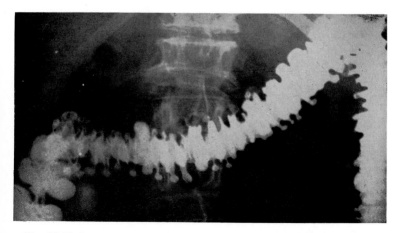

Fig. 19-21. Roentgenogram of diverticulosis of the colon. The diverticula are small and the stomas are narrow. (Courtesy Dr. H. Hunt and Dr. R. Moore.)

vary up to several centimeters in diameter. Microscopically their wall is found composed of a thinned mucosa and serosa between which may be a few connective tissue and muscle fibers.

When present without complications, the condition is known as *diverticulosis.* The common complication is inflammation or *diverticulitis.* This is promoted by the lodging of fecal matter in the sacs. Spread of inflammation to surrounding tissue *(peridiverticulitis)* may occur also. The chronic inflammatory process causes thickening of the bowel wall and adjacent tissues with constriction of the lumen of the bowel. The gross appearance may closely simulate that of carcinoma.

Pneumatosis cystoides intestinalis

Pneumatosis intestinalis is characterized by gas-filled cysts in the submucosa and/or subserosa of the small bowel, and sometimes of the colon. Ranging in size up to several centimeters, the cysts may be lined by flattened endothelium-like cells, forming pseudolymphatic spaces, or if the cysts have been recently formed, by mononuclear cells and multinucleated giant cells. The cysts appear to develop most frequently as a result of respiratory disease and pneumomediastinum, which is decompressed by the gas being forced into the abdomen. Other origins, as from obstruction and ulceration, have been considered.

Stricture of the rectum

A variety of inflammatory processes, scar contractions, and tumors may cause rectal stricture. It is particularly common as a complication of lymphogranuloma inguinale in females. This infection spreads by lymphatics from the primary lesion on the genitalia. The distribution of lymphatics in females is such as to involve perirectal tissue, whereas in the male the spread is usually to inguinal lymphatics. The rectal involvement is a chronic progressive granulomatous inflammation, which leads to serious stricture. Spread to the rectum by means other than by the lymphatics is believed to occur also.

Pilonidal sinus

Pilonidal sinus, or sacrococcygeal sinus, is a very common lesion, which in some cases may be a remnant of the neurenteric canal or an infolding of the epithelial layer of skin. Commonly, however, it is an acquired condition caused by the penetration

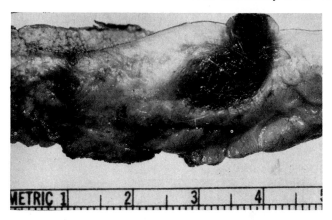

Fig. 19-22. Pilonidal sinus.

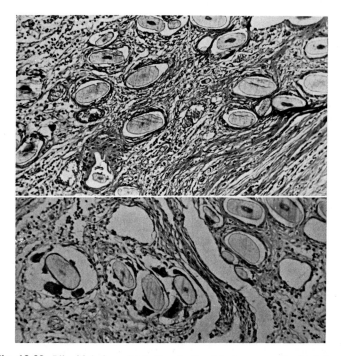

Fig. 19-23. Pilonidal sinus. Note the shafts of hairs, some of which have foreign body giant cells around them, and the infiltration of chronic inflammatory cells.

of hairs into subcutaneous tissues, with chronic mild infection. It occurs in the midline a few centimeters posterior to the anus, the sinus extending inward toward a cystic cavity in the subcutaneous tissue above the sacrococcygeal vertebrae. Microscopically the usual features are hair shafts, multinucleated giant cells of the foreign body type, and abundant lymphocytes and plasma cells. Troublesome recurrence is likely to follow incomplete removal or infection in adjacent tissue. Cancer in a pilonidal sinus is extremely rare.

Intestinal obstruction

Complete obstruction to the passage of intestinal contents either by a mechanical obstruction of the lumen or by a paralysis of the bowel wall bring about death in a relatively short period of time unless relieved. Such complete obstructions may be called acute to distinguish them from the partial mechanical obstructions of bowel lumen, which are compatible with life for long periods and hence are termed chronic obstructions.

The *chronic* partial mechanical obstruction of the intestine may be caused by a large variety of conditions, such as tumors in the bowel or pressure on it from the outside, adhesive or fibrous bands, impacted feces, etc. Perforation of an inflamed gallbladder into the intestinal tract with extrusion of a large gallstone may lead to intermittent upper intestinal obstruction *(gallstone ileus)*. Above a point of chronic partial obstruction the bowel is distended, and there is hypertrophy of the muscular wall. There is, of course, danger that the obstruction may become complete and acute at any time.

An *acute* obstruction may be a simple mechanical obstruction, or there may be an associated interference with the blood and nerve supply of the intestine, in which case it is said to be strangulated. Interference with the blood supply to a segment of intestine, as in thrombosis of mesenteric vessels, results in a paralytic obstruction, although there may be no mechanical blockage. Neurogenic factors may produce an *adynamic (paralytic) ileus,* e.g., after operations or as a result of peritonitis, severe pain (renal colic), or systemic infection. Obstructions with strangulation occur in hernias and as a result of volvulus (twisting) or intussusception. Necrosis or infarction of the bowel wall occurs unless the blood supply is promptly restored. The involved portion of intestine becomes congested, edematous,

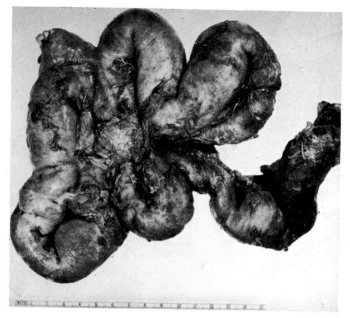

Fig. 19-24. Fibrous peritoneal adhesions of the bowel.

hemorrhagic, and finally gangrenous. Ulcerations occur in and above obstructed portions of intestine (stercoral ulcers).

The actual *cause of death* in intestinal obstruction has been a matter of much study and debate. The effects vary, depending upon the site and type of obstruction. High up in the intestinal tract, obstruction causes excessive vomiting with dehydration and chemical disturbances because of the great loss of water and chlorides. In experimental obstructions life can be greatly prolonged simply by replacing these substances. In low intestinal obstructions, dehydration and electrolyte loss may or may not be great, and death appears to be caused rather by the absorption of toxic substances. The exact nature of the toxic material is not clear. Part of the toxicity appears to be caused by histamine or a related substance, although multiple toxins probably are involved. The toxicity may result from bacterial action on injured intestinal tissue.

Hernia. An abdominal hernia is an abnormal protrusion of abdominal viscera outside the usual confines of the abdominal wall. Such protrusion may be through the inguinal canal, through the femoral canal, at the umbilicus, through a weak scar of an abdominal wound (ventral hernia), or through the diaphragm. Internal hernias are protrusions into intra-abdominal pouches.

A hernia becomes strangulated when there is a tight constriction of the loop of bowel at the neck of the sac. The constriction first compresses veins in which the pressure is low, causing congestion and swelling of the herniated loop. This in turn increases the constriction until eventually the arterial supply is cut off as well, and the involved tissue soon becomes gangrenous.

Diaphragmatic hernia. Herniation through the diaphragm may be congenital, i.e., caused by abnormality of development or by trauma or wounds of the diaphragm.

Congenital diaphragmatic hernia is quite frequently encountered in newborn or young children. It is about ten times more frequent on the left side. The hernia may be *true,* with the existence of a hernial sac composed of peritoneum and pleura. More commonly the hernia is *false,* with no hernial sac existing as the pleura and peritoneum are absent over the opening. Congenital false hernia is caused by abnormal persistence of the pleuroperitoneal canal, which connects the primitive pleural region with the abdominal region and normally becomes covered by a membrane about the seventh or eighth week of fetal life. An excessive mobility of the intestinal tract is usually associated because of the abnormal attachment of mesenteries.

Herniation may also occur through the esophageal hiatus. Other types of intra-abdominal hernias may occur, most commonly in or about the paraduodenal fossae, into the transverse mesocolon, or through the foramen of Winslow.

Volvulus. Volvulus is a twisting or rotation of a loop of bowel, which by its occlusion of blood vessels may result in strangulation. The coil of intestine becomes obstructed and gangrenous.

Intussusception. The invagination or passage of one portion of intestine into another segment is known as intussusception. The invaginated part tends to be carried along by peristaltic activity, dragging with it mesentery and blood vessels, which eventually become obstructed, so that congestion, edema, hemorrhage, inflammation, and adhesions occur. These changes may make reduction very difficult. Necrosis of the invaginated seg-

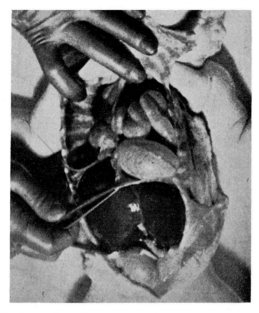

Fig. 19-25. Congenital diaphragmatic hernia. Note the stomach and loops of bowel in the left thoracic cavity. The diaphragm is held in the forceps.

ment eventually develops. The condition is more common in young children, usually beginning in the ileocecal region. Sometimes polyps or other tumors of the intestine are dragged along by peristalsis and start an intussusception. Multiple small intussusceptions of the small bowel are common at autopsy. They are caused by irregular intestinal contractions at the time of death and, being without inflammatory changes, are easily reduced.

Congenital megacolon. Megacolon, or Hirschsprung's disease, is a marked dilatation of the large intestine, usually throughout its entire length, with hypertrophy of the muscle fibers. The condition is congenital. Its exact etiology is unknown, although imbalance of the nerve supply to the colon and sphincters has been postulated. The distended bowel produces considerable abdominal enlargement, and fecal evacuations occur after abnormally long intervals.

Intestinal lipodystrophy (Whipple's disease)

Rare cases have been described in which there appears to be a disturbance of fat excretion and reabsorption from the intestines. The two chief hypotheses of pathogenesis are (1) the mechanical or inflammatory concept, which suggests that the primary lesion is an obstructive process involving some portion of the efferent lymphatic system, and (2) the chemical concept, according to which a defect in fat or carbohydrate metabolism is primary. Histochemical studies have suggested that there may be a disturbance resulting in abnormal production of a polysaccharide protein complex. Fatty diarrhea, accompanied by chylous ascites, a slight hypochromic anemia, and progressive emaciation proceed to a fatal ending. The mucosa of the small intestine is thickened, with clubbing of villi, and shows dilated lymphatics and infiltration with large foamy macrophages; mesenteric lymph nodes are enlarged, have lost their normal architecture, and show dilated spaces and sinuses filled with amorphous fat or large foamy macrophages and some multinucleated giant cells. Histiocytes contain abundant mucopolysaccharide demonstrable by periodic acid–Schiff staining. Some of the material in the cells is in the form of sickle-shaped particles, which electron microscopic evidence suggests are derived from mitochondria. Such evidence has suggested that Whipple's disease might be an intracellular defect within his-

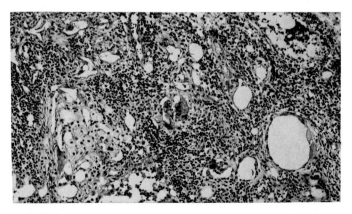

Fig. 19-26. Lymph node in Whipple's disease. Clear areas represent sites of lipid. Foam cells and some giant cell reaction are shown.

tiocytes or reticuloendothelial cells. Other evidence as well suggests that Whipple's disease is a systemic condition.

Celiac disease and sprue

Primary malabsorption syndromes or steatorrhea include celiac disease in infants and children, nontropical sprue in adults, and tropical sprue. Macrocytic anemia may be severe in tropical sprue (p. 563).

In celiac disease and nontropical sprue there is a genetic metabolic disturbance, which often manifests an intolerance to gluten in the diet. The small intestine shows villous atrophy, appearing flattened. Treated cases and also tropical sprue show less villous atrophy, and villi may show clubbing. The changes are greatest in the jejunum, which is a site used for biopsy.

Melanosis coli

Melanosis coli is a symptomless condition of brown or black discoloration of the mucosa of the large intestine caused by a melanin-like pigment held in large mononuclear cells. The pig-

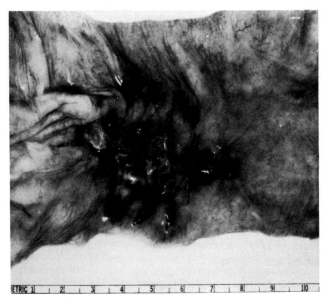

Fig. 19-27. Hemangioma of the intestinal mucosa.

ment may also be found in the submucosa and sometimes in mesenteric lymph nodes.

Tumors of the small intestine

Tumors are uncommon in the small intestine. Various benign tumors such as fibromas, myomas, and lipomas may involve the small bowel, but carcinoma is rare. Brunner's gland adenomas occur rarely. They may cause gastrointestinal hemorrhage. Multiple polyposis of the stomach and small bowel may be associated with focal melanin pigmentation of the lips and mouth (Peutz-Jeghers syndrome) inherited as an autosomal dominant trait. Such polyps rarely, if ever, become malignant. The polyps in Peutz-Jeghers syndrome contain more than one type of cell e.g., columnar cells and goblet cells, and the possibility that they are hamartomas has been considered. Malignant lymphomas may involve the ileum, as well as the region of the cecum or ascending colon. In some cases a malignant lymphoma of the small bowel is focal in nature and may be cured by complete excision. Angiomatous lesions of the alimentary tract are rare except in association with vascular lesions elsewhere as part of one of the hereditary vascular dysplasias.

Carcinoid tumors. Carcinoid tumors (argentaffinomas) are distinctive neoplasms, which have infiltrative and metastasizing potentialities but are of a low grade of malignancy. The tumor cells are believed to arise from Kultschitsky cells, argentaffin and chromaffin cells found at the base of Lieberkühn's glands, which produce serotonin (enteramine, 5-hydroxytryptamine). A small proportion of carcinoid tumors may have liver metastases which produce excess serotonin and a distinctive clinical syndrome (the carcinoid syndrome). Other substances, such as bradykinin, have

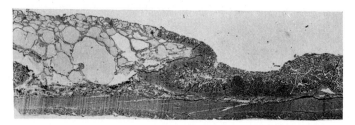

Fig. 19-28. Angioma of the intestinal mucosa.

been identified, which may contribute to the symptoms of this syndrome.

About 60% of carcinoid tumors occur in the appendix and most often near the tip, where they may form a yellowish annular thickening which encircles the lumen. In the appendix carcinoid tumors have a biologically benign course. They are not circumscribed, may infiltrate the muscularis, and in rare cases metastasize to lymph nodes, but distant metastases do not occur. Carcinoid tumors of the appendix do not give rise to the clinical carcinoid syndrome.

About 40% of carcinoid tumors arise from the remainder of the gastrointestinal tract, any part of which may be involved, although the ileum is the most frequent site. They most often occur as small yellowish or grayish submucosal masses with intact overlying mucosa and only uncommonly form large ulcerating or fungating masses. They are often multiple (25%). Infiltration of the muscularis and spread to lymph nodes are common, and about 15% metastasize to the liver. In all cases the degree of malignancy is low, and the natural course of the disease tends to be long and slow. Carcinoid tumors have also been described in the lung, gallbladder, and pancreas.

The cells composing a carcinoid tumor are remarkably uniform, and only very rarely are there mitoses or cells of polymorphous or giant form. The compact uniform cells have distinct nuclei but ill-defined borders and occur in solid clusters, sheets, islands, or cords with a variable but usually scanty stroma. Distinct gland formation is not commonly seen. Chrome and silver salts stain granules in the cytoplasm. A small proportion of carcinoids, particularly those of the rectum and colon, fail to stain with silver and are considered to arise from pre-enterochrome cells.

The carcinoid syndrome occurs in some of the cases in which there are metastases in the liver, presumably caused by the production of large amounts of serotonin. It is characterized by episodic flushing of the skin (beginning in the face and spreading over the trunk and extremities), a plethoric coloration or cyanosis, intestinal hyperperistalsis with diarrhea, asthmalike bronchoconstrictive attacks, and cardiac symptoms resulting from tricuspid and pulmonary valve involvement. In late stages there may be much wasting, weight loss, and cutaneous telangiectases or pellagra-like lesions.

The cardiac lesions are a fibrous thickening of tricuspid and pulmonary valves with pulmonary stenosis. The thickening appears to be caused by a fibrous tissue growth without elastic fibrils, superimposed on an intact valve cusp. It has been postulated that these changes are caused by exposure to large quantities of serotonin from the hepatic carcinoid metastases but that this substance tends to be destroyed in the lungs so that the left side of the heart is usually not similarly exposed. However, instances of left-sided heart involvement have been described.

Serotonin (5-hydroxytryptamine, enteramine) is derived from tryptophan and is a smooth muscle stimulating and vasoconstrictive substance carried normally by the blood platelets. The large amount of serotonin produced by a functioning carcinoid tumor results in an excess of 5-hydroxy-3-indole acetic acid in the urine, a valuable laboratory diagnostic test.

Although the carcinoid syndrome is produced most often from a carcinoid tumor of the ileum which has metastasized to the liver, it appears that the carcinoid type of bronchial adenoma may have a similar effect.

In rare examples a functioning carcinoid tumor, composed of nongranular argyrophil cells, appears to produce 5-hydroxytryptophan, a precursor of serotonin.

Carcinoma of the appendix. Apart from carcinoid tumors,

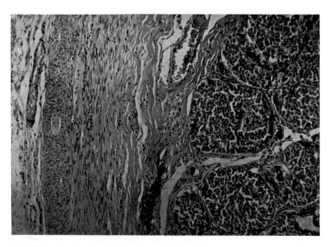

Fig. 19-29. Carcinoid tumor of the appendix. The muscular layers of the appendiceal wall are seen in the left.

the appendix is rarely a site of primary carcinoma. Malignant mucocele of the appendix is a type of carcinoma in which the dilated appendix is filled with gelatinous material, and the mucosa has prominent papillary folds of mucus-secreting epithelium. Peritoneal spread with production of pseudomyxoma peritonei may result from rupture or spillage at the time of surgical excision. A colonic type of carcinoma, similar in structure to tumors of the large bowel, is the rarest variety of carcinoma of the appendix. Carcinoids of the appendix must be distinguished from the rare true adenocarcinoma of the appendix by (1) situation in the distal rather than the proximal part of the appendix, (2) the distinct yellow color, (3) argentaffin and chromaffin granules in the cytoplasm, (4) lack or paucity of metastases, and (5) absence of glandular arrangement.

Tumors of the colon and rectum

Unlike the small bowel, the colon and rectum are common and important sites of carcinoma. The incidence is greatest in the sigmoid and rectum (55 to 70%), in the transverse colon and flexures (20%), and in the cecum and ascending colon (25%). They may begin as polypoid, sessile, or ulcerated neoplasms. The infiltrating ulcerative type may spread to

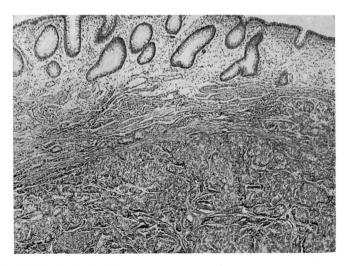

Fig. 19-30. Carcinoid of the rectum.

lymph nodes while at an early and small stage. The tumors vary in rate of growth and degree of malignancy, but in some cases metastatic spread is late and cure is possible by excision. Grading by Dukes' method based on degree of spread is helpful in prognosis. The age of greatest incidence is after 50 years, but younger ages are not exempt. Carcinoma of the colon is significantly (six to eight times) more common in patients with chronic ulcerative colitis than in the general population and

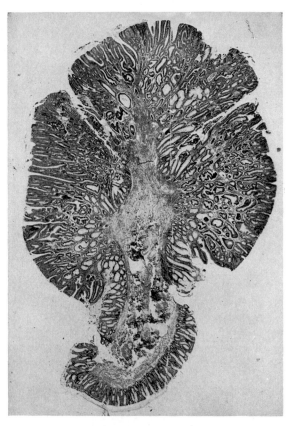

Fig. 19-31. Pedunculated benign polyp of the large bowel. (From Ackerman, L. V., and del Regato, J. A.: Cancer, ed. 3, St. Louis, 1962, The C. V. Mosby Co.)

occurs at a younger average age (p. 627). Carcinoma of the rectum is slightly more frequent in males, and carcinoma of the colon is more frequent in females. Carcinoids are less frequent tumors of the rectum and colon and may metastasize. Other uncommon rectal or anal tumors are benign lymphoma (benign lymphoid polyp), basaloid carcinomas, mucoepidermoid tumors, and malignant melanoma of the anorectal region.

Adenoma and polyposis. Polyposis of the colon and rectum is common. Most of these (60% or more) occur in the descending colon, sigmoid, and rectum, i.e., the same areas in which carcinoma is most frequent. The polyps are true adenomatous tumors and are to be distinguished from the inflammatory and hyperplastic areas of mucosa that simulate them in chronic dysentery and ulcerative colitis. There are two types of polypoid disease of the intestine: (1) diffuse polyposis, in which large numbers of polyps involve the colon and rectum, and (2) localized or solitary polyposis, in which there is only one or a few polyps present. Familial polyposis is hereditarily transmitted as an autosomal, nonsex-linked dominant trait. This diffuse mul-

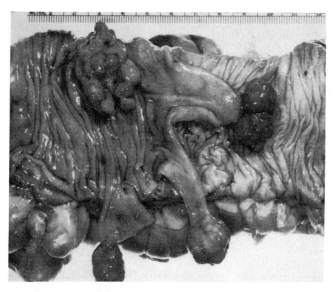

Fig. 19-32. Sigmoid colon with multiple polyps and a carcinoma.

tiple polyposis is present in early life and often is complicated by carcinoma at an early age.

Some of the confusion regarding the malignant potentialities of the polypoid tumors results from the failure to differentiate clearly different types of polypoid lesions of the bowel. The term *polyp* simply refers to an outgrowth from a mucous membrane.

Adenomatous polyps are characterized by a relatively normal covering epithelium over a mass of elongated, bizarre-shaped mucosal glands, often with goblet cells. Usually those lesions have a stalk, i.e., are pedunculated. They are very common, and

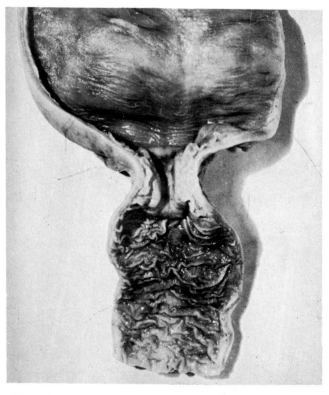

Fig. 19-33. Adenocarcinoma of the sigmoid colon. The tumor encircles the bowel and constricts the lumen. Note the dilatation of the colon proximal to the region of chronic obstruction.

estimates of their incidence have ranged from 10 to 50% of adults. Apart from diffuse multiple polyposis, the importance of the ordinary adenomatous polyp as a precursor of carcinoma is debatable. Arising as a local hyperplasia of mucosal glands, often it shows focal areas of atypical cells, but carcinoma arising in such lesions is probably rare.

Villous polyps, also called papillary adenomas, villous adenomas, and villous papillary adenomas, are composed of branching, fingerlike processes of surface origin. They are usually broad based or sessile rather than pedunculated, and the villi have cores of vascularized connective tissue. They may be multiple but also occur in solitary fashion in the rectum of older adults. They are distinguished by their broad attachment to the bowel wall, a villous architecture resulting from a disproportionate growth of surface epithelium, and a great tendency to recur after local removal. They are potentially malignant, and carcinomatous change may develop in any part. Mucus-secreting villous adenomas occasionally cause hypokalemia, hyponatremia, and dehydration caused by profuse secretion from the mucosa of the tumor. The electrolyte imbalance may be severe, with sudden collapse and death.

Juvenile or childhood polyps are characterized by a prominent stromal growth and eosinophilic cell exudate. The surface may be ulcerated and covered by granulation tissue. The glands in the polyp show cystic dilatation with intraluminal epithelial projections. Juvenile polyps remain benign.

Differentiation of benign polyps from those that have become malignant or from small polypoid carcinomas may be difficult. Tendency to ulceration is greater in the malignant polyps. Since malignant change can occur in any part of a polyp, sections from various portions must be examined before cancer can be ruled out. Sections from the base and from the tip are particularly likely to show malignancy. The important criteria of malignancy are (1) invasion of underlying tissue (muscularis mucosa) or of lymphatics or blood vessels, (2) anaplasia of the epithelial cells, and (3) disorderly arrangement of glands.

Less common benign tumors of the large intestine are lipomas and leiomyomas. Lymphoid polyps occur in the rectum and are benign.

Carcinoma of the colon and rectum.

Gross features. The two main gross types are (1) annular constricting and (2) papillary. The *annular constricting* type is

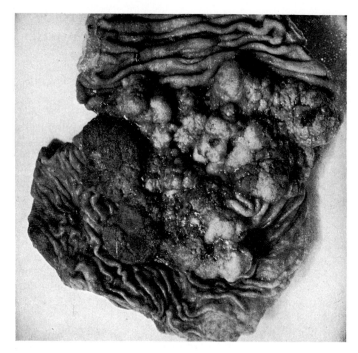

Fig. 19-34. Adenocarcinoma of the cecum. The fungating tumor is projecting into the lumen.

often ulcerative. It grows around the bowel, thickening and contracting the wall and narrowing and obstructing the lumen. The *papillary* variety grows as a bulky mass projecting into the bowel lumen, thus giving rise to symptoms of obstruction. Necrosis and infection of the tumor mass and inflammatory lymphadenitis are common with this type.

Histologic features. Histologically the tumors nearly always show some tendency to gland formation and hence may be termed adenocarcinoma. When this tendency is slight, the tumor cells form solid masses with scanty alveolar formation and hence the tumor is of a medullary type. Stroma is often scanty or moderate in amount, but it may be so abundant that the tumor is scirrhous. Mucinous degeneration is found in about 5%. This may be a mucoid change in individual cells so that they have a signet-ring appearance, or the mucoid material may be formed

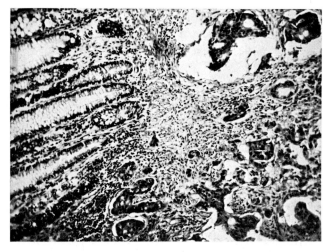

Fig. 19-35. Adenocarcinoma of the rectum. The edge of the tumor is shown, with the transition from normal to malignant epithelium. Note the invasion of the submucosa and the mucoid character in some areas.

by the tumor alveoli, with mucinous deposition in a considerable area in which only a few tumor cells are evident.

Grading. Classification according to degree of malignancy is important for prognostic and therapeutic purposes. There are two main methods of grading and these methods can be combined for greatest effectiveness. The histologic method is based on the criteria of invasiveness, glandular arrangement, nuclear polarity, and frequency of mitosis and indicates rate of growth of the tumor. Grade I is characterized by well-differentiated, compact glandular structure, nuclei of the cells close to the basal portion, little tendency to invasion of surrounding tissue, and infrequent mitoses. These tumors most nearly resemble adenomas and are sometimes termed "malignant adenomas." Grade II tumors have the glandular arrangement preserved but irregular, the nuclei in variable positions, a greater invasive tendency, and more frequent mitoses. In Grade III the glandular structure is almost completely gone, cells grow in solid masses, the cell polarity is lost, invasion is irregular, and mitoses are numerous. The practical value of the system of grading, if used alone, has been questioned.

The mucoid carcinoma of the signet-ring type tends to be of

high malignancy, Grade II or III, while those not of the signet-ring type are of lower malignancy, Grade I or II.

Dukes' method of classification is based on the degree of spread and appears to be more valuable for prognostic purposes. In group A are placed the carcinomas that have not spread through the rectal wall; in group B, those that have penetrated the rectal wall but have not invaded the adjacent lymphatics; and in group C, those that have invaded the local lymphatics.

Spread and metastasis. Spread tends to be earlier in the flat, sessile growths than in the papillary type. It occurs by growth laterally around the bowel and outward through the wall. Local lymphatics then become affected. From a rectal cancer this lymphatic involvement may be downward, lateralward, or frequently upward along the superior hemorrhoidal vessels by way of the retrorectal lymph nodes to the nodes of the pelvic mesocolon. Spread by bloodstream most commonly produces metastasis in the liver. Next to the liver and regional lymph nodes, the peritoneum and lungs are the most frequent sites of metastasis.

Effects. The disturbances produced by carcinoma in the colon and rectum depend upon the type and location of the growth. Because the symptoms are often slight until a late stage, the condition must be kept in mind and investigation made on the least suspicion. Ulceration is usually accompanied by slight bleeding, so that blood is detectable in the stools. Chronic obstruction is often a late development, usually in the annular stenosing type of carcinoma. The bowel above the obstruction is dilated.

Lymphoma of the rectum. Benign lymphoma of the rectum (lymphoid polyp) is more frequent than primary malignant lymphoma of the rectum, which is rare. Most occur in the lower rectum or anal region. Lymphoid tumors of the large intestine proximal to the rectum are more likely to be malignant than benign.

Malignant melanoma of the rectum. Melanoma of the rectum occurs predominantly at the anorectal junction or in the anus itself. It is often polypoid or pedunculated. The tumor is highly malignant, and the prognosis is poor.

PERITONEUM

The peritoneum is a closed sac in the male, but in the female it communicates with the genital tract by openings at the ends of the fallopian tubes. The smooth, shiny peritoneal lining is composed of flattened mesothelial cells, beneath which are a basement membrane and a small amount of connective tissue containing abundant blood vessels and lymphatics. The total surface area is very large, and through the peritoneum there is ready absorption with equal facility in all parts. The omentum actively functions to wall off inflamed areas and to retard the spread of peritonitis. Inflammation is the most important lesion of the peritoneum. Ascites is the accumulation of excessive fluid in the peritoneal cavity. Primary tumor (mesothelioma) of the peritoneum is rare, but metastatic growths involving peritoneum are common. Mesotheliomas may have epithelium-like structures, but they do not secrete mucin. Primary retroperitoneal tumors are of various histologic types, and some may arise from remnants of the urogenital fold. Most of the tumors are sarcomas, but epithelial cysts, lipomas, and other benign tumors also occur. Fibromatous and other solid tumors occur uncommonly in mesentery and omentum.

Peritonitis

Infection of the peritoneum may result by spread (1) from a ruptured viscus (e.g., perforated peptic ulcer or gangrenous appendix); (2) through an injured but unruptured bowel wall (e.g., in infarct of the bowel); (3) from or by way of the internal genital organs (e.g., in puerperal endometritis and primary pneumococcal peritonitis); or rarely (4) through the bloodstream. The peritoneal infection may be walled off so as to be limited to a localized area, as in periappendiceal abscess or subphrenic abscess, or there may be generalized involvement. Death may be caused by the absorption of toxins or by paralytic obstruction of a portion of intestine.

Acute peritonitis has been described as occurring in hyperemic, exudative, and plastic stages. These changes may be found locally or diffusely. In the hyperemic stage one sees great dilatation and congestion of peritoneal vessels, which gives the peritoneal surfaces a pinkish blue color. This stage occurs early, probably within an hour after the perforation of an ulcer. It is rapidly followed by the exudative stage in which inflammatory cells and fibrin accumulate on the surfaces, and there is an increase in the amount of fluid in the peritoneal sac. In the plastic stage the exudate forms adhesions walling off the affected region or joining peritoneal surfaces. Organization or fibrosis may occur.

Fecal peritonitis. Fecal peritonitis is caused by colon bacilli, which are common causative organisms in peritonitis. There is usually an abundant purulent exudate, which may have a fecal odor.

Streptococcal peritonitis. Streptococcal peritonitis is often a fulminating infection, in which only a thin, serous exudate is found. It is one of the most serious types of puerperal infection.

Gonococcal peritonitis. Gonococcal peritonitis is usually localized to the pelvis and has origin from an infected fallopian tube. It tends to become chronic and forms fibrous adhesions.

Pneumococcal peritonitis. Pneumococcal peritonitis may be primary in female children, the organisms reaching the peritoneum through the fallopian tubes, or it may be secondary to

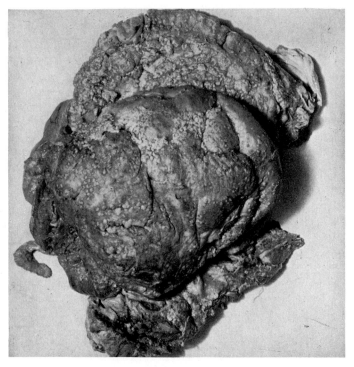

Fig. 19-36. Tuberculous peritonitis. The viscera are bound together by dense tuberculous exudate and granulation tissue.

pneumococcal infection in the lung or elsewhere. It is a common complication of the nephrotic syndrome in children.

Biliary peritonitis. Biliary peritonitis is caused by chemical irritation of the peritoneum by bile, most often as a result of rupture of a common bile duct after a surgical procedure involving the gallbladder or biliary tract. In some cases the bile is infected, and bacterial irritation is added.

Tuberculous peritonitis. Tuberculous peritonitis commonly results from local spread of the infection from the fallopian tube, intestine, or a mesenteric lymph node, but hematogenous infection from distant sources may occur. Tiny tubercles may fleck all peritoneal surfaces. They appear as yellowish opaque spots surrounded by a reddish zone. The exudate may be very abundant and serous so that a large amount of fluid accumulates in the peritoneal cavity. This is the moist form. A dry or plastic type also occurs, which is characterized by the matting together of abdominal viscera by firm adhesions or by a dense granulomatous tissue.

Various rare types of peritonitis, such as the rheumatic and actinomycotic forms, also occur. Periodic peritonitis is a peculiar hereditary disorder that occurs in repetitive episodes among persons of Armenian, Arabic, or Jewish extraction. A mild, sterile inflammatory process involves the walls of the appendix and gallbladder.

Ascites

In ascites (edema of the peritoneal cavity) very large amounts of transudate may accumulate. This is seen in conditions in which edema is generalized, as in congestive heart failure, nutritional edema, nephritis, and obstructions to the portal circulation, as in cirrhosis of the liver. The watery fluid has a low specific gravity (usually less than 1.015) and a low protein content (less than 2 or 3%). Fluid accumulation in the abdomen also may be an exudate resulting from inflammation, as in the moist form of tuberculous peritonitis. In such cases the fluid has a higher cellular and protein content and a higher specific gravity. Tumor metastasis to the peritoneum also may be associated with abundant fluid, particularly with ovarian cystadenocarcinomas. It is often possible to identify tumor cells in the centrifuged sediment of such fluid.

Chapter 20

The endocrine glands

PITUITARY GLAND (HYPOPHYSIS)
Structure and function

The pituitary is a small endocrine structure (0.5 to 0.9 gram) situated in the sella turcica. Its main divisions are into anterior and posterior lobes. At the posterior part of the anterior lobe is the pars intermedia, although in man this has no distinct histologic separation from the anterior lobe. The important anterior lobe arises from Rathke's pouch (craniopharyngeal duct), an evagination of the roof of the posterior nasopharynx. From there the cells migrate upward to reach their final position in the sella turcica. Small portions of pituitary tissue may be left along this course and give rise to epithelial tumors (Rathke's pouch tumors) or simply remain as small remnants of pituitary tissue. Such ectopic nests of pituitary tissue are most often found in the pharyngeal mucosa (pharyngeal pituitary gland) or in the body of the sphenoid bone. Cells of the anterior lobe extend upward over the stalk toward the base of the brain as the pars tuberalis. The posterior lobe develops as a downgrowth from the floor of the third ventricle and hence is of nervous origin. The posterior lobe becomes enveloped anteriorly by the anterior lobe. It is directly continuous with the neural tissues of the pituitary stalk, which carries the supraopticohypophysial tract of nerve fibers. These fibers from the supraoptic and paraventricular nuclei ramify throughout the posterior lobe.

The blood supply of the anterior lobe is by a portal system of large thin-walled vessels. This vascular link with the nervous system may convey trophic substances from the hypothalamic area, providing a neurohumoral mechanism regulating anterior lobe hormones.

Anterior lobe. The anterior lobe contains three main types of cells distinguishable by the ordinary hematoxylin and eosin (H and E) tissue stains. Although proportions vary slightly with age and sex, about 50% are *chromophobe* cells, which have a cytoplasm devoid of specific granulation. The chromophobes give rise to the other two types, *acidophils* (40%) and *basophils* (10%), by the accumulation of specific cytoplasmic granules,

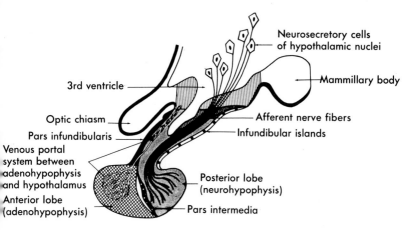

Fig. 20-1. Pituitary gland represented by a diagram showing neural and vascular relationships.

which respectively stain red with acid dyes and blue with basic dyes. Newer histochemical staining methods, using the periodic acid-Schiff (PAS) stain with orange G and methyl blue as counterstains and also using an aldehyde-fuchsin method, enable the three main varieties to be further subdivided. Such methods give promise of better correlation between categories of cells and the hormones they produce, although there is some confusion because of varying terminologies and interpretations. Table 20-1 indicates some of these names, varied proportions according to newer histochemical methods, and possible functions. It should be considered tentative rather than final.

The anterior lobe elaborates a number of principles, although it is uncertain how many of these may be distinct hormones. These may be listed as a growth-promoting (somatotropic) hormone (STH), a diabetogenic hormone, a thyrotropic hormone (TSH), an adrenocorticotropic hormone (ACTH), a lactogenic hormone, melanin-stimulating hormone (MSH or intermedin), and gonodotropic hormones, which are follicle-stimulating (FSH) or luteinizing (LH). Principles controlling parathyroid activity and water metabolism appear to be present but are established with less certainty. While the type of cells that elaborate these principles are not identified with certainty, current ideas are outlined in Table 20-1.

Table 20-1. *Cells of the anterior pituitary*

Types of cells	Staining reactions	Recent terminology	Function
Chromophils Acidophils 26-36%	Orange granules stained by orange G counterstain PAS-negative	Alpha cells	Somatotropic (growth) hormone (STH) ? Diabetogenic hormone ? Lactogenic hormone
Basophils 23-38%	PAS-positive granules Mucoid cells (mucoprotein-containing)	Beta cells PAS-positive (red) granules	? Thyrotropic hormone (TSH) ? Follicle-stimulating hormone (FSH) ? Luteinizing hormone (LH) ? Slow manufacture and release of adrenocorticotropic hormone (ACTH)
		Delta cells Amphophils PAS-positive purple granules by special counterstain	Dark delta cells ? Storage ACTH and release under stress Light delta cells ? Rapid formation and release of ACTH under stress
Chromophobes 34-42%	No granules in the cytoplasm by H & E or PAS	Gamma cells	No secretory function ? Precursors of chromophils

The endocrine glands 665

Posterior lobe. The posterior lobe is composed of neuroglial cells (pituicytes), nerve fibers, and some hyaline bodies. This portion of the pituitary is connected by nerve tracts with supra-optic and paraventricular nuclei of the floor of the third ventricle, forming an important endocrine unit, the neurohypophysis. Extracts of the posterior lobe contain a pressor factor, an antidiuretic factor, and an oxytocic factor. The pressor factor (vasopressin) causes peripheral vasoconstriction and raises blood pressure. The antidiuretic factor controls resorption of water by the renal tubules. The oxytocic factor (oxytocin or pitocin) stimulates uterine contractions. These hormones appear to be formed by neurons of the hypothalamic nuclei. This neurosecretory material reaches the posterior lobe by the supraoptico-hypophysial tract, where it is stored as an extracellular deposit demonstrable by aldehyde-fuchsin and other stains.

Pars intermedia. The indistinct pars intermedia contains the same cells as the anterior lobe, although basophils are more numerous. A few small cystic spaces containing pink-staining colloidlike material are usually present at the junction with the posterior lobe. A few basophils are sometimes found in the adjacent posterior lobe, especially in males over 50 years of age. In animals with a pars intermedia that is more distinct than in man, this area is considered to be the site of formation of MSH. In man, the site of origin of this hormone is not definitely known, although it is suggested that it may be the anterior lobe.

Diseases of the pituitary

Pathologic changes in the pituitary may be (1) adenomas or hyperplasias, which may result in pituitary hyperfunction, pressure effects, or both; and (2) destructive lesions, as a result of inflammation, thrombosis, embolism, atrophy, or pressure from adjacent tumors. These changes are associated with hypofunction of the gland.

Pituitary adenomas. Tumors developing from cells of the anterior lobe of the pituitary are usually benign adenomas. Some, however, develop local invasive characteristics consistent with malignancy and have considerable nuclear variability and mitoses. Carcinomas with distant metastases rarely develop from pituitary cells. Other rare pituitary tumors are teratomas, including those called "ectopic pinealomas," which resemble tumors arising in the pineal body.

Chromophobe adenoma. Chromophobe adenoma is the most

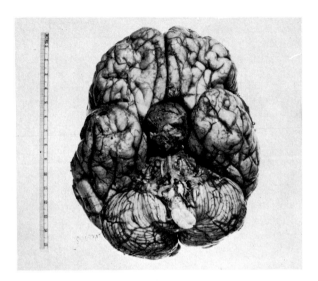

Fig. 20-2. Chromophobe adenoma of the pituitary.

common type of pituitary tumor. It varies from less than a millimeter to several centimeters in diameter. Since the chromophobes elaborate no specific hormone, the effects are simply caused by pressure of the expanding growth. Such pressure effects are on the surrounding glandular tissue of the pituitary, the bony and membranous walls of the sella turcica, and the optic chiasm. Pressure on the surrounding normal glandular tissue may produce various symptoms of hypopituitarism. The tumor tissue is soft, grayish, white, and susceptible to hemorrhage, degeneration, necrosis, and cyst formation. Occasional chromophobe adenomas may involve the nasopharynx, and rarely invasion of the nasal cavity occurs.

In rare cases adenomas of parathyroid and pancreatic islet cells have been associated with pituitary chromophobe or acidophil adenomas (pleuriglandular adenomatosis).

Acidophil adenoma. Tumors composed predominantly of acidophils cause clinical syndromes prominently featured by overproduction of growth hormone. If the adenoma develops within the growing period before ossification is complete, *giantism* results; if after bone growth is completed, *acromegaly* is produced. Acromegaly is characterized by overgrowth and thickening of bones, conspicuous in the skull, face, mandible, and peripheral portions of extremities. Overgrowth of the heart, tongue, and viscera and fibrous hyperplasia of the skin and subcutaneous tissue also occur. Other disturbances usually present are sexual disorders of impotence or amenorrhea and glycosuria. Eventually pressure effects result from continued growth of the adenoma, although these tumors tend to be smaller than chromophobe adenomas and are frequently confined to the sella. The pressure first may be on other portions of the gland, giving rise to evidence of hypopituitarism, and then on suprasellar regions where pressure on the optic chiasm or optic nerves produces visual disturbances. Microscopic foci of hyperplasia of acidophils are quite common and are not usually associated with hormonal disturbances.

Basophil adenoma. The least common type of pituitary adenoma is composed of basophilic cells. It is sometimes found associated with the clinical condition of *Cushing's syndrome,* clinical features of which are obesity (confined to the face, neck, and trunk), hypertension, polycythemia, a dusky cyanotic tinge of the skin, purplish striae on the breast and abdomen, hirsutism, and sexual disturbances. In 1932 Cushing pointed to the frequent association of this syndrome with a pituitary basophilic adenoma or hyperplasia. Later studies have shown that the association is not constant and that the condition is an adrenal cortical condition of hypercortisolism (p. 712). However, the clinical syndrome does seem to be quite constantly associated with a change in the pituitary basophils in which there is replacement of the cytoplasmic basophilic substance by a hyaline material, as described by Crooke. A similar change in the pituitary basophils has been described after the use of large doses of adrenal cortical steroids.

Hypopituitarism. Injuries or destructive lesions of the pituitary are not frequent. Pressure effects may be produced by tumors in or around the sella. Syphilis may cause a diffuse fibrosis of the pituitary. Tuberculosis, sarcoidosis, and other granulomas sometimes involve the pituitary, as may amyloid deposit in secondary amyloidosis. The anterior pituitary cells contain mucopolysaccharide in gargoylism (Hurler's disease). In xanthomatosis of the Hand-Schüller-Christian type the neurohypophysis is commonly involved. Lymphomas and metastatic carcinomas sometimes involve the gland. Diabetic patients who develop destructive lesions of the pituitary may show the Houssay phenomenon (hypoglycemia and an increase in sensitivity to insulin). Septicemia and embolism occasionally affect the hypophysis.

The commonest type of severe injury is a necrosis that occurs after childbirth, particularly in those cases in which there have been severe postpartum hemorrhage and collapse. The necrotic area undergoes fibrosis, and if it is extensive, hypopituitarism results.

Simmonds' disease. Simmonds' disease is the result of severe hypopituitarism in the adult. The condition is uncommon in men, as most cases appear to be the late effects of a postpartum necrosis of the pituitary. The condition is characterized by loss of sexual function, low metabolic rate, weakness, cachexia, loss of hair, pigmentation of the skin, and premature senility. Not only is there atrophy or destruction of the anterior lobe of the pituitary but also fibrosis or atrophy of the thyroid, parathyroids, adrenals, ovaries, and endometrium. Low blood pressure, hypoglycemia, and evidence of myxedema are usually present. Cachexia is not invariably present and is not a necessary feature of hypopituitarism. The cachexia is dependent mainly on loss of appetite and subsequent undernutrition. An unrelated condition, *anorexia nervosa,* is characterized by severe cachexia resulting from undernutrition. It has some of the clinical features of Simmonds' disease, but changes in the pituitary and other endocrine glands are lacking.

Sheehan has emphasized the danger and frequency of postpartum ischemic necrosis of the pituitary in women who suffer hemorrhage and circulatory collapse at the time of parturition. The anterior pituitary normally hypertrophies during pregnancy and involutes rapidly during the puerperium. A sudden reduction of blood flow to the gland results from hemorrhage at the time of delivery, and if in addition there is severe general circulatory collapse, the blood flow to the pituitary may be reduced sufficiently to cause focal ischemic necrosis. The type of hypopituitarism or Simmonds' disease that subsequently develops is often called *Sheehan's syndrome.* It varies in severity with the amount of pituitary tissue that has been destroyed by infarction. Atrophy of the supraoptic and paraventricular nuclei may be found when there is atrophy of the posterior lobe, and in severe cases there is loss of nerve fibers in the stalk.

Progeria. Progeria (Hutchinson-Gilford syndrome) is a condition of dwarfism and premature senility. A decreased number of eosinophils in the anterior pituitary has been described, but the primary cause is unknown.

Other pituitary syndromes. Various other clinical syndromes are related to disturbances of pituitary function. They are less clear-cut and their pathologic basis is less definite. *Dystrophia adiposogenitalis* (Fröhlich's syndrome) is characterized by adiposity of the trunk and a feminine configuration. It is probably a hypopituitarism and is often related to pressure on the pituitary by tumors. *Dwarfism* of the Lorain-Levi syndrome may be attributable to hypopituitarism. Failure of sexual development is a common accompaniment.

Conditions in which a pathogenetic relationship to the pituitary is rather questionable include the Laurence-Moon-Biedl syndrome, mongolism, and Morgagni's syndrome. The *Laurence-Moon-Biedl syndrome* is characterized by obesity, hypogenitalism, polydactylism, pigmentary retinal changes, and failure of proper mental development. There is a genetic basis, and various endocrine changes have been found, including increase of pituitary basophils. Also *mongolism,* a prenatal developmental disorder caused by the presence of an additional small acrocentric chromosome, shows evidence of pituitary involvement with secondary changes in the thyroid, adrenals, and gonads. *Morgagni's syndrome* is an endocrine disturbance occurring mainly in women after the menopause. It is characterized by *hyperostosis frontalis interna,* virilism with hirsutism, and obesity. The underlying endocrine changes are imperfectly known. It has been suggested that displacement of the brain by the bony thickening strains the pituitary stalk, providing a basis for the various changes that could be of pituitary or hypothalamic origin, although there may be no demonstrable lesion of the pituitary.

Diabetes insipidus. Diabetes insipidus is characterized by an excessive output of urine, which is of low specific gravity and without sugar. Excessive thirst and intake of fluid accompany the condition. Secretion of antidiuretic hormone is apparently by the cells of the hypothalamic nuclei, with storage in the posterior lobe of the pituitary. The antidiuretic hormone conserves water by increasing reabsorption of water by the renal tubules, and particularly by the loops of Henle and distal convoluted tubules. Interruption of the supraopticohypophysial tract anywhere from the nuclei in the floor of the third ventricle downward to the posterior lobe may bring about the condition. The most com-

mon causes are trauma, neoplasms, granulomatous inflammations, xanthomatosis, and lymphomas. Either hypothalamic or
pituitary injury may result in diabetes insipidus, although injury
of the posterior lobe alone may not do so. The anterior lobe
must be functioning for development of diabetes insipidus,
although the relationship is obscure. Hereditary diabetes insipidus
also occurs.

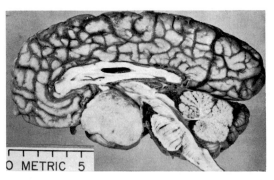

Fig. 20-3. Craniopharyngioma.

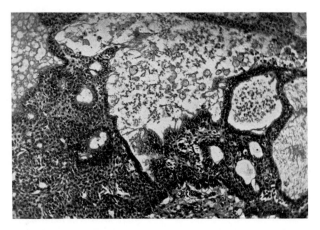

Fig. 20-4. Cystic craniopharyngioma (adamantinoma of the hypophysial
duct).

Craniopharyngioma. Remnants of Rathke's pouch or the craniopharyngeal duct may give rise to cystic tumors (craniopharyngiomas, pituitary adamantinomas, suprasellar cysts). Being composed of epithelium derived from the mouth cavity, the tumors consist of a squamous type of epithelium. This epithelium resembles the ameloblasts of the developing enamel organ, and consequently the tumor is sometimes similar in its microscopic appearance to the adamantinoma (ameloblastoma), which arises in the jaw (p. 584). A few cystic tumors of the pituitary have been lined by ciliated epithelium. Calcification is common in the tumor and may be sufficient to be of value in radiologic diagnosis.

Many of the craniopharyngeal tumors develop from the region of the hypophysial stalk, are cystic, and lie above the diaphragm of the sella, although a few are intrasellar. Hence the term *suprasellar cyst* is common. They constitute about 3% of intracranial neoplasms. Being of congenital origin, they may be found in early age periods, often before 15 years of age. They are benign growths, their serious effects being caused by pressure. Various types of hypopituitarism and stunting of growth may result, including Fröhlich's syndrome, dwarfism, and diabetes insipidus.

Tumors of the neurohypophysis. Tumors of the neurohypophysis are very uncommon. Atypical teratomas ("ectopic pinealomas"), lymphomas, and gliomas are all quite rare. In the posterior lobe and stalk small masses of rounded cells with granular cytoplasm have been termed choristomas. They appear to be of glial origin and without known significance.

Infundibuloma is a term used for a rare tumor that appears to be of neurohypophysial derivation and that simulates the structural pattern of the infundibulum. Occurring in children, it grows slowly in the floor of the third ventricle, causing pressure effects on neighboring structures. The cells resemble pituicytes, and the tumor has a distinctive vascular pattern.

THYROID GLAND
Development, structure, and function

The thyroid develops as a downgrowth from the region of the primitive pharynx. A mass forms at the base of the tongue and extends downward as a long tube, the thyroglossal duct, its final position being in front of the trachea and thyroid cartilage. The upper end of the thyroglossal duct is marked by a small depression at the root of the tongue, the foramen cecum. Normally the duct is obliterated during fetal life. Failure of the complete downgrowth and disappearance of this tissue leave aberrant thyroid tissue at the base of the tongue (lingual thyroid) or in the neck anywhere along the course of the thyroglossal duct. These nests of thyroid tissue may give rise to midline (thyroglossal duct) cysts, which must be distinguished from the lateral (branchial cleft) cysts of the neck.

The units of thyroid tissue are glandular follicles or acini. They are lined by a layer of epithelial cells, whose function is to synthesize thyroglobulin and secrete it in an apical direction toward the colloid in the follicle lumen. The number of follicular cells influences the rate of synthesis and secretion. The colloid in the follicular lumen is predominantly the mucoprotein, thyroglobulin. In the colloid, presumably by the action of an oxidizing enzyme also secreted by the cells, iodine is incorporated into the thyroglobulin molecules, initiating the synthesis of the thyroid hormones, thyroxin and triiodothyronine. Factors that influence the activity of the thyroid include the amount of iodine available for synthesis and the thyrotropic hormone of the pituitary. As necessary, the colloid is resorbed and secreted into the bloodstream. Cyclic activity of colloid formation and resorption occur. Colloid resorption appears to be brought about by the thyrotropic hormone of the pituitary. A deficiency of iodine from any cause promotes hyperplasia and enlargement of the thyroid. The thyroid has a specific iodine-trapping action.

The thyroid controls the rate of general body metabolism. Its proper secretion is necessary for normal physical, sexual, and mental development and function. Abnormalities of thyroid function may be in the direction of deficiency (hypothyroidism) or excess (hyperthyroidism). Hypothyroidism gives rise to cretinism in infants and children and myxedema in adults. Hyperthyroidism may occur in severe form with a diffuse enlargement of the thyroid (Graves' disease, exophthalmic goiter) or in a milder form in which the thyroid enlargement is nodular (toxic adenoma). The thyroid hormone acts to accelerate oxidation or rate of metabolism of cells or of the whole organism. The protein-bound iodine of the blood is an index of the amount of circulating thyroid hormone and closely correlates with thyroid function in hyperthyroidism or hypothyroidism.

Since the histologic structure of the thyroid reflects its func-

tional activity, a condition of underactivity or overactivity sometimes may be judged by microscopic examination. It must be
borne in mind, however, that the activity of the normal
thyroid tissue is cyclic and that in diseased thyroids different
portions of the gland may show different stages or degrees of
activity.

The type of epithelium lining the follicles is the most important criterion of thyroid activity. The height of acinar epithelium
acts as an index of functional activity and probably also of the
action of thyrotropic hormone of the pituitary. Secretory activity is charàcterized by cellular hypertrophy with a change
of resting low cuboidal epithelium to a columnar type. When
activity becomes excessive, epithelial proliferation (hyperplasia)
also occurs. Infoldings of the follicle wall result from the cellular
increase and may be simply slight elevations or definite lacelike
papillae. Increase in thyroid activity is also accompanied by
changes in the mitochondria and Golgi apparatus, demonstrable
only by special cytologic methods. The nature of the colloid
content of the follicles may also indicate the degree of activity.
Under conditions of glandular activity and active resorption into
the circulation, the colloid is very pale staining and vacuolated,
particularly about its periphery. Apparently this represents the
transformation of the intrafollicular colloid into a thinner, more
soluble form. Continued preponderance of resorptive activity
over colloid formation eventually produces exhaustion of the
gland. When iodine is administered to an individual with a
hyperactive thyroid, colloid storage is promoted and for a time
may predominate over resorption, with resulting clinical improvement. The improvement, however, is only temporary, since
the tendency to excessive resorptive activity still exists, and more
colloid has been made available.

The pituitary produces a thyroid-stimulating hormone, of
protein nature, administration of which to animals has reproduced many of the changes seen in human hyperthyroidism
(Graves' disease). It has been postulated that there exists normally a balance between the pituitary and the thyroid, any
deficiency of the thyroid stimulating the pituitary to produce
more of its thyrotropic hormone and, conversely, any overade-
quate supply of thyroid hormone reducing the pituitary production of the thyroid-stimulating factor. Disturbances of this normal
balance may be a factor in some cases of hyperthyroidism and
hypothyroidism.

Goiter

The term *goiter,* or struma, refers to an enlargement of the thyroid gland. Such enlargement may be related to several different etiologic factors, it may be diffuse or nodular (adenomatous), and it may be associated with a deficient, normal, or excessive production of hormone. A large variety of classifications of goiter have served to confuse the subject unnecessarily. Five main types may be recognized.

Simple (colloid) goiter, which is endemic to certain regions and has
    its origin in iodine deficiency
Diffuse goiter with hyperthyroidism (exophthalmic goiter, Graves'
    disease, Basedow's disease)
Nodular (adenomatous) goiter
    With hyperthyroidism (toxic adenoma)
    With hypothyroidism (cretinism, myxedema)
Inflammatory goiter
    Subacute (granulomatous) thyroiditis
    Lymphadenoid goiter (struma lymphomatosa)
    Riedel's struma
    Lymphocytic thyroiditis
Neoplastic goiter
    Benign (adenoma)
    Malignant (carcinoma)

Simple or endemic goiter. In certain regions of the world goiter is endemic and occurs with great frequency. Such regions occur particularly about great mountain ranges, but in North America a goiter belt also occurs around the Great Lakes and St. Lawrence Valley. The thyroid enlargement is a response to insufficient iodine intake, resulting from a deficiency in the soil and water in these regions. Bacterial contamination of water supplies may interfere with availability or absorption of iodine and give rise to goiter. Endemic goiter may be prevented by the addition to the diet of minute amounts of iodine, as by the use of iodized salt. The condition occurs more commonly in females and is particularly likely to develop at a time when the thyroid is subjected to extra functional stress, as in adolescence or pregnancy.

Gross examination of simple goiters shows great variation in size. The whole gland may be involved diffusely, or it may be nodular with patchy "adenomatous" areas. Probably the enlargement is always diffuse in the beginning, but successive cycles of uneven hyperplasia and involution give rise to the nodularity. The cut surface of the gland has a highly translucent appearance because of the abundant colloid. Degenerative changes are often

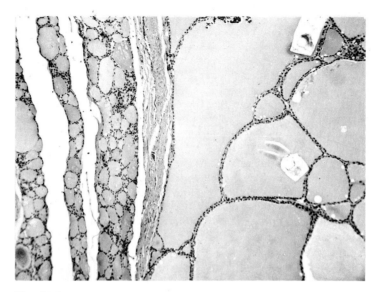

Fig. 20-5. Nodular colloid goiter. Note flat epithelium, abundant colloid, and fibrous band separating nodule. (×85.) (Courtesy Dr. S. E. Gould; from Anderson, W. A. D., and Winship, T.: Thyroid gland. In Anderson, W. A. D., editor: Pathology, ed. 5, St. Louis, 1966, The C. V. Mosby Co.)

evident, particularly in the nodular type, and there may be hemorrhage, cyst formation, and calcification. Coarse, irregular connective tissue trabeculae separate the adenomatous nodules.

Microscopically the goiter may be composed of large distended follicles, filled with abundant, deeply staining colloid and lined by a low cubical or flattened inactive type of epithelium. Such a "colloid goiter" is in an involutional phase and has been preceded by a stage of hyperplasia in response to the iodine deficiency. Subsequent flare-ups of hyperplasia, followed by involution and colloid accumulation, produce a nodular colloid goiter.

In some cases of simple goiter the gland is composed of small inactive follicles without excess colloid accumulation. This variety is termed by some the parenchymatous or microfollicular type.

Hyperthyroidism. Hyperthyroidism is the result of a hyperplastic, overactive thyroid, which secretes an excess of hormone into the circulation. Hyperthyroidism may be of all grades of severity; those cases that have diffuse thyroid hypertrophy and hyperplasia (exophthalmic goiter) are in general more serious than those with nodular goiters. There appears to be no fundamental difference between the diffuse and the nodular hyperplastic goiters as far as the thyroid factor itself is concerned. Histologic changes of hypertrophy and hyperplasia within the thyroid indicate excessive secretory activity. The quantitative concept must be borne in mind, however, in any attempt at functional interpretation from a tissue section. In the diffuse goiter of Graves' disease such functional interpretation may be fairly accurate. In nodular goiter there is great variation in activity in different portions of the gland and hence also in the microscopic picture. This precludes accuracy in any attempted estimation of function. Laboratory determinations that may be helpful in the diagnosis of hyperthyroidism include (1) the basal metabolic rate, (2) the protein-bound iodine level of the serum, (3) the uptake of radioactive iodine by the thyroid, and (4) the rate of conversion of radioactive iodine into iodine bound by protein.

Diffuse goiter with hyperthyroidism. Diffuse goiter with hyperthyroidism (exophthalmic goiter, Graves' disease) is the most acute and severe type of hyperthyroidism. It occurs particularly in adults of young and middle age. The incidence is sporadic and not limited to the goiter belts. There is evidence that the condition is a constitutional nervous and hormonal imbalance. In this imbalance the hyperthyroidism is only one part, although often the predominant, manifestation. The actual stimulus for the hyperactivity of the thyroid may be an excess of the pituitary thyrotropic hormone, although there is evidence that the thyroid-stimulating hormone does not have a primary pathogenetic role. Consideration has been given to the possibility that thyroid stimulators other than those of pituitary origin may be involved. A generalized hyperplasia of lymphoid tissue is a common accompaniment.

While usually associated with diffuse goiter, the thyroid enlargement is often slight and does not necessarily parallel the severity of the clinical symptoms. Exophthalmos, or protrusion of the eyes, is an inconstant feature. It is apparently not a direct result of hyperthyroidism and cannot be reproduced by thyroid extract. Exophthalmos has been produced experimentally

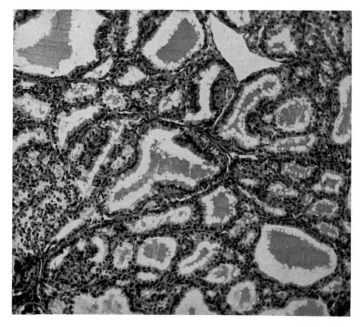

Fig. 20-6. Hyperactive thyroid (Graves' disease). Note the tall epithelium lining the acini and the vacuolation and scantiness of the colloid.

by injection of pituitary extract containing thyrotropic hormone. Recently the thyroid-stimulating hormone has been fractionated into two components, one of which has an effect on orbital contents but does not stimulate the thyroid. Increased metabolic rate, tachycardia, and nervous excitability are prominent features more closely related to the thyroid hyperfunction. A negative iodine balance is present. The condition may develop slowly or suddenly and proceed through a course that may be rapid or may be prolonged by a series of exacerbations and remissions. The end result is an exhausted condition of the gland, with actual hypothroidism. Cardiac damage usually occurs, often marked by disturbances of rhythm, such as atrial fibrillation.

The gross appearance of the thyroid gland is similar in all parts. Although it may not be much enlarged, it is highly vascular and has a characteristic meaty and firm consistency. The cut surface has a solid, firmly lobulated appearance, without the translucence imparted by a rich colloid content. By the promotion of colloid accumulation, preoperative iodine administration may change the aspect to a glistening translucence not unlike that of the normal gland.

Microscopically, characteristic features of thyroid hyperactivity are evident throughout the gland. The epithelial cells of the follicles are tall and columnar, and their nuclei are closely packed and basal in position. Papillary epithelial proliferation with lacelike projections into follicular lumina is often considerable. Hypertrophy of the Golgi apparatus is demonstrable by silver staining. New follicles with small lumina may be formed. The colloid is decreased in amount, thin, pale, and vacuolated or scalloped around the edges. Accumulations of lymphocytes, often with distinct germinal centers, are frequently prominent. By itself the lymphoid hyperplasia is not good evidence of thyroid hyperfunction.

The preoperative administration of iodine usually causes a change in this picture before it is seen in the laboratory. The epithelium is changed to a cuboidal form, the acini becoming larger, with less infolding of epithelium and containing a more deeply stained colloid. This involutional change is not diffuse, and patchy areas still exhibit hyperplastic character. The lymphoid accumulations are not influenced by the iodine medication.

Thiouracil and other thiourea derivatives have been found therapeutically effective in relieving hyperthyroidism. However, there may be an increase in size of the gland, which microscopically may show a very great degree of hyperplasia and little colloid content. The effect in this case does not appear to be preventable by iodine. It is postulated that thiouracil prevents oxidation of iodide to iodine. Meanwhile the thyroid gland itself is increasingly stimulated to hyperplasia by the unopposed pituitary thyrotropic hormone or by a decrease of stored iodine within the gland. The extreme degrees of hyperplasia of thyroid tissue that may be seen as a result of thiouracil or thiocyanate therapy must be distinguished with care from neoplastic lesions of the thyroid. Cobalt compounds, used in the treatment of anemia, have produced in children goiters that are characterized by severe hyperplasia but depressed function.

Exophthalmos associated with goiter appears to result mainly from swelling and edema of the orbital contents. There is an increase of fat in the orbits and lids, and the fatty tissue becomes swollen and edematous. The extrinsic muscles of the eye also may be swollen. Compression of orbital veins by increased contraction of ocular muscles may be a factor in the increased accumulation of fluid. The severity of the exophthalmos is not correlated with the degree of hyperthyroidism. Secondary ulceration of the cornea may complicate severe exophthalmos.

Various other organs may show changes in severe hyperthyroidism. Lymphoid hyperplasia is generalized, not simply in the thyroid itself. The thymus is often enlarged, and even the blood may show a relative lymphocytosis. The heart shows few changes, despite the frequent occurrence of cardiac complications. There may be cardiac hypertrophy and some myocardial degeneration and fibrosis. Voluntary muscles, such as the quadriceps, also may show degenerative changes. Some skeletal osteoporosis is common. The liver is affected by hyperthyroidism and in severe cases may show fatty degeneration and necrosis. The adrenal glands also may be involved by degenerative and atrophic changes.

Nodular goiter with hyperthyroidism. Hyperthyroidism with a nodular goiter (toxic adenoma) is probably fundamentally the same condition as Graves' disease. The nodularity is the result of recurring cycles of hypertrophy and hyperplasia affecting the gland in irregular fashion. Because the hyperactivity may appear in a previously existent simple goiter, it is sometimes termed secondary Graves' disease. The condition tends to occur in later life, the degree of hyperthyroidism is milder, and exophthalmos is usually absent. Large nodular goiters may cause disturbance by pressure on surrounding structures, e.g., the trachea.

Both the gross and microscopic appearance is extremely variable. The enlargement of the thyroid may be great and irregular. Areas of degeneration are often present. Nodular or adenomatous areas of varying size may show fibrosis around them. Their cut surface may be meaty and firm, indicating hyperplasia, or it may be soft and translucent, because of colloid storage. The appearance is often quite variable in different portions of the gland, both grossly and microscopically. Hence there is difficulty of evaluation in terms of function, which evidently depends upon the total balance of hyperplasia and involution.

Hypothyroidism. Insufficient function of the thyroid produces the condition of cretinism in early life and myxedema in the adult. While fundamentally the same, the clinical syndromes

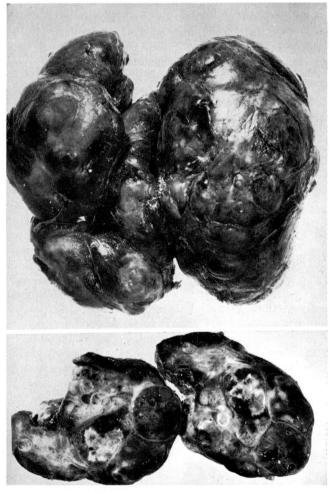

Fig. 20-7. Nodular goiter, with fibrosis, hemorrhage, and necrosis evident on the cut surface.

differ because of the retardation and distortion of physical, sexual, and mental development in the childhood form. Skeletal growth is stunted and distorted, the skin is thick and coarse, hair is scanty, metabolism is depressed, and both sexual and mental development are of low degree.

Cretinism. Cretinism occurs sporadically. It is caused by a hypoplasia or failure of proper development of the thyroid. The thyroid may be absent or may consist of only a few glandular remnants set in connective tissue. Cretinism also commonly occurs in regions where goiter is endemic.

In goitrous sporadic cretinism there is evidence of a genetic basis for a biochemical abnormality with a defect in the synthesis of thyroid hormone. The goitrous glands in these cases show severe epithelial hyperplasia, with irregular and pleomorphic epithelial cells and adenoma-like nodules.

Myxedema. Myxedema is the antithesis of Graves' disease. The general metabolism is low, heat tolerance is increased, and physical and mental activities are retarded. The skin becomes dry, coarse, and thickened by subcutaneous accumulation of a mucoid material. This results in the appearance of a nonpitting edema, particularly prominent on the face, neck, and hands, which feature has given origin to the term myxedema. Specific cytologic changes may be found in the exocrine sweat glands, with PAS-positive granules in the large pale cells of the secretory coil. The hair tends to become coarse and scanty. Loss of sexual desire and impotence or amenorrhea are common. The condition responds readily and effectively to thyroid administration.

Mild degrees of myxedema may follow operative removal of most of the thyroid gland or result from exhaustion of the gland after severe hyperthyroidism. Pituitary deficiency may be associated with a secondary thyroid deficiency caused by a lack of the thyrotropic hormone. Prolonged ingestion of iodides as medication has been known to produce goiter and myxedema. Most primary cases are of unknown etiology. Circulating antibodies to thyroglobulin are demonstrable in the sera of about 80% of patients with primary myxedema. This and other histologic evidence suggest that the condition may be a late stage of chronic diffuse thyroiditis. The thyroid tissue is atrophic and inactive often displaying severe fibrosis. Vacuolization and mucoid degeneration of skeletal muscle fibers have been noted. A similar degeneration in the media of the aorta, leading to dis-

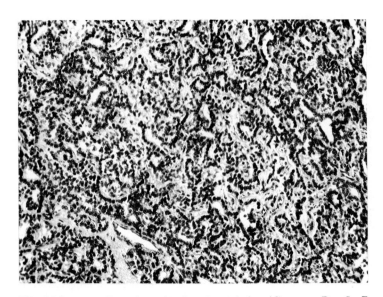

Fig. 20-8. Sporadic goiter showing hypoplasia. (Courtesy Dr. S. E. Gould; from Anderson, W. A. D., and Winship, T.: Thyroid gland. In Anderson, W. A. D., editor: Pathology, ed. 5, St. Louis, 1966, The C. V. Mosby Co.)

secting aneurysm and fatal rupture, has been described in induced hypothyroidism. The heart is dilated, there is a loss of muscle tone, and interstitial edema and some scarring may be present. Mucoid (basophilic) degeneration has been observed in myocardial fibers. Atherosclerosis of advanced degree may be present in young adults with myxedema.

Inflammation of the thyroid. Since the thyroid appears quite resistant to most infections, inflammatory processes in the thyroid are uncommon. Direct spread may occur from neighboring tissues. Thyroiditis may also be produced by trauma or radiation. However, distinctive types of supposedly inflammatory conditions are termed subacute (granulomatous) thyroiditis, lymphadenoid goiter, and Riedel's struma.

Subacute (granulomatous) thyroiditis. Subacute (de Quervain's) thyroiditis occurs predominantly in adult women. The clinical onset may be acute, with sore throat, pain on swallowing, pain and tenderness in the thyroid, and some fever. The effects are often mild, and local pressure symptoms are not prominent. The sedimentation rate is elevated. Serum protein-bound iodine is near the upper limit of normal or is elevated, but the uptake of radioiodine by the gland is depressed. The $alpha_2$ globulin fraction of the serum may be elevated, probably because of colloid entering the bloodstream from destruction of follicles.

The thyroid is slightly to moderately enlarged, and involved areas are firm and yellowish white. Some degree of perithyroiditis is frequent. The microscopic changes are focal, with degeneration of follicles, infiltration of leukocytes, lymphocytes, and plasma cells, and variable amount of fibrosis. Groups of histiocytes and giant cells produce a tuberculoid appearance, but caseous necrosis is not present. The giant cell formation often appears to be a reaction to altered colloid, and some giant cells seem to be formed by fusion of follicular cells around colloid masses.

The etiology is obscure, but a viral infection has been suggested. Some cases have shown evidence of a relation to the virus of mumps. It is usually a self-limited disease, commonly persisting for one to three months.

Lymphadenoid goiter. Lymphadenoid goiter (Hashimoto's disease, struma lymphomatosa) is a condition in which excessive lymphoid tissue develops in the thyroid, often with prominent lymphoid follicles and a crowding out and replacement of thyroid acini. A characteristic feature is alteration of thyroid epithelium with enlargement, an abundant oxyphilic cytoplasm, and nuclei that may be hyperchromatic and of variable size and shape. The associated change of thyroid parenchyma is accompanied by a varying degree of interstitial fibrosis. The thyroid tissue is usually diffusely and symmetrically enlarged, with uniformly firm rubbery consistency and a white to yellowish brown color. The occurrence may be at any age, but most cases seem to be in women over 40 years of age. Moderate diffuse enlargement of the thyroid is usual. Functional disturbance is usually not a prominent feature, but mild hypothyroidism (myxedema) may be present in later stages. Basal metabolism is usually in the low normal range. The serum protein-bound iodine values usually are in the hypothyroid range.

The inflammatory nature of the condition has often been

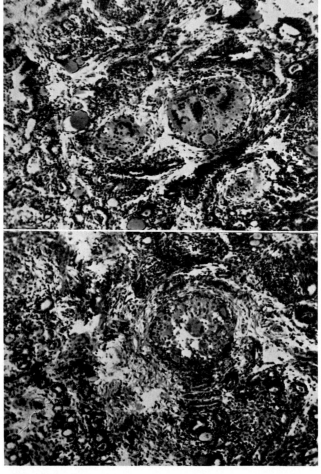

Fig. 20-9. Subacute (granulomatous) thyroiditis: multinucleated giant cells, fibrosis, lymphocytes, and a few thyroid follicles.

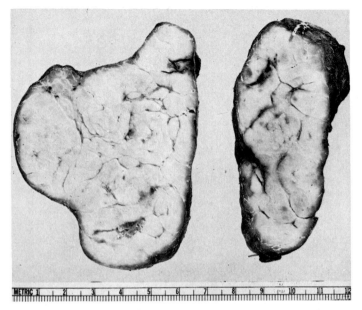

Fig. 20-10. Thyroid, Hashimoto's disease.

in doubt. A lesser degree of lymphoid involvement is common in hyperfunctioning thyroid glands (e.g., exophthalmic goiter). Some consider lymphadenoid goiter a functional disturbance in which the basic cause is an excess of thyrotropic hormone. An excessive involutional change, either idiopathic or after mild hyperthyroidism, is a possible explanation. Others have considered that lymphadenoid goiter is only an early stage of Riedel's struma and that slow progressive replacement by fibrous scar tissue will produce the hard goiter of this latter condition, but this opinion is not now commonly held. Experimentally a somewhat similar lymphoid type of goiter may be produced by prolonged thiouracil administration. Recent evidence indicates that the condition may be an autoimmunization of the patient against his own thyroid protein material. An initial injury to the thyroid (e.g., a viral infection) leads to the inflammatory release of thyroglobulins. Freeing of thyroglobulin from thyroid acini attracts cells that form antibodies. The pathologic changes may result from progressive interaction of the antibody with thyro-

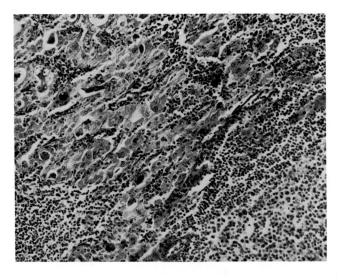

Fig. 20-11. Hashimoto's thyroiditis. In addition to the lymphoid infiltrate the atrophic follicular cells show a granular oxyphilia. (From Anderson, W. A. D., and Winship, T.: Thyroid gland. In Anderson, W. A. D., editor: Pathology, ed. 5, St. Louis, 1966, The C. V. Mosby Co.)

globulin in the gland, the destruction of cells freeing more thyroglobulin. Lesser degrees of lymphoid infiltration in other thyroid lesions may also represent a localized immune response. Particularly in females over 50 years of age, complement-fixing antibodies may be detectable in the serum and are associated with some lymphocytic infiltration and Hürthle cell change in the thyroid (i.e., enlargement of follicular cells and oxyphilic alteration of their cytoplasm).

Riedel's struma. Riedel's struma (struma fibrosa, woody thyroiditis, invasive fibrous thyroiditis) is a rare condition characterized by a thyroid of very firm consistency. Its essence is a slow progressive replacement of thyroid tissue by dense scar tissue and extension of the fibrous tissue to involve surrounding structures. Sometimes only a portion of the gland is affected. It occurs at any age, but usually in adults, and almost as frequently in men as in women. It may be associated with mild hypothy-

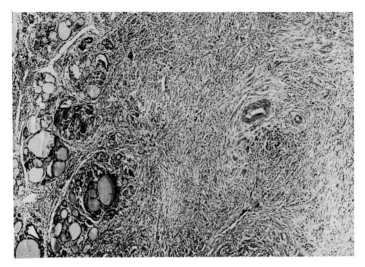

Fig. 20-12. Riedel's struma. A dense but irregular fibrosis involves the thyroid tissue. (From Anderson, W. A. D., and Winship, T.: Thyroid gland. In Anderson, W. A. D., editor: Pathology, ed. 5, St. Louis, 1966, The C. V. Mosby Co.)

roidism and is easily confused clinically with carcinoma. Clinical manifestations are mainly severe pressure symptoms.

Although extensive fibrosis is the essential microscopic feature, lymphoid accumulation is frequently prominent, and forms occur that have suggested a transition from lymphadenoid goiter to Riedel's struma. The fibrous thyroid tissue is hard, gritty, white, and often without any gross resemblance to normal thyroid tissue. Capsular involvement is an important and distinctive feature. Extensive involvement of adjacent structures of the neck by the dense fibrous tissue makes surgical resection difficult.

Lymphocytic thyroiditis (lymphoid thyroiditis). Sporadic cases of goiter in children and young women have been characterized by extensive lymphocytic infiltration, but without the oxyphilic changes in follicular epithelium that occurs in Hashimoto's struma. By some, however, this is considered an early phase or a form of lymphadenoid goiter. The gland is diffusely enlarged and there is an intact capsule. The cut surface of the tissue is grayish white or yellowish white. Clinical evidence of mild hypothyroidism is present in some cases. Serum protein-bound iodine levels are variable but sometimes elevated. Radio iodine uptake shows no significant change.

Tumors of the thyroid

The common neoplasms of the thyroid are adenomas and carcinomas. Some carcinomas of the thyroid are believed to originate in a benign adenoma. Atypical adenomas and adenomas with atypical foci are probably precancerous lesions. In reported cases, proportions of solitary thyroid nodules varying from 6 to 20% have been found to be carcinomatous.

Adenoma of the thyroid. The so-called "adenomas" of nodular goiters are not true tumors but are localized areas of hyperplasia or involution. Criteria for true thyroid adenomas are (1) complete encapsulation, (2) homogeneous texture throughout, although degenerative changes may be present, (3) definite variation of the tissue of the adenoma from that outside the capsule, and (4) evidence of compression of adjacent thyroid tissue.

Papillary adenoma is a variety composed of papillary or cystadenomatous structures. Active or cellular papillary adenomas are difficult to distinguish from papillary carcinomas unless invasion is seen. Some believe that it is not possible to classify papillary thyroid tumors into benign and malignant tumors on histologic grounds. *Colloid adenoma* is composed of differentiated thyroid follicles containing colloid. Their distinction from areas of colloid involution in a nodular goiter may be difficult. *Embryonal* and fetal *adenomas* are so called because of resemblances to embryonic or fetal thyroid tissue. The embryonal type is composed of cords and trabeculae of cells with little tendency to gland formation. The fetal adenoma consists of small follicles lined by low epithelium and often separated by abundant hyaline colloidlike material or abundant and edematous stroma. From a practical standpoint the colloid, embryonal, and fetal adenomas may all be classed together as *follicular adenomas*.

Hürthle cell tumor. Hürthle cell tumors are composed of large, polyhedral cells, with prominent granular nuclei and abundant pale eosinophilic cytoplasm. The cells are arranged in solid-looking masses and clumps, but with formation of small alveoli. Stroma is usually small in amount. The origin of the distinctive cells is uncertain, but they are generally considered to be retrogressive variants of thyroid follicular cells. The microscopic resemblance to parathyroid adenoma may be very striking, but the functional disturbances characteristic of parathyroid tumors are lacking. Benign and malignant forms occur. Criteria for malignancy are the same as those in other thyroid tumors, vascular invasion being most important. In general the Hürthle cell change tends to be associated with a decreased growth capacity and a more favorable prognosis.

Hürthle cells are frequently seen in thyroid glands, apart from tumors, apparently as an involutional change in thyroid cells as a result of injury (e.g., by radiation) or exhaustion after overstimulation. Various thyroid tumors may show a Hürthle cell change in focal areas.

Carcinoma of the thyroid. Carcinoma of the thyroid may arise from a benign adenoma and may be histologically well differentiated, so that diagnosis and prognosis are often very difficult. Invasion, particularly vascular invasion, may be the only evidence of malignancy. Some of the well-differentiated tumors that invade blood vessels and produce secondary growths in other organs have been given the anomalous name of "benign

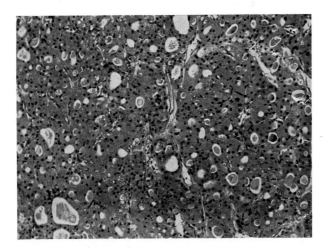

Fig. 20-13. Thyroid, Hürthle cell tumor.

metastasizing struma." Although invasion of blood vessels, lymphatics, or capsule is the most reliable microscopic evidence of malignancy, in many cases cellular anaplasia is present and the usual histologic criteria of malignancy can be applied. Hyperfunction is rarely an accompaniment of thyroid cancer, even though well-differentiated cancer cells may show evidence of function and take up radioactive iodine.

Malignant tumors of the thyroid are, with rare exception, of epithelial nature (carcinomas). Fibrosarcoma and lymphosarcoma are relatively very uncommon. Carcinoma of the thyroid occurs in all age periods, but the highly malignant undifferentiated carcinomas almost all occur after the age of 40 years. Thyroid carcinomas occurring in childhood have often been in children who have received irradiation to the area during infancy, usually for an enlarged thymus.

The different histologic varieties of thyroid carcinoma show extreme variation in their natural history. Some papillary carcinomas may exist over a period of several decades, while many undifferentiated carcinomas may cause death within six months or a year. Between the extremes are follicular cancers of varying degrees of differentiation and malignancy. Mixed papillary and follicular carcinomas are common.

Papillary adenocarcinoma. The tumor epithelium is arranged on fibrovascular stalks projecting into cystic spaces. Metastatic deposits show a similar architectural pattern. Psammoma bodies may develop from the hyalinized stroma of the papillae. The presence of psammoma bodies may be considered evidence of malignancy. Areas of squamous metaplasia are often present, but squamous metaplasia in the thyroid is not ordinarily a precancerous lesion. Papillary carcinomas of the thyroid are usually of a low grade of malignancy, grow slowly, and may exist over many years. They have a tendency to local infiltration and spread to cervical lymph nodes, but distant metastasis tends to be uncommon or late. Death from papillary carcinoma usually results from infiltration of the trachea.

Follicular carcinoma. Follicular carcinomas of the thyroid are of varying degrees of undifferentiation and malignancy. Many of them appear as encapsulated adenoma-like tumors, are distinguishable only by vascular or capsular invasion, and have a relatively good outlook. Some are small, nonencapsulated, and sclerosing (variously called "nonencapsulated sclerosing tumor" and "occult sclerosing thyroid carcinoma"). Some follicular

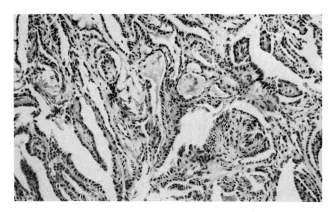

Fig. 20-14. Papillary adenocarcinoma of the thyroid.

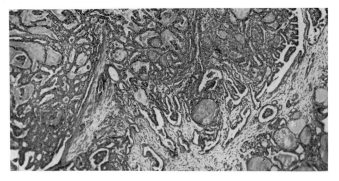

Fig. 20-15. Follicular adenocarcinoma of the thyroid.

carcinomas show a Hürthle cell change, in some parts or as a whole, which is usually an indication of slow growth. The more undifferentiated follicular carcinomas may show solid masses of cells, with relatively little formation of distinct follicular lumina, great cellular and nuclear variability, and numerous mitoses. Such tumors are of a relatively higher grade of malignancy. Some of these form medullary (solid) carcinomas of sheetlike and trabecular growth. They lack the anaplasia, frequent mitoses, and high malignancy of undifferentiated carcinomas.

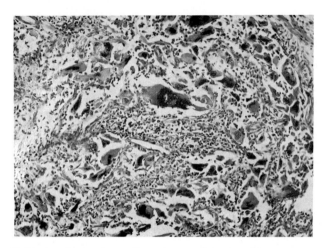

Fig. 20-16. Anaplastic giant cell carcinoma of the thyroid.

Amyloid may be present in the stroma. Metastases occur in cervical lymph nodes as well as in distant organs.

Undifferentiated carcinoma. Undifferentiated carcinomas may be of small cell, spindle cell, giant cell, or epidermoid varieties. They are of high malignancy. The highly anaplastic carcinomas may arise from a change in malignant character occurring in papillary or follicular carcinomas.

A unique type of thyroid carcinoma is a solid medullary tumor with amyloid in the stroma. Although variable in its course, most have a better outlook than the undifferentiated carcinomas but one that is less favorable than the pure follicular tumors.

Spread of thyroid cancer may be to adjacent tissues and lymph nodes, but bloodstream metastasis to the lungs and skeleton is common. Papillary carcinomas characteristically spread to cervical lymph nodes, often before the primary tumor is clinically evident, and may remain long periods in such nodes before wider extension occurs. Such metastases as these have been mistaken for foci of *lateral aberrant thyroid* tissue. Well-differentiated thyroid tissue in metastases will take up radioactive iodine, whereas undifferentiated thyroid tumor tissue does not store the tagged iodine.

Struma ovarii. Struma ovarii is a teratoma of the ovary, in

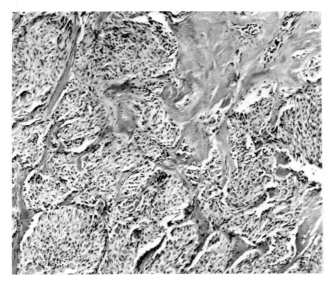

Fig. 20-17. Undifferentiated carcinoma, medullary type. The stroma of the tumor contains amyloid. (From Anderson, W. A. D., and Winship, T.: Thyroid gland. In Anderson, W. A. D., editor: Pathology, ed. 5, St. Louis, 1966, The C. V. Mosby Co.)

which thyroid tissue is the sole or chief constituent. Malignancy and metastasis may occur rarely. Functional activity of the tissue seldom is sufficient to produce clinical hyperthyroidism.

PARATHYROID GLANDS
Structure and function

The parathyroid glands are usually four in number and are situated on the posterior surface of the thyroid, or they are embedded in the thyroid tissue but separated from it by a connective tissue capsule. There is considerable variation in their position, particularly in the site of the lower pair, which are derived from the third branchial pouch in close association with portions of the thymus. One or both of the lower parathyroid glands may be found in the mediastinum in or near the thymus.

Histologically the gland contains three main types of cells: (1) small dark chief cells, (2) clear chief cells (*wasserhelle* or water-clear cells), and (3) oxyphilic cells. The clear chief cells have a clear nongranular cytoplasm and a large pale nucleus. The oxyphilic cells, which do not appear to secrete parathormone, are larger and have a granular acidophilic cytoplasm and a small dark nucleus. The eosinophilic granules by electron microscopy appear as mitochondria, and secretory granules are absent from the cytoplasm. The small dark cells have a finely granular cytoplasm, which stains faintly with eosin, and a small dark nucleus. Glycogen is found in considerable quantity in the parathyroid tissue, particularly in the chief cells. The cellular elements in the normal gland may be diffuse or compact,, but usually they have a definite arrangement in irregular strands or trabeculae. There may be occasional acinar arrangement. Fat cells are often quite abundant between the parenchymal cells. The parathyroid glands are important in the regulation of calcium and phosphorus metabolism. Parathyroid regulation maintains the diffusible ionized portion of serum calcium (i.e., the portion of serum calcium not bound to protein) within a narrow normal quantitative range. The mechanism of regulation appears

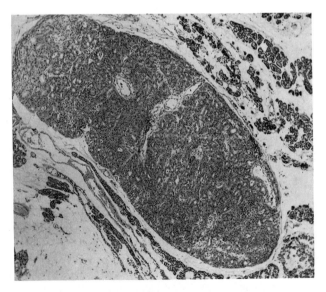

Fig. 20-18. Small oxyphilic adenoma of the parathyroid.

to be by promotion of renal phosphate excretion and through mobilization of calcium from bones by stimulation of osteoclasts. It is thus evident that disturbances of parathyroid hormone production may be expected to produce changes in calcium and phosphate regulation, with lesions not only in the parathyroids themselves but also in bones and kidneys. Hypoparathyroidism, or insufficient hormone production, is associated with tetany (neuromuscular irritability). Hyperparathyroidism, in which there is excessive hormone, may result in the skeletal changes of osteitis fibrosa cystica, calcium deposits in soft tissue (metastatic calcification), and renal calculi. Hypercalcemic crises (calcium intoxication) may occur in hyperparathyroidism and be rapidly fatal unless recognized and treated.

Dietary hypercalcemia, known as the Burnett or milk-alkali syndrome, may simulate primary hyperparathyroidism with secondary renal damage. It is usually caused by prolonged excessive intake of milk and absorbable alkalies. There is hypercalcemia without hypercalciuria, ocular calcinosis known as "band keratopathy," pruritus, azotemia, and mild alkalosis.

Diseases of the parathyroid glands

Hyperparathyroidism. Hyperparathyroidism may be primary or secondary. The primary form originates in the parathyroid glands either as a tumor (adenoma) of one gland or rarely as an idiopathic hypertrophy and hyperplasia of all glands. In secondary hyperparathyroidism there is diffuse hyperplasia of all glands. A mild degree of such secondary parathyroid hyperplasia occurs in chronic renal disease, osteomalacia, and rickets and may be produced experimentally by phosphate injections. Longstanding chronic renal insufficiency may produce pronounced parathyroid hyperplasia and in turn skeletal changes (renal dwarfism, renal hyperparathyroidism, p. 393). Pancreatitis is an occasional complication of hyperparathyroidism.

Parathyroid adenoma. Parathyroid adenoma is a benign tumor involving a single gland or portion of a gland. It is most commonly composed of dark chief cells and less commonly of large water-clear cells or oxyphils. The oxyphil cell adenomas may not cause hyperparathyroidism. The cellular elements are compactly disposed, with loss of trabecular arrangement of cells and decrease of fat and connective tissue. Acini are often numerous, but there is variability of cellular arrangement. Individual cells may be increased in size and contain multiple nuclei.

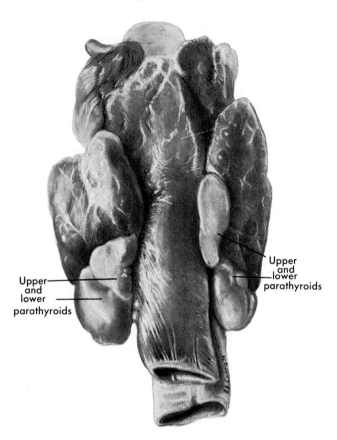

Upper and lower parathyroids

Upper and lower parathyroids

Fig. 20-19. Parathyroid hyperplasia. Considerable enlargement of all parathyroids in a case of renal dwarfism.

Variations in cell morphology or invasion of the capsule do not necessarily indicate malignancy. Malignancy is rare, but functioning metastases have been reported.

Primary idiopathic hypertrophy and hyperplasia. In this condition all the parathyroid glands are enlarged and of uniform structure, being composed of extremely large cells having a very clear cytoplasm (water-clear cells). This type of hyperparathyroidism is very rare.

Secondary hyperparathyroidism. Secondary hyperparathyroidism is characterized by enlargement of all the glands because of increased numbers of normal small dark chief cells. The various glands are not necessarily enlarged to the same degree, but all show a decrease of interstitial fat.

Hyperparathyroidism is characterized clinically by weakness, polyuria, pain in the bones, skeletal changes, and increased serum calcium and phosphatase and decreased serum phosphate. The bony changes seen on x-ray film may appear as a uniform osteoporosis, or the decalcification may be associated with cyst formation. Renal or skeletal disease is usually prominent. Renal disease in association with hyperparathyroidism is discussed on p. 393, and the hyperparathyroid skeletal disease, osteitis fibrosa cystica, on p. 834.

Hypoparathyroidism. Manifested clinically by tetany, hypoparathyroidism is most commonly seen after operations upon the thyroid gland, in which the parathyroid glands have been accidentally removed or had their blood supply disturbed. Idiopathic cases also occur.

Tetany. Tetany is a manifestation of neuromuscular hyperirritability caused by low blood and tissue calcium; it occurs also in conditions other than hypoparathyroidism, such as rickets, osteomalacia, and hyperventilation.

Pseudohypoparathyroidism is a rare genetic disorder characterized by short stature, mental retardation, hypocalcemic tetany unresponsive to parathyroid extract, and osseous abnormalities (Albright's hereditary osteodystrophy).

Polyendocrine disease. Several syndromes that have a strong familial incidence are characterized by functioning adenomas in more than one endocrine gland. Pancreatic islets, parathyroid glands, the anterior lobe of the pituitary, adrenal glands, and the thyroid may be involved with varying frequency and combinations. Peptic ulcer is a frequent manifestation. Some cases of the Zollinger-Ellison syndrome (p. 604) may have a polyendocrine background.

THYMUS
Structure and function

The thymus is an epithelial and lymphoid structure prominent during childhood. Its relative size is greatest at birth, when it weighs about 13 grams, and its absolute size is greatest at puberty, when the average weight is about 30 grams. In adult life it undergoes atrophy and replacement by fatty tissue.

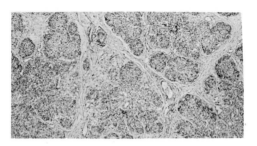

Fig. 20-20. Thymic alymphoplasia.

The epithelial elements are derived from the third branchial cleft, and the lymphoid structures develop later in fetal life. The epithelial cells form concentric collections known as Hassall's corpuscles.

The thymus appears to be an important source of small lymphocytes. In adition to this lymphopoietic function it also appears to have erythropoietic and myelopoietic activity, at least during fetal life. Its important function appears to be related to immune mechanisms. At birth it is presumed to be the carrier of the immunologically competent cells, and it is essential in the development of immunologic defenses.

Thymic alymphoplasia, a congenital anomaly, has been described in association with congenital agammaglobulinemia, lymphocytic hypoplasia, and lymphopenia. The hypoplastic thymus consists of a small number of poorly developed lobules separated by thick fibrous septa. Small lymphocytes and Hassall's bodies are absent.

Pathologic changes in the thymus

Pathologic changes in the thymus are rare and consist of atrophy, hyperplasia, and cyst and tumor formation.

Atrophy. In addition to the physiologic atrophy that occurs after puberty, an atrophy occurs in most serious illnesses or infections of childhood.

Hyperplasia. Hyperplasia of the thymus occurs in hyperthyroidism (Graves' disease), acromegaly, some cases of Addison's disease, and in eunuchs.

Status thymicolymphaticus. The concept of status thymicolymphaticus is that of a constitutional abnormality in certain persons characterized by an enlarged thymus, generalized lymphoid hyperplasia, hypoplasia of the aorta, atrophy of the adrenals, and underdevelopment of testes or ovaries. Such persons are supposedly subject to sudden death as a result of relatively trivial stimuli, e.g., mild trauma, anesthesia, etc. It is probable that the thymus plays no role in the condition other than being part of the generalized lymphoid hyperplasia. That such a condition actually exists is often doubted.

Tumors. Tumors of the thymus are uncommon, although they are one of the important types of anterior mediastinal neoplasms. Although the histologic pattern varies considerably, they are collectively termed thymomas. Some are well circumscribed or encapsulated, but many extend or infiltrate locally, although distant metastasis is rare.

Histologic classifications of thymomas are numerous and variable. A simple classification is into three groups: (1) epithelial (most frequent), (2) lymphoid, and (3) teratomatous (least frequent). Among the epithelial group of thymomas the tumors may contain epidermoid cells or may be composed of oval or spindle cells. Commonly there is a mixed or granulomatous picture, with combinations of epithelial cells, multinucleated giant cells, fibrous tissue, lymphocytes, and eosinophils, a picture simulating Hodgkin's disease. Undifferentiated epithelial thymomas may show numerous mitoses and are most likely to spread by metastasis. Some of these histologically resemble testicular seminomas or ovarian dysgerminomas and so have been called mediastinal seminomas or germinomas. Lymphoid thymomas are lymphosarcomas similar to those arising from lymphoid tissue elsewhere. Anterior mediastinal teratomas are considered by some to arise mainly from the anlage of the thymus. Lipomas of the thymus occur only rarely but may be of large size.

The relation of thymic enlargement or thymic tumors to myasthenia gravis is still uncertain, and a causal relationship has not been clearly established. *Myasthenia gravis* is a condition of weakness or abnormal fatigability of muscles. It is believed to be caused by some interference with the transmission of impulses across the myoneural junction, a condition that is temporarily overcome by the administration of neostigmine (Prostigmin) and is simulated by curare poisoning. Lymphocytic infiltrations (lymphorrhages) are found in affected muscles. It has recently been proposed that myasthenia gravis is an auto-

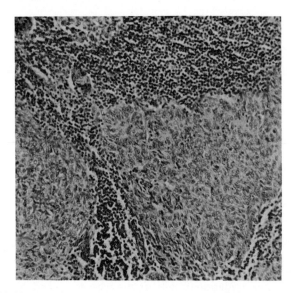

Fig. 20-21. Thymoma with lymphoid and epithelial-appearing areas. (From Anderson, W. A. D.: Thymus. In Anderson, W. A. D., editor: Pathology, ed. 5, St. Louis, 1966, The C. V. Mosby Co.)

immune disease, and cross reactions have been demonstrated between antimuscle antibodies in the sera of myasthenic individuals and certain cells of the thymus. The reactive elements in the thymus may be actual muscle cells rather than entodermal reticular elements.

The incidence of thymoma among patients with myasthenia gravis has been reported as from 15 to 30%. Conversely about 75% of patients with thymoma show symptoms of myasthenia gravis. In most cases removal of a thymoma in a patient with myasthenia gravis does not relieve the condition, and myasthenia gravis has been reported as developing after removal of an asymptomatic thymoma. Female patients with myasthenia gravis without thymomas have been reported to be improved by thymectomy. Thymomas in patients with myasthenia gravis show large pale epithelial cells arranged in cords or clusters around vessels and loosely mixed with lymphocytes. Foci of myocardial degeneration and of necrosis and myocarditis have been observed in some instances of myasthenia gravis, especially associated with thymoma.

The association of thymoma and aregenerative anemia has been noted in a few cases and, more rarely, the association of thymoma and pancytopenia. Excision of the thymoma has relieved the anemia in some cases, but not all have responded. The thymomas associated with blood dyscrasia have been found to be of spindle cell type with apparent frequency.

Cysts of the thymus may be congenital, inflammatory, or neoplastic. *Dubois' abscess* is a cyst of the thymus caused by persistence of the embryonic duct, which gives rise to the epithelial structures. It may be associated with congenital syphilis.

PINEAL BODY
Structure and function

The function of the pineal body is as yet unknown. There is some evidence that it has a secretory function, although it is not essential to life, pregnancy, or parturition. Several neurohumoral substances (e.g., serotonin and histamine) as well as a skin-lightening agent (melatonin), which appears to be an antagonist of the pituitary melanocyte-stimulating hormone, have been reported in bovine pineal tissue. There is also some evidence that the pineal body may produce an adrenotropic hormone affecting aldosterone secretion.

At about the time of puberty regressive structural changes are initiated in the pineal body. There is an increase in interstitial connective tissue, which accentuates fibrous trabeculae and gives the gland a lobulated appearance in microscopic section. Calcareous concretions (acervuli) also begin to form about puberty and are almost constant after the sixteenth year. In adult life they are sometimes sufficiently dense to be evident on an x-ray plate.

Areas of neuroglial hyperplasia often with irregularly cavitated centers, are quite commonly present in the pineal. True cysts also occur, usually lined by ependymal cells.

Tumors

Tumors of the pineal body constitute its only important lesion. Pineal tumors are of three types: (1) pinealomas, (2) teratomas, and (3) gliomas.

Pinealomas are tumors composed of pineal parenchymal cells

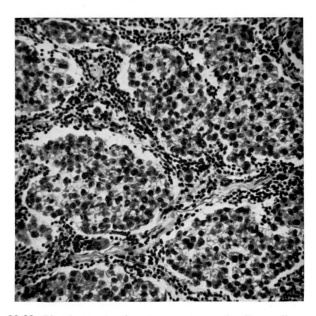

Fig. 20-22. Pinealoma, showing the two types of cells usually present.

and have a microscopic appearance similar to that of some stage of embryonic development of the pineal body. Two types of cells are usually present: large pale cells with prominent rounded nuclei and indefinite cytoplasm, resembling cells of the adult period, and fewer small, round, dark cells, resembling lymphocytes. The tumor is locally invasive and malignant. Pinealomas also may have a structure resembling the adult pineal body. While some evidence has suggested that the usual pinealoma is really an atypical teratoma, there are also *teratomas* of the pineal which are similar to teratomas elsewhere and contain bone, teeth, cartilage, epithelium, hair, etc. *Gliomas* of the pineal usually closely resemble the ependymomas that arise in other areas of the brain, but spongioblastic pineal tumors also occur.

Because of their situation, pineal tumors soon obstruct the aqueduct of Sylvius, producing internal hydrocephalus and considerable increase of intracranial pressure. Certain pineal tumors in preadolescent boys have been associated with precocious sexual development (pubertas praecox or macrogenito-somia praecox). A similar condition of hypergenitalism has been associated with midbrain lesions or tumors as well as with various endocrine disturbances.

ADRENAL GLANDS
Structure and function

The adrenals consist of two distinct glands, cortex and medulla, which have different origins and functions. The cortex is of mesodermal origin from the urogenital ridge and is thus closely related to gonads and other urogenital organs. The medulla originates from the neural crest in common with sympathetic nerve cells. While anatomically associated in man, the cortex and medulla are quite separate in their function and pathology and are best considered as separate glands. The cortex, which is essential for life, is associated with salt and water (electrolyte) metabolism, with protein and carbohydrate metabolism, and with development and maintenance of secondary sexual characteristics (androgen production). The adrenals are essential for adjustment to changes in internal and external environment. The adrenal medulla secretes epinephrine (adrenaline), the effects of which simulate sympathetic stimulation. Survival is possible in the absence of the medulla. Accessory adrenal tissue may be found between the origins of the celiac and superior mesenteric arteries.

The adrenals are relatively largest at time of birth, when they are usually one third the size of the kidney. The large size results from a highly vascular inner cortical tissue, which degenerates soon after birth and disappears almost entirely during the first year of life. In adult life the adrenals are about one thirtieth the size of the kidney.

Adrenal cortex

Although numerous steroids have been isolated from adrenal tissue, three are recognized as principal cortical hormones in man: cortisol, corticosterone, and aldosterone. The first two, which have an effect on carbohydrate metabolism, are called glucocorticoids. Aldosterone has its main effect on salt and water metabolism and is termed a mineralocorticoid.

The adrenal cortex is divided into zones descriptively named from without inward, the glomerulosa, fasciculata, and reticularis. Internal to these the highly vascular zone that exists at birth is replaced by a thin juxtamedullary zone. Some brownish pigment, of no known significance, is often present in the inner part of the cortex.

The outer zone, the zona glomerulosa, is composed of rounded clusters of cells. It appears to be the zone mainly concerned with the group of adrenal steroids termed mineralocorticoids and is concerned principally with the control of water and electrolyte metabolism. The naturally occurring hormone is aldosterone, and its synthetic relative is called desoxycorticosterone. These hormones bring about reabsorption of sodium and chloride by the renal distal convoluted tubules, with a corresponding loss of potassium, and provide the mechanism by which sodium, potassium, and extracellular fluid are maintained in normal osmotic balance. Output of aldosterone appears to be regulated by changes in the relations of sodium, potassium, and extracellular fluid and is not under control of the anterior pituitary. Aldosterone also antagonizes the activity of hydrocortisone (cortisol), which inhibits inflammatory reactions and produces a decrease of circulating eosinophils. Urinary excretion of aldosterone provides an index of the amount of circulating hormone. The electrolyte composition of sweat serves as an index of the effect of the mineralocorticoid on the sodium content of the tissues. An increase of the hormone (secondary hyperaldosteronism) may be brought about by a prolonged low sodium intake, and also it occurs in conditions of generalized edema or persistent hypertension. Primary hyperaldosteronism occurs from the activity of certain adrenal cortical tumors and hyperplasias. Selective hypoaldosteronism appears to be rare.

The thick middle zone of the cortex, the zona fasciculata, is composed of parallel cords of cells that are rich in lipids and appear pale or vacuolated. It is a site of formation of the glucocorticoids, which influence intermediate carbohydrate metabolism. The production of the glucocorticoids is under the control of the anterior pituitary adrenocorticotropic hormone (ACTH), and in turn the glucocorticoid level controls the adrenocorticotropic activity of the anterior pituitary. The main glucocorticoids are cortisol (compound F) and corticosterone. Synthetic derivatives used therapeutically are prednisone and prednisolone. The glucocorticoids cause acceleration of gluconeogenesis from protein and deposition of liver glycogen, with related effects on the metabolism of carbohydrates, protein, and fat. They suppress inflammatory response (antiphlogistic activity) and cause eosinopenia, lysis of lymphoid cells, and atrophy of lymphoid tissues. The glucocorticoids are important in resistance to nonspecific stress. They are not without some mineralocorticoid activity, just as aldosterone has some weaker glucocorticoid action. Prolonged medication with cortisone or its relatives may produce the phenomena seen in Cushing's syndrome.

The inner zone, the zona reticularis, is usually narrow and made up of an interlacing network of "compact" cells, which are eosinophilic and contain abundant phosphatase and ribonucleic acid. It appears to be the site principally concerned with the androgenic sex hormones (nitrogen hormones). These hormones are involved in masculinization (androgenic function) and also are anabolic, increasing the synthesis of amino acids and protein from nitrogen. Their amount is reflected in the urinary excretion of 17-ketosteroids. Some estrogen production also may occur. According to some views the zona reticularis is also the ordinary site of formation of glucocorticoids, with additional formation in the zona fasciculata when there is unusual stimulation.

The assignment of separate functions to the different zones is provisional, and it is uncertain as to how distinct may be the functional separation. Ascorbic acid is stored in the reticularis and inner part of the fasciculata, and its concentration parallels the lipid content of the cortex. Lipid material is present throughout the cortex but is most abundant in the zona fasciculata. The shift of lipid patterns gives some indication of adrenal cortical activity caused by pituitary adrenotropic hormone. When ACTH is administered, the cells of the inner part of the zona fasciculata have a decrease of their lipid and become similar to the "compact" cells of the zona reticularis. Increasing the amount of ACTH stimulation extends this change outward in the zona fasciculata. The lipids in adrenocortical cells consist of doubly refractile cholesterol, anisotropic neutral lipids, and steroids. The lipids tend to be depleted as the gland becomes exhausted.

Lesions in the adrenal cortex may roughly be grouped as (1) regressive and destructive changes, and (2) hyperplasia and tumors.

Regressive and destructive lesions. Adrenal cortical tissue is most commonly injured or destroyed by hemorrhage, infarction, metastatic tumors, infections, and amyloid deposits.

Hemorrhage and necrosis. Extensive hemorrhage into adrenals or thrombosis of adrenal vessels may produce acute adrenal insufficiency. Hemorrhage is particularly common in newborn infants, in some cases from trauma incident to birth. Adrenal hemorrhage or focal necrosis may also occur with extensive burns or in various infections. Small areas of hemorrhagic necrosis may occur in eclampsia. In newborn infants the highly vascular inner zone of the cortex may be mistaken for hemorrhage unless carefully examined.

Various acute infections may severely damage the adrenal cortex, the necrosis of cells transforming the solid cords of cells of the zona fasciculata into apparent tubular structures containing inflammatory exudate. The adrenal damage may bear some relation to the circulatory collapse that occurs in some of these patients. Small focal areas of inflammation or necrosis are common with generalized infections or toxemias. Histoplasmosis and blastomycosis quite commonly involve the adrenal glands.

Massive bilateral hemorrhages of the adrenal glands may occur in cases of fulminating meningococcemia, in which rapid death occurs, often before there is any great involvement of the meninges (Waterhouse-Friderichsen syndrome). The fatal outcome appears to result from the overwhelming meningococcemia, acute adrenal insufficiency having only a minor role. The hemorrhages in the adrenals, skin, and elsewhere appear to be the result of toxic injury of capillary endothelium. Only about 2 to 4% of meningococcal infections have the complication of the Waterhouse-Friderichsen syndrome.

Atrophy of the adrenal cortex may be produced by continued administration of cortisone. Loss of lipid occurs first, particularly in the zona fasciculata, and the glands decrease in weight and show narrowing of the cortex and loss of color. The changes seem to be reversible in most cases and appear to be caused by suppressed endogenous production of corticotropin by the pituitary. Basophils of the anterior pituitary may show loss of granularity of their cytoplasm.

Addison's disease. Chronic adrenal cortical insufficiency produces the clinical condition of Addison's disease. Symptoms appear when about 80% of adrenal cortical tissue has been destroyed. In about 70% of cases the bilateral destruction of the adrenal glands formerly was caused by tuberculosis. In most of the remaining cases there was atrophy or destruction from un-

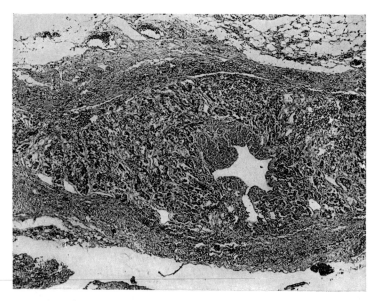

Fig. 20-23. Adrenal gland in Addison's disease showing cortical loss. Only medulla is seen, which is focally infiltrated with lymphocytes. (From Anderson, W. A. D., and Cleveland, W. W.: Adrenal glands. In Anderson, W. A. D., editor: Pathology, ed. 5, St. Louis, 1966, The C. V. Mosby Co.)

known causes, by some thought to result from unsuspected chemical or drug poisoning. In the United States, cortical necrosis or atrophy now appears to account for about 50% of cases. The incidence of tuberculosis as a cause of Addison's disease apparently is decreasing. In the case of the tuberculous lesions, both cortex and medulla of the glands are usually destroyed. With cortical necrosis or simple atrophy the medulla may be unaffected. The pathogenesis of the cortical destruction or atrophy is usually unknown. Autoantibodies to adrenal tissue have been suggested as a possible mechanism. The medulla evidently is unimportant in the pathogenesis of this entity. Amyloidosis, inflammatory changes, fibrosis, histoplasmosis, and torulosis of the cortex are sometimes causative of Addison's disease, but bilateral metastatic tumors or gummas only rarely are a cause. In the tuberculous type of adrenal destruction, active tuberculous lesions usually are found elsewhere.

Addison's disease is characterized by extreme weakness, low blood pressure, and pigmentation of the skin. The pigmentation is caused by excessive melanin, presumably from the increased secretion of the melanocyte-stimulating hormone of the pituitary, which results from lack of inhibition by the adrenal cortical hormones. It may be irregular in distribution and often is best seen in the mucous membranes of the lips or mouth or in scars. Urinary excretion of ketosteroids is decreased to a low level. Salt metabolism is disturbed, there being excessive loss of sodium salt in the urine with low sodium and chloride levels and a rise in potassium in the plasma. High sodium and low potassium intake relieves many of the symptoms. Adrenal cortical extracts successfully replace the hormonal deficiency.

Schmidt's syndrome is the concurrence of nontuberculous Addison's disease and chronic lymphocytic thyroiditis. It has been found mainly in females, and generally the adrenal insufficiency has preceded recognizable thyroid disease. Circulating antibodies against thyroid tissue and also against adrenal tissue may be present. Some cases also have had diabetes mellitus, and it has been suggested that such cases may be a polyendocrinopathy and that the basis may be immunologic.

Anencephaly. The adrenal glands have frequently been reported as defective or absent in anencephalic monsters. Usually they are present but atrophic and histologically of the adult rather than the infantile type. The adrenal atrophy is believed to be secondary to pituitary changes.

Hyperplasia and tumors. Hyperplasia in the adrenal cortex may be diffuse but more often takes the form of small circumscribed nodules, which vary in size from microscopic to a diameter of several centimeters. In *nodular hyperplasia* there are small nodules, with or without distinct encapsulation, which occur as an incidental finding (without an associated endocrine syndrome) in a considerable proportion of autopsies on adults. They probably are developmental in origin or represent a regenerative process after infection or other injury of the adrenals. Microscopically they consist of columns of adrenal cells like those of the fascicular zone. *Diffuse hyperplasia* of the adrenal cortex is relatively infrequent and often is associated with a clinical endocrine syndrome. This may be the adrenogenital syndrome, Cushing's syndrome, or a condition having mixed features of these two. Hyperplasia is not found with feminization of adrenal cortical origin and only rarely is diffuse hyper-

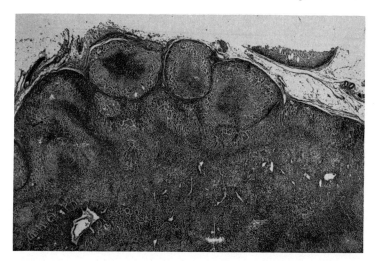

Fig. 20-24. Nodular hyperplasia of the adrenal cortex. The low-power photomicrograph shows multiple nodules with varying degrees of encapsulation.

plasia the lesion accompanying hyperaldosteronism. Diffuse hyperplasia may be produced by ACTH administration. *True adenoma* also occurs as a yellowish mass, which is usually 1 or 2 cm. in diameter but may grow to considerable size. It is usually single and unilateral. Although well circumscribed and having a definite capsule, it may press upon and deform the remainder of the gland. *Carcinomas* are similar to the adenomas but contain areas of atypical and malignant-looking cells. Invasion of veins or the capsule may be seen, and metastasis occurs readily to distant organs and to the opposite adrenal gland. *Myelolipoma* is a tumorlike nodule of adipose and hematopoietic tissue, resembling bone marrow. It has been found as an incidental finding in the adrenal glands of adults.

In persons having a functioning adrenal cortical adenoma or carcinoma, the opposite adrenal gland may be atrophic and insufficient to meet sudden functional demands. Consequently an acute adrenal insufficiency may develop after surgical removal of the tumor.

Adrenal cortical hyperfunction. Hyperplasias, adenomas, or carcinomas of the adrenal cortex may be associated with ex-

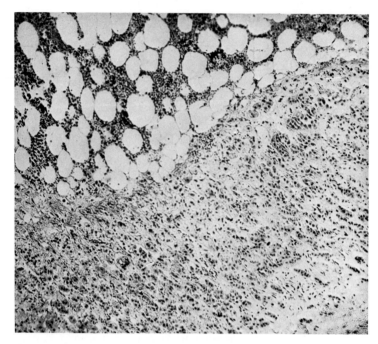

Fig. 20-25. Myelolipoma of the adrenal gland. The fatty and myeloid tissue, resembling bone marrow, formed a tumorlike nodule enclosed by adrenal cortical tissue.

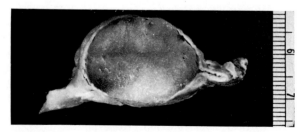

Fig. 20-26. Lipoma of the adrenal gland.

cessive hormonal production and clinical effects, although more commonly these lesions are encountered without apparent hormonal effects. Those that are associated with excess hormone production may result either in a clinical syndrome in which the effects of one type of adrenal cortical hormone are dominant or in a mixed picture in which the effects of excess of more than one hormonal principle are evident. Although the varying excesses of the different hormones produce gradations in the clinical features, with some exceptions cases may be grouped into three classes: the adrenogenital syndrome, Cushing's syndrome, and primary aldosteronism.

Adrenogenital syndrome. The adrenogenital syndrome is an adrenal virilism in which an excess of androgenic hormones produces the dominant effects. Overgrowth of cortical tissue that produces male hormone causes a variety of sexual disturbances, depending upon the age at which it occurs. Congenital virilism appears to be an inborn metabolic fault in which incompletely oxygenated steroids instead of hydrocortisone are secreted into the bloodstream. The resulting lack stimulates excess production of pituitary corticotropin, which in turn causes a large out-

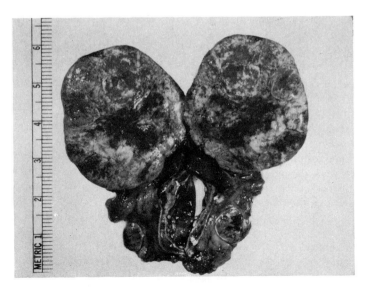

Fig. 20-27. Adrenal carcinoma associated with Cushing's syndrome.

put of androgens. The condition often starts in utero and in female infants produces pseudohermaphroditism. Occurring in childhood, it is commonly the effect of an adrenal cortical tumor. In boys it is characterized by precocious sexual and muscular development with genitalia of adult size and secondary sexual characteristics. In girls pseudosexual precocity with masculinity occurs, with the appearance of pubic hair and hypertrophy of the clitoris. Adult females become masculinized, the change being characterized by hirsutism, enlarged clitoris, atrophy of breasts, amenorrhea, deepening of the voice, and various masculine characteristics. Urinary excretion of 17-ketosteroids is excessive. The adrenal lesion in adults may be hyperplasia, adenoma, or carcinoma. The hyperplastic gland in virilism is composed of "compact" cells extending up to the zona glomerulosa, an appearance consistent with excessive stimulation by ACTH. The virilization must be distinguished from that which may be produced by certain ovarian tumors. Rarely an adrenal carcinoma may produce excess estrogen and cause feminization of males or precocity in young females.

Cushing's syndrome. Cushing's syndrome is produced by excessive secretion of cortisol and is more commonly caused by adrenal cortical hyperplasia and less often by adrenal adenoma or carcinoma. A few cases show no apparent adrenal lesion. Occasional instances of Cushing's syndrome have been associated with carcinoma of the lung, apparently resulting from the production of a corticotropic substance by the tumor. It is more common in women (3 or 4:1). Clinical characteristics are obesity of the face, neck, and trunk; polycythemia and a dusky color of the skin; purplish striae of the skin of the abdomen, buttocks, and flanks; hypertension; osteoporosis; a tendency to diabetes mellitus; weakness and fatigue; and sexual impotence or amenorrhea. Most of these clinical effects can be reproduced by the administration of an excess of glucocorticoids. Associated pituitary changes may be hyalinization of basophils (Crooke's change) or less commonly a basophilic hyperplasia or adenoma. There is an overproduction of ACTH by the anterior pituitary, but the primary site and cause of the regulatory disorder is uncertain.

Primary aldosteronism. Primary aldosteronism (Conn's syndrome) results from excess mineralocorticoid, which is usually caused by an adenoma or carcinoma of the adrenal cortex or, less often, by hyperplasia. The tumors are 1 to 5 cm. in diameter,

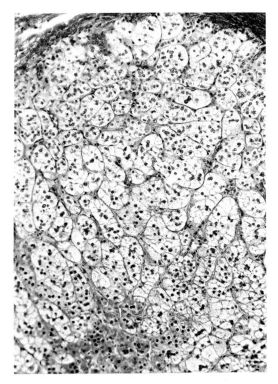

Fig. 20-28. Large, clear, lipid-laden adrenal cortical cells associated with hyperaldosteronism. (×125.) (Courtesy Dr. S. E. Gould; from Anderson, W. A. D., and Cleveland, W. W.: Adrenal glands. In Anderson, W. A. D., editor: Pathology, ed. 5, St. Louis, 1966, The C. V. Mosby Co.)

bright yellow in color, and composed of large, clear, lipid-containing cells. They usually are in the outer part of the cortex and probably arise in the zona glomerulosa. Aldosteronism is characterized clinically by periodic severe muscular weakness, intermittent tetany and paresthesia, polyuria, polydipsia, and hypertension. Edema is not present. There is excessive loss of potassium in the urine, and the blood levels of potassium are low. Alkalosis is present, manifested by the elevation of pH and carbon dioxide combining power. The urinary aldosterone level is high. Before recognition of their true nature, some of these cases have been called "potassium-losing nephritis." Conn has noted that in certain cases of primary aldosteronism the potassium level in the blood may be normal, at least initially in the disease.

Overproduction of aldosterone and suppression of plasma renin activity are diagnostic of an aldosterone-secreting adrenal cortical tumor. Some of the cases of normokalemic primary hyperaldosteronism may masquerade as essential hypertension but have as their basis aldosterone-secreting adrenal cortical adenomas.

Increased aldosterone secretion is frequently present in advanced stages of hypertensive disease and in malignant hypertension. The increased rate of aldosterone secretion appears to be secondary to and to correlate with increased plasma renin levels.

Adrenal glands in eclampsia. The adrenal cortex may have a role in the toxemias of pregnancy, although specific changes may not be present. A hyperadrenalism involving mineralocorticoids and glucocorticoids appears to produce some of the features accompanying pregnancy, but enzymes of the placenta normally suppress or inactivate certain of the effects of the adrenal hormones. Ischemic placental lesions may interfere with this mechanism and result in preeclampsia or eclampsia with convulsions.

Adrenal medulla

The medulla of the adrenal has an origin from ectoderm, in common with sympathetic nerve tissue. The cells of the medulla stain with chrome salts as do certain other tissues, such as abdominal paraganglia and the carotid body. Their function, production of epinephrine and norepinephrine, is not essential for life. Epinephrine causes contraction of some vessels and dilatation of others (e.g., the coronary arteries), tachycardia, and increased cardiac output. Norepinephrine constricts vessels and causes increased peripheral resistance. Epinephrine has a greater effect upon oxygen consumption and glycogenolysis. Functional disturbances caused by destructive lesions of the medulla are overshadowed by the associated involvement of the cortex, as in the tuberculous type of Addison's disease. The only lesions of the adrenal medulla that are of practical importance are tumors.

Tumors. Tumors of the adrenal medulla or other parts of the sympathetic nervous system are composed of immature or mature cell types comparable to those that occur in embryonic development of medullary and sympathetic nerve tissue. The most immature form, the precursor of the other types, is the sympathogonia, a small dark lymphocyte-like cell, which differentiates into neuroblasts (sympathoblasts and pheochromoblasts). The sympathoblasts mature as ganglion cells, and the pheochromoblasts develop into pheochromocytes, the mature cells of the adrenal medulla. Tumors composed of the immature forms (sympathogonioma and neuroblastoma) are highly malignant, while those composed of mature forms (ganglioneuroma and pheochromocytoma) are benign.

Sympathogonioma. Sympathogoniomas usually develop during intrauterine life or in early infancy, are highly malignant and invasive, and metastasize early. They are composed of small dark cells resembling lymphocytes, some of which group to form rosettes. No neurofibrils are formed.

Adrenal neuroblastoma. The adrenal neuroblastoma (sympathoblastoma) is a highly malignant tumor that occurs almost exclusively in infants and young children. It arises either

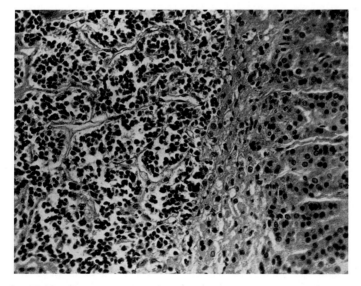

Fig. 20-29. Adrenal neuroblastoma (newborn infant). (From Anderson, W. A. D., and Cleveland, W. W.: Adrenal glands. In Anderson, W. A. D., editor: Pathology, ed. 5, St. Louis, 1966, The C. V. Mosby Co.)

in the adrenal medulla or the immediate neighborhood. Microscopically it is extremely cellular, is composed of small rounded dark cells resembling lymphocytes, and has the characteristic feature of rosette formation (circular grouping around a fine fibrillar network). It differs from the sympathogonioma only in its somewhat greater maturity, and some differentiated ganglion or pheochrome cells may be present. The cells tend to be larger and irregular or oval in shape, and they may have elongated cytoplasmic processes. Tumors having similar histologic structure are the medulloblastoma of the midbrain and the retinoblastoma of the eye. They also arise from undifferentiated neural elements and occur in childhood.

Rare examples of neuroblastoma have given evidence of secretion of epinephrine or norepinephrine. However, there usually is evidence of abnormalities of tyrosine metabolism, with formation of excessive 3,4-dihydroxyphenylalanine (dopa). The excess dopa is metabolized through dopamine to homovanillic acid (HVA) or through dopamine and norepinephrine to vanilmandelic acid (VMA). The urinary excretion of these terminal metabolites may be detected and measured, providing an effective method for diagnosis and for following results of treatment. Increase of these urinary metabolites has also been reported with ganglioneuromas and ganglioneuroblastomas. It appears that 95% of patients with neuroblastoma, ganglioneuroblastoma, or ganglioneuroma will show elevation of urinary HVA, VMA, or both.

Adrenal neuroblastoma spreads early and widely, and the clinical picture largely depends on the metastases. Tumors of the right adrenal tend to metastasize to retroperitoneal lymph nodes and liver, producing the Pepper syndrome. Metastasis to bones, particularly of the skull and around the region of the orbits, produces the Hutchison syndrome, likely to result from a tumor of the left adrenal medulla. The two classic types frequently overlap. In rare instances the tumor cells mature to ganglion cells, producing a benign ganglioneuroma.

Ganglioneuroma. Ganglioneuroma is a benign tumor composed of differentiated, large sympathetic ganglion cells and often a few nerve fibers. It may occur in either a child or an adult. While the common origin is from the adrenal medulla, it may arise in any part of the abdominal sympathetic system or very rarely is found in the central nervous system. It produces symptoms only by virtue of the large size to which it may grow.

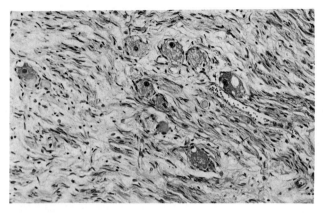

Fig. 20-30. Ganglioneuroma. The tumor is composed of an irregular jumble of nerve cells and fibers.

A form also occurs in which undifferentiated or incompletely differentiated cells are mixed with some ganglion cells and nerve fibers (ganglioneuroblastoma).

Pheochromocytoma. Chromaffinoma (pheochromocytoma) is a rare tumor composed of a differentiated mature type of cell, resembling those that normally compose the adrenal medulla. About 90% of these tumors arise in the adrenal, somewhat more frequently on the right, and about 10% of cases with adrenal origin are bilateral. Some 10% or less arise in extra-adrenal sites, usually near the kidneys, adrenals, aortic bodies, organs of Zuckerkandl, or rarely, in the urinary bladder. Those arising from extra-adrenal chromaffin tissue have been called para-gangliomas. The tumors are usually less than 10 cm. in diameter, circumscribed, yellowish brown in color, and frequently with cystic, necrotic, or hemorrhagic areas. The tumor cells are large, irregular or polyhedral, and occur in groups surrounded by a vascular fine connective tissue stroma. Mitoses are absent. Some of the cells are stained brown by fixation in bichromate. Most pheochromocytomas are benign, and malignancy should not be considered in the absence of invasion or metastasis. The rare malignant pheochromocytomas tend to have a spindle cell growth pattern predominating.

The tumor usually occurs in persons of middle age or beyond. In some cases there is evidence of familial occurrence, and

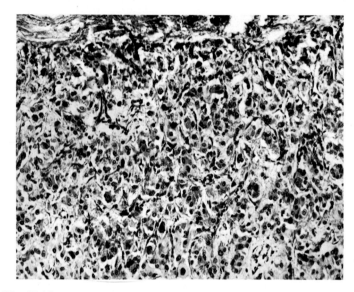

Fig. 20-31. Pheochromocytoma of the adrenal gland.

association with thyroid carcinoma of the medullary type has been noted. It occurs also with somewhat greater than usual frequency in patients with multiple neurofibromatosis. Although some pheochromocytomas are clinically asymptomatic, many produce symptoms as a result of catecholamine content (epinephrine and norepinephrine). Paroxysmal attacks characterized by hypertension, tachycardia, hyperglycemia, sweating, and trembling are most characteristic, and are particularly epinephrine effects. Tumors in which persistent secretion of norepinephrine predominates may give rise to persistent hypertension. Extra-adrenal pheochromocytomas may secrete only norepinephrine. Catecholamines or their metabolites may be demonstrated in urine or blood as a diagnostic procedure. Catecholamines may be assayed also in the fresh tumor tissue. Surgical resection of a functioning tumor may be followed by hypotension and shock.

Glomic tissue tumors (chemodectomas or *nonchromaffin paragangliomas)* may arise in the carotid and aortic bodies, the glomus jugulare, and retroperitoneal space. Some examples have been found to secrete norepinephrine.

Chapter 21

The female genital organs

The important pathologic conditions of the female genitalia are inflammations, endocrine disturbances, tumors, and cysts. Many gynecologic diseases are closely related in both functional and morphologic aspects to hormonal imbalance. The endocrine factors important in gynecologic pathology are the pituitary gonadotropic principles and the ovarian and placental hormones.

HORMONAL RELATIONSHIPS

Pituitary gonadotropic hormones. There are two pituitary principles that act on the ovaries: (1) a follicle-stimulating hormone, which controls maturation of the ovarian follicles, and hence in turn the production of follicular hormone (estrogen); and (2) a luteinizing hormone, which controls luteinization of the ruptured follicle, and hence in turn the production of the luteal hormone (progesterone). The nature and chemical structures of these pituitary principles are still unknown.

Ovarian hormones. The two ovarian hormones that normally are controlled in this fashion by the pituitary are of known chemical nature and structure, and they exert pronounced effects on the endometrium, vagina, and other tissues. Menstrual changes and periodicity are dependent on these hormones.

Maturing ovarian follicles produce a hormone, estrogen (theelin). This has been isolated in a number of closely related forms, all characterized by the ability to produce estrus (heat) in castrated animals. Various names given to these estrogens are estradiol, estrone, and estriol. Certain estrogenic substances can be derived synthetically (e.g., stilbestrol). The basic chemical structure of estrogens is the phenanthrene ring system. Thus there is a chemical structural resemblance to certain naturally occurring sterols and to some potent carcinogenic materials, a relationship that has caused much interesting speculation.

Estrogen, formed by the mature ovarian follicle, is a sexual growth-stimulating substance that acts especially on the uterus and vagina. It brings about the proliferative endometrial growth characteristic of the first half of the menstrual cycle (p. 749). In addition it controls the rhythmic activity of the uterine musculature and causes cornification of the vaginal epithelium and growth of the duct system of the breast. At puberty estrogen is responsible for the appearance of the various secondary sexual characteristics.

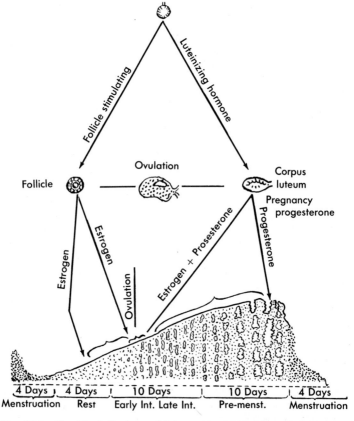

Fig. 21-1. Simplified diagram of hormonal relationships of the anterior pituitary, ovary, and endometrium. (From Faulkner, R. L., and Douglass, M.: Essentials of obstetrical and gynecological pathology, ed. 2, St. Louis, 1949, The C. V. Mosby Co.)

The ovarian follicle ruptures about the middle of the menstrual cycle and then forms the corpus luteum. This luteinized follicle produces not only estrogen but also a new and characteristic hormone, progesterone. This latter substance also is a sterol, of known chemical formula, and has been isolated, crystallized, and synthesized. It has a close structural relationship to the male sex hormone, testosterone.

Progesterone also affects the endometrium, vagina, and breast. In the endometrium it brings about a secretory phase (p. 750). The endometrium remains hypertrophied, but the glands become very irregular in outline and secretory in function. The stromal cells of the endometrium begin a decidua-like change. These changes are in preparation to receive the fertilized ovum. If conception fails to occur, the corpus luteum atrophies, the endometrium breaks down, and menstruation occurs. However, if pregnancy occurs, the corpus luteum continues to develop and produces progesterone, its effects being important in maintenance of the pregnancy in its early phases.

In addition to its effect on the endometrium, progesterone inhibits contractility of the uterus, suppresses ovulation and menstruation, and causes a mucus-secreting phase in vaginal epithelium and a lobular proliferation of the breast.

Hormones of pregnancy. During pregnancy chorionic gonadotropic hormones are produced and are found in the urine (urinary prolan). The biologic pregnancy tests (Aschheim-Zondek, Friedman) are based on demonstration of such hormones in the urine. These substances are anterior pituitary-like (APL) in their action. The placenta also seems capable of producing progesterone, an action important in the maintenance of later stages of pregnancy.

OVARIES
Development and structure

The ovaries, as well as the testes, first appear as *genital ridges* (thickenings of celomic epithelium and underlying mesenchyme) on the medial side of the mesonephros. Soon primordial cells migrate from the yolk sac into the genital ridges. In this indifferent stage it is not possible to make a distinction between the ovaries and the testes. Enormous numbers of primitive follicles develop as the ovary differentiates. The cortex of the ovary is composed of these primitive graafian follicles and a dense connective tissue stroma. The so-called epithelial cells of the follicles (i.e., granulosa cells) and the stromal cells (including theca cells, which are specialized stromal cells around follicles) have a common mesenchymal origin. Their close relationship is evident in certain tumors (e.g., granulosa–theca cell tumors). The primordial follicles consist of a central ovum surrounded by a layer of low cuboidal epithelium, the granulosal membrane. As the follicle matures and enlarges under the influence of the pituitary follicle-stimulating hormone, the granulosa becomes more cuboidal and several layers thick. A central cavity appears, the ovum being at one pole, surrounded by a pile of granulosa cells, the discus proligerus. Around the follicle is a specialized layer of connective tissue cells, the theca interna. Call-Exner bodies are small, rounded, clear, glandlike areas found in the granulosa layer, and similar structures appear in tumors composed of granulosa cells. About the middle of the menstrual cycle the follicle ruptures, and the ovum is extruded. The ruptured follicle develops into a corpus luteum under the influence of the luteinizing hormone of the pituitary.

At the time when the follicle ruptures, many other follicles are approaching maturity. Their further development is stopped by the hormone of the corpus luteum, and they undergo regression. These atretic follicles form cysts, and in some cases the cysts reach a considerable size. Usually the cystic stage is promptly followed by fibrosis, forming a small hyalinized area, the corpus fibrosum.

In the development of the corpus luteum after follicular rupture, the granulosa is vascularized, and the cells become large and polyhedral with abundant vacuolated cytoplasm. They are then called lutein cells and form a bright yellow zone. Hemorrhage into the follicular lumen usually occurs, and in some cases this is abundant. The mature corpus luteum is much larger than the follicle, measuring up to 10 or 15 mm. in diameter.

If fertilization does not occur, regression of the corpus luteum begins shortly before menstruation. Fatty change of the lutein cells is followed by atrophy, fibrosis, and hyalinization. This results in a convoluted hyalinized mass, the corpus albicans, which slowly regresses further and disappears. Occasionally the corpus luteum fails to regress but develops into a cyst (corpus luteum cyst). Also, if pregnancy occurs, the corpus luteum does not regress but becomes even larger and more prominent.

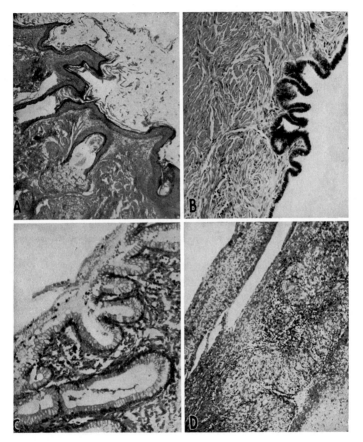

Fig. 21-2. Ovarian cysts, showing characteristic linings. **A,** Dermoid cyst, with keratinizing squamous epithelium and sebaceous glands. **B,** Serous cystadenoma, lined by dark-staining cuboidal cells. **C,** Mucinous cystadenoma, lined by pale columnar cells with basal nuclei. **D,** Corpus luteum cyst, lined by a thick layer of large luteal cells. (From Berman, J. K.: Synopsis of the principles of surgery, St. Louis, 1940, The C. V. Mosby Co.)

Inflammation (oophoritis)

Inflammation of the ovary is secondary to inflammation elsewhere, most commonly spreading from the tube. Oophoritis secondary to tubal infection is usually caused by the gonococcus, streptococcus, or tubercle bacillus. Occasionally there is hematogenous infection of the ovary, as in mumps. Inflammatory reactions in the ovary are similar to those elsewhere. Acute and chronic abscesses are common. An abscess often involves a corpus luteum, the organisms apparently gaining entrance to the ovary through a ruptured follicle. Oophoritis is followed by fibrosis and adhesions to surrounding structures.

Tuberculous oophoritis is almost always secondary to tubal tuberculosis. Tuberculous peritonitis is usually present as well. The microscopic picture is the same as in tuberculosis elsewhere.

Cysts

Cysts of the ovary are of two main groups : (1) retention cysts, i.e., dilated glandular structures; and (2) neoplastic cysts, i.e., cystic tumors. The latter will be considered with other ovarian tumors.

Ovarian retention cysts sometimes rupture and cause intraperitoneal hemorrhage. The clinical aspects depend on the amount of intraperitoneal hemorrhage, which in rare cases may be quite massive. Clinical differentiation of such cases from other acute abdominal conditions may be difficult. Nonneoplastic cysts are of four main types.

Follicular cyst. A follicular cyst is caused by the distention of an unruptured graafian follicle. They are extremely common and usually remain small in size, but occasionally they reach several centimeters in diameter. Lining granulosa cells are evident in the smaller cysts, but the larger cysts may be lined by a single layer of low cuboidal epithelium. Hemorrhage into the cyst occasionally occurs.

Luteal cyst. A luteal cyst is the result of dilatation of a corpus luteum. They are less frequent than the follicular type and must be distinguished from the normal corpus luteum hematoma, the large corpus luteum of pregnancy, and the hemorrhagic cysts of endometriosis. Luteal cysts are recognized microscopically by remnants of granulosa-lutein cells found in the wall.

Theca-lutein cyst. Theca-lutein cysts are found in the ovaries in association with choriocarcinoma and hydatidiform mole

(p. 763). These cysts are multiple, bilateral, and lined by theca-lutein cells; i.e., the lutein cells lining the cyst are believed to arise from the theca interna rather than the granulosa.

Endometrial cyst. Endometrial cysts, or chocolate cysts of the ovary, are caused by endometriosis. They may reach a size of several centimeters, are often bilateral, and may be associated with endometriosis elsewhere (p. 753). Hemorrhage into the cyst cavity results in a thick chocolate-like content. This is not a distinctive feature, however, as a similar content may be found in hemorrhagic luteal cysts. Identification is by finding endometrial glands in some part of the cyst wall. Beneath the lining there is often a layer of swollen mononuclear phagocytic cells, which contain blood pigment and are easily confused with luteal cells.

Stein-Leventhal syndrome. Multiple bilateral cystic follicles with hyperplasia of the theca interna cells may be associated with the Stein-Leventhal syndrome. This is a clinical syndrome characterized by sterility, hirsutism, and menstrual irregularities, which may progress to oligomenorrhea or amenorrhea. The ovaries have thickening of the tunica albuginea in addition to the cysts. Although androgenic activity is evident, various hormonal patterns are found. However, the normal cyclical fluctuations of hormonal levels are lacking. Endometrial hyperplasia may be present, and endometrial carcinoma occurs with increased frequency in association with this syndrome.

Hyperthecosis (thecomatosis) is characterized by nests of lipid-containing lutein cells in the ovarian stroma, which is often hyperplastic and dense. It may be associated with clinical syndromes similar to those with polycystic ovaries, with virilism, or with obesity, hypertension, and a disturbance in glucose tolerance.

Tumors

Classification of ovarian tumors has been modified by the recognition of the endocrine function of various tumors. Herein they will simply be grouped into cystic and solid varieties, each group having both benign and malignant components. Those tumors with endocrine function are found among the solid tumors. A number of very rare types of ovarian tumors and many histologic variants of the commoner varieties have been described but will not be considered here.

Cystic ovarian tumors
Cystic ovarian tumors may be further classified as follows:

```
                        simple
              serous <              benign
                        papillary <
Cystadenoma <                       malignant (cystadenocarcinoma)
                        benign
              mucinous <
                        malignant (cystadenocarcinoma)
```

Dermoid cyst

Cystadenoma. Cystadenoma is the commonest variety of ovarian tumor.

Serous cystadenomas may be unilocular or multilocular and sometimes reach enormous size. There may be a smooth lining of epithelial cells, but frequently there are papillary projections into the cavities. This papillary growth may be so great that the tumor appears almost solid. The lining cells of the cyst are cuboidal or columnar epithelium, and sometimes are ciliated. Calcium deposits are common in the papillary masses.

The simple cysts are benign, but the types with papillary overgrowth are frequently malignant. Invasive growth through the cyst wall results in papillary masses on the outer surface of the cyst. These may break off and implant throughout the peritoneal cavity. The cyst cavity contains a clear fluid with a rich content of serum proteins. The origin of the cysts is believed to be from germinal epithelium covering the ovary.

Serous cystadenocarcinoma is the commonest type of ovarian cancer, constituting about 60% of malignant ovarian tumors. Some of these have a tubal type of epithelium, often showing cilia, are sometimes termed endosalpingiomas, and have a low degree of malignancy. Others have a greater degree of anaplasia and are often seen only in later stages of disease when extension has occurred and operability is poor, and so the prognosis is poor. Psammoma bodies may be present.

Mucinous cystadenomas contain a mucoid material. They are thin walled and multilocular and have a smooth lining without papillary growth. The cysts are lined by a single layer of tall columnar epithelial cells with basal nuclei and a clear secretory cytoplasm. Mucinous cystadenomas do not become malignant as

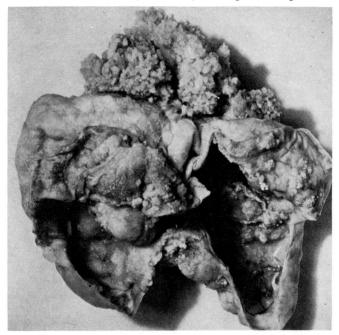

Fig. 21-3. Papillary cystadenocarcinoma of the ovary. Note the papillary masses growing on the external surface of the cyst.

commonly as do the serous cystadenomas, but occasionally a proliferative adenocarcinomatous change occurs.

Rupture of a mucinous cystadenoma implants the secretory epithelium over the peritoneal cavity. Continued secretory function of the implants causes an accumulation of large quantities of gelatinous material in the abdomen, the condition called *pseudomyxoma peritonei*. It may be difficult to find the epithelial elements on biopsy of the peritoneal tissue.

The exact origin of mucinous tumors is debatable, but a common theory is that they are teratomatous, with overgrowth of entodermic tissue to the exclusion of other types. Another theory is that they arise from germinal epithelium.

Dermoid cyst. Cystic teratomas constitute about 10% of ovarian cystic tumors. They are rounded masses of any size up to that of a grapefruit, with an opaque, grayish wall. The cyst

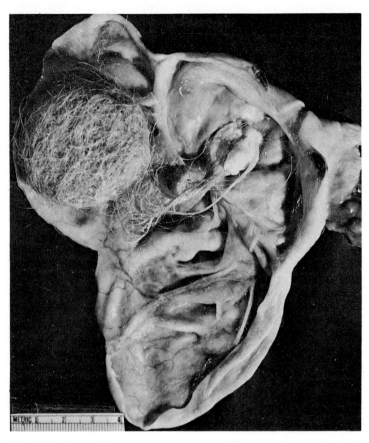

Fig. 21-4. Dermoid cyst of the ovary, showing hair and dermoid tubercle. (Courtesy Dr. J. F. Kuzma.)

content is a greasy, grayish yellow sebaceous material mixed with a variable amount of hair. The cyst lining tends to be rough or granular and at one point is a small, raised or thickened area from which the hair arises. Section through this dermoid tubercle shows skin tissue and appendages, which give rise to the cyst contents. In addition to squamous epithelium, sebaceous glands, and hair follicles, a variety of other tissues may be found, such as cartilage, bone, teeth, thyroid, glands, and intestinal tissue.

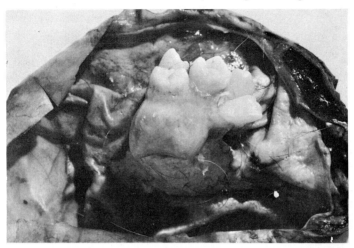

Fig. 21-5. Dermoid cyst of the ovary, showing teeth, hair, and dermoid tubercle. (Courtesy Dr. J. F. Kuzma.)

Dermoids of the ovary are benign tumors, but in about 2% one element may become malignant. This is most frequently the squamous epithelium. Other complications are torsion with hemorrhagic infarction and, infrequently, a granulomatous peritonitis resulting from a leakage of cyst contents. The most popular theory of their origin is that they represent spontaneous growth of a totipotential ovum, i.e., it seems to be an attempt of a germ cell to form a new individual under unfavorable circumstances.

Teratoma of the ovary is the counterpart among the solid tumors of the dermoid cyst. It is rare and, unlike the dermoid cyst is usually malignant.

Solid ovarian tumors

While less common than cystic neoplasms, the solid tumors of the ovary are of wide variety, some forms being quite rare. They may be classified into three groups: (1) benign solid tumors, (2) tumors with endocrine function, and (3) malignant tumors. Among the endocrine tumors, some are biologically benign, while others have a low grade of malignancy.

Benign solid ovarian tumors. The only two common varieties in this class are fibromas and Brenner tumors.

Table 21-1. *Classification of endocrine syndromes associated with pathologic findings in the ovary***

Hormone status	Syndrome	Clinicopathologic findings	Associated ovarian pathology
Estrogen excess (or prolonged uninterrupted estrogen)	Estrinism 1. Precocious puberty 2. Metropathia hemorrhagica (or other menstrual disorders) 3. Postmenopausal bleeding	Metrorrhagia, amenorrhea Enlargement of breasts and secondary sex development Hyperplasia of endometrium (? carcinoma) and tubal epithelium Hypertrophy of myometrium (? myomas) Cornification of vaginal mucosa	Single follicle cysts Polycystic ovaries Granulosa-theca cell tumors Rare Sertoli-Leydig and lipoid cell tumors
Estrogen lack (or slight androgen excess)	Defeminization (or failure of feminization)	Oligomenorrhea, amenorrhea Breast atrophy and regression of secondary sex characteristics Atrophy of endometrium, myometrium, tubal epithelium, and vaginal mucosa	Ovarian atrophy (or agenesis) Polycystic ovaries Germinomas Masculinizing ovarian tumors
Androgen excess	Masculinization (with or without defeminization)	Hirsutism Enlargement of clitoris Temporal hair recession and baldness Enlargement of larynx and voice changes Masculine habitus	Polycystic ovaries with hyperthecosis Hilus cell hyperplasia Sertoli-Leydig cell tumors Lipoid cell tumors Rare granulosa-theca cell tumors
Corticosteroid excess	Cushing's syndrome (with or without masculinization)	Adiposity of trunk, striae Polycythemia Hypertension Diabetic tendency Osteoporosis	Lipoid cell tumors

Fibroma of the ovary. Fibroma is a firm, whitish, circumscribed tumor that may reach a considerable size. The cut surface is firm and may be homogeneous or trabeculated. Microscopically it is composed of well-differentiated, regular connective tissue, is of uniform pattern, and shows little evidence of active growth.

Ascites is sometimes associated with ovarian fibroma, and hydrothorax may be present as well (Meigs' syndrome) and disappear after removal of the tumor. Other solid ovarian tumors (theca cell, granulosa cell, and Brenner tumors) may have an associated ascites and hydrothorax. The fluid is a transudate, apparently originates in the peritoneal space, and reaches the pleural space by transdiaphragmatic passage.

Fibromas must be distinguished from theca cell tumors, which have an endocrine function. Although similar in many respects to fibromas, theca cell tumors have a more yellowish color grossly, and microscopically they exhibit a high fat content.

Brenner tumor. Brenner tumors are uncommon benign tumors usually found after the age of 50 years. As a rule, they are without hormonal function, but a few have been accompanied by hyperestrinism similar to that of granulosa cell tumors. They are small, firm circumscribed tumors that occur alone or in the wall of a mucinous cystadenoma. Grossly they resemble a fibroma. Microscopically they are characterized by islands or strands of epithelial cells set in a dense fibrous stroma. Frequently the nuclei of the epithelial cells have a characteristic longitudinal grooving or folding. Similar infolding may be evident in the nuclei of Walthard cell islands, giving them an appearance reminiscent of Puffed Wheat. Some of the epithelial islands may have cystic centers, which are sometimes lined by columnar mucus-producing cells. Their origin is debatable, but theories suggest derivation (1) from tiny masses masses of undifferentiated cells called Walthard islands; (2) from a teratoma, as suggested by frequent association with mucinous cystadenoma; (3) from displaced urogenital epithelium, similar to that of the renal pelvis or ureter; (4) from germinal epithelium of the ovary; or (5) from follicular tissue. The evidence indicates that they do not arise from Walthard nests but that their origin is from germinal epithelium of the ovarian surface or is follicular and similar to that of theca and granulosa cell tumors from ovarian mesenchyme. Very small Brenner tumors are commonly found near the hilum of the ovary.

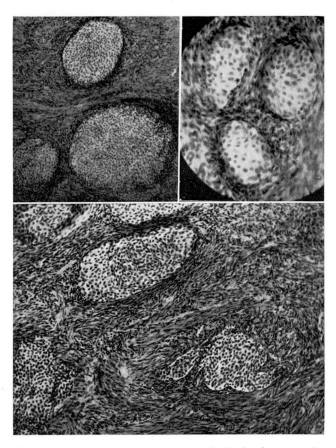

Fig. 21-6. Brenner tumor of the ovary. Small islands of tumor cells in a fibrous stroma.

The Walthard islands occur most frequently on the posterior aspect of the lateral portion of the fallopian tube, less frequently in the mesosalpinx, and only rarely in the ovary. These small nests of cells are focal areas of metaplasia of the serosa, and by central degeneration they may form small cysts. Similar nests are sometimes found in the serosa near the appendix testis in the male. They appear to have no significance as precursors of tumors.

Malignant solid ovarian tumors. A number of solid tumors of varying degree of malignancy but without endocrine effects arise in the ovary. Only the more important types—carcinoma, sarcoma, and dysgerminoma—are considered here. The Kruken-berg tumor is a bilateral solid tumor that is usually metastatic from the gastrointestinal tract.

Carcinoma. Primary solid carcinoma of the ovary is less common than the cystic type and is often bilateral. Probably many are cystic tumors in early stages. They are grayish brown, are variable in size, shape, and consistency, and often have areas of necrosis. Microscopically, malignant epithelial cells may form well-defined glands (adenocarcinoma) or solid sheets of cells (medullary form). Extension is commonly to the other ovary, to the peritoneum, and by lymphatics to lumbar and other lymph nodes. Occasionally spread by the bloodstream involves distant organs. An embryonal carcinoma of the ovary occurs mainly in young women and has a poor prognosis.

Sarcoma. Sarcoma of the ovary is much rarer than carcinoma. It may develop from malignant change in a fibroma or from the ovarian stroma. Grossly it is of moderate size and lobulated; it has a tendency to necrosis. Microscopically it is usually a spindle cell sarcoma.

Dysgerminoma. Dysgerminoma (seminoma) is believed to arise from the primordial germ cells of the sexually indifferent embryonic gonad. An entirely similar tumor (seminoma) occurs in the testicle. It has no hormonal effects, but it is often associated with congenital hypoplasia of internal genitalia or with pseudohermaphroditism. Such associated changes are not caused by the tumor and remain after its removal.

Most dysgerminomas occur before the age of 35 years and sometimes are found during childhood. The degree of malignancy is variable. They form fairly large encapsulated or nodular tumors of rubbery consistency, grayish pink color, and friable cut surface. They are often bilateral.

Microscopically they are composed of cords and nests of cells with round hyperchromatic nuclei and a small amount of indistinct pale cytoplasm. The cell cords are separated by loose fibrous trabeculae infiltrated with lymphocytes. Giant cells may be present. Mitoses are often numerous. Occasional cases show some choriomatous or teratomatous tissues.

Homologous tumors of ovary and testis. Teilum has presented evidence that there are two groups or series of homologous

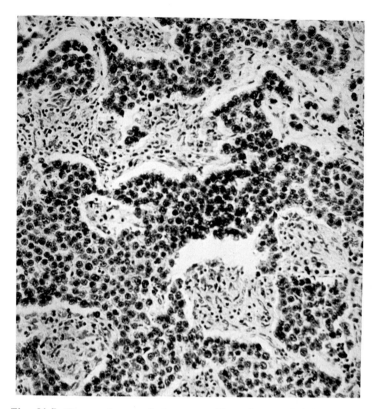

Fig. 21-7. Dysgerminoma of the ovary. Note the rounded hyperchromatic nuclei, the scanty and indistinct cytoplasm, and the lymphocytes infiltrating the stroma.

tumors of the ovary and testis. One group is composed of germ cell tumors (gonocytomas), which have their origin from early stages of germ cells in the testis or from homologous remnants of the medullary cords in the ovary. This includes seminomas (testis), dysgerminomas (ovary), and choriocarcinomas. The second series (androblastomas) includes the arrhenoblastomas, certain estrogen-producing tumors of the testis and ovary, the clear cell or hypernephroid tumors, and the masculinovoblastomas. Although the histogenetic theory is attractive, the classification has not yet achieved common usage.

Embryonal carcinoma. Embryonal carcinoma is a rare, specific, highly malignant ovarian tumor of germ cell origin. Morphologically it is analogous to the infantile form of embryonal carcinoma of the testis. Occurring mainly in young adults, the tumors average about 15 cm. in diameter, are cystic, and have a thin capsule, often with gross evidence of penetration. Microscopically they show a loose meshwork of moderately pleomorphic poorly differentiated cells. Cystic spaces and thin-walled vascular spaces are present. Round or oval hyaline globules are usually present. Some tumors may show areas resembling dysgerminoma or features of a teratocarcinoma.

Teilum has categorized the main type of embryonal carcinoma as an endodermal sinus tumor (mesoblastoma vitellinum) from overgrowth of the extraembryonic mesoblast and yolk sac endoderm. The histologic features are a vacuolated meshwork with an endodermal sinus pattern and primitive vitelline vesicles.

Mesonephroma. A rare malignant ovarian tumor appears to arise from mesonephric elements or remnants. The tumor cells have a tubular pattern formed by flattened or cuboidal cells with oval nuclei and scanty clear cytoplasm. The clear cell carcinoma (metanephroma) of the ovary belongs to this general group. Similar tumors of mesonephric origin may be found in the cervix, vagina, parametrium, broad ligament, or body of the uterus, and homologous tumors may be found in the male in the region of the epididymis, testis, and spermatic cord. According to Teilum, the tumor originally termed mesonephroma by Schiller may be a variant of a germinal tumor, one that recapitulates stages in the phylogenetic development of extraembryonic structures such as allantois and yolk sac.

Krukenberg tumor. Metastatic carcinoma of the ovaries caused by spread from gastrointestinal tract or pelvic organs is quite common. Krukenberg tumors are a particular type of metastatic ovarian cancer, usually bilateral, in which the tumor cells are mucus producing. The distended cytoplasm and flattened nuclei of individual cells produce a signet-ring appearance. The primary tumor is usually in the stomach (80%), intestinal tract, or gallbladder and often is inconspicuous. The possible modes of spread to the ovaries are by retrograde metastasis along lymphatics and by peritoneal implantation. In rare instances a strikingly similar or identical Krukenberg type of tumor is primary in the ovary.

Grossly the tumors are firm, solid, lobulated growths of mod-

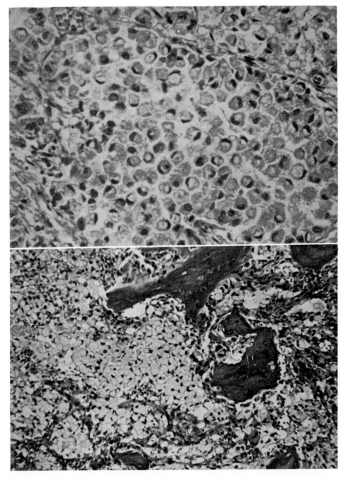

Fig. 21-8. Krukenberg tumor. The lower illustration shows a metastasis to the bone. Note the signet-ring cells.

erate size and have a variegated appearance on the cut surface. Microscopically there are mucoid epithelial cells having a signet-ring appearance and arranged in solid masses or small clusters. Occasionally there is a tendency to gland formation. The stroma may be abundant and cellular. Since the tumor is usually the result of metastatic spread, the prognosis is often hopeless.

Endocrine tumors of the ovary

Like other glands that produce hormones, the ovary gives rise to tumors whose cells have endocrine function as well as excessive growth energy and in this fashion exert far-reaching effects upon the body. The endocrine function of the ovary is the production of female sex hormones. The commonest endocrine tumors of the ovary are those that produce excess female sex hormones (estrogen). There are two such tumors, the granulosa cell and the theca cell types. Two other ovarian endocrine tumors produce masculinizing hormones. These latter tumors are the arrhenoblastoma and the masculinovoblastoma (hypernephroma) of the ovary. As might be expected, the masculinizing tumors are very rare. The arrhenoblastoma is believed to arise from rests of male-directed mesenchyme cells of the early embryonic undifferentiated stage of the ovary. The masculinovoblastoma has been presumed to arise from adrenal rests in the ovary.

Granulosa cell tumor. The granulosa cell tumor is the commonest ovarian endocrine neoplasm and is estimated to comprise 10% of solid ovarian carcinomas. Occurring at any age, it is characterized by production of excessive estrogenic hormone. In the child this causes precocious sexual changes, with the development of the breasts and onset of menstruation. These changes of precocious puberty disappear after removal of the tumor. During the reproductive period the tumor may cause either excessive menstrual bleeding or periods of amenorrhea. After the menopause the hyperestrinism causes resumption of menstrual bleeding. Endometrial hyperplasia is present in these cases as the result of the excessive estrogen. Granulosa cell tumors and thecomas are described as separate tumors here, but often elements of both are present in individual tumors, so that frequently they are considered as *granulosa–theca cell tumors.*

Since many granulosa cell tumors are relatively benign or of very low-grade malignancy, complete removal results in cure. Ten percent or more are obviously malignant and form metas-

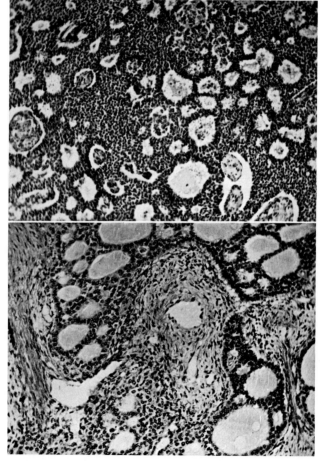

Fig. 21-9. Granulosa cell tumor of the ovary, folliculoid type.

tases. The origin of these tumors is believed to be from either (1) ovarian mesenchyme, perhaps containing embryonal rests of granulosa cells (progranulosa cells of ovarian mesenchyme), or (2) persistent granulosa cells of atretic follicles.

Granulosa cell tumors are unilateral, circumscribed tumors that have a smooth or slightly nodular surface and are a few millimeters to 30 cm. in diameter. The cut surface shows a fleshy, pale yellow or grayish tissue, sometimes with cystic areas. Gross features alone are not characteristic enough for diagnosis.

Histologic structure is widely variable, both in different specimens and in the same tumor. The main types are folliculoid, cylindromatous, and diffuse. In the *folliculoid type* there is formation of follicle-like structures, sometimes with surrounding stroma. Call-Exner bodies (p. 722) may be seen. The *cylindromatous form* has solid cords and strands of tumor cells, separated by a small amount of fibrous stroma. In the *diffuse* variety there may be solid, sarcoma-like patternless masses of tumor cells. Areas of luteinization are not uncommon, and when this is predominant, the designation "luteoma" has sometimes been used. Lipid-containing fibromatous areas such as characterize theca cell tumor also may occur, indicating their close relationship. Adenocarcinoma of the uterus has been observed to be

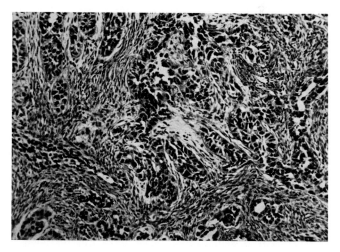

Fig. 21-10. Granulosa cell tumor of the ovary, cylindromatous type.

quite frequent in association with granulosa cell and theca cell tumors of the ovary. This suggests hyperestrinism as a possible contributing etiologic factor in endometrial carcinoma, although final proof is lacking.

Theca cell tumor (thecoma). Theca cell tumors are often considered a type of granulosa cell tumor, but usually theca cell tumors present distinctive morphologic features that warrant separate consideration. Rarer than granulosal tumors, these fibromatous neoplasms have a later age incidence and are characterized by a content of doubly refractive lipid (cholesterol). Excess production of estrogenic hormone results in irregular uterine bleeding with endometrial hyperplasia. Generally, the thecoma is benign; in rare instances it is malignant and has the character of a spindle cell sarcoma. There is evidence that the theca cell tumors have their origin in cortical stromal hyperplasia of the ovary.

Grossly they are unilateral, solid, encapsulated tumors, of firm consistency, and in general quite like the more common ovarian fibroma. The cut surface shows a yellowish fibrous tissue structure. Histologically of fibromatous appearance, they have bundles of broad spindle cells that irregularly interlace. Doubly refractive lipid within tumor cells and in surrounding connective tissue is the diagnostic feature.

Arrhenoblastoma. Arrhenoblastoma (Sertoli-Leydig cell tumor) is an uncommon solid ovarian tumor, which by hormone production causes loss of feminine characteristics and masculinization. It is thought to arise from rests of male-directed cells persisting from early stages of gonadal development. Most of these tumors occur between puberty and the menopause and exhibit moderate malignancy. Defeminizing changes of amenorrhea, sterility, and atrophy of breasts are followed by development of the masculine characteristics of hirsutism, deepening of the voice, and enlargement of the clitoris. Clinical differentiation must be from other causes of masculinization, such as adrenal cortical tumors. Arrhenoblastomas vary greatly in their degree of hormonal activity.

Grossly they are small or of moderate size, gray or yellowish, firm, and unilateral. Microscopically there is wide variation in appearance, with highly differentiated, intermediate, and undifferentiated varieties. The more undifferentiated types have the greatest clinical masculinization. The most differentiated type (testicular tubular adenoma) shows a pronounced tubular arrangement closely imitating the testicle. The undifferentiated type consists of sheets and masses of cells having a sarcomatous appearance. In the intermediate grades there are varying degrees of imperfect attempted tubule formation. An arrangement resembling sex cords and areas having cells similar to the interstitial (Leydig) cells of the testis may be present. Crystalloids of Reinke may be found in the Leydig cells. The tumor usually contains considerable lipid.

Hilus cell tumors of the ovary are rare benign neoplasms that produce a defeminizing and masculinizing syndrome. The ovarian hilus cells are slightly eosinophilic and granular and occur in close relationship to the sympathetic nerve trunks at the hilus of the ovary. They may contain hyaline inclusions, lipofuscin pigment, and Reinke crystalloids.

Gynandroblastoma. Ovarian tumors have been described that give rise both to masculinization and to evidences of hyperestrinism. The secondary sexual characters change in a male direction but with continuation of cycle menstrual bleeding. The microscopic pattern in such cases is not constant but usually presents combinations of the features found in arrhenoblastomas and granulosa cell tumors. It has been suggested that gynandroblastomas are of teratomatous nature.

Lipoid cell tumor. Lipoid cell tumor (masculinovoblastoma, adrenal tumor of the ovary, luteoma) is a rare tumor that produces masculinization with clinical effects similar to those of the arrhenoblastoma. The exact origin and proper terminology are still matters of debate. Origins suggested are (1) from luteal cells, (2) from rests of adrenal cortical tissue in the ovary, or (3) that it is a lipid form of arrhenoblastoma. It is unilateral, of small or moderate size, an orange-yellow color, and has a high fat content. Microscopically it is composed of large pale cells similar to those of the adrenal cortex. One type (stromal luteoma) appears to arise from luteinized stromal cells. *Hypernephroid tumors* of the ovary, similar to the clear cell adenocarcinoma of the kidney, also occur. These yellow malignant tumors do not produce masculinization.

FALLOPIAN TUBES

The fallopian tubes have a muscular wall covered on the outer surface by peritoneum and lined by a mucosa that is thrown up into intricate papillary arborescent folds. Some of the cells lining the mucosa are ciliated, while others are non-

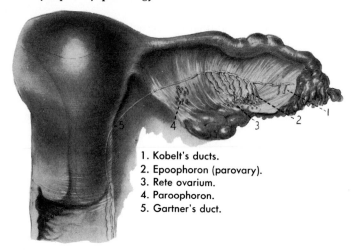

1. Kobelt's ducts.
2. Epoophoron (parovary).
3. Rete ovarium.
4. Paroophoron.
5. Gartner's duct.

Fig. 21-11. Vestigial structures of the broad ligament. (From Anderson, W. A. D.: Pathology, ed. 2, St. Louis, 1953, The C. V. Mosby Co.)

ciliated and appear to have a secretory function. The tubal epithelium undergoes some cyclic changes with the menstrual cycle. During menstruation or pregnancy, the epithelial cells are low or flat. A few days after menstruation the epithelium becomes tall, columnar, and compact. After ovulation the ciliated cells become lower, and the lining epithelium appears flattened and irregular or uneven. Activity of secretory cells becomes more prominent, and in later parts of the cycle they too become lower.

Salpingitis

Inflammation is the most common tubal lesion. In 60 to 80% of cases this is caused by gonococcal infection. The gonococcus reaches the tubes from an infection of the cervix, spread by way of the endometrium. Streptococcal or staphylococcal infection of the tube is commonly the result of postabortal or postpartum spread from an infected uterus. Less than 5% of cases of salpingitis are tuberculous.

Acute salpingitis. In acute salpingitis the tube is swollen, reddened, and has a purulent exudate in the lumen. Microscopically the mucosal folds are enlarged, edematous, and dif-

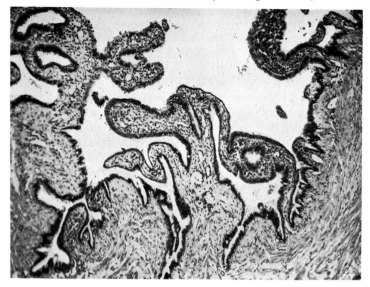

Fig. 21-12. Chronic salpingitis. Adherent mucosal folds give the appearance of glandlike follicles. (From Faulkner, R. L., and Douglass, M.: Essentials of obstetrical and gynecological pathology, ed. 2, St. Louis, 1949, The C. V. Mosby Co.)

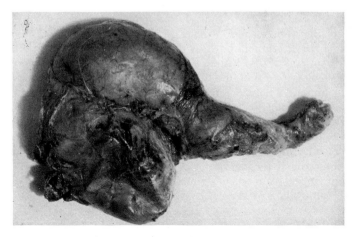

Fig. 21-13. Hydrosalpinx. Note the retort-shaped deformity of the fallopian tube.

fusely infiltrated by neutrophilic leukocytes. Later this inflammatory exudate involves also the muscularis and serosa of the tube. The fimbriated extremity may become adherent to the ovary, and extension of the infection to the ovary by way of a ruptured follicle produces a tubo-ovarian abscess. With subsidence of the inflammation to a subacute phase, a greater proportion of lymphocytes and plasma cells compose the exudate.

In nongonorrheal acute salpingitis there is greater enlargement of the tube, and the inflammatory infiltration is proportionately greater in muscular and serosal layers.

Chronic salpingitis. In chronic salpingitis the thickened mucosal folds are infiltrated by lymphocytes and plasma cells, and the muscularis and serosa may be similarly involved. Adhesions may be present between mucosal folds and, when great, result in a glandlike or follicular pattern (follicular salpingitis). The lumen often becomes blocked by adhesions. The purulent exudate may accumulate and greatly distend the blocked tube into a large retort-shaped mass (pyosalpinx). Resorption of the exudate ultimately leaves the cavity filled with a watery fluid (hydrosalpinx). The mucosal folds may be very atrophic and flattened (hydrosalpinx simplex), or because of adhesions the folds may form a number of distended compartments (hydrosalpinx follicularis).

Salpingitis isthmica nodosa. Salpingitis isthmica nodosa is a form of chronic salpingitis in which the medial portion of the tube is nodular. Microscopically one sees considerable thickening of the wall, because of increase of muscle, and a number of small irregular lumina lined by mucosal epithelium, which probably represent outpocketings of the tubal lumen. These epithelium-lined spaces must be distinguished from endometriosis and from tumor. A noninflammatory and even congenital origin has been suggested by some authors.

Tuberculous salpingitis. This inflammation is secondary to tuberculosis elsewhere, usually in the lungs, but is the primary site of tuberculosis in the female genitalia. From the tube, spread often occurs to endometrium and to peritoneum. The microscopic appearance is similar to that of tuberculosis elsewhere with epithelioid and giant cells and caseation.

Tumors

Primary carcinoma of the tube is a rare lesion. The tube is greatly enlarged and sausage shaped. Microscopically it is usually a papillary carcinoma. Metastatic carcinoma of the tube is more frequent than the primary form and is usually from the ovary or uterus. Sampson has demonstrated the method by which implantation of such tumors may occur in tubal mucosa.

Rare small benign tumors of distinctive appearance, which have been termed adenomatoid tumors, may be found in relationship to the fallopian tube or to the testicular tunic in the male. They are composed of large and small acini lined by flattened or cuboidal cells. Their genesis is obscure, and their mesothelial, epithelial, or lymphangiomatous origin is a matter of debate (p. 422 and Fig. 13-39).

Tubal pregnancy

Ectopic pregnancy results when a fertilized ovum becomes implanted in any site other than the endometrium. In most cases the ectopic site is in a fallopian tube. An important factor causing tubal pregnancy is the effect of chronic salpingitis, which prevents passage of the fertilized ovum into the uterus or delays it until the trophoblast is developed sufficiently for successful implantation. Chorionic villi penetrate the tubal wall. A decidua forms in the endometrium, similar to that which would form if the implantation were in the uterus.

In most cases of tubal pregnancy, death of the ovum occurs in a few weeks. Tubal rupture is common. This may be internal, with bleeding into the tube (hematosalpinx), or external bleeding into the abdominal cavity. In the latter case bleeding is usually profuse and sometimes fatal. Tubal abortion occurs when the ovum breaks away and is expelled from the tubal orifice. This usually causes hematosalpinx and often profuse bleeding into the abdominal cavity. Tubal pregnancy is the commonest cause of hematosalpinx. When the ovum dies, the uterine decidua may be discharged as a thick cast. In rare instances the abdominal cavity or the ovary may be the site of an ectopic pregnancy.

UTERUS

The uterus has a thick muscular wall, the myometrium, and a lining layer, the endometrium, composed of glands set in a connective tissue stroma. The main portion is the corpus or body of the uterus, while the smaller lower part, the neck or cervix of the uterus, protrudes into the upper part of the vagina. The cervical lining layer also contains glands; although distinctive from those of the body of the uterus, and surrounds a narrow canal. The portion of cervix that protrudes into the vagina is covered by squamous epithelium.

The uterus undergoes remarkable hypertrophic changes during pregnancy, followed after delivery by normal regressive and atrophic changes. One of the most serious complications of this process is infection, i.e., a puerperal endometritis and myometritis, which in severe cases may spread widely by lymphatics and veins.

The endometrium undergoes cyclic changes under the influence of ovarian hormones. These changes are in preparation for implantation of a fertilized ovum and, failing this, culminate in menstruation. Ovarian endocrine imbalance may disturb the endometrial cycles, so that pathologic hyperplasia or other abnormalities result. Tumors arising from the endometrium are most commonly adenocarcinomas. Endometritis is most often caused by abnormal retention of placental tissue, but tuberculous endometritis not uncommonly follows tuberculous salpingitis. Ectopic endometrial tissue (endometriosis) is quite frequent in various situations in the pelvis. Most commonly the misplaced islands of endometrium are in the muscular wall of the uterus, the condition here being termed adenomyosis.

The chief lesion of the myometrium is a benign tumor of smooth muscle, termed a leiomyoma, but because it often has abundant fibrous stroma, it is sometimes referred to as a fibromyoma or fibroid. These tumors are extremely common, particularly in the Negro race, are often multiple, and reach large sizes. A small proportion undergo sarcomatous change.

Fibrosis uteri is a frequently misused term for a diffuse hypertrophy of the uterus accompanied by abnormal bleeding, usually affecting multiparous women between the ages of 40 and 50 years. The symmetrically enlarged uterus is thick walled, smooth, and freely movable, but fibrosis is often not greater than can be accounted for by physiologic aging. Endocrine imbalance, parity changes with deficient involution, and chronic inflammation are probable causal factors.

Endometrium

Pathologic disturbances of the endometrium include abnormalities of the cyclic hormonal changes, inflammation, tumors, and ectopic endometrium (endometriosis).

Cyclic changes. The cyclic changes are controlled by the ovarian hormones of the maturing follicle (estrogen) and the corpus luteum (progesterone). The estrogenic effect is essentially to stimulate proliferation of endometrial glands. Progesterone promotes a secretory activity of the glands and a decidua-like change in the stromal cells. If pregnancy fails to occur, the corpus luteum degenerates, and there is a breakdown of the endometrium with hemorrhage and sloughing of all except the most basal layer (menstruation). Thus there are three main phases in the menstrual cycle: (1) the menstrual (first to fourth day); (2) the proliferative (fifth to fourteenth day of cycle), which is controlled by estrogen; and (3) the secretory (fifteenth to twenty-eighth day), in which progesterone as well as estrogen

Table 21-2. *Histology of the menstrual cycle*

Day of cycle	Ovary	Endometrial phase	Endometrial histology
1 to 4	Degenerating corpus luteum	Menstrual	Infiltration of leukocytes, degeneration and breakdown of endometrium; hemorrhage and sloughing of endometrium
5 to 12	Developing follicle Mature follicle	Proliferative (estrogen)	Regeneration of endometrium from basalis; glands rounded, regular, with piled-up cells; mitoses; stromal cells elongated spindly, with scanty cytoplasm
13 to 15	Ovulation		
16 to 28	Corpus luteum	Secretory (estrogen + progesterone)	Glandular epithelium lines up in single layer; subnuclear vacuolization, followed soon by peripheral vacuolization of glandular epithelium with basal nuclei; glands tortuous, saw-toothed; stroma edematous in early stages, later stromal cells swollen, rounded, finally decidua-like; congestion of blood vessels and infiltration of polymorphonuclears and lymphocytes in final stages

influences the endometrium. The beginning of the cycle is counted from the first day of menstruation, since that is a point most easily determined. Ovulation usually occurs near the middle of the cycle (fourteenth day) and is followed shortly by corpus luteum formation and a progesterone effect on the endometrium. The histologic changes summarized in Table 21-2.

Menstrual phase. During the menstrual phase (first to fourth day) there are denervation and breakdown of the endometrium, with thrombosis of blood vessels and infiltration of leukocytes. Except for a basal layer the endometrium is desquamated. From the remaining basal tissue there is rapid regeneration. The basal layer does not participate in the histologic changes of the cycle.

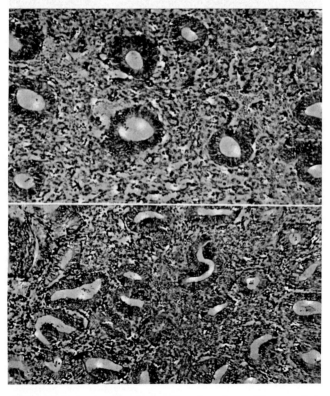

Fig. 21-14. Endometrium in the proliferative phase. The rounded and regular glands are lined by several layers of cells.

Proliferative phase. The proliferative phase (fifth to fourteenth day) extends from the end of menstruation to ovulation, and is controlled by estrogen from the developing ovarian follicle. It is characterized by active proliferation of cells and formation of straight tubular glands. At first the endometrium is 1 to 2 mm. in thickness and contains three or four glands per low-power field, set in a loose stroma. The lining epithelial cells

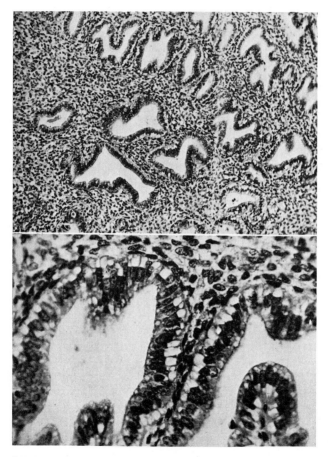

Fig. 21-15. Endometrium in the early secretory phase. The subnuclear vacuolization is a characteristic feature.

are columnar, have nuclei at all levels, and are crowded together or "piled up." In the latter part of this stage mitoses may be numerous in the glands. The glands in this phase appear very regular in outline and either elongated or round, depending upon the direction in which they have been sectioned. Toward the end of this phase the nuclei of the glandular cells are basal in position, and the cells become longer. The average number of glands now may be six or seven in a low-power field, and the endometrium is 2 to 2.5 mm. in thickness. The stromal cells are elongated, spindly, and have scanty cytoplasm.

Secretory phase. The secretory (differentiative or progestational) phase (fifteenth to twenty-eighth day) extends from ovulation to the beginning of menstruation. Its characteristic features are the effect of progesterone produced by the corpus luteum. Hence when these changes are present, ovulation may be assumed to have occurred. The main features are tortuosity of the glands, evidence of secretory activity, and in later days of the phase a swelling and rounding up of the stromal cells so that they resemble decidual cells.

Early in the secretory phase the columnar glandular cells become more regularly arranged into line, no longer appearing

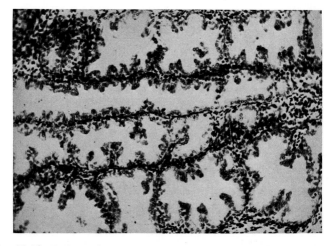

Fig. 21-16. Endometrium in the secretory phase. Note the irregularity of the glandular linings.

"piled up." Clear vacuoles of glycogen appear at the base of the cells, pushing the nuclei into a more central position. This subnuclear vacuolization is one of the important early indications of this phase. It is soon followed by vacuolization of peripheral parts of the cells and sinking of the nuclei to a basal position. The glands become twisted and have a very irregular, sawtoothed appearance. In early days of this phase the stroma is loose and very edematous, particularly in its central portions, so that a spongy layer may be distinguishable between a lining compact layer and the basal portion. Late in the phase the stromal cells become swollen and rounded, possess abundant cytoplasm, and are young decidual cells. The endometrium at this time may be 4 to 7 mm. in thickness. The blood vessels are congested, and there may be small hemorrhages. At the end of this phase there is an infiltration of polymorphonuclear leukocytes and lymphocytes in the stroma.

Endometrial hyperplasia. Cystic glandular hyperplasia of the endometrium is an exaggeration of the changes of the proliferative phase of the menstrual cycle. It may be caused by excessive estrogen production, either absolute or relative, because of failure of ovulation and corpus luteum formation. Follicular retention cysts are usually present in the ovaries. Most cases occur after the age of 35 years, and it is most common around the menopausal period. Its chief symptom is irregular and persistent bleeding (functional uterine bleeding). The bleeding is believed to occur when there is a sharp drop or withdrawal of estrogenic hormone, and hence it is not correlated with the degree of hyperplasia, nor is it a regular and invariable accompaniment. Endometrial hyperplasia also accompanies tumors having excess estrogenic hormone production, such as granulosa cell and theca cell tumors. During reproductive years it is a benign lesion, but after the menopause endometrial hyperplasia may predispose to adenocarcinoma.

The hyperplastic endometrium is thickened, velvety, and often roughened by folds or irregular polypoid projections. Curettage produces abundant endometrial fragments, which are firm, smooth, intact, nonnecrotic and nonfriable, and hence usually distinguishable grossly from the abundant but friable and necrotic masses obtained when there is carcinoma of the uterus.

Microscopically the endometrium has the features of proliferative endometrium, with the addition of much irregularity in the size of the glands. Some glands are small, some are medium

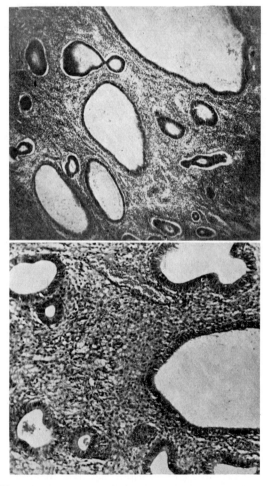

Fig. 21-17. Endometrial hyperplasia. "Swiss cheese" appearance resulting from the cystlike dilatation of the endometrial glands.

sized, and others show cystic enlargement. When the latter are abundant, the endometrium has a characteristic Swiss cheese appearance. Proliferative activity (mitoses) is sometimes evident in the stroma as well as in the glandular epithelium. The endometrium appears similar at all levels without layering. Small focal areas of degeneration and necrosis with thrombosis of small vessels are sometimes present.

Endometrial polyp. Endometrial polyps are localized areas of benign overgrowth of endometrium, attached by a narrowed pedicle or base. Endometrial hyperplasia may be polypoid in form, but polyps also occur singly and without generalized endometrial change. They may undergo cyclic changes with the rest of the endometrium, but often they show a proliferative type of change only, with cystic glandular dilatation and a picture similar to that of endometrial hyperplasia. Such polyps may be composed of endometrium, which responds to estrogenic stimulation but not to progesterone. Large polyps often ulcerate and bleed or show considerable inflammation. Malignant change in a polyp is uncommon.

Endometritis. Inflammation of the endometrium may result from puerperal infection (streptococcal, staphylococcal, etc), gonorrhea, or tuberculosis. The most severe form is the acute puerperal infection, which is often associated with myometritis, infective thrombophlebitis, and lymphangitis. Hence, the infection may spread throughout the pelvis and to other parts of the body. Gonococcal endometritis is usually less important than the tubal and cervical inflammation. Tuberculous endometritis is secondary to tuberculosis of the fallopian tube and shows the usual microscopic picture of epithelioid and giant cells. Postabortive endometritis is commonly seen in curettings sent to the laboratory and is identified by finding remnants of retained chorionic villi.

Endometriosis. Endometriosis refers to the condition of ectopic endometrium, endometrial tissue in an abnormal position. The commonest abnormal site is a muscular wall of the uterus, there having been direct invasion of myometrium. Here the condition is termed adenomyosis or internal endometriosis. Other common sites are the ovary, fallopian tube, or peritoneal surfaces any place in the pelvis. Occasionally the condition involves laparotomy scars or the umbilicus. It also occurs infrequently in the cervix uteri, vagina, vulva, urinary bladder, and rectum. Rarely, distant sites are involved. Endometriosis in any situation

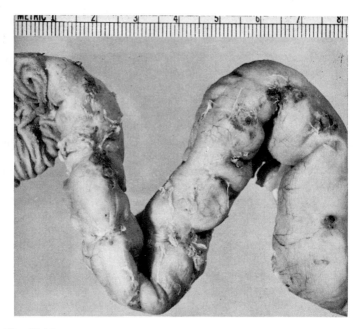

Fig. 21-18. Endometriosis of the ileum.

is found only in the female and during the period of ovarian activity.

There are two main theories regarding endometriosis, neither of which satisfactorily explains all cases. Sampson presented evidence that it is caused by retrograde menstruation, i.e., viable fragments of endometrium that pass through the fallopian tube at the time of menstruation and implant on serosal surfaces. The second theory is that it is caused by coelomic heteroplasia, i.e., an abnormal differentiation of certain areas of coelomic epithelium. The serosal cells of the peritoneum and the mucosa of the uterus, tubes, and vagina have a common origin, and some hormonal factor may stimulate the metaplasia in extrauterine sites. Spread of endometrial fragments by lymphatics and blood vessels has also been suggested, especially for distant foci of endometriosis. Adenomyosis appears to be best understood as an exaggerated invasiveness of the endometrium. There is usually a direct continuation of the uterine mucosa with the endometrial

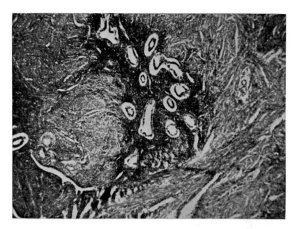

Fig. 21-19. Adenomyosis (endometriosis) of the wall of the uterus. Islands of the endometrial glands and stroma are surrounded by myometrium.

areas in the myometrium. Adenocarcinoma only rarely develops in adenomyosis.

The extrauterine endometrial masses are usually small cysts, often only a few millimeters in diameter, containing a thick, chocolate-like fluid and possessing a hemorrhagic lining. In the ovary these chocolate cysts may be several centimeters in diameter but in rare cases are very large. They are easily confused with hemorrhagic corpus luteum cysts. When endometrial implants of pelvic peritoneum are numerous, they cause considerable irritation and development of pelvic adhesions. The aberrant endometrial tissue may respond to ovarian hormonal stimuli with periodic "menstrual" bleeding, hence the cystic dilatation by accumulation of chocolate-colored hemorrhagic material. Rupture of the cysts causes peritoneal irritation, fibrosis, and adhesions. Very rarely malignant change may supervene in ovarian endometriosis, resulting in adenocarcinoma or in adenoacanthoma if there is also squamous metaplasia.

Identification of endometriosis depends on microscopic recognition of endometrial glands and stroma. In the larger endometrial cysts, as in the ovary, this may be difficult because of atrophy of much of the endometrial lining of the cysts. The symptoms caused by endometriosis are often those of chronic pelvic inflammation, although dysmenorrhea may be prominent.

Tumors of the corpus uteri

Tumors arising from the body of the uterus include the following:

> Leiomyomas (fibroids) arising from myometrium and occasionally, by malignant change, resulting in sarcoma
>
> Adenocarcinoma arising from endometrial glands and its variant, adenoacanthoma
>
> Sarcoma derived from endometrial stroma
>
> Mixed tumors of mesodermal origin
>
> Hydatidiform mole and choriocarcinoma, which, respectively, are caused by cystic degeneration and malignant change in chorionic villi

Rare tumors of the uterus include hemangioma, lipoma, and rhabdomyosarcoma. Hemangiomas of endometrium or myometrium may be a source of vaginal bleeding. Hemangiopericytomas of the uterus also occur and have been confused with stromal myosis.

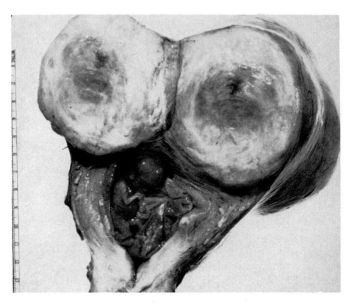

Fig. 21-20. Gravid uterus with a large intramural leiomyoma.

Leiomyoma (myoma, fibroid). The commonest tumor of the uterus is a benign smooth muscle growth of the muscular wall. Some evidence has suggested that it may arise from the smooth muscle of blood vessel walls rather than from uterine muscle fibers. It occurs during the reproductive age and tends to regress after the menopause, even if artificial or induced. It is said to occur in 20% of women over 35 years of age and has a much higher incidence in the Negro race. The tumors are frequently multiple, grow to large size, and are subject to degenerative changes on account of their poor blood supply. They distort the uterus, have secondary effects on the endometrium, and interfere with pregnancy and delivery. A small proportion become malignant. A variant form of myoma of the uterus may be very vascular, and is sometimes termed angiomyoma.

Etiology. The etiology of uterine myomas is unknown, although a relationship to hyperestrinism has been postulated. Evidence for this is incomplete. Sterility is quite common with leiomyomas, probably as an effect rather than a cause.

Gross appearance. Most leiomyomas involve the body of the uterus, but a troublesome small proportion are in the cervix. The tumors begin in the myometrium as *intramural* (or "interstitial") growths. With continued expansive growth they may take up a position beneath the peritoneum (*subserous* fibroids) or beneath the endometrium (*submucous* fibroids). In either case they can become pedunculated and attached by a narrow pedicle or neck, which carries their blood supply and which is easily twisted. *Intraligamentous* fibroids are those that extend out between layers of the broad ligament. In rare cases the omentum becomes adherent to a pedunculated fibroid and provides a new blood supply. The uterine attachment may be lost, and it becomes a *wandering*, or *parasitic*, fibroid. The tumors are always well circumscribed and easily shelled out from their surrounding pseudocapsule. They are usually multiple and vary in size from a few millimeters to enormous growths many centimeters in diameter, and weights up to 100 pounds have been reported. On being cut, a fibroid tends to bulge outward as a result of retraction of surrounding myometrial tissue. The cut surface is firm and has a characteristic whorled, trabeculated appearance because of interlacing bundles of muscle fibers.

Microscopic appearance. Microscopically the bundles of smooth muscle cells can be seen running in all directions and producing the whorled pattern. When cut longitudinally, the

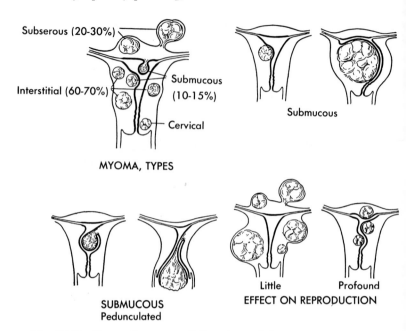

Fig. 21-21. Types of myomas of the uterus. Submucous myomas cause enlargement of the surface area of the endometrium, which tends to bleed. Myomas disturb pregnancy when they distort and encroach upon the endometrium and the uterine cavity. (From Mengert, W. F.: J. Mich. Med. **49:**1302, 1950.)

muscle cells are spindle shaped with elongated rodlike nuclei. When the bundles are cut across, the cells appear rounded with central round nuclei. The fibrous stroma may be slight but is variable in amount. Mitoses are rare, and there is little variation in the size, shape, and staining properties of the cells. A rare clear cell leiomyoma has been described.

Degenerative changes. Degenerative changes in fibroids are very common, mainly because of their poor blood supply. These secondary changes include hyaline degeneration (most common), necrosis and red degeneration, calcification, and cystic degeneration. Telangiectatic and fatty changes occur but are unusual. Infection of a fibroid is commonest in the submucous type. Sarcomatous change affects only a small proportion of fibroids (probably less than 2%) and often may be suspected grossly

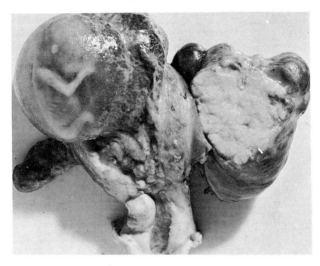

Fig. 21-22. Carcinoma in the pregnant uterus and the ovary. (Courtesy Dr. J. F. Kuzma.)

when the cut surface of the tumor is soft, white, and brainlike in consistency and appearance. Rare cases of uterine leiomyomas, which appear benign microscopically, metastasize and appear to be low-grade myosarcomas.

Effects. The more important effects on the uterus are caused by the interstitial and submucous fibroids. They may result in great distortion of the uterus and its cavity, so that growth and accommodation of a fetus or its delivery may be impossible. With submucous fibroids the overlying endometrium becomes thin and atrophic. Infection, endometrial inflammation, and sometimes bleeding result from submucous growths. Associated with large myomas, a few cases of polycythemia have been reported, the erythrocytosis disappearing on removal of the tumor.

Adenocarcinoma. Carcinoma of the body of the uterus is an adenocarcinoma arising from endometrial glands. It comprises about 10% of uterine carcinomas, being much less common than carcinoma of the cervix. Its peak incidence is after the menopause at about 55 years of age. It appears to have a greater frequency in infertile women and to have some genetic and endocrine dysfunctional basis. Ovarian stromal hyperplasia, presumably associated with increased estrogen production, is found with abnormal frequency in women with endometrial carcinoma. The chief symptom is postmenopausal bleeding, the diagnosis being made, except in advanced cases, by curettage and microscopic examination of tissue fragments. Postmenopausal hyperplasia of the endometrium appears to have some relationship to the development of adenocarcinoma. There is evidence that carcinoma of the endometrium is often preceded by hyperplasia, which may appear atypical or adenomatous. Some of the focal or polypoid atypical hyperplasias may be considered as carcinoma in situ.

Gross appearance. The tumor may involve the endometrium diffusely, making it thick, rough, and polypoid, before there is much myometrial invasion. The tumor tissue tends to be bulky, friable, and often with areas of necrosis. In other cases the tumor tissue is localized to one part of the fundus and may be polypoid in form.

Microscopic appearance. Microscopically there is usually a well-differentiated glandular structure but with considerable irregularity and lawlessness of pattern. Often the glands are closely and irregularly placed, with little stroma between them. Actual invasion through basement membranes may not be seen except in the more malignant examples. The cells show varying degrees of differentiation. There may be great variation in size, shape,

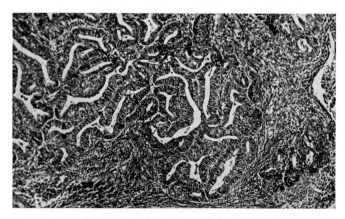

Fig. 21-23. Adenocarcinoma of the endometrium.

and staining of cells and many typical and atypical mitoses in the highly malignant types. Histologic grading, on the basis of the proportion of differentiated and undifferentiated cells, gives some indication of prognosis.

Spread. Spread of adenocarcinoma of the uterus is chiefly by lymphatics to involve the lumbar glands at the lower end of the aorta and sometimes the inguinal glands. There is a variable degree of direct invasion of the myometrium, and extension to the cervix occurs readily. In some cases there is implantation on the tubes, ovaries, or peritoneum. Blood vessel spread is a late event.

Adenoacanthoma. Adenoacanthoma of the uterus is a type of adenocarcinoma in which there are areas of squamous epithelium among the gland-forming tumor cells. The squamous metaplasia is from certain "indifferent" cells beneath the columnar epithelium, which possesses the ability to form squamous epithelium.

Sarcoma. Sarcoma of the uterus is relatively uncommon, constituting about 3% of uterine cancers. It is commonest during the fourth and fifth decades. Sarcoma may arise from leiomyomas or de novo from muscle or connective tissue elements of the uterus. Its symptomatology does not easily distinguish it from other uterine malignancies. Rhabdomyosarcomas rarely

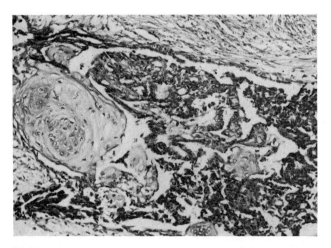

Fig. 21-24. Adenoacanthoma of the endometrium. Areas of glandular and squamous epithelium are intermixed.

occur in the uterus in pure form but sometimes as part of a mixed mesodermal tumor.

The gross appearance may suggest the diagnosis but often is not distinctive. In malignant myomas the firm consistency and whorled appearance of fibroids are lacking, and the tissue is soft, rubbery, and fleshy.

Microscopically the tumor may be of spindle cell, round cell, or mixed type. The degree of malignancy rather accurately parallels the number of mitoses. Metastasis is mainly by bloodstream to the lungs and liver and to a lesser extent by direct extension and lymphatics.

Endometrial sarcoma is often polypoid. It is relatively rare and often of complex composition. In addition to frank endometrial sarcoma, there also occurs a lesion suggestive of endometriosis but composed only of stromal cells. Such lesions of "stromal endometriosis" have also been considered neoplastic, either low-grade stromal sarcomas or hemangiopericytomas. The clinical course is prolonged, and extensive spread or recurrences are common.

Mesodermal mixed tumor. The mixed tumors of the uterus are probably caused by inclusion and persistence in the müllerian organs of mesenchymal cells, which have a capacity for differentiation into various mesodermal tissues. Most cases arise in the body of the uterus and occur about the fifth decade. Those arising in the cervix occur at an earlier age. The mesodermal mixed tumors are highly malignant and have a poor prognosis.

The growth begins in the mucosal layer and assumes a polypoid form. While not distinctive clinically, it is very constantly manifested by a sanguineous discharge from the vagina. Portions of the tumor are sometimes passed per vaginam.

Various types of tissue occur in these tumors, but myxomatous tissue and cartilage are most constant. Striated muscle fibers are frequent constituents. Myxosarcomatous and undifferentiated sarcomatous elements also are common. The solitary uterine tumors with intermingled carcinomatous and nonspecific sarcomatous components are often designated carcinosarcoma. Homologous carcinosarcomas, not of the mesodermal mixed tumor type, are rare.

Sarcoma botryoides is sometimes classified with mixed tumors of the uterus, although it appears to be a distinct entity. Grossly it is a nodular (grapelike) growth, most often involving the upper vagina and occurring almost exclusively in infancy or

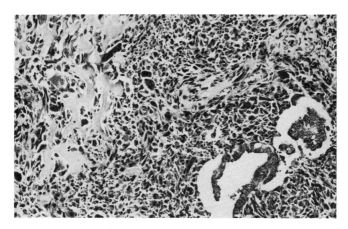

Fig. 21-25. Mixed mesodermal tumor of the uterus. Glandular, cartilaginous, and undifferentiated areas are evident.

early childhood. It is probably a form of embryonal myosarcoma originating in the subepithelial tissues. Fusiform cells, striated cells, and tumor giant cells commonly compose the tumor. Nodular protruding growths in the vagina and vulva are characteristic, but spread may occur also to the cervix and pelvic organs, with eventual widespread metastases.

Hydatidiform mole and choriocarcinoma. These tumors arise from fetal membranes rather than from the tissues of the mother, but they have the ability to invade and destroy maternal tissues extensively. Determination of the degree of malignancy and prognosis from microscopic examination is a difficult procedure with many pitfalls.

The normal chorionic villus is covered by two layers of trophoblastic cells. The inner layer of Langhans cells is composed of cuboidal cells with a pale nucleus and cytoplasm. The outer or syncytial layer consists of masses of cytoplasm having multiple very dark nuclei. These trophoblastic cells are normally invasive and even in normal pregnancy may be found invading myometrium and even blood vessels. Some trophoblastic cells may be carried to the lungs but always regress and disappear. This normal event may cause confusion in diagnosis, being mistaken for malignant invasion. The benign invasion (infiltration with syncytium only) is sometimes called *syncytial endometritis,* or *syncytioma.* Occasionally a part of the placenta fails to be detached after abortion or delivery and remains implanted in the endometrium. Such a *placental polyp* may be a cause of abnormal bleeding.

Park* has outlined a concept of degrees of primary trophoblastic abnormality that enables a classification according to varying severity.

1. *Simple dysfunction* causing death of the embryo, but with no histologic change in the villi
2. *Dysfunction causing oversecretion of fluid* into the villous stroma, with death of the embryo (hydropic abortion)
3. *Benign neoplasia with oversecretion of fluid*—hydatidiform mole
4. *Locally malignant neoplasia with oversecretion of fluid*—chorioadenoma destruens
5. *Metastatically malignant neoplasia with oversecretion of fluid*—choriocarcinoma that follows a hydatidiform mole
6. *Metastatically malignant neoplasia without villous disturbance*—choriocarcinoma that follows an abortion or term pregnancy

Hydatidiform mole is a hydropic degeneration of chorionic villi, which become enlarged into clusters of grapelike vesicles. Blood vessels are scanty, and there is some proliferation of trophoblastic cells. This abnormality occurs about once in every 2,000 pregnancies, and although it is benign, the patient must be carefully followed, as some cases (1.25 to 2.5%) progress to malignant choriocarcinoma. Various gradations occur between the benign hydatidiform mole and the malignant choriocarcinoma. Greater degrees of trophoblastic proliferation in moles appear to indicate a correspondingly greater risk of development of choriocarcinoma.

Some degree of hydatidiform degeneration of chorionic villi is found in two thirds of spontaneously aborted pathologic ova, apparently caused by the absence or defectiveness of fetal circulation. The typical hydatidiform mole appears to be derived from a pathologic ovum in which the embryo was absent or defective but which failed to abort at the usual time.

Choriocarcinoma is a very malignant and rare tumor (about one per 160,000 normal term pregnancies). There is massive overgrowth of both Langhans and syncytial cells, which exhibit many of the atypical features of malignant cells elsewhere.

---

*Adapted from Park, W. W. In Collins, D. H.: Modern trends in pathology, New York, 1959, Paul B. Hoeber, Inc., Medical Book Division, Harper & Row, Publishers, p. 191.

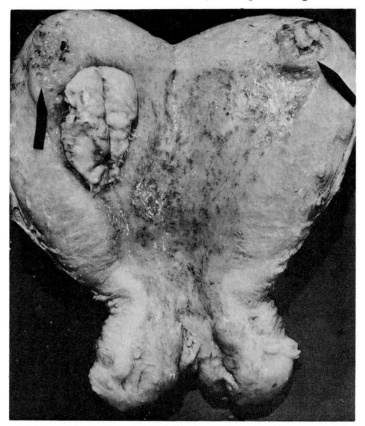

Fig. 21-26. Chorioadenoma destruens, with invasion of the uterine wall. (Courtesy Dr. J. F. Kuzma.)

Nevertheless, histologic interpretation or diagnosis is frequently difficult or unreliable. Invasion occurs freely in the pelvis, and spread by the bloodstream occurs to the lungs, brain, and other organs. The ovaries are involved by multiple lutein cysts that reach a large size.

Chorionic gonadotropin may be demonstrated in blood and urine when living trophoblastic tissue is present in the body and hence is often important in the diagnosis and management of hydatidiform mole and choriocarcinoma. Quantitative tests are even more useful than the ordinary qualitative procedures. It has been noted that spinal fluid gives a positive qualitative test in the presence of mole or choriocarcinoma, but not in normal pregnancy. Spontaneous regression of metastases has been noted in rare cases. Chemotherapy with folic acid antagonists (Methotrexate) has produced significant regression of metastases and good results in some cases.

Choriocarcinoma occurs also in the ovary (rare) and in the male, as a form of teratomatous tumor of the testis. Its microscopic features and malignancy in such cases are similar, and also the hormone titers are elevated.

Benign placental tumors are rare, and almost all are hemangiomas (chorangiomas). They are usually a vascular nodule, 2 or 3 cm. in diameter, with varying proportions of capillary proliferation and stromal cells. In some cases there is a clinical association of hydramnios and prematurity.

CERVIX UTERI

The cervix or neck of the uterus connects the vagina with the uterine cavity. It has an internal os, a canal lined with mucosa having high columnar epithelium and racemose glands, an external os, and a vaginal portion. At the external os there is a rather sharp line dividing columnar epithelium of the endocervix from the squamous epithelium that covers the portion that protrudes into the vagina. The main lesions of the cervix are inflammation (cervicitis), polyp formation, and carcinoma. Carcinoma of the cervix is a frequent and highly important tumor. In most cases it is a squamous cell carcinoma arising from epithelium of the vaginal portion. Adenocarcinoma of the endocervix is uncommon, and when it occurs, it is often difficult to be sure that its origin has not been from endometrium.

Cervicitis

Acute cervicitis. Acute cervicitis is commonly the result of gonococcal infection, although it may be caused by other organisms.

Chronic cervicitis. Chronic cervicitis may be caused by traumatic or mechanical factors in addition to bacterial causes. It is one of the commonest gynecologic lesions and is the usual cause of vaginal discharge or leukorrhea. In chronic cervicitis the chief microscopic change is an infiltration of plasma cells and lymphocytes.

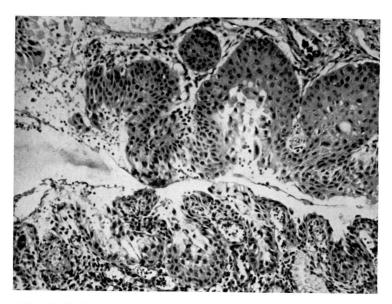

Fig. 21-27. Squamous metaplasia in the cervix. Squamous epithelial cells of benign appearance replacing glandular linings. (From Faulkner, R. L., and Douglass, M.: Essentials of obstetrical and gynecological pathology, ed. 2, St. Louis, 1949, The C. V. Mosby Co.)

Erosion. Erosion of the cervix is a lesion in which there is an area of loss of the squamous covering of the cervix and eventual replacement by columnar epithelium of the endocervix. This is to be distinguished from *ectropion* or eversion of the endocervical mucosa caused by laceration of the cervix. In cervicitis inflammatory obstruction of the outlets of endocervical glands often result in their cystic dilatation (nabothian cysts).

Epidermidization (squamous metaplasia). Epidermidization is a common change in the cervix, particularly in the healing phase of erosions. Squamous epithelium invades beneath the lining of cervical glands, with a gradual lifting up and replacement of the cylindric epithelium by squamous epithelium. This process is benign and is distinguished from carcinoma by the normal appearance of the squamous epithelial cells, the infrequency of mitoses, and the absence of invasion of interstitial tissues.

Tuberculous cervicitis. Tuberculous cervicitis is rare and usually secondary to tuberculosis in the fallopian tube. Although the gross appearance may simulate carcinoma, the usual picture of tuberculosis is seen microscopically.

Cervical polyp

In benign cervical polyp there is a localized overgrowth or heaping up of cervical mucosa, which becomes pedunculated and inflamed. It is often associated with inflammation of the cervix. A polyp tends to cause intermenstrual spotting or bleeding, and hence clinically it must be differentiated from carcinoma. Epidermidization is common in cervical polyps, but carcinomatous change occurs in very few.

Carcinoma

Carcinoma of the cervix is one of the most important and frequent forms of cancer affecting women. About 95% are squamous cell carcinomas, the remainder being adenocarcinomas arising from the cervical canal or from remnants of Gartner's duct. Mixed squamous cell and adenocarcinoma also may occur. The peak incidence occurs in persons from 40 to 50 years of age, but many cases occur in the thirties. The most important factor in prognosis is the degree of extension when treatment is instituted and, secondarily, the histologic type of malignancy. Disregarding stage or type, 35 to 54% of cases show a five-year survival. Since early cases often are not distinctive grossly, early diagnosis depends on cytologic study and biopsy of suspicious areas. Regular cytologic examination of cervical or vaginal smears enables early diagnosis and curative treatment. Spread is mainly by lymphatics. Involvement of the bladder and ureters frequently occurs, and uremia is a common terminal event.

Etiology. Little is known concerning etiologic factors in cervical carcinoma. The chronic irritation of untreated lacerations from childbirth and other types of chronic cervicitis have been considered predisposing factors, but even these have been somewhat discredited. Epidemiologic studies have shown an association with early and frequent coitus, particularly where there is lack of circumcision and poor penile hygiene. Early cases have been recognized that exhibit characteristic cytologic changes of malignancy, but without invasion. They have been variously termed intraepithelial carcinoma, preinvasive carcinoma, carcinoma in situ, etc.

Carcinoma in situ. Carcinoma in situ is a lesion in which an area of the squamous epithelial surface is replaced by anaplastic cells similar to those of invasive cancer but with no stromal invasive penetration demonstrable. The entire thickness of the epithelium is more or less involved, with loss of normal stratification. The anaplastic cells show altered polarity, an increased number of mitoses, and relatively large, hyperchromatic and irregular nuclei. The cytologic features are thus indistinguishable from invasive cancer, but evidence for the presence or absence of invasion sometimes may be inconclusive, and occasionally invasion is shown only by multiple or serial sections. Rounded buds of cells pushing into and displacing the underlying stroma from the basal layer of the surface epithelium do not constitute evidence of invasion. Likewise, extension of the anaplastic cells may occur into the underlying glands, even appearing to replace such glands, but without extension through a basement membrane and so without definite stromal or lymphatic invasion.

The anaplastic or atypical cervical epithelium may involve only the basal part of the surface epithelium or less than the full thickness, without loss of stratification. Such "dysplasia," "atypical epithelium," or "basal cell hyperplasia" is to be distinguished from carcinoma in situ. Its significance is uncertain,

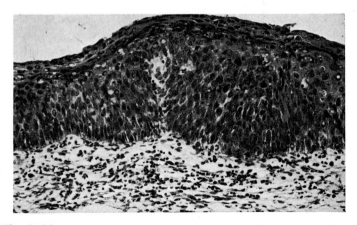

Fig. 21-28. Dysplasia of the cervical mucosa. Stratification is evident, with a flattened surface layer.

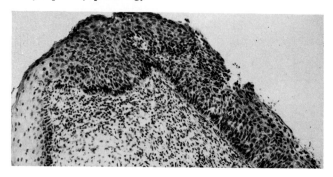

Fig. 21-29. Carcinoma in situ of the cervix. The margin is shown, with normal mucosa on the left. There is no invasion into underlying subepithelial tissues.

and although it may sometimes be only a temporary disturbance, there is evidence also that there may occur transformation to carcinoma in situ. In such transformation there may be stages in which distinction between the two lesions is unreliable or a matter of individual judgment. Basal cell hyperactivity or dysplasia is sometimes present on the periphery of areas of carcinoma.

The significance of carcinoma in situ also is not entirely clarified. The site of the change is most often the squamocolumnar junction of the cervix or the transitional zone. It may arise from subcylindric cell anaplasia or from anaplastic squamous epithelium that arose from subcylindric cell anaplasia. Carcinoma in situ appears to develop from a field of abnormal cells rather than from a single cell. A certain proportion of cases progress to invasive cancer after a latent interval of months or years. A microinvasive stage is sometimes recognized. The average age of women with carcinoma in situ appears to be about 10 years younger than the average of those with invasive cervical carcinoma.

Gross appearance. Carcinoma in situ usually presents no gross changes. The gross appearance of invasive carcinoma of the cervix is not distinctive in early stages. It presents a small, hardened, granular, or friable area at the margin of the external os. Later the tumor may grow outward, forming an everting growth of cauliflower appearance, or it may be inverting, extensively invading the cervix and vaginal wall, which are hardened and thickened. The Schiller test is of clinical value in bringing early suspicious areas into prominence when iodine is painted on the cervix. Normal cervical epithelium, because of its glycogen content, stains brown with iodine, whereas carcinomatous cells are deficient in glycogen and remain unstained.

Microscopic appearance. Microscopically the tumor is composed of squamous epithelial cells showing varying degrees of differentiation and atypicalness in their size, shape, staining reactions, polarity, and pattern. Invasiveness is evident except in the earliest or in situ cases. Some keratin pearl formation may be present in the more highly differentiated examples.

Grading and prognosis. In the cervix, as elsewhere, the degree of malignancy of a tumor may be estimated from its growth activity and the immaturity or undifferentiation of the cells.

The system of Broders is applicable in other situations as well and has been discussed on p. 261. The tumors are classified into four grades. Grade I tumors have less than 25% undifferentiated cells; Grade II, 25 to 50% undifferentiated cells; Grade III, 50 to 75% undifferentiated cells; and Grade IV, more than 75% undifferentiated cells. The Grades I and II tumors are less malignant and less radiosensitive; the Grades III and IV are more malignant and more radiosensitive.

Martzloff divided the tumors into three groups according to the predominant cell type, designated as (1) spinal cell, (2) transitional cell, and (3) spindle cell.

The Broders and the Martzloff systems of grading have not been found of very dependable prognostic value. Wentz and Reagan have divided cases into three histologic groups: a large cell nonkeratinizing type, a keratinizing cancer, and a small cell carcinoma. These types appear to have significant differences of survival time, persons with the large cell nonkeratinizing cancer having a high rate of survival, and the small cell carcinoma being associated with the lowest rate of survival.

Histologic grading indicates rate of growth and degree of radiosensitivity but is probably less important in prognosis and as a guide to treatment than is the degree of extension of the tumor at the time examined. In this regard certain clinical stages of the disease have been designated as a guide.

Group 0—carcinoma in situ; 100% have five-year cures.

Group I—carcinomas (invasive types) are limited to the cervix; the uterus is mobile; about 80% obtain five-year cures.

Group II—carcinoma spreads upward into the uterus and downward into the vagina; the uterus is partially mobile; about 40% have five-year cures.

Group III—carcinoma extends outward into the parametrium, with beginning fixation of the uterus; about 20% have five-year cures.

Group IV—carcinoma massively invades parametrium and extends to the wall of the pelvis, with complete fixation ("frozen pelvis"); less than 10% have five-year cures.

Combined consideration of the histologic grade or type and the degree of extension leads to the most accurate prognosis.

A diagnosis of cervical or endometrial carcinoma can often be made by expert examination of a vaginal smear, but it should be confirmed by biopsy or curettage (p. 268).

Extension and metastasis. Direct extension of cervical carcinoma occurs in a radical manner and may massively involve the vagina and body of the uterus. Involvement of the parametrium may be by direct extension or by lymphatic permeation. Lymphatic extension is important, with metastasis developing in the periaortic, iliac, and hypogastric nodes and sometimes in the sacral, obturator, lumbar, and inguinal nodes. In late stages there may be some spread by the bloodstream. The cause of death is often obstruction in the urinary tract (e.g., blocking of ureters), leading to uremia, or hemorrhage resulting from erosion of a large vessel. Uremia and infection are more often the cause of death than is wide or distant spread of the cancer.

Carcinoma of the vagina. Primary cancer of the vagina is usually a squamous cell carcinoma. It may arise in any part of the vagina, but it most commonly involves the posterior wall. Metastasis may occur to inguinal lymph nodes.

VULVA

The vulva, which includes the structures from the pubis to the perineum, is subject to inflammatory lesions, atrophic changes, and tumors. Being covered by skin, the vulva is involved by the same inflammatory and neoplastic lesions that affect skin elsewhere, and many vulvar lesions are such skin conditions. In addition, venereal lesions occur frequently, including gonorrhea, syphilis, chancroid, lymphogranuloma venereum, and granuloma inguinale.

Venereal lesions

Gonorrheal inflammation. Gonorrhea of the vulva affects particularly the urethra, periurethral Skene's ducts, and Bartholin glands. The squamous epithelium of adult vulvar and vaginal mucosa is resistant to gonorrheal infection, although the thin mucosa of infants is not. Bartholinitis is most commonly the result of gonorrheal infection, and in acute stages there is much swelling of the gland caused by purulent exudate. In chronic phases there may be blockage of the duct and cystic distention of the gland. Chronic gonorrheal infection may linger long in Skene's ducts and Bartholin's glands.

Syphilis. The primary chancre of syphilis may involve the vulva, and in the secondary stage flat condylomas occur there (p. 185).

Granuloma inguinale. This is a spreading ulcerative granulomatous lesion affecting the vulvar region. There is a subcutaneous infiltration of neutrophils, plasma cells, and characteristic large, foamy mononuclear cells, which contain in their cytoplasm the encapsulated causative organisms, the Donovan bodies (p. 199).

Lymphogranuloma venereum. Lymphogranuloma venereum is caused by an agent of the psittacosis-LVG group. Ulceration and productive lesions (elephantiasis) involve the vulva, and spread occurs to pararectal lymphatics (p. 203).

Kraurosis

Kraurosis is a shrinkage or atrophy of the vulva. A mild degree of such atrophic change is common after the menopause, but in kraurosis the change is extreme. It is probably caused by withdrawal of ovarian hormones.

Leukoplakia

Leukoplakia of the vulva may be localized or may affect the whole vulva. It begins with hypertrophic changes in the epithelium, which are followed by atrophy and shrinkage. Cellular atypism and dyskeratosis are present. Chronic inflammatory cells are present in the subepithelial tissues. A collagenous layer develops beneath the epithelium, but there is an absence of elastic tissue. The condition has associated serious symptoms, and there is a great tendency to the development of carcinoma. A variety of distinct conditions of the vulva that produce flat white lesions have probably been included under the term *leukoplakia*.

Carcinoma

The most important tumor of the vulva is epidermoid carcinoma. It occurs in elderly women, usually after 60 years of age and in one half or more of all cases is preceded by leukoplakia. The microscopic features are similar to those of epidermoid carcinoma elsewhere on the skin. There is early lymphatic extension to the superficial inguinal nodes, and later to the deep inguinal, hypogastric, and iliac nodes; therefore, successful surgical removal is difficult.

In rare instances adenocarcinoma arises from Bartholin's gland. Some of these have a cylindromatous architecture. Squamous carcinoma may arise from a Bartholin gland duct. Hidradenoma of the vulva is an uncommon benign tumor of apocrine sweat gland origin. The epithelium shows papillary and glandular structures. It is easily mistaken for adenocarcinoma (Fig. 21-30). Also rare are tumors of the clitoris, which have a more sarcomatous appearance.

TOXEMIA OF PREGNANCY

The etiology of the toxemias of pregnancy (eclampsia, preeclampsia) is still uncertain. The main theories are that it is (1) a form of hypertensive cardiovascular renal disease, modified and colored by the metabolic disturbances of pregnancy, (2) an endocrine dysfunction, in which the pituitary plays the main

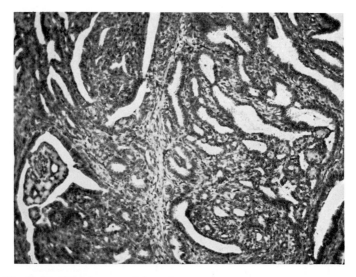

Fig. 21-30. Hidradenoma of the vulva.

part, or (3) a result of a toxic material absorbed from the placenta, particularly from areas of infarction.

One view (Browne) is that the normal protective enzyme (oxidase of trophoblastic origin) of the placenta becomes ineffective when the placenta is rendered ischemic from any cause and its oxygen tension is lowered. The enzyme normally inactivates excess adrenal cortical pressor hormones produced normally in pregnancy by placental corticotropin secretion and by increased pituitary corticotropin secretion. When the placental-inactivating enzyme becomes ineffective, hypertension results, with the clinical manifestations of preeclampsia. Eclampsia, with its characteristic convulsions, appears to be a manifestation of hypertensive encephalopathy.

Lesions are found in the kidneys, liver, placenta, and sometimes in other organs. The changes in the kidney have been described (p. 399). Glomerular capillaries frequently show occlusions. Narrowing of capillary loops of glomerular tufts, mainly by thickening or swelling of the basement membranes, subendothelial deposits of electron dense material, and focal endothelial proliferation, is common. Hyaline droplets may be found in glomerular epithelium Degenerative changes in convoluted tubules are the usual findings.

The liver may show gross lesions that, while not constantly found, are so characteristic as to be diagnostic. Irregular large and small areas of hemorrhage may be evident on both the capsular and cut surfaces (Plate 3, p. 492). Areas of hemorrhagic or anemic necrosis are common. Microscopically there are hemorrhages and necroses of hepatic cells. These lesions are particularly in periportal areas, although any part of the liver lobule may be involved. The lesions have been attributed by some to thrombi in periportal venules. Diffuse degenerative changes are present in hepatic cells, and sometimes destructive changes are so severe and widespread as to be classed as acute yellow atrophy.

Necrotic and hemorrhagic areas similar to those of the liver are occasionally found in other tissues, such as adrenal cortex. Areas of infarction very constantly occur in the placenta. The pituitary has been described as having increased numbers of basophils that may show hyaline degenerative changes. Basophilic invasion of the posterior lobe of the pituitary probably has no significance as far as eclampsia is concerned.

Intracellular retention of sodium and fluid may be important in eclampsia, accounting for some of the clinical symptoms. Intravascular fibrin deposition in arterioles and capillaries throughout the body appears to be responsible for the necroses and hemorrhages seen in eclampsia and for the uncommon bilateral renal cortical necrosis and pituitary necrosis associated with pregnancy. It has been suggested that the mechanism underlying the fibrin deposition is similar to that in the generalized Schwartzman reaction.

Chapter 22

The breast

The breasts have an origin from the skin similar to that of sweat or sebaceous glands and like them are branched tubular glands. They are composed of a number of separated subdivisions, or lobes, each of which is drained by a duct. The various ducts come together and open at the nipple. The inner ends of the various ducts branch and rebranch, the beginning of the ducts being small glands or acini.

During fetal development and until about four months after birth the breast develops a duct system of fifteen to twenty-five branching epithelial channels. Quiescence then follows until puberty, when there is renewed growth of the ducts. This developmental period is transient in males and is followed by quiescence and involution. In females the ductal development continues during adolescence and is accompanied by increase in the surrounding fibrous and fatty tissue and by development of buds of cells at the ends of the tubules or ducts. Acinar structures differentiate from these buds under hormonal stimulation as sexual maturity is reached. With the occurrence of pregnancy and lactation there is maximum acinar development. Proliferation of acinar buds appears to be a response to estrogenic stimulation, differentiation into acini is promoted by luteal hormones, and secretory activity is initiated by the pituitary. Throughout life the breast tissue is under the influence of pituitary and ovarian hormones. Mild cyclic changes involving hyperplasia followed by involution occur with each menstrual cycle. Luteal hormones influence epithelial hyperplasia in the breast in the latter part of the menstrual cycle. Regression occurs in the breast at the onset of the menstrual phase of the cycle, with involution and desquamation of epithelial cells and infiltration of a few lymphocytes in the periglandular connective tissue.

During pregnancy the breast undergoes a tremendous proliferative activity. There is great increase in number of glandular acini and a relative decrease in connective tissue, which ap-

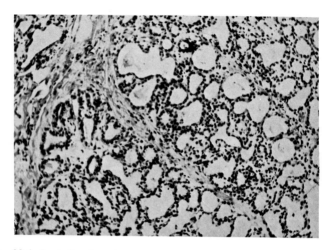

Fig. 22-1. Lactating breast.

parently results from the uninterrupted influence of luteal hormone. After parturition, the placental hormone being withdrawn, secretory activity and lactation follow stimulation by the pituitary hormone, prolactin. The dense glandular structure and hyperactive epithelium of the breast during pregnancy and lactation are a revelation of the power of physiologic hormonal stimulation. After the menopause, involutionary changes occur; connective tissue gradually replaces the glandular tissue, and the breasts decrease in size.

Pathologic changes in the breast consist of disturbances of the cyclic (hormonal) activity, the irritant effects of retained secretions, acute and chronic infections, and tumors.

HYPERTROPHY

Excessive development of the breasts is usually associated with endocrine disturbances. Hypertrophy in the male, gynecomastia, most commonly is associated with teratomatous tumors of the testicle and less often with tumors of the adrenal cortex or pituitary. Precocious puberty in female children usually has associated an excessive mammary growth and is found with granulosa cell and theca cell tumors of the ovary, adrenal cortical disturbances, and certain destructive lesions of the hypothalamus.

Overgrowth of the breasts during adolescence (virginal hypertrophy) or during pregnancy (gravid hypertrophy) appears to be an excessive response to hormonal stimuli on the part of abnormally sensitive mammary tissue.

Gynecomastia. Gynecomastia is an enlargement of the breast tissue of males, which is usually caused by proliferation of connective tissue and ducts. It is more often unilateral than bilateral. Endocrine disturbance, particularly with increase of estrogenic substances, is an important etiologic factor. Testicular tumors, particularly teratomas, choriocarcinomas, and interstitial cell tumors, may be associated with gynecomastia, as may adrenal cortical hyperplasia and tumors. Hepatic disease (cirrhosis) and dietary deficiency also may bring about gynecomastia. The breast lesion also occurs in the aged, probably the result of decreased androgenic hormone influence. Gynecomastia does not predispose to tumor formation. Pseudogynecomastia is an enlargement of the mammary regions caused by the deposition of fat.

MAMMARY DYSPLASIA

Mammary dysplasia is characterized by varying degrees of proliferative change in the epithelium and connective tissue of the breast, often with cystic dilatation of the ducts. The term *chronic cystic mastitis,* although commonly used, has evident defects in that the condition is not a chronic inflammation in the usual sense and is not always cystic. The following terms referring to various phases or forms of this condition may be encountered: fibrocystic disease, fibrocystic mastitis, cystic hyperplasia, chronic cystic mastopathia, Schimmelbusch's disease, mazoplasia, cystipherous desquamative hyperplasia, cystoplasia, cystic disease of the breast, adenosis of the breast, and adenofibrosis.

Etiology. The etiology of mammary dysplasia appears to be an imbalance of hormones (estrogen and progesterone) influencing the breasts, or an irregular and abnormal response of the breast tissue to these endocrine influences. The irritative effects of retained secretions and desquamated material have been considered another causative factor.

Mild degrees of the condition are very common, being usually a tender or painful area of breast tissue of increased density (mazoplasia). The pain and swelling may be mainly premenstrual and caused by vascular engorgement. In such cases there may be diffuse *fibrosis* and relatively little epithelial activity. In more severe cases the breasts are diffusely nodular or "shotty." Such nodularity is mainly caused by epithelial hyperplasia, fibrosis, and microscopic cyst formation, and this stage has been referred to as *adenosis* and *adenofibrosis*. In a more advanced stage, one or more large cysts may result from secretory changes *(cystic* or *fibrocystic disease)*. Firm, freely movable masses varying in size are sometimes palpable. When the nodularity is not diffuse, the condition must be distinguished from carcinoma. The age of greatest incidence is between 35 and 45 years.

Gross appearance. The gross appearance of the sectioned breast is often distinguished by the presence of cysts. Involved areas are grayish, of rubbery consistency, and not sharply outlined. The cysts may be of varying size and number, but they are not always present. The colorless content of the cysts shining

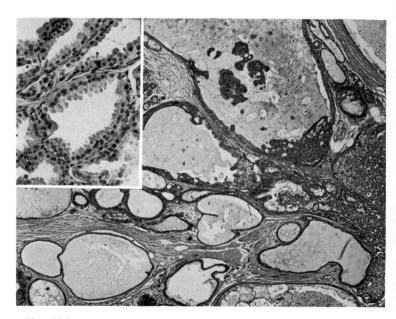

Fig. 22-2. Chronic cystic mastitis with atrophy, intracystic epithelial proliferation, and duct carcinoma. Inset shows high magnification of apocrine type of epithelium. (×40.) (From Kuzma, J. F.: Breast. In Anderson, W. A. D., editor: Pathology, ed. 5, St. Louis, 1966, The C. V. Mosby Co.)

through their tense, translucent walls gives them a bluish color (blue-domed cysts). Occasionally the contents of the cysts are brown or yellow from altered blood pigment. The cut ends of dilated ducts may release casts of grayish desquamated material.

Microscopic appearance. The microscopic features consist of (1) epithelial changes, (2) cyst formation, (3) fibrous hyperplasia, and (4) lymphocytic infiltration. These features exist in varying combinations and proportions, and some may be entirely absent. The cysts, which vary from microscopic size to several centimeters in diameter, are believed to be dilated ducts rather than glands. They are lined by a single layer of flattened or cuboidal epithelium. Obstruction of ducts by epithelial debris and retarded involution have been offered as explanations of the cyst formation.

Hyperplastic epithelial changes are usually present in ducts and glands. Solid buds of epithelial cells may be formed, or localized proliferations of the lining of ducts cause irregular papillary projections into the lumen. Bridges of epithelial cells may unite opposite walls, or the lumen may be completely filled by the proliferative epithelium. Sometimes the hyperplastic epithelial cells are large, clear, or eosinophilic and of a type suggesting apocrine sweat gland epithelium. Irregular atrophic changes may be present in the epithelium, instead of hyperplasia. In those cases where intraductal proliferation is great and papillary masses fill the lumen (intraductal papillomatosis) or solid epithelial overgrowth occludes ducts, differentiation from carcinoma may be difficult. Such distinction must be based on the histologic character of the cells and the presence or absence of invasion beyond the ductal basal membrane.

Fibrous hyperplasia with increase in connective tissue stroma is usual, and occasionally the stromal overgrowth is great enough to simulate the appearance of a fibroadenoma. Infiltration of lymphocytes in the stroma is a common but inconstant finding. Their presence originally suggested that the condition was of inflammatory nature, but they are now known to be part of the involutionary phase of cyclic activity.

Sclerosing adenosis is a term commonly applied to a lesion that is easily and frequently misinterpreted as carcinoma. A localized and somewhat lobular area of glandular hyperplasia undergoes fibrosis. The dominant overgrowth of hyalinizing connective tissue, by constricting the epithelial cells, produces variability in their shape and pattern. Thin isolated epithelial columns result, and microscopically there is a simulation of invasiveness and pleomorphism. However, in this benign lesion mitoses are absent except in the florid stage, and nuclear staining is regular. Electron microscopic studies in sclerosing adenosis show that the cells resemble those of the normal mammary gland, possessing intact basement membranes, evidences of secretory activity, well-formed mitochondria, etc. Infiltrating duct carcinoma cells, on electron microscopy, lack intact basement membranes and other structural refinements.

Myoepithelial cell proliferation. Myoepithelial cell proliferations in the breast, either alone or in cases of cystic mastopathy or adenofibrosis, if not recognized are easily misinterpreted as malignant.

Mazoplasia. The term *mazoplasia* was introduced to refer to a diffuse nodularity of the breasts, without cyst formation but with pain, usually related to menstrual periods. This condition is considered more physiologic than pathologic, has no etiologic relationship to carcinoma, and should be sharply distinguished from the cases of mammary dysplasia in which cysts or papillomas occur. The condition is common in women between 30 and 40 years of age. This condition of painful mammary tissue is also referred to as mastodynia.

The changes in mazoplasia are desquamation of epithelial cells filling and distending terminal ducts and acini, hyperplasia of connective tissue about the ducts and acini, and accumulation of lymphocytes.

Relationship to carcinoma. The relationship of mammary dysplasia to carcinoma has been a greatly debated point and obviously is of importance. That it is not precancerous and that it causes no great likelihood of malignant change has been the view of some. At the other extreme it is considered that at least 20% of breast carcinomas have passed through a type of chronic cystic mastitis. Whether or not chronic cystic mastitis should be considered a truly precancerous lesion, several statistical studies have shown that it is associated with a definitely greater likelihood of development of breast cancer. The incidence of carcinoma in women with cystic disease is about three to five times that of the general female population. Although this risk is insufficient to justify bilateral mastectomy for chronic cystic mastitis, subsequent careful watching is warranted.

Galactocele. Galactocele is a cyst containing milk, which results from a duct obstruction during lactation. It is a rare lesion.

FAT NECROSIS OF THE BREAST

The uncommon condition of fat necrosis in the breast is usually the result of trauma. The necrotic areas are opaque and are grayish yellow or chalky in appearance. The microscopic appearance is characterized by areas of necrosis and multinucleated foreign body giant cells and hence at times may be confused with tuberculosis.

MASTITIS AND ABSCESS

Acute infection in the breast is most commonly caused by staphylococci or streptococci, which gain entrance via a cracked nipple during the period of lactation. By one of the main ducts, spread occurs into the breast substance where a localized abscess forms. Chronic periductal or plasma cell mastitis is an inflammation in and about larger ducts near the nipple, usually found in older women near menopausal age. It may simulate carcinoma on gross examination.

TUBERCULOSIS

Tuberculous mastitis, although rare, may give difficulty in clinical differentiation from carcinoma. Most cases are secondary to tuberculosis elsewhere in the body, the spread to the breast commonly being from infected axillary or mediastinal lymph nodes or by the bloodstream. Microscopic diagnosis is necessary. Since fat necrosis and plasma cell mastitis can produce a somewhat similar microscopic picture, demonstration of the organisms is necessary for positive diagnosis.

BENIGN TUMORS

Fibroadenoma. Fibroadenomas are compound epithelial and connective tissue tumors in which growth of fibrous tissue is associated with hyperplasia of glandular cells. There are two types: pericanalicular, in which fibrous overgrowth surrounds the glandular spaces, and intracanalicular, in which proliferated connective tissue projects into the ducts as polypoid masses. Fibroadenoma of the breast is not a precancerous lesion. Its occurrence does not increase the chances of carcinoma developing in the breast.

The fibroadenomas are firm, lobulated, encapsulated tumors, easily movable in the breast, and usually remain quite small. Microscopically the pericanalicular form shows great proliferation of connective tissue around the acini, so that each tubule

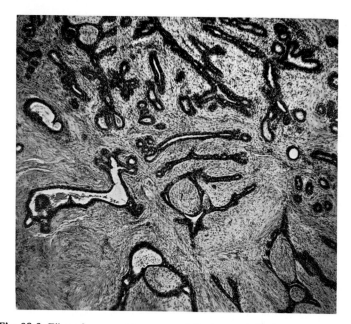

Fig. 22-3. Fibroadenoma of breast, partially intracanalicular.

appears surrounded by a ring of fibrous tissue. The innermost portion of the fibrous sheath frequently shows a myxomatous change. In the intracanalicular form a more diffuse growth of the connective tissue draws out and distorts the acini, so that polypoid masses of connective tissue covered by a layer of epithelium project into the lumen. If the pedicles of these masses are not included in the section, the duct lumina appear filled by rounded masses of connective tissue covered by a layer of epithelium. Occasionally, the epithelial component of a fibroadenoma is so prominent that the lesion is regarded as an *adenoma*.

Duct papilloma. Duct papilloma (adenocytoma, intracystic papilloma) is a papillary epithelial tumor that projects into a dilated duct, often quite close to the nipple. It occurs most commonly in the fourth or fifth decade and is often multiple. The tumor may or may not be palpable clinically, but discharge from the nipple, often bloody, is a common symptom. Grossly the papilloma forms a soft arborescent papillary growth, pro-

Table 22-1. *Tumors of mammary gland*

Benign
  Epithelial
    Papillomas
  Mixed epithelial and mesenchymal
    Fibroadenoma
      Intracanalicular
      Pericanalicular
      "Adenoma"
  Mesenchymal—breast tumors only by geography and in no way distinctive in the mammary gland; viz., lipoma, angioma, fibroma, myoma, chondroma, osteoma
Malignant
  Mammary ducts
    Noninfiltrating tumors
      Papillary carcinoma (intraductal)
      Comedo carcinoma (intraductal)
    Infiltrating carcinoma
      Paget's disease
      Papillary carcinoma
      Comedo carcinoma
      Carcinoma with productive fibrosis (scirrhous, simplex)
      Adenocarcinoma
      Medullary carcinoma
      Colloid carcinoma
  Mammary lobules
    Noninfiltrating—in situ
    Infiltrating—lobular adenocarcinoma
  Epithelial or mesenchymal origins such as tumors of the skin, skin appendages, and supporting tissues of breast; these are the same as found elsewhere in body—sweat gland tumors, basal or squamous cell carcinoma of skin, liposarcoma, lymphosarcoma, etc.

jecting into a cystic space that contains a clear or hemorrhagic fluid.

Three microscopic forms are sometimes differentiated: fibrous, glandular, and transitional. The fibrous type consists of ramifying stalks of connective tissue covered by epithelium, projecting into the dilated duct. Fusion of the stalks results in pseudoglandular structures. The glandular type shows hyperplastic or adenomatous acini invaginated into a duct or cyst. The fibrous and glandular types are benign. The transitional cell type resembles in appearance a papilloma of the bladder. Although histologically benign, there is greater danger of carcinoma developing on the basis of this transitional cell type.

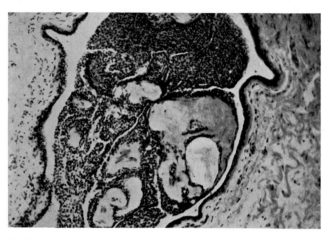

Fig. 22-4. Intraductal papilloma of the breast.

Malignancy in an intracystic papillary tumor is suggested by great variation in size, shape, and staining of cells and their nuclei, frequent mitoses, and invasion. Penetration of the basement membrane and invasion of stroma are the most important indications of malignancy (p. 791).

CANCER

The breast is one of the common sites of carcinoma in women, but it is rare as a site in males. It may occur at any adult age but is most common between 40 and 60 years of age. As in other carcinomas, the etiology is incompletely known. Certain factors, however, are believed important. These include hereditary susceptibility, irritation of retained secretion because of inadequate drainage by lack of nursing after pregnancy, endocrine (estrogen) disturbances, trauma, and fibrocystic disease. Whereas injection of large quantities of the ovarian hormone estrogen frequently produces mammary cancer in susceptible exeperimental animals, the relationship, if any, to human breast carcinoma is still not clear. Many women with breast cancer appear to have endocrine dysfunction manifested by thyroid atrophy, increase in the pituitary gland of sparsely granulated basophils (amphophils), ovarian stromal hyperplasia, and associated continuous estrogen stimulation of breast epithelium. The relationship of fibrocystic

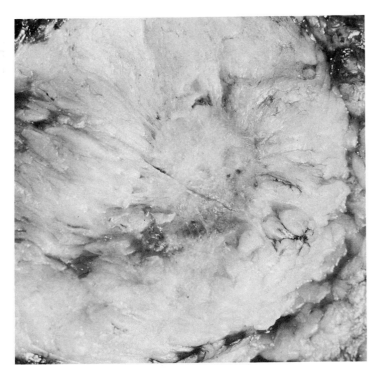

Fig. 22-5. Scirrhous carcinoma of the breast. (Courtesy Dr. J. F. Kuzma.)

disease (cystic hyperplasia) to cancer is likewise debatable (p. 782). This lesion appears to predispose to development of breast carcinoma, but there is no certain means of determining which case will develop malignancy and which will not. Trauma is rarely an important etiologic factor.

Classification into the various anatomic and histologic types of breast carcinoma is a useful procedure that may be one of the factors in determining prognosis. Such classifications cannot always be strict, however, as different portions of the tumor may show a different condition. Likewise, the degree of differentiation of the tumor cells—in size, shape, arrangement, and staining—also indicates the degree of malignancy. In prognosis, however, such anatomic considerations are only one factor to be considered in conjunction with the size of the tumor, the presence or absence of metastases, the age and condition of the patient, pregnancy, lactation, etc. Methods of classification that combine histologic grading and stage (degree of progression or spread) appear most useful for prognosis. Histologic features important in grading are tubule formation; regularity in size, shape, and staining of nuclei; and hyperchromatic nuclei and mitoses. Tubule formation is a favorable indication. The greater the irregularity in size, shape, and staining of nuclei or the greater the number of hyperchromatic nuclei and mitoses the worse the prognosis.

Carcinoma of the male breast accounts for less than 1% of breast cancers. As in women, it is found at an average age of about 56 years, occasionally is bilateral, and a history of trauma is not usually found. It is most often an infiltrating duct carcinoma. Gynecomastia is not in itself a precursor, but some reported cases of cancer have followed prolonged massive therapy with female hormones, which also may cause the development of gynecomastia. Orchiectomy has been effective in some cases in producing remissions, particularly in the presence of bone metastases.

Scirrhous carcinoma. Scirrhous carcinoma forms a hard

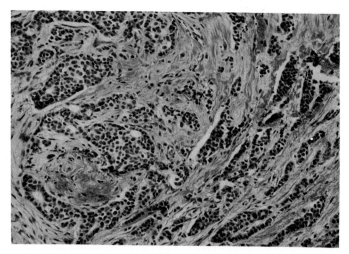

Fig. 22-6. Infiltrating scirrhous carcinoma of the breast.

nodule, which is most frequent in the upper and outer quadrant of the breast. The tumor is not encapsulated and soon becomes adherent to skin or deep fascia. The cut surface is composed of a hard, gritty, grayish, translucent tissue, with occasional opaque, yellowish areas of necrosis. There is no definite margin, but irregular lines of fibrous tissue radiate out into the surrounding tissue.

Microscopically there are thin masses and columns of epithelial cells, separated by an abundant dense fibrous stroma. Gland formation is slight; mitoses are infrequent. Scirrhous carcinoma tends to progress more slowly than the medullary type and with less tendency to ulcerate or form a bulky tumor but has a poor prognosis.

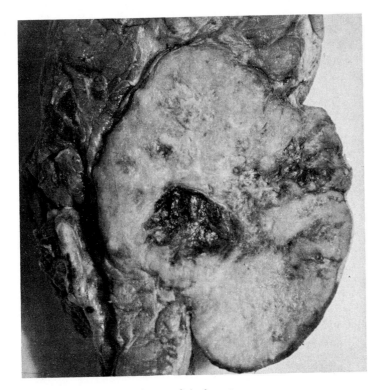

Fig. 22-7. Medullary carcinoma of the breast.

Medullary carcinoma. Medullary carcinoma forms a soft, massive tumor of relatively rapid growth, which tends to ulcerate and form a fungating mass on the surface. Microscopically it shows masses of malignant epithelial cells, separated by a scanty stroma. There is often some tendency to gland formation. Medullary carcinomas have a relatively favorable prognosis as compared to most other types of mammary cancer.

Adenocarcinoma. Some degree of differentiation into glandu-

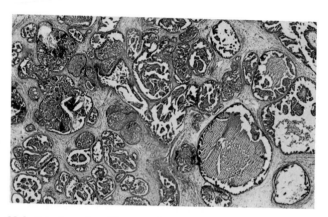

Fig. 22-8. Intraductal papillary carcinoma of the breast.

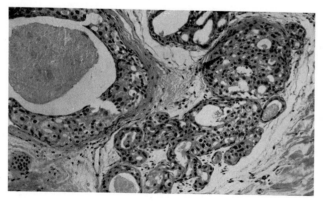

Fig. 22-9. Intraductal carcinoma of the breast.

lar structures is not uncommon in the scirrhous and medullary forms and in the papillary tumors arising in ducts. The true adenocarcinoma, in which gland formation is predominant, is much less common. It forms a soft bulky tumor of slow growth and relatively low-grade malignancy.

Intraductal carcinoma. Intraductal carcinoma includes two types of tumors: (1) *malignant papillary tumors,* arising from ducts and sometimes representing a malignant change in a duct papilloma; and (2) *comedo carcinoma,* so called because on the cut surface plugs of tumor cells may be expressed from ducts, giving an appearance similar to that when a comedo is expressed from a blackhead. Small dark-staining oval cells proliferate within the ducts, forming there a thick lining or wall. The tumor cells grow diffusely along ducts and for a long time remain within the ducts so that evidence of invasion may be absent. The tumor grows slowly, metastasizes late, and has a relatively favorable prognosis.

Papillary carcinomas, particularly if well differentiated, may give difficulty in differentiation from benign intraductal papillomas. Features distinguishing a papillary carcinoma are a single type of epithelial cell covering the papillary projections, nuclear hyperchromatism, a cribriform glandular pattern, a delicate or

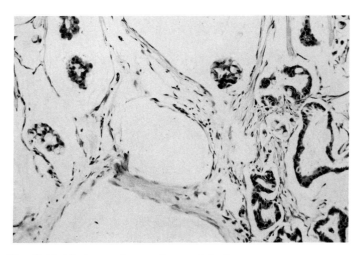

Fig. 22-10. Mucinous adenocarcinoma of the breast.

absent connective tissue stroma, epithelial invasion of stroma, intraductal carcinoma in adjacent ducts, and usually absence of sclerosing adenosis in adjacent breast tissue. Subsequently, the intraductal carcinomas invade the stroma of the breast beyond the ducts (infiltrating types).

Mucoid (gelatinous) carcinoma. Mucin-producing carcinoma of the breast is an infrequent tumor, which remains small for a long period, is likely to cause protrusion and enlargement of the nipple, and has a cystic character on palpation. The mucoid nature is evidenced grossly in the tumor by a gray, translucent appearance, which may be diffuse throughout or involve only a portion of the tumor. When the gelatinous change occurs in a papillary cancer or adenocarcinoma, the change is likely to be diffuse. Those showing partial mucin-producing change are usually of the scirrhous type. The mucinous material is secreted by the tumor cells, which by electron micrographic study show elaborate organelle structure. Microscopically there are nests of tumor cells surrounded by loose stroma distended with mucoid material. The survival rate of patients with mucin-producing carcinomas is better than that associated with the more common infiltrating duct or scirrhous carcinomas.

Inflammatory carcinoma. In occasional cases signs of inflammation in the breast (edema, redness, and heat) may arise simultaneously with the development of the breast cancer or

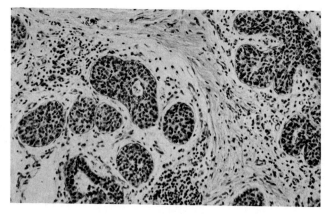

Fig. 22-11. Lobular carcinoma of the breast.

after the tumor has been present for some time. The inflammatory signs are caused by lymphatic blockage and congestion by cancer cells. The cancer cells grow in lymphatic spaces and veins, disseminate rapidly throughout the breast, and tumor nodules appear in the skin. Such "inflammatory" or "acute" carcinomas progress rapidly and have a poor prognosis.

Lobular carcinoma. Lobular carcinoma is a proliferative pattern that centers in one or more lobules without forming a distinct tumor mass. Epithelial cells that normally line the acini in two regular layers proliferate and fill up the acini. The general pattern of the lobule is maintained, although the acini may be closely packed with little intervening stroma. The proliferating cells may be fairly regular and are normal in appearance, or they may be larger, variable in size and shape, with some hyperchromatism and occasional mitoses. An infiltrating type has also been described.

The true nature of the lesion is uncertain, and its natural history is not well documented. It has been considered a precancerous lesion or a true carcinoma of slow evolution.

Paget's disease of the nipple. Paget's disease begins as a chronic eczematous lesion of the nipple, often with extension to adjacent skin of the breast, and associated with a duct carcinoma in the underlying breast. Section of the involved skin shows characteristic clear, hydropic "Paget" cells in the epidermis. The exact relationship of the epidermal change to the underlying duct cancer has been a matter of debate. The Paget cells have been considered by some as degenerated epidermal cells, possibly melanocytes, and interpreted by others as tumor cells arising from the underlying duct cancer. The carcinoma associated with Paget's disease of the nipple has a relatively higher age incidence. A similar epidermal change in other parts of the body (extramammary Paget's disease) occurs in the axillary or anogenital regions, associated with a tumor of an underlying apocrine gland. Paget's disease of the nipple may be simulated clinically in the presence of a benign adenoma of the nipple, which histologically may resemble a sweat gland adenoma.

Sarcoma. Sarcoma is an uncommon tumor of the breast. It may arise from the connective tissue stroma, from a preexisting fibroadenoma, from fat, or from underlying muscle tissue. Stromal sarcoma may show fibrous, myxoid, or fatty patterns, and has a better outlook than that of other types of sarcoma or carcinoma of the breast.

Adenosarcoma, which represents a malignant form of adenofibroma, is the most frequent type. The malignant transformation of the connective tissue is accompanied by epithelial elements. The tumor tends to remain circumscribed until a considerable size is reached, but there is a distinct tendency to recurrence after local removal.

Cystosarcoma phyllodes (giant mammary myxoma) is a very large bulky tumor of slow growth derived from a fibroadenoma. Grossly it has a cauliflower-like appearance, with multiple frond-like masses or cystic spaces into which project polypoid masses. Microscopically myxomatous connective tissue is the predominant feature, forming polypoid masses covered by a layer of epithelium. Although generally benign in nature and successfully treated by wide local excision, malignant (sarcomatous) variants have been described. The latter tumors appear to be sarcomas that develop in the fibroepithelial tumors, but only the mesenchymatous elements appear to be malignant and are found in metastases.

Carcinosarcomas are rare cancers of the breast, in which both carcinomatous and sarcomatous elements occur. They appear to be carcinomas in which the stroma has undergone sarcomatous change.

Spread of cancer of the breast. Direct invasion and metastasis by lymphatics and by the bloodstream are all important in breast cancer. Scirrhous carcinoma particularly tends to invade adjacent tissues and often involves pectoral muscles. Spread by lymphatics may be by direct growth along the channels (lymphatic permeation) or more commonly by tumor emboli. Lymphatic spread to axillary nodes is most common, but occasionally there is early involvement of mediastinal nodes. Spread to supraclavicular nodes is usually a late feature. Pleural and lung involvement may be by direct extension through the pectoral fascia to subpleural lymphatics, or it may be from mediastinal nodes. The liver occasionally is invaded by a spread through lymphatics of the coronary ligament. Spread by bloodstream gives rise to metastases in the red marrow of bones.

Lymphangiosarcoma may complicate chronic edema of an arm after mastectomy for cancer of the breast, although metastases in the edematous tissue from the original carcinoma also may occur and may simulate such tumors.

Chapter 23

The skin

The general principles of inflammations, infections, and neoplasms apply in involvement of the skin as elsewhere, modified in some instances by the position and structure of the skin.

STRUCTURE

The skin is composed of two main layers, the epidermis and the corium. The **epidermis,** or outer portion, has a well-defined basal layer of columnar cells next to the corium, which dip down between papillae of the corium to form interpapillary processes. The cells of the basal layer undergo a gradual change to the flattened, resistant, cornified squamous cells found on the surface. In the intermediate layers of the epidermis the so-called prickle cells have prominent protoplasmic threads forming intercellular bridges. The outer cornified layer of epidermis may undergo excessive growth (hyperkeratosis), be imperfectly cornified (parakeratosis), undergo degeneration or abnormal cornification (dyskeratosis), or be atrophic with diminished cornification. Tumors arising from epidermal cells are common. Inflammatory lesions involving epidermis frequently produce vesicles and bullae (edema), pustules, and finally ulcers.

Small masses of "sex" chromatin may be identifiable in the nuclei of epidermal or buccal epithelial cells. Those chromatin structures are found in 30 to 80% of nuclei in females and in 0 to 9% of nuclei in males. Sex determination from skin biopsy or buccal smear by this method may be useful in pseudohermaphroditism.

The *corium,* or **dermis,** is the inner layer of the skin beneath the epidermis. It is a fibrous layer, consisting of collagenous, elastic, and reticular fibers, that contains hair follicles, sebaceous glands, blood vessels, lymphatics, and nerve endings. Beneath the dermis is an adipose tissue layer, actually the deeper continuation of the dermis but sometimes described as a third layer of the skin, which is often referred to as the **hypoderm,** or

795

subcutaneous tissue. In inflammations of the skin it is usually in the corium that cellular, vascular, and degenerative changes are most prominent. Hypertrophy, atrophy, and neoplasia are types of pathologic change that affect elements of the corium. Sebaceous glands are small racemose glands that occur in association with hair follicles. They may undergo hypertrophic, atrophic, cystic, and neoplastic changes. The sweat glands are tubular glands that form a coil. The common type is a small gland that discharges through a spiral duct passing through the epidermis. Larger sweat glands, known as apocrine glands, open into hair follicles and are found mainly in the axillary and genital regions. Sweat glands may be diminished in number, but functional disorders are more common than anatomic changes. Rarely tumors may arise from sweat glands (spiradenoma, carcinoma). Blood vessels, lymphatics, and nerves of the corium, in addition to being involved in inflammatory processes, may give rise to tumors. Disturbances of a fatty nature in the skin usually take the form of an abnormal deposit of lipid (xanthoma) or a neoplasm of adipose tissue (lipoma, liposarcoma). Changes in the pigment deposits in the skin occur in a number of local and internal conditions (e.g., Addison's disease), and pigmented cells give rise to tumors (pigmented nevi and malignant melanomas).

INFECTIONS AND INFLAMMATIONS

A variety of inflammatory skin lesions of infectious or noninfectious origin, both nonspecific and granulomatous, have already been considered in previous chapters (e.g., bacterial, fungous, viral, and rickettsial infections; rheumatic nodules; tophus of gout; fat necrosis with foreign body reaction; etc.). In this section a few more examples will be considered. The majority of the lesions that follow are of the granulomatous type. Psoriasis is presented as an example of a nonspecific dermatitis and is of interest because it is common, has a characteristic histologic appearance, and is associated with other systemic disorders.

Tuberculosis. Tuberculosis of the skin, or *lupus,* occurs in a wide variety of forms, the common type being a localized form known as *lupus vulgaris.* The granulomatous inflammation is found mainly in the deeper layers of the corium. The cellular changes are similar to those of tuberculosis elsewhere, with the accumulation of epithelioid cells, multinucleated giant cells, and lymphocytes. Caseation is uncommon, however, and it is difficult to demonstrate tubercle bacilli in the tissues. The overlying epidermis may be unchanged, atrophic, or irregularly hypertrophic. Other skin lesions in which a tuberculous origin is suspected include scrofuloderma and erythema induratum.

Granuloma annulare. Granuloma annulare is a chronic dermatitis of unknown cause, characterized by a group of nodules arranged in a ringlike or circinate fashion. There is an intradermal zone of fibrinoid necrosis, surrounded by palisaded epithelioid cells, lymphocytes, and fibroblasts. An occasional giant

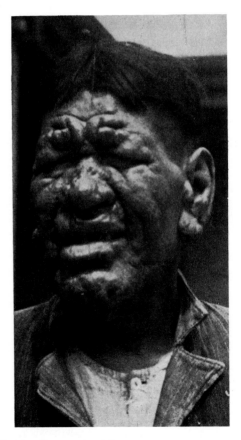

Fig. 23-1. Nodular (lepromatous) leprosy.

cell of the foreign body type may be seen. It is similar to rheumatic or rheumatoid nodules, which differ in being subcutaneous. Also the lesion may be mistaken for necrobiosis lipoidica, which is sometimes associated with diabetes mellitus.

Leprosy (Hansen's disease). The leprosy bacillus *(Mycobacterium leprae)* most commonly affects the skin, nasal mucosa, and peripheral nerves, although lesions may also be found in the liver, spleen, lymph nodes, testicles, and elsewhere. Duration of life with the disease is often twenty years or more, and secondary amyloidosis is common. Renal insufficiency from amyloidosis is a frequent cause of death. Secondary bacterial infections may complicate the disease and cause death. Only the two principal types of leprosy *(lepromatous* and *tuberculoid)* are considered here.

In the lepromatous type, the more progressive form, the skin is most commonly involved, with irregular nodules or elevations

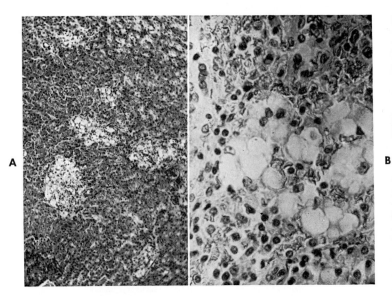

Fig. 23-2. A, Lepromatous leprosy. Miliary lepromas in the liver, composed of vacuolated histiocytes, often containing lepra bacilli. (×80.) **B,** Same as **A,** higher magnification. (×360.) (From Koppisch, E.: Leprosy. In Anderson, W. A. D., editor: Pathology, ed. 4, St. Louis, 1961, The C. V. Mosby Co.)

and more diffuse infiltrating lesions affecting the face, hands, and feet, and less commonly the trunk. The resultant thickening and wrinkling of the skin produces a characteristic "leonine facies." Sections from these nodules show an atrophy and flattening of the epidermis and characteristic changes in the corium. In this latter situation there occurs a peculiar granulomatous reaction, characterized by histiocytes (lepra cells), some of which contain abundant intracytoplasmic lipid. In ordinary sections the lipid in the latter cells is dissolved out, and the cells exhibit a pale, vacuolated, and foamy cytoplasm (Virchow's cells). The histiocytes vary in size and occasionally are multinucleated, and they contain clusters of the causative bacilli within them. The lepra bacillus multiplies within these cells. Globular masses of the bacteria, within or outside cells, are known as *globi*. Because organisms are abundant in lesions of the skin and nasal mucosa, lepromatous leprosy is the more infectious type. An abundant network of loose connective tissue and blood vessels is present in the lesion.

In the tuberculoid type the histologic picture closely simulates that of tuberculosis. However, in the United States the tuberculoid form is much less frequent than the lepromatous type. Histologically, noncaseating tubercles are characteristically seen, and organisms are difficult to find or not demonstrable. Maculopapular lesions of the skin occur, but the considerable nodular thickening is absent.

Lepra bacilli and tubercle bacilli are distinguished by the following points: The lepra bacilli are numerous in the lesions (at least in the lepromatous type), are intracellular, and are arranged in masses or bundles; they are straight, plump, and contain coarse granules. The tubercle bacilli are scarce in skin lesions, occur singly, or in small groups, and are slender, bent, and finely granular.

Peripheral nerve lesions occur in both types of leprosy but are especially prominent in the tuberculoid type. Anesthesias of the skin commonly occur, and subsequently trophic and traumatic lesions develop in the anesthetic areas. Paralyses result in deformities (e.g., claw hands). Neural involvement also leads to gradual atrophy and resorption of bone with resultant shortening of digits.

Sarcoidosis (Besnier-Boeck-Schaumann disease). Originally described as sarcoma-like nodular lesions of the skin, sarcoidosis is now recognized as a generalized systemic granulomatous disease in which there is most commonly involvement of the lymph nodes, lung, bone marrow (phalanges), spleen, liver, eye, parotid gland, and other organs. The lesions consist of nodular accumulations of epithelioid cells similar in appearance to the epithelioid cells in tuberculosis, with which the condition is most easily confused. Necrosis is absent or minimal, and when present, it is not true caseation necrosis. The clinical manifestations depend upon the organs involved. Most patients are between 20 and 40 years of age and have a benign but sometimes prolonged course. Death from sarcoidosis per se is uncommon. Death usually results from extensive lung involvement with pulmonary insufficiency and cor pulmonale. Occasionally frank tuberculosis supervenes. The frequency of the disease appears greater in the southeastern than in other areas of the United States, and the incidence is higher in Negroes.

Etiology. The etiology of sarcoidosis is unknown. It frequently has been considered an atypical form of tuberculosis, although characteristically it is impossible to demonstrate the tubercle bacillus in the lesion by staining or animal inoculation, and the patients often do not react to tuberculin injection. It may be an exaggerated nonspecific response to a lipid fraction of varied organisms or other irritants.

Recent epidemiologic studies have led to the investigation of forest products as possible etiologic factors in sarcoidosis. Pollen from pine (and other gymnosperms) has been shown to contain waxes similar to those of tubercle bacilli and to produce similar epithelioid lesions on injection. Direct evidence of a possible etiologic relationship is awaited. A common opinion is that an immunologic abnormality, involving sensitivity to a variety of agents, is responsible.

Clinical features are variable. In addition to pulmonary manifestations, already mentioned, there may be the following: lymphadenopathy, involving any group of nodes, especially intrathoracic and cervical; radiolucent lesions in bones, particularly in the phalanges, as seen by x-ray examination; involvement of the uveal tract of the eye and parotid gland (uveoparotid fever or Heerfordt's syndrome); skin lesions (papules, nodules, infiltrating plaques, and erythema nodosum); hepatomegaly caused by lesions in the liver; symptoms resulting from direct myocardial involvement, although less common than cor pulmonale related to lung disease; and sometimes constitutional symptoms

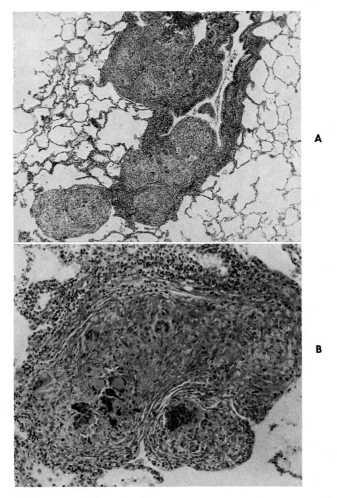

Fig. 23-3. Sarcoidosis of the lung. **A,** Nodular granulomas surround a bronchiole and small vein (low magnification). **B,** Giant cells and other cellular components of a fused cluster of nodules, shown at higher magnification. (From Gunn, F. D.: Lung. In Anderson, W. A. D., editor: Pathology, ed. 4, St. Louis, 1961, The C. V. Mosby Co.)

with no significant evidence of organ involvement (e.g., fever, weight loss, malaise, etc.).

Structure. The sarcoid lesion consists of dense nodular accumulations of the epithelioid type of large mononuclear cells. Necrosis is absent or minimal, reticulum remains relatively intact throughout the nodule, and giant cells are few. Inclusions, often of stellate (asteroid body), conchoidal (Schaumann body), or irregular bizarre shape, sometimes are seen in the giant cells. Fibrosis develops with aging and healing of the lesions. The Nickerson-Kveim skin test, using a suspension of human sarcoidal tissue, is positive when a papule develops, which histologically consists of a sarcoidlike granuloma. Lesions of berylliosis and the granulomatous reaction to silica crystals simulate those of sarcoidosis.

The points differentiating sarcoid from tuberculosis are (1) caseation is absent; (2) giant cells are relatively scarce, larger,

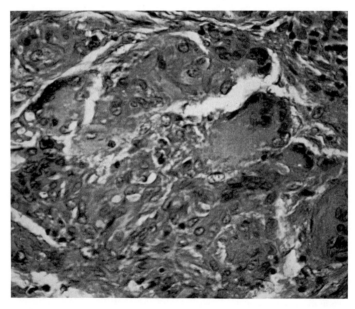

Fig. 23-4. Silica granuloma. Sarcoidlike nodule with multinucleated foreign body giant cells, which occasionally contain small crystalline structures. (From Haukohl, R. S., and Anderson, W. A. D.: Pathology seminars, St. Louis, 1955, The C. V. Mosby Co.)

and contain more nuclei that are evenly distributed throughout the cell; (3) a delicate reticulum is demonstrable in the lesion by silver staining, whereas in tubercles the reticulum is destroyed by caseation; and (4) there is no evidence of active tuberculosis elsewhere in the body.

Biochemical changes in Boeck's sarcoid include hyperproteinemia, hyperglobulinemia, and elevated serum calcium and blood alkaline phosphatase. Hypercalcemia is thought by some to result from increased sensitivity to vitamin D.

Rhinoscleroma. Rhinoscleroma is a rare granulomatous inflammation of the nose that has specific histologic features. The subepidermal tissue is packed with plasma cells, among which are characteristic large pale cells, having a small nucleus and foamy cytoplasm and known as Mikulicz cells. Causative bacilli, *Klebsiella rhinoscleromatis,* are found in the cytoplasm of the Mikulicz cells. Hyaline (Russell) bodies are present in the cytoplasm of some of the plasma cells. The area undergoes a gradual fibrosis.

Weber-Christian disease. Weber-Christian disease (relapsing, febrile, nodular, nonsuppurative panniculitis) is characterized by

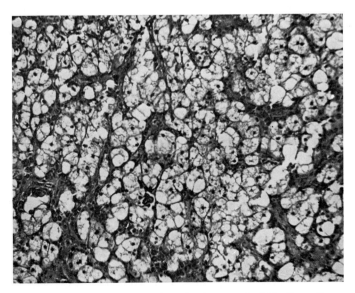

Fig. 23-5. Rhinoscleroma, showing the large pale Mikulicz cells.

crops of subcutaneous painful nodules and is accompanied by fever and systemic manifestations. In some cases lesions in the internal fat areas have been described (e.g., perivisceral, mesenteric). The characteristic lesion consists of lobules of fat, which show degenerative changes, lymphocytic infiltration, and sometimes giant cell granulomas. Neutrophils, according to some authors, may be seen in an early stage of the lesion. Vasculitis also may be noted. Septa between the fatty lobules show relatively little change in early stages. A somewhat similar panniculitis may be seen in erythema nodosum, erythema induratum, and fat necrosis caused by trauma or chemical agents.

Sclerema neonatorum. A generalized form of sclerema neonatorum occurs in the first few weeks of life and is characterized by widespread patchy hardening of subcutaneous tissue. The visceral fat may also be involved. There is a foreign-body type of granulomatous inflammatory reaction of the subcutaneous adipose tissue associated with precipitation of fatty acid crystals. Death usually occurs in a few weeks. A localized self-limited form also exists. A deficiency in the composition of the fat and birth trauma are considered to be factors in sclerema neonatorum.

Scleredema. Scleredema is an uncommon benign condition characterized by firm nonpitting edema, which may affect the face, neck, thorax, or arms. Effusions into pleural, pericardial, and joint spaces also may occur. Young women are most frequently affected. Recovery occurs spontaneously after a course of several months to years. Inflammation in the tissues is not striking, usually evidenced as a slight lymphocytic infiltration. The disease is not to be confused with *sclerema neonatorum* and must be distinguished from *scleroderma*. The cause of scleredema is unknown, but it often occurs after an upper respiratory infection.

Psoriasis. Psoriasis is a chronic, recurrent disorder of unknown cause, characterized by papules and plaques, which are dry and usually covered by thin silvery scales. The extensor surfaces of the extremities, e.g., elbows and knees, are common sites of involvement, but the scalp, nails, back, buttocks, and anogenital regions are often affected also.

The microscopic features, which are characteristic, include (1) acanthosis (thickening of the epidermis because of hyperplasia of stratum malpighii) with regular downward prolongations of the interpapillary processes that are rounded at the ends;

(2) thinning of the suprapapillary portion of the epidermis; (3) prominent parakeratosis; (4) absence of stratum granulosum; (5) nonspecific inflammation with edema of the upper dermis, especially of the papillae that contain dilated venules; and (6) foci of neutrophils in the epidermis ("Munro microabscesses").

Patients with psoriasis sometimes develop a form of arthritis similar to rheumatoid arthritis. In psoriatic arthritis, however, serologic tests for the rheumatoid factor are usually negative, and the terminal interphalangeal joints are involved rather than the proximal interphalangeal joints as in rheumatoid arthritis. The incidence of diabetes mellitus and a positive family history of this metabolic disorder are said to be higher among those with psoriasis.

Collagen diseases

In recent years a concept has evolved of certain diseases as primarily disturbances of connective tissues of the body, with certain clinical and morphologic similarities. A grouping together of these conditions as *collagen diseases* has been popular and productive, although the conditions are not necessarily related to the same cause. Commonly grouped as collagen diseases are systemic lupus erythematosus, dermatomyositis, systemic scleroderma, polyarteritis nodosa, thrombotic thrombocytopenic purpura, rheumatic fever, and rheumatoid arthritis. Such widespread or diffuse collagen diseases are to be distinguished from the localized connective tissue disturbances of the skin, such as keloids, balanitis xerotica obliterans, acrodermatitis chronica atrophicans, granuloma annulare, and necrobiosis lipoidica.

Connective tissue is composed of fibrous connective tissue cells or fibroblasts, intercellular fibers, and an amorphous ground substance that lies between them. The intercellular fibers are of three kinds: (1) collagen, (2) elastic, and (3) reticulin fibers. The collagen fibers are generally most abundant and easily seen, but the elastic and reticulin fibers can be differentially stained, the latter being argyrophilic. The homogeneous, viscid ground substance is composed of mucopolysaccharides and is generally inconspicuous, but condensations form the basement membranes of such structures as bronchi, renal glomeruli and tubules, and appear as thin hyaline membranes. In the collagen diseases the ground substance may undergo conspicuous alteration. Among the components of connective tissue, only the fibroblasts are living structures. The inert fibers and ground substance may be acted upon and undergo change but are incapable of active response to injury.

In the collagen diseases the connective tissues show varying combinations of degeneration and fibroblastic proliferation. The most characteristic change is a localized "fibrinoid" degeneration of connective tissue. The ground substance becomes increased in quantity and prominence, the collagen fibers become swollen and fragmented, and the debris becomes fused into a prominently eosinophilic area lacking normal structural detail and taking on staining reactions similar to those of fibrin. The fibrinoid formation has been considered characteristic of an allergic reaction, but it is probably not specific for injury of any particular type (p. 73).

Dermatomyositis. Dermatomyositis is an inflammatory and degenerative condition of the skin, subcutaneous tissue, and striated muscles. Although many features suggest an infective origin, no organism has been found and the cause is unknown. In some cases (7 to 15%) there is an associated malignant neoplasm somewhere in the body. Inflammatory changes in small blood vessels of involved tissues often appear as an important feature. The histologic changes are not specific for dermatomyositis but are similar to those of scleroderma and other conditions; resemblances to disseminated lupus erythematosus have been noted.

The skin shows atrophy of the epidermis, edema, swelling of endothelial lining of small vessels, and perivascular and diffuse infiltration of lymphocytes and plasma cells. Muscle fibers show focal lymphocytic infiltration and degenerative changes varying from swelling and loss of striations to hyaline or vacuolar changes and necrosis. Sarcolemmal nuclei may be increased. Creatinuria usually occurs. Vital muscles of deglutition and respiration may be affected and promote terminal pneumonia. Heart muscle as well as skeletal muscle may be involved.

Scleroderma. Scleroderma may be circumscribed *(morphea)* or systemic *(progressive systemic sclerosis)*. Although both are similar histologically, the systemic disease is more serious. The latter consists of diffuse thickenings of the skin that are often associated with pigmentations and vascular phenomena similar to those of Raynaud's disease. The pathogenic changes are mainly collagenous fibrosis and changes in small arterioles leading to narrowing of their lumina. Inflammatory cell infiltration, chiefly lymphocytic, is usual in the early stages. These changes involve viscera, such as esophagus, gastrointestinal tract, heart, lungs, and kidneys, as well as skin. Atrophic changes occur in voluntary muscles.

Disseminated lupus erythematosus. Disseminated lupus erythematosus has been recognized to be associated with important systemic and visceral manifestations involving particularly the heart and kidneys. It occurs most commonly in middle-aged persons, particularly women. The duration may be a few weeks to several years, but the prognosis is poor. The cause is unknown. Some evidence suggests that the condition may be an allergic reaction of tissues, apparently an autoimmune disease. There appears to be a disturbance of cellular nucleic acid metabolism, and hyperglobulinemia is constantly present. This increase in globulin is chiefly in the gamma fraction. The essence of the condition has been stated to be a widespread and characteristic alteration or fibrinoid degeneration of collagenous tissue, with a special predilection for injury to collagen of the heart, glomeruli, blood vessels, skin, spleen, and retroperitoneal tissues. The histologic change is thought to result from DNA depolymerization.

Patients with active disseminated lupus erythematosus may

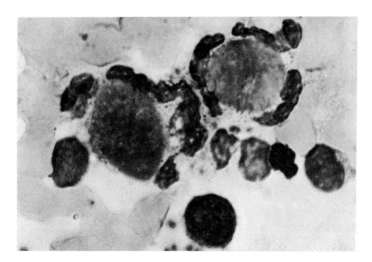

Fig. 23-6. LE cells in a blood smear. (Courtesy Dr. J. F. Kuzma.)

show a distinctive cell (the LE cell) in bone marrow smears. This LE cell appears to be a mature polymorphonuclear leukocyte, which has phagocytized a homogeneous purple-staining mass of chromatin (nuclear) material. A factor (the LE factor) present in the gamma globulin fraction of plasma or serum of such patients is capable of reacting with nuclear constituents of normal neutrophils in vitro, transforming the nuclei to homogeneous rounded masses, which are rendered susceptible to phagocytosis, usually by granulocytes, forming the LE cells (LE cell phenomenon). The LE factor sometimes induces formation of rosettes of clumped leukocytes, which surround the altered nuclear material (LE rosette phenomenon). Similar hematoxylin-staining bodies may be seen in sections of various tissues in acute lupus erythematosus. These "hematoxylin bodies" contain partially depolymerized DNA. In addition to the LE factor a variety of other antinuclear autoantibodies, as well as antibodies to cytoplasmic constituents, have been described.

The histologic changes in the skin lesions consist of hyperkeratosis and edema of the epidermis and dilatation of lymphatic and small blood vessels of the corium with perivascular lymphocytic and neutrophilic infiltration.

Nonbacterial atypical verrucous endocarditis, as described by Libman and Sachs, occurs in a considerable proportion of cases (p. 338). Renal changes also are frequent but not constant. The kidneys are of normal size or are enlarged. Glomerular capillaries have a characteristic "wire-loop" appearance because of hyaline thickening of the basement membrane and subendothelial fibrinoid deposits, and endothelial proliferation in the glomerular tufts is frequent. The spleen shows a characteristic periarterial fibrosis of central arteries, assuming a pattern of thick concentric rings of collagen fibers.

TUMORS OF THE SKIN
Benign tumors

Verruca vulgaris. The common wart, or verruca vulgaris, is apparently infective in origin and caused by a filtrable virus. Electron microscopic studies have shown virus particles associated with nucleoli of cells of the stratum spinosum. The virus particles appear related to basophilic inclusions seen in ordinary sections. Certain investigators have reported seeing also, on occasion, cytoplasmic virus particles in cells containing particles in the nucleus. There is hypertrophy of both the outer keratinized layer and of the prickle cell layer, and irregular down-ward prolongations of the interpapillary processes are seen. There may be some infiltration of chronic inflammatory cells about blood vessels of the corium. The lesion occurs most often in children and appears commonly on the fingers and the hands, although it may occur elsewhere.

Condyloma acuminatum. There are several other forms of verrucae, including the *verruca plana* (flat wart), *verruca plantaris* (plantar wart), and *condyloma acuminatum* (venereal wart), which are caused by the same or allied strains of virus as that causing verruca vulgaris. Condyloma acuminatum occurs on the glans penis, on the mucosal surfaces of the vulva, and about the anus. It consists of groups of verrucous nodules that coalesce to form a cauliflower-like lesion. Microscopically there is papillomatosis of severe degree with acanthosis, slight hyperkeratosis, spotty parakeratosis, and vacuolization of the upper epidermal cells. In the dermis there are dilated capillaries and inflammatory cell infiltration, usually mononuclears. The lesion must be differentiated from condyloma latum resulting from syphilis.

Pigmented papilloma (seborrheic keratosis). Pigmented papilloma, also known as *basal cell papilloma,* occurs most commonly on the trunk and less often on the arms, neck, and face. It is brown or black, has a greasy surface and appears "stuck on" the skin. Clinically it may be mistaken for malignant melanoma. Microscopically the lesion consists of thickened epidermis in which are cystic areas containing keratin. The cells resemble basal cells; those about the keratin cysts are more mature squamous cells. The cysts appear to form from invaginations of the horny layer. Melanin is usually present in the cells of the tumor. The lower limit of the tumor is on a level with the adjacent normal epidermis, thus accounting for the gross "stuck on" appearance. The surface is covered with varying amounts of keratin, which causes the greasy appearance grossly (Fig. 23-7).

Keratoacanthoma. Keratoacanthoma (molluscum sebaceum) is a rapidly growing, keratotic, papular lesion of the skin that undergoes spontaneous resolution. It is commonest on the face and probably arises from the pilosebaceous apparatus. Histologically it is characterized by a superficial crater containing a keratin mass, surrounded by papillary hyperplastic squamous epithelium. The epithelial cells may suggest the appearance

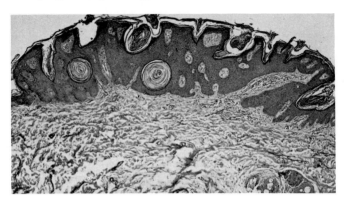

Fig. 23-7. Seborrheic keratotic lesion of the skin.

of a low-grade squamous cell carcinoma. Some regular extensions may be seen at the margins, but irregular invasive activity is absent. Similar multiple self-healing keratoses and carcinoma-like lesions of the skin have been described.

Acanthosis nigricans. Although acanthosis nigricans is not itself a neoplasm, in adults it is frequently associated with a visceral carcinoma. It is characterized by patchy, warty pigmented lesions, particularly occurring in the axilla, groin, mammary region, or on knees or elbows. It is a papillary hyperkeratosis of the skin with underlying acanthosis and considerable melanin pigmentation of the basal layer.

Benign tumors of skin appendages. Benign tumors may arise from the sweat glands, sebaceous glands, or hair follicles. Sweat gland tumors (spiradenomas or syringomas and hidradenomas) are somewhat more common than sebaceous adenomas. A verrucous, papillary, and sometimes cystic tumor of sweat gland origin (syringadenoma papilliferum) may grow rapidly and to a considerable size. The majority occur on the scalp or face, and a few are associated with basal cell carcinoma. The syringomas are mainly localized malformations of sweat glands (hamartomas). Hidradenomas arising from the vulva have a distinctive appearance, with narrow, branched, anastomosing, papillary fronds. (See Fig. 21-30.) The lesion arising from hair follicles (trichoepithelioma) is discussed later (p. 816).

Mesenchymal tumors. Fibromas, lipomas, leiomyomas, and

neurofibromas may occur. These are discussed in Chapter 11 (p. 275). Hemangiomas, lymphangiomas, and glomus tumors are considered in Chapter 12 (p. 315).

Precancerous lesions

A variety of skin and mucosal conditions, although not themselves neoplastic, give rise to carcinoma so frequently that they may be termed precancerous. These are (1) the keratoses—senile or solar, localized (cutaneous horn), and arsenical; (2) occupational dermatoses (from tar products); (3) x-ray and radium dermatitis; (4) xeroderma pigmentosum; and (5) leukoplakia.

Keratoses. The precancerous keratoses are characterized by a hyperkeratosis or thickening of the outer cornifying layers of epithelium. This may be accompanied by atrophy of remaining portions of the skin. A striking feature is the presence of atypia in the cells of the lower layers of the epidermis, i.e., hyperchromatic nuclei, irregular size and shape of nuclei, loss of polarity, and mitotic activity. Exposure to sunlight appears to be a causative factor (thus called *actinic,* or *solar, keratosis*). It is also known as *senile* keratosis; but while it tends to occur in persons past middle life, it is not limited to old age. A localized hyperkeratosis may produce a fingerlike projection, or *cutaneous horn. Arsenical keratosis,* a lesion that is similar to actinic keratosis histologically, develops usually on the palms or soles from continued absorption of the drug.

Occupational dermatoses. The occupational dermatoses are chronic inflammatory conditions or hyperkeratoses caused by long-continued irritation by certain chemicals. Tar and mineral oils and their products and derivatives are most important in this respect.

Radiation dermatitis. Dermatitis resulting from overexposure to radium or roentgen rays is particularly likely to occur in certain sensitive skins and often has carcinoma as a late sequel. The carcinomatous change usually is preceded by hyperkeratoses, fissures, ulcers, or scars.

Xeroderma pigmentosum. In xeroderma pigmentosum there is abnormal sensitivity of the skin to sunlight. The condition usually appears in infancy or early childhood and ends in death from carcinoma before adult age. Exposed areas of skin develop spotty pigmentations, warty hyperkeratoses, atrophy, and telangiectasia, and multiple carcinomas appear. The disease appears to be inherited with an incomplete sex linkage rather than as a simple recessive.

Leukoplakia. Leukoplakia is a localized lesion of mucous membrane epithelium characterized by white thick patches. (See Fig. 19-1.) It is the counterpart of senile keratosis of the skin and is apparently caused by a local chronic irritation. The histologic picture is similar to that of senile keratosis, except there is parakeratosis instead of hyperkeratosis. Leukoplakia predisposes to the development of carcinoma.

More rarely carcinoma also may develop in other skin lesions, such as the scars of burns, chronic varicose ulcers, chronic discoid lupus erythematosus, etc. Certain authors consider such lesions as *Bowen's disease* of the skin and *erythroplasia of Queyrat* of the glans penis as precancerous. Others, however, regard them as carcinoma in situ, and they are discussed as such here.

Carcinoma of the skin

In the epidermis the two innermost layers are most active, i.e., the basal layer and the spinous cell layer. The outer layers that undergo physiologic degeneration and death (keratinization) have little or no growth activity. Hence the main types of carcinoma of the skin arise from or simulate the inner active layers of epithelium and are known as (1) basal cell carcinoma and (2) squamous cell carcinoma (spinous cell carcinoma). There are also mixed forms, in which the fundamental types of basal and squamous cells are present in varying proportion. Finally there occasionally occurs a carcinoma arising from special structures of the skin, such as hair follicles and sebaceous or sweat glands.

Carcinoma of the skin develops usually in persons after middle age. It occurs particularly on exposed and unprotected parts of the skin, i.e., face, neck, arms, etc. Injury by excessive exposure to sunlight, heat, wind, roentgen rays, arsenicals, and other chronic irritants seems to be important in causation. The development of actual cancer is often preceded by benign keratoses or other precancerous lesions. Being readily accessible, treatment usually results in cure if the lesion is recognized in time. Size when first treated is important in prognosis. The histologic grade of malignancy is next in importance in prognosis.

Basal cell carcinoma (**rodent ulcer**). Basal cell carcinoma is the most frequent type of skin cancer. It is particularly common on the upper two thirds of the face and about the nose and eyelids. It is a tumor of low-grade malignancy and slow growth. It rarely metastasizes but erodes its way into surrounding tissues with ulceration and much local tissue destruction. This is the "rodent ulcer" form. It may also have a nodular or fungating form. The origin of some of the tumors of basal cell type appears to be from hair follicles or the anlage of hair follicles.

Microscopically the tumor is composed of cords and masses of cells with deeply basophilic nuclei. Each mass of cells tends to have a definite margin composed of a palisaded row of cells

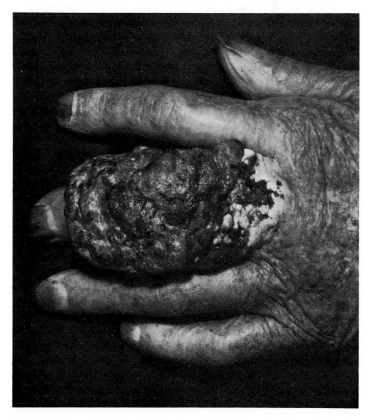

Fig. 23-8. Squamous cell carcinoma of the finger.

that stain deeply with hematoxylin. Mitotic figures are not abundant. There is ordinarily no keratinization or prickle cell formation. However, in about 10% there is some prickle cell formation or a few nests of keratinization. Occasionally the pegs of basal cells tend to form a glandular or adenoid picture. Since excessive pigment is sometimes present, the tumor is easily confused with a melanoma on gross examination.

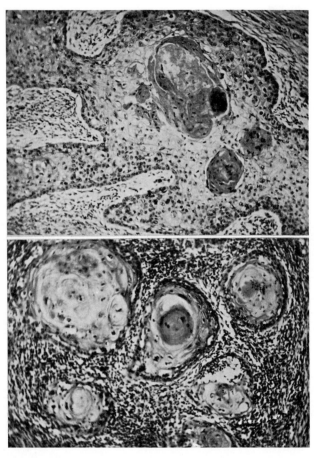

Fig. 23-9. Squamous cell carcinoma. Note the rounded masses of keratinized material.

Squamous cell carcinoma. Squamous cell carcinoma occurs not only in the skin but also wherever squamous or transitional epithelium is found. Hence it may involve the lip, mouth, tongue, larynx, cervix uteri, bladder, and esophagus. It may also arise in other situations, e.g., bronchial mucosa or gallbladder, presumably by a metaplastic change of the lining epithelium.

Squamous cell carcinoma of the skin, like other types, is commonest in persons after the fifth decade and is frequently related to some chronic injury or irritation. The tumor may appear as a projecting nodular mass or as an ulcer. Growth is more rapid than in the basal cell type, and metastasis occurs to regional lymph nodes. Distant metastases are rare.

Microscopically there is much greater irregularity than in the basal cell type. It is composed of irregular downgrowths and masses of enlarged epithelial cells, which show great variations and irregularities. Mitoses may be numerous and often are atypical. The amount of keratinization is variable. The keratinized cells are seen in concentric nests, or "pearls." The masses of keratin and the presence of prickle cells are the chief differential features for this type of tumor.

The squamous cell carcinoma that arises from the lip, tongue, intraoral mucosa, glans penis, or vulva tends to grow, penetrate, and metastasize more rapidly than the squamous cell carcinoma of the skin.

The lower lip is a particularly common site for carcinoma. These lesions are nearly all of the squamous cell type. The less frequent carcinomas of the upper lip are usually of the basal cell variety. Chronic irritation, as from excessive exposure to sunlight, pipe smoking, or bad oral hygiene, may be a predisposing factor. Leukoplakia may precede the formation of a carcinoma. The tumor may be papillary or ulcerative. Metastasis to submental and submaxillary nodes readily occurs (p. 582).

Epidermal hyperplasia, which develops in certain chronic ulcers or chronic inflammatory processes, may imitate the appearance of squamous cell carcinoma (pseudocarcinomatous hyperplasia), and differentiation may be difficult. In this reactive hyperplasia the epidermal cells are usually limited by a definite basement membrane, and there is less irregularity of cells and architectural arrangement. The clinical features are often an aid in the differentiation.

Epithelioma adenoides cysticum (Brooke's tumor). Brooke's tumors are single or multiple, small, often familial, and occur mainly in early adult life. Histologically they may resemble basal cell carcinoma, but characteristically the epithelial strands have cystic spaces filled with hyaline or keratinized material. Some of the structures, especially in the solitary lesions, resemble abortive hair follicles, and thus the lesions are considered to be *trichoepitheliomas*. Their behavior is benign. Carcinomatous change rarely occurs in these lesions, and they must be differentiated from true basal cell carcinomas.

Basosquamous (metatypical) carcinoma. The mixed cell type of carcinoma of the skin contains prominent features of both basal and squamous carcinoma.

Malignant tumors of skin appendages. Basal cell carcinomas may arise from the epithelium of hair shafts. Sebaceous carcinoma, which is rare, may be confused with basal cell or squamous carcinoma, but it resembles sebaceous gland tissue in at least some portion. Carcinoma of sweat gland origin is uncommon. Extramammary Paget's disease may be associated with an adenocarcinoma arising in an apocrine gland, as in the vulva. Malignant change rarely occurs in a trichoepithelioma, a tumor arising from hair follicles.

Intraepidermal carcinoma. Intraepidermal carcinoma is limited to the epidermis, but spread beyond this layer develops only occasionally or in late stages. One variety is known as Bowen's disease, which involves the skin. A similar lesion is erythroplasia of Queyrat which affects the glans penis.

Bowen's disease. Bowen's disease appears as a dull red patch of skin on the trunk or extremities, often with areas of crusting. Microscopically all layers of the epidermis show large, hyperchromatic nuclei surrounded by halos in the cytoplasm. Mitotic figures are seen in the affected cells. Acanthosis, hyperkeratosis, and parakeratosis are evident. Bowen's disease is associated with internal cancer in a significant number of cases. Sometimes the visceral cancer appears several years after the diagnosis of Bowen's disease has been made.

Malignant mesenchymal tumors

Dermatofibrosarcoma protuberans. Dermatofibrosarcoma protuberans may appear as a plaque or protuberant mass, which histologically resembles a low-grade fibrosarcoma. It grows slowly and with recurrence unless widely removed, but metastasis is unusual.

Fibrosarcoma. Fibrosarcoma of the skin also may form protuberant masses. It grows more rapidly and has a more serious outlook.

Kaposi's disease. Multiple idiopathic hemorrhagic sarcoma, or Kaposi's disease, is an infrequent condition, of unknown origin, and of uncertain nature. Its incidence in the Negro population in Africa is relatively frequent. A large majority of cases occur in men. The lesions are multiple and variable in form, but usually they are hemorrhagic and pigmented. They tend to involve the extremities, particularly the lower, in symmetric fashion. Mucous membranes also may be affected, and rarely viscera may be involved without external lesions. Temporary spontaneous regressions occur, but eventually lesions may develop in lymph nodes and internal organs, particularly the gastrointestinal tract and lungs. There is a controversy as to whether the lesions in the lymph nodes and viscera represent metastases or multicentric foci of origin. Lymph node involvement is common in the African cases. It has been debated whether the condition should be classed as a chronic granulomatous inflammation or as a true tumor (angiosarcoma). Current opinion favors regarding Kaposi's disease as a neoplasm of

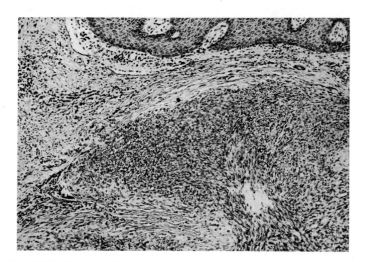

Fig. 23-10. Kaposi's disease. An irregular area of thin spindle cells and small vascular slits occupies the dermal tissue.

the vascular system with multifocal origin, although evidence also has suggested it is a disease of the reticuloendothelial system, probably related to the lymphomas.

The lesions involve corium and are characterized by irregular fascicles or bundles of spindle-shaped cells, which intertwine and are irregularly interrupted by vascular slits. The vascular spaces are often congested by red blood cells, but they do not appear to be lined by identifiable endothelium. The spindle-shaped cells are often poorly defined, and their nuclei are fusiform, oval, or round. Varying amounts of focal hemorrhage, deposits of blood pigment, and fibroblastic proliferation may be present. The late stage is characterized by obliteration of the

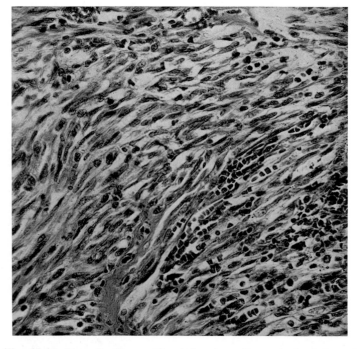

Fig. 23-11. Kaposi's disease. The lesion is a disorganized mixture of vascular slits and thin spindle cells. (From Haukohl, R. S., and Anderson, W. A. D.: Pathology seminars, St. Louis, 1955, The C. V. Mosby Co.)

vascular spaces, increased mitoses, and larger nuclei, the appearance changing to that of an angiosarcoma, fibrosarcoma, or undifferentiated sarcoma. The occurrence of Kaposi's disease with leukemia or malignant lymphoma (e.g., lymphosarcoma, Hodgkin's disease, mycosis fungoides) in the same patient has been reported by several investigators.

Mycosis fungoides (**granuloma fungoides**). Mycosis fungoides is considered by most authors to be a variant of malignant lymphoma, rather than a granuloma, involving principally and primarily the skin. The term *mycosis* is a misnomer, since the lesion is not a fungous disease. In early stages there is an eczematoid eruption, followed by a tumor phase in which there may be ulceration. In the tumor stage there is a dense massive accumulation of cells in the corium, with thinning and flattening of the overlying epidermis. In the cellular tumorlike mass the cells are polymorphic, appearing as mononuclear cells, lymphoblasts, and plasma cells. Some neutrophilic leukocytes, eosinophils, and giant cells may be present. The lesion may closely resemble Hodgkin's disease. There may be occasionally an involvement of internal organs, in addition to the skin.

Pigmented nevi and malignant melanomas

Both benign and malignant tumors may arise from melanoblasts, i.e., cells capable of producing melanin pigment. The pigment actually produced in a particular tumor may be small in amount or abundant. The extremely common benign form is called a pigmented nevus. The relatively rare malignant form is referred to as a melanocarcinoma, or malignant melanoma. Melanomas occur most commonly in the skin but also are found in the mouth, rectum, eye, meninges, and rarely in other sites.

The melanoblast is thought to be a modified basal cell of the epidermis and is capable of producing a pigmented material from 3,4-dihydroxyphenylalanine (dopa) by means of an oxidizing ferment that it contains. Melanin probably is produced by oxidation of some substance closely allied to dopa and to epinephrine.

The nevus cells that compose the benign tumor are believed to arise from two possible sources, the melanoblastic cells of the basal layer of the epidermis and the Schwann cells of the sheaths of dermal nerves.

Pigmented nevi. Pigmented nevi are found in almost every person. They occur in early years of life, grow to a certain size, and then remain stationary or become fibrotic. They are flat or raised pigmented lesions, with or without hair. Nevi on the hands, feet, and genitalia are particularly susceptible to malignancy. It is usually considered advisable to excise these and also others whose situation subjects them to constant irritation or trauma.

Allen* has classified the nevi into the following types:

1. Junctional nevus (dermoepidermal nevus)
2. Intradermal nevus (common mole, or neuronevus)
3. Blue nevus (Jadassohn-Tièche nevus)
4. Compound nevus
5. Juvenile melanoma

The *junctional nevus* is particularly important, as evidence suggests that it may be a forerunner of the malignant melanoma. It is characterized by clusters of enlarged, rounded, loosened cells of the basal layer of the epidermis. In the *intradermal nevus,* or common mole, the clusters and cords of the nevus cells are found only in the dermis. Histologically the epidermis is thinner than normal and may be flat or papillary. Beneath the epidermis are nests of rounded or polygonal, pale-staining "nevus cells," which contain variable amounts of melanin. The cells occur in islands, separated by connective tissue, but there is no sharp line of separation or encapsulation, and the cells may extend somewhat irregularly into subcutaneous tissue. The *compound nevus* is a combination of the junctional and the intradermal nevus. The *juvenile melanoma,* which occurs in children before puberty, is a special form of compound nevus with distinct histologic features that distinguish it from the malignant melanomas of adults. Juvenile melanomas do not metastasize or run a malignant course.

The *blue nevus* is a benign, bluish black, flat or slightly raised lesion. It is composed of interlacing bundles of elongated or spindle cells, abundantly pigmented and usually situated quite deep within the dermis.

Malignant melanoma. Malignant melanoma (melanocarcinoma) most frequently develops on the face, neck and extremities. The incidence is greatest in persons between 30 and 60 years of age. Clinical malignancy is rare before puberty. The tumor is relatively less frequent in the Negro race. Many cases appear to develop from a previously benign nevus, i.e., a junc-

---

*Allen, A. C.: The skin, St. Louis, 1954, The C. V. Mosby Co.

tional nevus or the junctional component of a compound nevus.

Malignant melanoma is one of the most malignant of tumors. It invades blood vessels and lymphatics early, metastasizes widely, and is very radioresistant. The first metastases are often seen in the skin around the periphery of the tumor. Regional lymph nodes are involved early. Melanuria may occur when there are widespread metastases. The urine turns brown or black a short time after being voided.

The possibility of malignant change in a pigmented nevus should be entertained when there have been repeated irritations, a noticeable increase in size or pigmentation, pain, or ulceration. In suspected malignant melanoma the entire growth should be widely excised, rather than a portion biopsied. Histologic evidence of malignancy includes mitotic activity, loss of architectural arrangement of the nests of nevus cells, as well as the cytologic criteria used in other cancers. There is often an inflammatory reaction in the stroma of the tumor. Metastatic nodules may be more highly pigmented than the primary tumor.

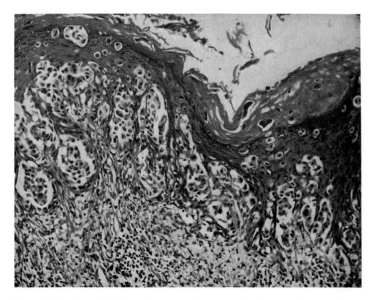

Fig. 23-12. Superficial malignant melanoma showing evidence of epidermal origin. (Courtesy Dr. A. C. Allen.)

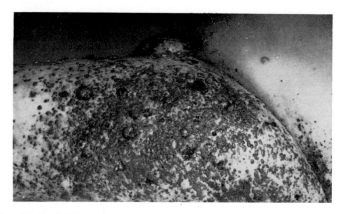

Fig. 23-13. Malignant melanoma showing spread in the skin of the upper thigh and abdomen.

Pigmented papillomas (seborrheic keratoses) of the skin are benign epithelial tumors easily mistaken clinically for pigmented nevi or malignant melanoma but containing no nevus cells. Sclerosing hemangiomatous tumors may be highly pigmented by hemosiderin and must be distinguished from melanotic tumors. A familial disorder characterized by melanin-pigmented spots of the lips and mouth (and to a lesser degree of the skin), associated with intestinal polyposis, is known as the Peutz-Jeghers syndrome (p. 648).

Tumorlike conditions of the skin

Keloid. Keloids are fibroma-like lesions developing in the corium, usually as the result of trauma but sometimes spontaneously. They occur in persons having a constitutional factor predisposing to their development and are relatively more common in the Negro race. Various types of minor or severe traumatism initiate their growth. They are particularly common after burns, are frequently multiple, and may reach a considerable size.

Histologically they are composed of thick, intertwining, hyalinized bands of collagen fibers. Mitoses are unusual except in early stages. Skin appendages are absent, and the overlying epidermis may be thinned out and its processes flattened. An ordi-

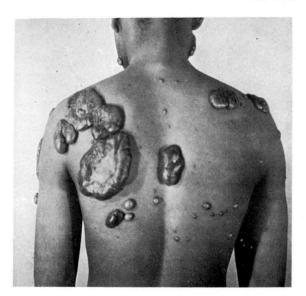

Fig. 23-14. Keloids.

nary scar tends to be more cellular and contains thinner collagen fibers.

Xanthoma. Xanthomas are plaquelike or nodular lesions characterized by the presence of lipids in a localized area of the corium. They are usually multiple and occur in various situations and quite commonly on the eyelids (xanthelasma). They may occur in association wth diabetes or hypercholesterolemia, but not necessarily so. Probably they should not be considered true neoplasms (p. 559).

Histologically the characteristic feature is the presence in the corium of lipid-containing histiocytic foam cells and connective tissue proliferation. Lipids can be demonstrated in the xanthoma cells, and crystals of lipoid material may lie in the tissues. Giant cells are sometimes present. Inflammatory reaction is usually evident in the diabetic xanthomas, particularly about the margins of the nodule.

Pyogenic granuloma. Pyogenic granuloma is an ulcerating, projecting, tumorlike mass of exuberant granulation tissue with abundant, enlarged blood vessels. The lesion resembles a capil-

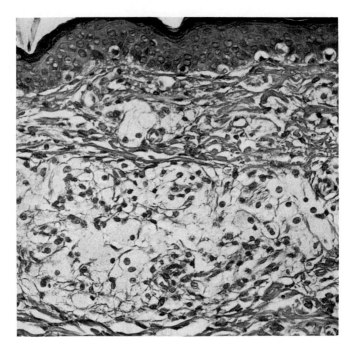

Fig. 23-15. Xanthoma of the skin. The lipid-containing foam cells form a poorly circumscribed mass in the dermis.

lary hemangioma and is frequently referred to as "granuloma telangiectatum." The so-called pregnancy tumor, or granuloma gravidarum, arising on the gums during pregnancy, is a similar lesion.

Sebaceous cysts, dermoids, and epidermoids. Certain lesions, of epithelial origin, are cystic tumorlike formations in the skin, varying in size from a few millimeters to several centimeters. Within the cyst is a cheesy, grayish white substance composed of keratinized material, desquamated partially cornified cells, and granular debris. (See Fig. 11-16.) The walls are composed of epidermis (epidermoid or epidermal cysts) or may have skin appendages as well, i.e., sweat glands, sebaceous glands, and hair (dermoid cysts). Epidermoid cysts have a tendency to familial and hereditary occurrence, but some are of traumatic origin, as a result of implantation of some surface epithelium in the corium. The dermoid cysts are congenital inclusions of the skin. The term *sebaceous cyst* is often loosely used in referring to almost any cyst of the skin having soft, semisolid contents. However, true retention cysts of sebaceous glands do occur and have sebaceous gland cells as part of the lining. Sebaceous cysts and epidermal cysts, which may not be distinguishable clinically, are often called *wens*.

Chapter 24

The bones, joints, and tendons

T **BONES**

he bones are not inert matter but are active living substance influenced by vascular and biochemical factors, endocrine and nutritional changes, infections, and trauma. The bone marrow has the important function of blood formation.

Bone formation occurs by a process of ossification and calcification. In long bones there is ossification in cartilage (endochondral ossification); i.e., there is first a growth of cartilage, which later degenerates, disappears, and is replaced by bone formed by osteoblastic activity. In flat bones of the skull, bone is formed in membrane (intramembranous ossification) by differentiation of connective tissue cells into osteoblasts, which progressively lay down bone. A long bone increases in length by progressive ossification on the diaphyseal side of the growing epiphyseal cartilage. Increase in width of a bone occurs by the formation of new bone on the surface under the periosteum. With increase in width, the marrow also increases in size because of resorption of adjacent bone by osteoclasts.

In the formation of bone a proper supply of calcium and phosphorus is essential. For this there must be a sufficiency of dietary mineral intake, sufficient vitamin D to promote absorption of calcium, and proper function of the parathyroid glands. The calcium is laid down in bone in the form of a complex calcium phosphate and calcium carbonate compound with the assistance of an enzyme, phosphatase, which hydrolyzes phosphoric esters to form inorganic phosphate. Phosphatase is found in high concentration in growing bone. Vitamin C also is essential for bone formation. Skeletal growth is controlled by the anterior lobe of the hypophysis.

Once deposited in bone, the calcium is not necessarily there permanently but is in a storehouse from which it may be quickly and easily withdrawn. Mobilization of calcium from the bones is brought about by parathyroid hormone. Excess of this hormone will raise the level of calcium in the blood at the expense of the bones. The calcium and phosphate concentration of the blood is very stable and delicately balanced by storage or removal from bones. Bone resorption is generally associated with activity of osteoclasts (bone phagocytes). They may be multinucleated and are similar to foreign body giant cells.

Disturbances of circulation

Like other tissues, bone is dependent on adequate blood supply for preservation of its structure and function. Certain circulatory malformations, e.g., arteriovenous fistula, sometimes affect the circulation of a limb and cause overgrowth of the bone. Necrosis (infarction) occurs in bone when the circulation is seriously reduced. This is commonly a result of trauma, and in fracture some necrosis usually occurs near the ends of the fragments. Fracture or dislocation of the hip may interrupt the blood supply through the ligamentum teres and result in aseptic necrosis of the head of the femur. Blockage of circulation in bone in adults may cause infarction.

Osteodystrophy

The osteodystrophies are a group of conditions in which there is abnormality of development, form, or structure of bone. Some are congenital (achondroplasia), others are caused by endocrine disturbances (osteitis fibrosa cystica) or dietary deficiency (rickets), and yet others are of obscure or unknown origin.

Giantism. The effects of endocrine factors on skeletal growth are well illustrated by the occurence of giantism and dwarfism as a result of endocrine disturbance. Overproduction of the growth hormone of the anterior pituitary during the period of growth produces the most extreme cases of giantism (p. 666). Acromegaly is a skeletal overgrowth resulting from hyperpituitarism in adult life.

Dwarfism. Failure of proper development of the long bones during the growth period may result from hypopituitarism (pituitary dwarfism), hypothyroidism (cretinism), and chronic renal insufficiency (renal dwarfism). In this latter condition hyperplasia of the parathyroids is probably a factor (p. 393). Various other abnormalities of bone development, such as oxycephaly or "tower skull," are more obscure in their cause and pathogenesis.

Chondrodystrophy. Chondrodystrophies (chondrodysplasias) are disturbances in skeletal growth found at birth or developing during childhood and adolescence. Although numerous entities are included under the term, some are specific disorders with a genetic basis, a metabolic defect, and definite sites of involvement.

Most chondrodystrophies can be classified into two groups, those characterized by epiphyseal dysplasia and those with metaphyseal dysplasia. The epiphyseal dysplasias include achondroplasia, spondyloepiphyseal dysplasias (several forms including Morquio's disease), gargoylism (Hunter-Hurler disease), chondroectodermal dysplasia (Ellis–van Creveld disease), and dysplasia epiphysealis punctata. The metaphyseal dysplasias include metaphyseal dysostosis, enchondromatosis (Ollier's disease), and osteochondromatosis (hereditary multiple exostosis).

Achondroplasia. Achondroplasia (chondrodystrophia fetalis) is one of the most frequent forms of dwarfism. There is extreme shortness of the bones of the extremities, while the bones of the trunk and head have developed to normal size. Since endochondral growth and ossification have been deficient, the bones are short but disproportionately thick. The condition is often evident at birth. Intelligence is not affected. There is usually dominant transmission, but some cases occur from spontaneous mutations.

Spondyloepiphyseal dysplasias. Spondyloepiphyseal dysplasias comprise a group of chondrodystrophies in which the disturbances are of the osseous centers of vertebrae, carpal and tarsal bones, and the epiphyses of long bones. They occur in various genetic forms, the autosomal recessive form being known as Morquio's disease, or Morquio-Ullrich disease. A disturbance of mucopolysaccharide metabolism has been demonstrated in the latter disease.

Gargoylism. Gargoylism is characterized by a hereditary, abnormal metabolism of mucopolysaccharides. Various forms of the syndrome were described by Hunter (1917) and Hurler (1919). Gargoyle facies and hepatomegaly are the most constant features, followed by mental retardation; flexion contractures, corneal cloudiness, splenomegaly, and lumbar kyphosis.

Chondroectodermal dysplasia. (Ellis-van Creveld disease) and *dysplasia epiphysealis punctata* are relatively rare genetic chondrodystrophies.

Enchondromatosis. Enchondromatosis (Ollier's disease) is essentially a hamartomatous growth of cartilage cells within the metaphysis of several bones, causing thinning of the overlying cortices and distortion of growth in length. Considerable growth of those cartilage masses occurs mainly in the hands and feet.

Osteochondromatosis. Osteochondromatosis (hereditary multiple exostoses) is transmitted as a dominant trait. A disturbance in proliferation and ossification of bone-forming cartilage results in multiple cartilaginous and osteocartilaginous growths, usually benign and often roughly symmetric. Secondary distortions and deformities of the skeleton may occur, such as inequality of length of limbs.

Osteogenesis imperfecta. Osteogenesis imperfecta (fragilitas ossium) is a hereditary and familial disease in which there is mesenchymal hypoplasia. Blue sclerotics are often present, the sclerotics being thinner than normal and defective in fibrous tissue so that the underlying pigmented choroid shines through. The bones have thin cortices with a decrease in the cancellous elements. The trabeculae of the medulla are delicate and widely separated. The delicate bones fracture with extreme ease, and

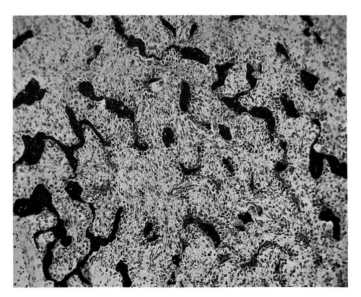

Fig. 24-1. Osteogenesis imperfecta. Very delicate, well-calcified bone trabeculae within fibrous tissue. Osteoblasts of irregular shape and arrangement. (Courtesy Dr. W. H. Bauer.)

affected infants are often born with multiple fractures. In other cases fractures and deformity develop later. Healing occurs with abundant callus but poor ossification. There is an increase of the acid mucopolysaccharide content of the cartilage of the epiphyses and the long bones, which may inhibit ossification. There is a characteristic disturbance of dentine, similar to that in the bones. Deafness caused by otosclerosis develops in many cases. Aminoaciduria and low blood creatinine may also be found.

Osteopetrosis. In osteopetrosis (marble bone or Albers-Schön-berg disease) great increase occurs in the thickness and density of the bones, and profound anemia (osteosclerotic anemia) develops because of encroachment on the hemopoietic tissue of the marrow. The ultimate cause is unknown, but there seems to be a familial factor. The vertebrae, pelvic bones, base of the skull, proximal ends of the femora, and distal ends of the tibiae are most affected. Although of increased density, the bones are chalky and tend to fracture more easily than normal.

Skeletal lesions in nutritional deficiencies. Skeletal lesions form a prominent feature in *scurvy* caused by vitamin C deficiency (p. 250), in *rickets* caused by vitamin D deficiency (p. 253), and in *osteomalacia*. Osteomalacia is the adult counterpart of rickets caused by a deficient supply of calcium and vitamin D. It is rare except in countries where undernutrition is great, occurs almost exclusively in women, and is aggravated by the high calcium demand of pregnancy. The lumbar vertebrae, pelvis, and long bones of the lower limbs are most affected, and severe pelvic deformities may interfere with childbirth. The changes are less limited to growing ends of bones than in rickets. A large proportion of poorly calcified osteoid tissue composes the soft bones, so that they are gradually bent and deformed by muscles and tendons. The bone marrow is fibrous, gelatinous, and sometimes hemorrhagic, and, as in rickets, the parathyroids are often found to be enlarged.

Osteoporosis. Osteoporosis is a reduction in the amount of calcified bone mass per unit volume of skeletal tissue. The commonest form, *senile osteoporosis,* occurs in the aged. The spine, pelvis, and peripheral limb bones are affected earliest and most severely. The cause is uncertain. Although lessened physical activity has been considered to have a role, hormonal changes such as diminished estrogen or androgen appear to be more important. Deficiency of dietary calcium intake does not appear to

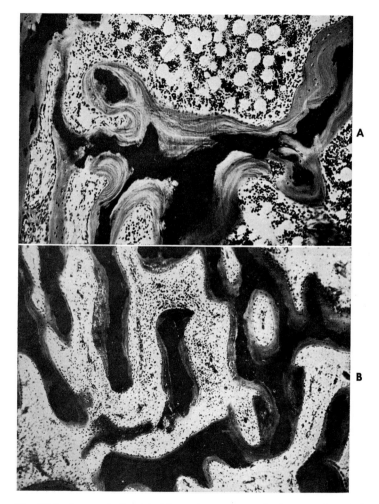

Fig. 24-2. Osteomalacia and rickets. **A,** Osteomalacia (symphysis pubis). Well-calcified remnants of old bone are coated with extremely wide osteoid tissue. **B,** Rickets. Note the broad osteoid zones surrounding well-calcified bone trabeculae.

be an important factor. There is increased liability to fractures and deformity.

In the *postmenopausal osteoporosis* of women, hypoestrinism appears to be the cause. A lack of estrogen leads to an inadequate formation of bone matrix because of insufficient stimulation of osteoblasts. Excess of corticosteroids, as in *Cushing's syndrome* or after the administration of *cortisone or ACTH,* also leads to inadequate stimulation of osteoblasts. Generalized osteoporosis is also seen in clinical states characterized by decreased formation of matrix because of an insufficient amount of available protein and vitamin C, as in *nutritional deficiency states,* or because of an increased catabolism of protein, as in *hyperthyroidism* and *diabetes mellitus.* A local osteoporosis involving individual bones may be seen; e.g., osteoporosis in a single bone after immobilization or localized osteoporosis (atrophy) in an area of a bone being compressed by a tumor or an aneurysm.

Fibrous dysplasia. Polyostotic fibrous dysplasia of bone (osteitis fibrosa disseminata) appears to be a defect of development involving mainly bone but sometimes extraskeletal tissues as well. Symptoms of pain, disability, and deformity of a limb usually begin in childhood, and the disease runs a slow and protracted course. The skeletal lesions, usually multiple, are entirely or predominantly unilateral and are commonest in the femur and tibia. The lesions are roentgenologically similar to those of osteitis fibrosa, but uninvolved skeletal areas show no decalcification. Serum calcium is normal or only slightly elevated, calcium balance and serum phosphorus are normal, and serum phosphatase is increased. In some cases there are pigmented areas of the skin. In another small group of cases in girls, precocious skeletal and sexual maturation occur in addition to the cutaneous pigmentation and fibrous dysplasia of bone (Albright's syndrome).

A monostotic form of fibrous dysplasia is also described that has none of the clinical or metabolic features of the polyostotic form. Some investigators consider the monostotic form as an entity distinct from polyostotic fibrous dysplasia.

The lesions show a thinning of the cortex of the bone and a replacement of the spongiosa and marrow by a rubbery whitish fibrous tissue, which is gritty from the presence of spicules of newly formed bone. Cyst formation is absent, although there may be small areas of focal cystic degeneration. Micro-

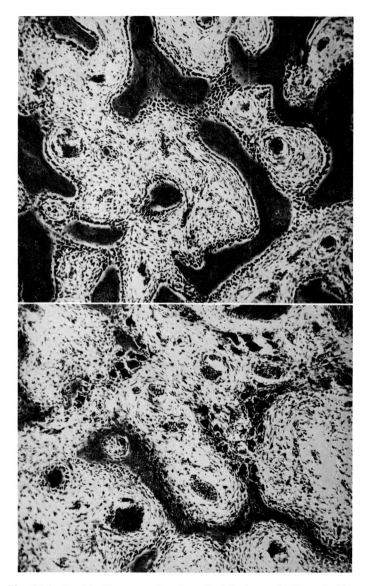

Fig. 24-3. Osteitis fibrosa cystica (von Recklinghausen's disease). Note the irregular arrangement of newly formed bone trabeculae, which exhibit narrow osteoid zones and osteoclastic resorption. The marrow is fibrous and hyperemic.

scopically, fibrous tissue replaces the spongiosa and fills the marrow cavity and is irregularly traversed by tiny trabeculae of primitive, poorly calcified new bone. Small islands of hyaline cartilage may be present.

Generalized osteitis fibrosa cystica. Osteitis fibrosa cystica (von Recklinghausen's disease) is caused by hypersecretion of parathyroid hormone, usually the result of an adenoma in one gland. It is characterized by distortion of the skeleton because of the lack of sufficient mineralization and replacement of the osseous tissues and marrow spaces by fibrous tissue. In advanced cases there are so-called giant cell tumors and cysts. Associated with the disease one finds decreased neuromuscular sensitivity to galvanic stimulation, hypercalcemia and hypophosphatemia, increased serum phosphatase, and often metastatic calcification in other tissues, particularly the kidney.

The change in osteitis fibrosa is essentially an osteoclastic resorption of bone and its replacement by connective tissue in which there are abortive attempts at new bone formation. This may be of any degree. When mild, the gross change in the bones is merely a slight porousness and, microscopically, mild generalized osteoporosis and marrow fibrosis. With progression of the condition there is more and more loss of osseous tissue, which is replaced by connective tissue. Immature, poorly calcified bone develops in the connective tissue. The newly formed bone soon may again undergo resorption. Osteoclasts are abundant. Large fibrous scars develop in the place of the original spongy bone. Some of the lesions are brownish and are often called brown or giant cell tumors, although they are not true neoplasms. The brown tumors are areas of round and spindle cells, fibroblasts, and giant cells. The giant cells show phagocytosis of red cells or hemosiderin, which imparts the brown color to the lesion.

Cysts are not always formed, and the presence of neither cysts nor brown tumors is necessary for the diagnosis. The cysts may be minute or large, single, multilocular, or multiple. They result from degeneration or hemorrhage and are lined by connective tissue.

When osteitis fibrosa is severe, the involved bones are soft, easily deformed or cut, and the skeletal lesions may be varied, with extreme decalcification, deformities, cysts, and giant cell formation. The long bones and spine are most involved, followed by the pelvis, skull, and jaw. The degree of functional stress and strain apparently is a factor in localization.

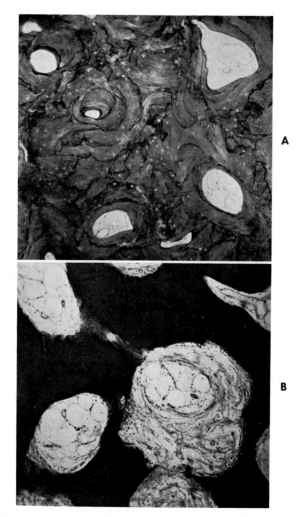

Fig. 24-4. Paget's disease of the bone. **A,** Note the mosaic structure. **B,** Fibrosis of the fatty marrow is proceeding from the periphery of the marrow space.

Hypertrophic pulmonary osteoarthropathy. In hypertrophic pulmonary osteoarthropathy there is symmetric enlargement (clubbing) of the distal phalanges of the fingers and toes, with swelling of the joints. Subperiosteal deposition of bone is increased, with thickening of connective tissue around the bone and joint. These changes are usually associated with conditions of chronic anoxemia or with some toxemia. Chronic lung abscess, bronchiectasis, empyema, pulmonary tumors, and congenital cardiac defects are conditions with which this phalangeal lesion is often associated.

Osteitis deformans (Paget's disease of bone). Paget's disease of bone is a curious condition which usually occurs in persons after the age of 50 years. It is characterized by osteoclastic resorption of bone and simultaneous overgrowth of new, poorly calcified, irregular bony spicules. There is also excessive periosteal growth of bone with deficient calcification. The result is an increase in thickness of bones with simultaneous distinct softening, so that severe bowing or other deformities occur. The spine, sacrum, femur, cranium, sternum, pelvis, tibia, and jaws are most commonly involved. The blood phosphatase is high, but blood calcium and phosphorus concentrations are not changed. The calcium balance is positive, and the parathyroid glands are apparently uninvolved. Osteogenic sarcoma may be a late feature of some cases and has a very poor prognosis.

Grossly the thickened bones are often extremely soft, light, and porous, although in late stages a more hardened state may develop. Microscopically there is evidence of osteoclastic resorption and formation of new bony trabeculae. Between the new trabeculae there is an excessive amount of loose connective tissue. Irregularly shaped plates of new and old bone stain with varying degrees of density and are separated by irregular lines of ground substance, a feature that imparts a mosaic appearance to the bony tissue. This mosaic arrangement is the diagnostic characteristic of the microscopic appearance of the bone in fully developed Paget's disease. Increased vascularity often appears in the lesions, and this may behave in the manner of an arteriovenous fistula, resulting in cardiac hypertrophy and failure.

Aseptic necrosis

One form of aseptic necrosis of bone is the result of an interruption of the circulation such as occurs at the site of a fracture, which was mentioned previously. A second form is idiopathic aseptic necrosis, which occurs most commonly in the epiphyses of growing children. *Osteochondritis deformans* (Legg-Perthes disease, coxa plana) is a caries and rarefaction of the head of the femur in children 5 to 10 years of age. A similar rarefaction of bone affects the tibial tubercle in *Osgood-Schlatter disease,* the tarsal scaphoid in *Köhler's disease,* and the semilunar bone of the wrist in *Kienböck's disease. Osteochondritis dissecans* is an aseptic necrosis involving subchondral bone, with secondary changes in adjacent cartilage, which may show softening and degeneration. The involved tissue may be extruded, forming a loose body in the joint. Most cases occur in young adults, the knee being most often involved. Trauma is usually considered a causative factor.

Inflammatory lesions

The skeletal tissues, like the soft tissues of the body, respond to injuries by a process of inflammation. In many cases the injurious agent is of bacterial nature, as in osteomyelitis caused by staphylococci, but other inflammatory processes are of more obscure etiology. In the acute inflammation it is the periosteum, the contents of the haversian canals, and the bone marrow that are mainly involved. In the more chronic processes changes in the osseous portions are also prominent, as in this case there is time for changes to occur in the hard tissues.

Osteomyelitis. Bacteria may reach bone directly through a wound (e.g., a compound fracture), may spread to bone from an adjacent tissue (e.g., from a suppurative infection of a tooth or of the middle ear), or may be brought to bone by the bloodstream from a distant focus of inflammation (e.g., in tonsillitis). When the inflammation is restricted to periosteum, it is properly called a periostitis, and when involving bone substance, an osteitis. In most cases bone and marrow tissue are involved as well as periosteum, and the term *osteomyelitis* is commonly used.

Acute hematogenous osteomyelitis is mainly a disease of childhood and is rare after the age of 30 years. It is usually caused by the *Staphylococcus aureus,* but in rare cases it is caused by streptococci or typhoid bacilli. The original focus of the organisms is often not discoverable, although sometimes it is an obvious furuncle or carbuncle. At the onset, fever, local pain, and leukocytosis occur. Radiologic changes in the involved bone are not discernible in the early acute stage.

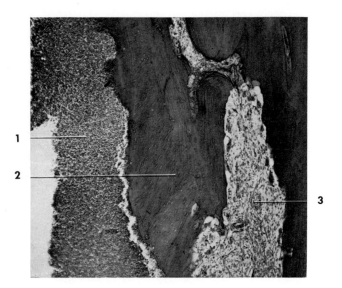

Fig. 24-5. Acute osteomyelitis with the formation of a sequestrum: **1,** pus; **2,** formation of sequestrum; **3,** granulation tissue. (From Weinmann, J. P., and Sicher, H.: Bone and bones, ed. 2, St. Louis, 1955, The C. V. Mosby Co.)

The affected focus is usually in a long bone of an extremity and situated close to the end of the diaphysis near the epiphyseal cartilage, or it is more superficial and lying just beneath peri-osteum. These are situations in a growing bone that have rel-atively high vascularity and are subject to trauma. Spread of the infection may be outward to form a subperiosteal abscess and inward to reach the central canal and thence spread widely in the bone. In most cases the epiphyseal cartilage opposes spread to the epiphysis. Purulent exudate forms and may be seen in the haversian canals, marrow spaces, and beneath the peri-osteum. Fragments of bone become necrotic, influenced by thrombosis of haversian vessels. This dead bone (sequestrum) undergoes digestion and removal only very slowly and with great difficulty. Its continued presence prolongs the inflamma-tion and prevents healing. An irregular casing of new bone (involucrum) may form around the sequestrum. Occasional complications of acute osteomyelitis include extension into a joint, formation of fistulous tracts, and pyemia. Some cases become chronic and persist for years with draining fistulous tracts. Amyloidosis may occur in such cases.

Brodie's abscess is a circumscribed focal chronic osteomyelitis. In most cases the chronic abscess is found in the upper end of the tibia. It may be the sequel of an acute osteomyelitis with organisms of low virulence.

Nonsuppurative nonspecific inflammation. There sometimes occurs a localized condition which is apparently of inflammatory nature but in which specific etiology is unknown. *Sclerosing osteitis* (Garré's disease) is an example and is characterized by intense pain in a local area of dense cortical bone.

Syphilis. Syphilis, either congenital or acquired, may produce a chronic osteitis, osteochondritis, or periostitis. In congenital syphilis, osteochondritis of a long bone is particularly characteristic. The epiphyseal line is irregularly widened, opaque, and yellowish gray in color. Microscopically there is great irregularity of bone formation in this area, with a chronic inflammatory reaction and severe endarteritis and periarteritis. In acquired syphilis there may develop an actual gumma or a chronic fibroproliferative periosteal infection of bones with spread into the subjacent bony tissue. Periarteritis and endarteritis are also prominent in the skeletal lesions.

Tuberculosis. A chronic granulomatous form of osteomyelitis is caused by the tubercle bacillus. Children are the victims more frequently than adults. The bovine form of the organism accounts for a small proportion of cases. The infection is brought to bone by the bloodstream in most cases, although the primary focus is often insignificant and may be difficult to find. The vertebrae, ends of the long bones of the legs, and bones of the hands and feet are the most frequent sites. Bony trabeculae are gradually destroyed and replaced by tuberculous granulomas or by caseous and creamy material. In long bones either the epiphysis or the diaphysis is involved, and spread often occurs to the adjacent joint.

Tuberculosis of the vertebrae (Pott's disease of the spine). This disease usually occurs during childhood. Several vertebrae may be involved. The lesions start in the bodies, produce bony destruction, and spread similarly to destroy adjacent intervertebral discs. Thus weakened, the affected vertebrae tend to collapse, producing an acute anteflexion or angular kyphosis.

Complications include compression of the spinal cord and extension of the tuberculous pus to produce a "cold abscess," which may burrow beneath the psoas muscle and appears as a swelling in the inguinal region.

Eosinophilic granuloma

Eosinophilic or solitary granuloma of bone occurs mainly in children and adolescents. Although several bones may be affected, more commonly only one is involved. The lesion may be seen in almost any bone except those of the hands or feet and gives rise to local pain and tenderness. Systemic manifestations are usually absent. The blood may show a leukocytosis or eosinophilia in some cases.

The involved area of bone shows a soft brownish tissue, which may have yellowish streaks or regions of hemorrhage and cyst formation. Microscopically there are collections of phagocytic large mononuclear cells, among which are eosinophilic leukocytes and lesser numbers of multinucleated giant cells, lymphocytes, and plasma cells. In late stages the eosinophils may be scarce, the large mononuclear cells have abundant foamy cytoplasm, and fibrosis develops. The prognosis is good, as the lesions heal after radiation or curettement, or even spontaneously. It has been suggested that multiple eosinophilic granuloma is a variant of the basic process of histiocytosis, other examples of which are Hand-Schüller-Christian disease and Letterer-Siwe disease.

Traumatic injury

Minor injuries may cause a localized periostitis. In some cases this is accompanied by overgrowth of osteoid tissue (callus) in the injured area. More severe injuries may cause *fracture*. In children relative elasticity of the bone may allow bending without a complete break *(greenstick fracture)*. In elderly persons bones are relatively brittle and fracture with slight trauma. In other cases very minor trauma may cause a *"spontaneous" fracture* when the bone is weakened by tumor growth or systemic disease. *Compound fractures,* in which there is communication with the exterior, are often complicated by infection. In *comminuted fractures* the bone is broken into more than two fragments.

Healing of a fracture occurs readily if the broken ends are in apposition and movement is limited. Muscle or other structures between the broken ends may prevent healing, infection

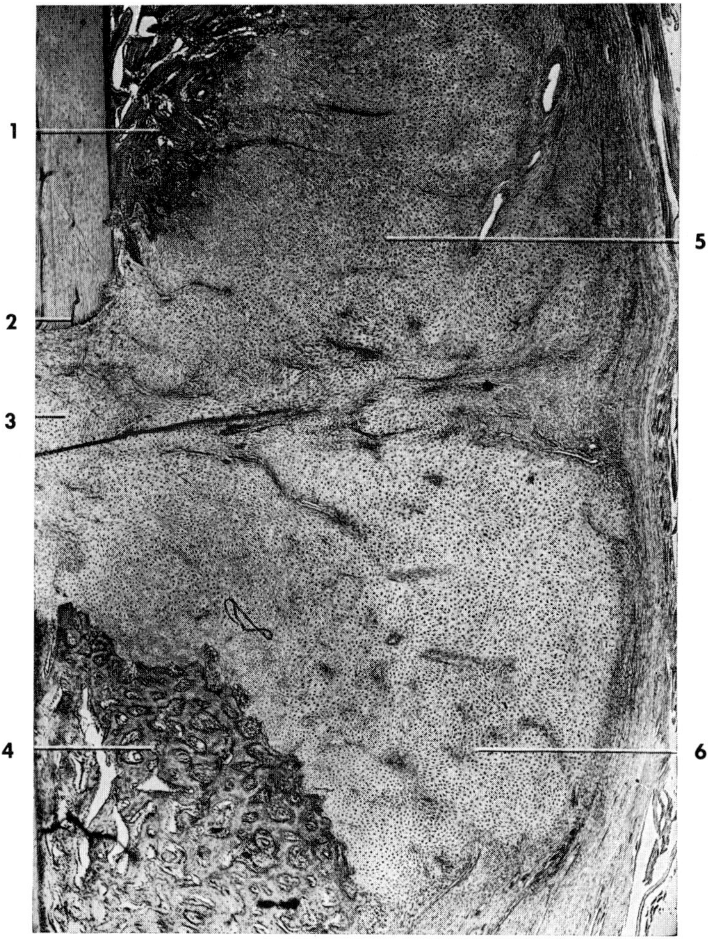

Fig. 24-6. Callus two weeks after an experimental fracture of the tibia of a cat: 1 and 4, anchoring callus; 2, fracture; 3, uniting callus; 5 and 6, bridging callus. (From Weinmann, J. P., and Sicher, H.: Bone and bones, ed. 2, St. Louis, 1955, The C. V. Mosby Co.)

retards repair, and excessive movement tends to promote fibrous and cartilaginous rather than bony union. When a bone is fractured, hemorrhage and exudation occur between and around the broken ends. This material becomes organized by granulation tissue growth. Osteoblastic activity in the periosteum and endosteum produces an overgrowth of osteoid tissue (callus) in the area. This becomes calcified and converted into bone. The excess callus in the medullary and external parts is gradually removed, and the new bone is knit and shaped by osteoclasts until healing is complete.

Tumors

Tumors arising in the skeletal tissues are of mesenchymal origin, and hence their malignant representatives are sarcomas. Most bone tumors tend to arise at the ends of bones near epiphyseal lines in areas where there are complexities of growth and function. Tumors of bone are uncommon. Malignancies of bone probably represent about 1% of all malignant tumors. The tumors may arise (1) from external parts of periosteal tissues (periosteal fibrosarcoma), (2) from the body of the bone (osteogenic tumors), or (3) from the medulla (myeloma, Ewing's tumor). From the standpoint of malignancy and prognosis there are likewise three classes: (1) benign curable tumors, which include exostosis, osteoma, chondroma of the phalanges, osteoid osteoma, fibroma, bone cyst, and most giant cell tumors; (2) tumors of borderline malignancy and hopeful prognosis, including central chondroma; and (3) malignant tumors, many of which are incurable, including myeloma, Ewing's tumor, etc. A modification of a commonly used classification will be used here and is as follows:

> Periosteal fibrosarcoma
> Osteogenic tumors
> > Benign
> > > Exostosis
> > > Osteoma
> > > Osteoid osteoma
> > > Chondroma
> > > Benign chondroblastoma
> > > Fibroma
> > Malignant (osteogenic sarcoma and chondrosarcoma)
> Giant cell tumor
> Angioma
> > Benign
> > Malignant

Periosteal fibrosarcoma. Periosteal fibrosarcoma is a very rare tumor, most frequent in males in early adult life. It arises from the fibrous layer of the periosteum and resembles sarcoma arising from other connective tissue structures. The tumor is single and is most frequent in long bones such as the femur and ulna. It forms a fairly large, firm, whitish, circumscribed tumor, the underlying bone usually showing destructive and sometimes reactive changes. Microscopically it is similar to fibrosarcoma arising elsewhere.

Osteogenic tumors. Osteogenic tumors are those that arise from mesenchymal cells having the power to differentiate into and form cartilage and bone. The differentiation may be of varying degrees of completeness. In the benign forms the differentiation is advanced, so that on a histologic basis such tumors may be termed osteomas, chondromas, fibromas, osteochondromas, osteochondrofibromas, etc. In the malignant forms (osteogenic sarcoma and chondrosarcoma) the formation of bone and cartilage may be very irregular and is atypical.

Exostosis. Exostoses (osteochondromas) are benign bony or cartilaginous and bony outgrowths from the surface near the end of a long bone. They occur usually in persons between the ages of 10 and 25 years. Microscopically they show normal laminae of bone beneath a zone of calcifying cartilage, which in turn is thinly overlaid by fibrous tissue. *Hereditary multiple exostoses* is a developmental disturbance in which bilateral and symmetric lesions appear in juxtaepiphyseal areas. Chondrosarcomatous change sometimes occurs in one of the exostoses.

Osteoma. Osteomas are rare benign tumors composed of compact bone. The term *cancellous osteoma* is sometimes used to refer to the exostosis or osteochondroma.

Osteoid osteoma. Osteoid osteoma is a small benign tumor that may be found in almost any bone but most frequently in the tibia or femur. It occurs mainly in adolescent children or young adults, and pain is the outstanding clinical feature. The tumor consists of a small, well-defined, rounded central nidus, sharply demarcated from a surrounding zone of bone thickening or sclerosis. The central nidus is only a few millimeters or up to a centimeter in diameter. It consists of a network of osteoid tissue and trabeculae of partly calcified osseous tissue set in a matrix of highly vascular osteogenic connective tissue containing abundant osteoblasts and some osteoclasts. Surgical removal relieves the pain, and there is no recurrence.

Chondroma. Chondroma (enchondroma) is a benign cartilaginous tumor occurring in the small bones of the hands and feet, ribs, sternum, and spine, usually in persons between the ages of 20 and 30 years. Most frequent in the phalanges of the hand, it produces a central area of rarefaction. Those arising in or about the sternum are larger tumors. Grossly they are lobulated or trabeculated, are pearly gray, and may be gelatinous or cystic. Microscopically they are composed of fairly normal cartilage, the cartilage cells lying in pairs or tetrads in small lacunae. Certain of the cartilaginous tumors that appear to have a benign histologic structure exhibit erratic or malignant behavior and should be considered chondrosarcomas.

Benign chondroblastoma. Benign chondroblastoma is a neoplasm characterized by cartilaginous and giant cell elements that has been variously called a "calcifying giant cell tumor" and Codman's tumor. It occurs in young persons, most frequently during the second decade, and most often involves the upper end of the humerus. Although often very cellular and sometimes causing considerable destruction of bone, it acts in benign fashion and is satisfactorily treated by curettement or local removal.

Fibroma. Fibroma is a rare tumor of bone, usually arising from periosteum in the nasopharyngeal (p. 587) or maxillary regions.

Mesenchymal chondrosarcoma. Recently described, mesenchymal chondrosarcoma is a multicentric tumor composed of an undifferentiated cellular stroma with focal areas of chondroid differentiation. Sometimes there are zones with a clustering of the small cells about capillary vessels. Arising in various bones in young adults or those of middle age, metastases develop in various and sometimes unusual locations. Recurrences are common after therapy. Death from the malignant lesion is after variable but sometimes long periods.

Chondrosarcoma. Chondrosarcoma may be primary or may result from a malignant change occurring in a benign chondroma. The presence of cellular areas consisting of atypical, ir-

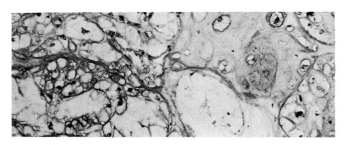

Fig. 24-7. Chondrosarcoma. The neoplastic cartilage cells are very irregular in their arrangement, size, shape, and nuclear staining.

regularly arranged cartilage cells with large, sometimes multiple, hyperchromatic nuclei, dispersed throughout a hyaline matrix, differentiates chondrosarcoma from the benign chondroma. Compared to osteogenic sarcomas as a whole, chondrosarcomas occur predominantly in adults between 30 to 50 years of age and have a relatively low degree of malignancy.

Osteogenic sarcoma. Osteogenic sarcoma is composed of osteoblastic (bone-forming) cells, which may be derived from the inner layer of periosteum or from the endosteum. It is the most frequent malignant tumor of bone. The greatest incidence is in young people between 10 and 30 years of age. The prognosis of this tumor is extremely poor. The common site is in the shaft of a long bone but near the epiphysis. About 50% occur around the knee. There is often a history of trauma to the area. Local pain at the site is followed by swelling. Osteogenic sarcoma is radioresistant.

The tumor begins quite superficially but extends both outward and inward, so that subperiosteal and endosteal growth occurs. In late stages the tumor produces a massive bulbous enlargement of the end of the bone. There may be a bone-destructive (osteolytic) action or a bone-forming (sclerosing or osteoplastic) reaction induced by the tumor. In an x-ray plate of the tumor, radiating spicules of newly formed bone may result in a ·characteristic "sun-ray" appearance. Histologically the picture is extremely variable and complex, and skeletal tissue in all stages of differentiation and development may be found. In some cases marked vascularity, hemorrhage, and necrosis are prominent features (telangiectatic type). The tumor, sometimes referred to as osteosarcoma, usually spreads by the bloodsteam

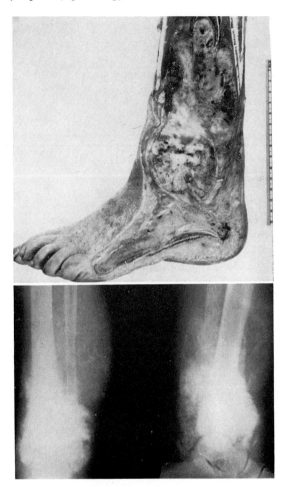

Fig. 24-8. Osteogenic sarcoma.

to many organs, especially the lungs, but seldom to other bones.

Osoteogenic sarcoma develops in extraskeletal soft tissues as a rare event. It must be distinguished from a similar, benign lesion, which is an atypical form of myositis ossificans. The malignant lesion is distinguished by its cellularity, cellular pleomorphism, mitoses, and atypical osteoid tissue.

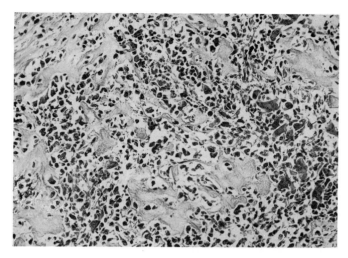

Fig. 24-9. Osteogenic sarcoma. The neoplastic cells are polymorphous with some multinucleated giant cell forms. Irregular areas of osteoid tissue are present.

In experimental animals, osteogenic sarcomas have been produced by radioactive calcium or strontium deposited in the skeleton.

Giant cell tumor. Giant cell tumor usually involves the epiphyseal region of a long bone. It occurs in early adult life but is uncommon before the age of 20 years. Pathologic fracture may occur. Grossly the affected skeletal area is expanded and outlined by a thin shell of bone. The tumor tissue is dark red or reddish brown in color and of a fleshy or friable consistency. Dark red areas of hemorrhage or yellowish areas of necrosis may be present. Hemorrhage and necrosis sometimes lead to a cystic change. The x-ray picture is characteristic, the tumor producing a rarefied, multilocular cystic or bubblelike appearance. Microscopically the tumor consists of spindle-shaped or ovoid cells, highly vascularized and resembling young connective tissue. Varying numbers of multinucleated giant cells are interspersed. The many nuclei of the giant cells tend to accumulate in the center of the cell.

There are differing theories of origin of these tumors. It is

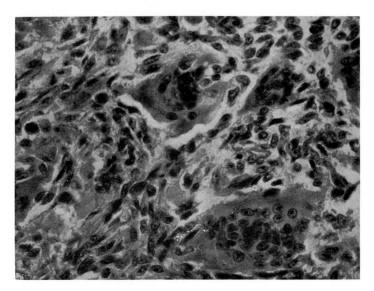

Fig. 24-10. Giant cell tumor of the bone. (AFIP No. 63505, courtesy Dr. G. A. Bennett.)

believed by some that the giant cells represent osteoclasts, and hence the tumor has been called an osteoclastoma. Others have suggested that it arises from undifferentiated supporting connective tissue of the marrow or that it is a tissue reaction to trauma and hemorrhage which may later acquire neoplastic character. Histologically similar tumors are the giant cell epulis (p. 582), the giant cell tumor of tendon sheaths (p. 862), and the so-called giant cell tumors that occur in osteitis fibrosa cystica (hyperparathyroidism).

Most of the giant cell tumors of bone are perfectly benign. The uncommon malignant examples are characterized by abundant compact stromal cells with marked anaplasia, pleomorphism, and a tendency to a whorled arrangement. However, occasional examples of malignant giant cell tumors have not been histologically distinguishable from the ordinary benign giant cell tumors. Some reported malignant giant cell tumors have contained osteoid tissue and appear related to osteogenic sarcoma.

Angioma. Angioma is an uncommon tumor of bone that

may be benign or malignant. It is similar to angiomatous tumors elsewhere. The malignant angiosarcoma is very uncommon. Rare cases of benign osseous angiomatosis have an associated "massive osteolysis" with progressive localized resorption of bone and resultant deformity.

Ewing's tumor (endothelial myeloma). Ewing's tumor occurs in childhood or adolescence and involves the shaft of a long bone. It is accompanied by severe pain, fever, and leukocytosis and hence is easily mistaken for acute osteomyelitis. Its growth in the shaft stimulates reactive formation of multiple new laminae of bone, presenting a layered, onionlike appearance in an x-ray picture. The tumor is highly radiosensitive, a characteristic often of diagnostic help, but cure by radiation therapy alone is rare.

The soft grayish tumor starts in the medulla but rapidly invades and expands the bone. The tibia, femur, humerus, fibula, and clavicle are the most frequent sites. Often more than one bone is involved. Microscopically it is composed of small, round uniform cells of lymphoblastic appearance, arranged in solid sheets and columns or around blood vessels. The lack of stroma is conspicuous. By silver stains reticulin can be demonstrated surrounding groups of cells.

The origin of this tumor was originally believed to be from vascular endothelium (i.e., an endothelial myeloma). It also has been considered to be derived from young reticular cells, although primary reticulum cell sarcoma of bone is said to be distinguishable by reticulin running between individual cells, or coarser collagenous material may separate the cells into small clusters or rows. Lymphocytes may be numerous in a reticulum cell sarcoma.

Adamantinoma. Adamantinoma is an epithelial tumor usually occurring in the jaw and having a histologic structure resembling the enamel body (p. 584). Rare examples of adamantinoma (so-called) have been found in the tibia or ulna, where they have been considered by some to be primary bone tumors showing synovial differentiation (synovial sarcoma), by others to be malignant angioblastomas, or to be derived from an embryonal rest of ectoderm. They grow slowly and are locally invasive.

Multiple myeloma. Multiple myeloma, or generalized myelomatosis, is a fatal disease of later life, more than 95% of cases being persons over the age of 40 years. After diagnosis the average length of life is 1½ to 2 years. Rarely persons have survived up to 10 years. Persons with Bence Jones proteinuria have a relatively unfavorable outlook. Bone pain, most often in the spine and ribs, is the most frequent beginning. The bone pains are severe, and the bones become weak and brittle, so that fractures occur easily. Roentgenograms may show osteolytic, punched-out lesions or generalized resorption of bone or both. Generalized resorption is only recognizable radiologically after 20 to 40% of calcium has disappeared and so usually is evident only in later stages of the disease. Numerous punched-out osteolytic lesions may be seen in the skull ("sieve skull"). Refractory anemia commonly occurs, and there may be some leukopenia. Hypercalciuria is present in about 50% of patients with multiple myeloma, but alkaline phosphatase is not increased. Renal complications and uremia are frequent. Depositions of amyloid (or paramyloid) occur in about 10% of cases.

Myelomatosis is a malignant proliferation of immature plasma cells. There is a generalized infiltration of bone marrow by plasmablasts. Localized tumorous overgrowth form grayish red soft tumors, surrounded by a thin shell of softened bone.

Myelomatosis is to be distinguished from plasmacytosis, an increase in the number of normal plasma cells. Bone marrow plasmacytosis occurs in diseases in which serum gamma globulin is increased, such as sarcoidosis, lupus erythematosus, hepatic cirrhosis, kala-azar, lymphopathia venereum. Increased numbers of mature plasma cells may also occur with some lymphomas, in severe drug reactions, and in cases of agranulocytosis. The immature plasma cells of myelomatosis are more readily differentiated in smears than in decalcified bone marrow sections. The nuclei of the myeloma cells are surrounded by an areola of brightly stained cytoplasm, one or more nucleoli are often seen, and mitoses or multinucleated cells are not infrequent. Hyaline vacuoles may be present in the cytoplasm, may fill the cytoplasm (Mott cells), and may extend to the outer limit of the cytoplasm, which becomes wavy and irregular ("grape cells" of Stich). The grape cells are said to be pathognomonic for multiple myeloma, and the vacuoles, which contain neutral mucoproteins, stain deeply with Giemsa or Wright stains. The cytoplasm of myeloma cells may also contain fuchsinophilic inclusions (Russell bodies), which consist mainly of gamma globulins rich in glycoproteins.

In multiple myeloma, abnormal proteins that are practically specific are demonstrable by electrophoretic methods in serum, urine, or both. Bence Jones protein, which is found in about 50% of cases of multiple myeloma, can also be found in macroglobulinemia. Bence Jones demonstrated the protein as a precipitate in urine made strongly acid and characterized by disappearance of the precipitate on boiling. Trace amounts may also be demonstrable in serum by immunoelectrophoresis.

In more than 60% of patients with multiple myeloma there is hyperglobulinemia, which is mainly an increase of gamma globulins. Gamma globulins are produced within the cytoplasm of plasma cells. The myeloma cells produce immunoglobulins or fragments of globulins (Bence Jones protein), not as a cellular response to antigenic stimulation but as products of the abnormal myeloma cells. In patterns produced by electrophoresis the increased globulin of myeloma produces a steep, high, and narrow-based spike ("church spire peak"). Gamma 2 globulins, which react as cryoglobulins, also may be present in myelomatosis.

In about 10% of cases of multiple myeloma an amyloid material (paramyloid) may be present, most often deposited in muscle, subcutaneous tissue, lymph nodes, and vessel walls. In viscera the paramyloid is mainly in blood vessel walls. The complication of paramyloid deposition occurs mainly in cases having Bence Jones protein in the urine but with little or no hyperglobulinemia. Deposition of paramyloid in the tongue may produce a striking macroglossia. Skin papules may result from subcutaneous accumulation, hoarseness from involvement of the larynx, and heart failure from myocardial deposition. Paramyloid deposition on the synovial membranes of joints is unique to myelomatosis.

Renal complications in myeloma patients with Bence Jones proteinuria are mainly caused by tubular obstruction by the precipitated protein. Proximal convoluted tubules as well as more distant parts of the nephrons may be obstructed and the tubular lining cells injured. Bence Jones protein casts often elicit a giant cell reaction. Nephrocalcinosis and renal stones also may develop.

Rare cases of benign plasmacytomas of bone have been observed, with the absence of Bence Jones proteinuria, no hyperglobulinemia, and absence of generalized involvement of bone marrow by plasma cells. Plasmacytomas outside the skeleton may occur, mainly in regions of the upper part of the respiratory tract and oropharynx.

Metastatic tumors. Certain tumors metastasize to skeletal tissues with particular frequency. These include hypernephroma of the kidney and carcinomas of the prostate, lung, ovary, breast, testis, and thyroid. A large proportion of metastatic tumors in the skeleton are from bronchogenic carcinomas. Spread is by the bloodstream, and the spine, pelvis, femur, skull, ribs, and humerus are the most frequent sites. The secondary tumors are often multiple, and pathologic fractures are not uncommon. The metastases are osteolytic or bone-destroying, except in the case of carcinoma of the prostate and some well-differentiated mammary carcinomas, which often stimulate an osteosclerotic or bone-forming reaction. The undifferentiated bronchogenic tumors may cause little or no bony reaction.

Inflammatory conditions simulating tumor. Some of the difficulties in differentiation of Ewing's tumor and osteomyelitis have been pointed out. *Myositis ossificans* is a condition in which bone develops in muscle tissue. It usually follows trauma and hemorrhage and occurs most frequently in the quadriceps or in muscle about the elbow. The ossification may be extensive and simulate osteogenic sarcoma, and in rare cases there is actual development of malignancy. Parosteal and periosteal forms of posttraumatic ossification also occur. *Osteoperiostitis* is a benign condition in which areas of ossification develop in granulation tissue or hemorrhage beneath a raised periosteum. It is usually of traumatic or syphilitic origin. *Osteitis fibrosa*, in which the lesions microscopically simulate giant cell tumor, is considered on p. 834. *Solitary bone cyst* occurs near the end of the shaft of a long bone, most often in the upper part of the shaft of the humerus. Of unknown etiology, it is seen most often in childhood or adolescence. The cyst is lined by fibrous tissue. Fracture through the weakened area of bone is a common complication.

Phosphatase

Phosphatase is an enzyme capable of hydrolyzing monophosphoric esters. It is present in highest concentration in renal tissue, intestinal mucosa, and growing bone. In the latter site it is important in the process of ossification. Phosphatases that exhibit maximum activity in alkaline and in acid media exist and, respectively, are called alkaline and acid phosphatase. Serum acid phosphatase often is increased in patients with carcinoma of the prostate. The level of alkaline phosphatase in the serum is fairly constant for age periods. It is increased in skeletal diseases associated with great osteoblastic activity and in certain other conditions (e.g., jaundice). See Table 24-1.

JOINTS

Movable joints have a capsule around cartilage-covered ends of bones and are lined by a synovial membrane, which encloses a cavity containing a small amount of lubricating fluid. The joint is formed of connective tissue derivatives. It functions as an organ of support and passive motion and is affected by mechanical, circulatory, neurologic, and inflammatory changes. Diseases of joints may be classified as (1) specific infectious arthritis, (2) arthritis of rheumatic fever, (3) rheumatoid arthritis (including Still's disease and Marie-Strümpell spondylitis), (4) osteoarthritis, (5) arthritis of traumatic origin, (6) arthritis

Table 24-1. *Calcium, phosphorus, and phosphatase of the blood in skeletal diseases*

Disease	Calcium	Phos-phorus	Alkaline phosphatase
Osteitis deformans (Paget's disease)	Normal	Normal	Very high
Osteitis fibrosa cystica (hyperparathyroidism)	High	Low	High
Rickets	Low	Variable	High
Osteoma	Normal	Normal	Normal
Chondroma	Normal	Normal	Normal
Chondrosarcoma	Normal	Normal	Normal
Osteolytic osteogenic sarcoma	High	Normal	Normal or slight increase
Osteoplastic osteogenic sarcoma	High	Normal	Increased
Ewing's tumor	Normal	Normal	Normal
Myeloma	Normal or high	Normal or high	Normal
Metastatic tumors of bone (except prostatic)	Normal	Normal	Normal or slight increase
Metastatic carcinoma of prostate in bone	Normal	Normal	High (both acid and alkaline phosphatase)

of gout, (7) tumors, and (8) miscellaneous forms, e.g., arthritis associated with other diseases.

The numerically most important diseases of joints are rheumatoid arthritis and osteoarthritis. Being of very common occurrence, they account for a tremendous total of pain, crippling, and disability. Rheumatoid arthritis is essentially an inflammation of synovial membrane, the cause of which is unknown. Osteoarthritis is a degenerative change affecting primarily articular cartilage with secondary hypertrophic changes in the underlying bone. It is often a senescent change and is possibly related to wear and tear and to changes in vascular supply.

Infectious arthritis. Infection of a joint by known organisms is usually the result of hematogenous spread in pyemia or septicemia. Less commonly the bacteria may reach the joint from an adjacent infection of bone such as osteomyelitis or tuberculosis of bone. Also there may be introduction from without by penetrating wounds. The common pyogenic organisms that thus infect joints are the staphylococcus, streptococcus, pneumococcus, and gonococcus. Metastatic infection of joints may occur in puerperal sepsis, bacterial endocarditis, meningitis, otitis media, pneumonia, and typhoid fever.

The joint becomes swollen and acutely inflamed. Fluid, at first serous but later purulent, accumulates in the joint cavity. The synovial membrane is greatly congested, swollen, and infiltrated with inflammatory cells. There may be considerable destruction of tissue, so that in healing there is formation of fibrous adhesions (fibrous ankylosis). In some cases this may be transformed into bone, and a disabling bony ankylosis results.

Gonorrheal arthritis. Gonorrheal arthritis is a complication that usually develops fairly early in an acute gonorrheal infection. Several joints may be affected, but major involvement is usually in one only.

Tuberculous arthritis. Tuberculous arthritis is commonly an extension from a tuberculous involvement of bone. It occurs mainly in children and most frequently affects the hip. The synovial membrane is greatly thickened by tuberculous granulation tissue. The inflammation may spread to erode the articular surface. Separation of flakes of cartilage or synovial fringes with adherent fibrin may form small, rounded, firm, loose bodies in the joint (melon seed bodies). Arrest may occur at any stage, or there may be rupture and sinus formation or an end result of fibrous or bony ankylosis.

Arthritis of rheumatic fever. Acute nonsuppurative arthritis is often a prominent feature of rheumatic fever, particularly in the acute cases arising in adolescence or early adult life. Several joints tend to be affected in succession. Acute tenderness and swelling occur, with an excess of turbid fluid in the cavity. The inflammation is predominantly in the synovial membrane, but nodules may develop in subsynovial and periarticular tissues. The histologic character of these may resemble that of the Aschoff bodies of the myocardium or rheumatic nodules elsewhere. The inflammation usually subsides completely and without residual disability.

Rheumatoid arthritis. Rheumatoid arthritis is also referred to as atrophic, proliferative, or chronic nonspecific infectious arthritis. It is a very common chronic and disabling disease, with a prevalence in the general population of about 4%. It

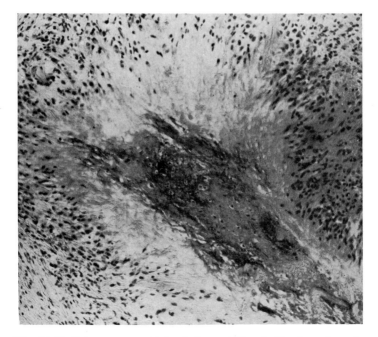

Fig. 24-11. Subcutaneous nodule of rheumatoid arthritis. A portion of a necrotic focus surrounded by palisades of proliferating cells. (AFIP No. 73941, courtesy Dr. G. A. Bennett.)

has its greatest incidence among women of the reproductive age and occurs about three times more frequently in women than in men. Although of unknown etiology, evidence suggests that it is a chronic inflammation resulting most likely from hypersensitivity or autoimmunity. It usually starts gradually, but it may begin acutely and is often accompanied by general symptoms, fever, leukocytosis, anemia, etc. The small joints of the hands and feet are most frequently affected, and larger joints are involved later. The affected joints show a spindle-shaped swelling, are very painful, and progress to deformity and limitation of movement. Subcutaneous nodules are present in some cases and show a histologic picture somewhat similar to that of rheumatic fever nodules. Rheumatoid disease is a systemic condition and may include visceral lesions such as granulomas of heart valves, pericardium, myocardium, and pleura. Biopsies of skeletal muscles often show focal accumulations of lymphocytes and macrophages with occasional plasma cells and eosinophils. Amyloidosis is present in some cases. Rheumatoid arthritis may be associated with keratoconjunctivitis and salivary gland swelling as part of Sjögren's syndrome (p. 587).

The first and essential change is in the synovial membrane, which is thickened by a granulation tissue pannus and is infiltrated by many neutrophils, lymphocytes, and plasma cells. The thickened synovial membrane may develop numerous villous processes, in which there may be necrosis, hemorrhage, or fibrosis. Adjacent surfaces form adhesions, so that fibrous ankylosis tends to occur and later may become bony. The joint cartilage is attacked, and there is extension of granulation tissue from the synovial membrane. Inflammatory edema and cellular infiltration are also found in periarticular tissues. An increased effusion of cloudy and highly cellular fluid is often present in the joint cavity. Vasculitis and perivasculitis are prominent features of both synovial and systemic lesions.

Still's disease is an acute form affecting children. It is accompanied by fever, leukocytosis, and enlargement of spleen and lymph nodes. *Felty's syndrome* is a somewhat similar condition in adults, in which chronic arthritis is associated with leukopenia and enlargement of lymph nodes and the spleen. In *Marie-Strümpell (or ankylosing) spondylitis* the arthritic changes mainly involve the spine, affecting particularly the intervertebral and costovertebral ligaments. Stiffness and ankylosis of the spine result from ossification of the ligaments and fusion of adjacent

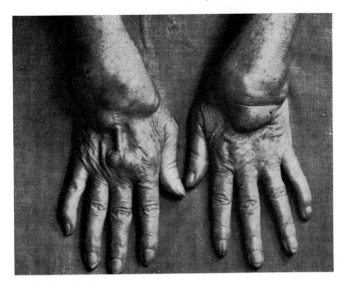

Fig. 24-12. Rheumatoid arthritis.

vertebrae. Severe kyphosis may be present. Most cases occur in males. Some investigators regard ankylosing spondylitis as an entity separate from peripheral rheumatioid arthritis because of certain distinctive features: (1) the very high incidence in men whereas peripheral rheumatoid arthritis occurs mainly in women; (2) it commonly exists without peripheral arthritic manifestations; (3) the serologic reaction for the "rheumatoid factor" is usually negative in the absence of peripheral joint involvement, and even when the latter is present, the incidence of positive tests is low; and (4) the cardiovascular disease associated with ankylosing spondylitis is usually an aortitis with aortic valvulitis and insufficiency mimicking syphilitic heart disease, in contrast to the cardiac granulomas of "rheumatoid heart disease."

Osteoarthritis. Rather than a primary inflammation, osteoarthritis (degenerative, hypertrophic, or senile arthritis) is essentially, a degenerative condition of joint cartilage, with reactive and hypertrophic changes in underlying bone. Affecting the sexes equally, it is a disease of later life, being common in persons after the age of 40 years. Large joints, including the hip, tend to be affected, and there is little local inflammation or pain. While there may be considerable deformity and limitation of movement, complete crippling of a joint is unusual. Trauma and changes because of excessive function are most prominent in the causation of osteoarthritis. Other types of injury to the joint, inflammations, synovitis, and endocrine disturbances also may be etiologic factors.

Changes begin in the articular cartilage. The cartilage cells degenerate, and the normally smooth surface becomes rigid, frayed, and fibrillated. The elasticity of the cartilage and its cushioning function become reduced. The subchondral bone is thus exposed to excessive functional stresses, and its marrow reacts to this chronic irritation by proliferative changes. Osteoclasts resorb the subchondral bone trabeculae, and blood vessels penetrate into the cartilage. The vascularization of the cartilage is followed by ossification, the bone so formed becoming highly polished (eburnated). Exostoses formed in this fashion at the margins of the joint and periosteal bone formation produce the characteristic bony "lipping" at the edges of the joint. This process occurs prominently in the fingers, forming painless Heberden's nodes. Osteoarthritic changes in the spinal column (spondylitis deformans) may produce kyphosis, extreme rigidity of the back ("pokerback"), and pain caused by the pressure of osteophytic growths on nerve roots. Although bony ankylosis may occur in this type of spondylitis, ankylosis is an uncommon result of osteoarthritis elsewhere.

Traumatic injury. Trauma to a joint may be followed by effusion of fluid into the joint cavity and by acute inflammation of surrounding soft tissues.

Charcot's joint. Charcot's joint is a condition that occurs in certain cases of tabes dorsalis, neuropathy (e.g., diabetic), and syringomyelia. Destruction of nerve fibers results in the loss of sensation in the joint, which is then subjected to unusual trauma. The painless joint is excessively mobile, and destructive changes occur in the joint cartilage and adjacent bone.

Protrusion of intervertebral discs. Protrusion of an intervertebral disc is a common cause of low back pain and sciatica. The intervertebral discs have a semifluid central matrix (nucleus pulposus) surrounded by circumferentially laminated fibrous tissue and fibrocartilage (annulus fibrosus). Protrusion may involve (1) a bulging disc without detachment from the bone and without a rent in the annulus fibrosus; (2) a herniated disc that extends through a rent of the annulus fibrosus into the spinal cavity; or (3) a slipped disc that has been freed from its an-

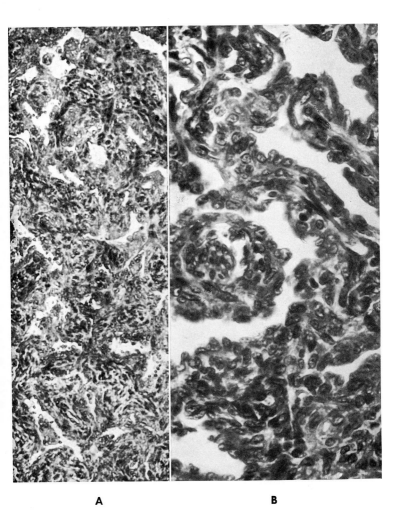

A   **B**

Fig. 24-13. Synovial sarcoma. **A,** Malignant tumor of synovial membrane origin showing characteristic structure. **B,** Higher power of tumor in **A.** (AFIP No. 90623; courtesy Dr. G. A. Bennett.)

chorage and slipped backward·as a result of trauma involving the cartilaginous epiphyseal plate. This sometimes is accompanied by a chip fracture of the vertebral rim. Symptoms are caused by pressure of the protrusion on the spinal cord or one of its branches. Trauma is believed to be the initial cause of herniation or slipping of the disc rather than primary disease of the disc itself.

Arthritis of gout. Gout is a disease of genetic nature that is connected in some fashion with a disturbance of purine (protein) metabolism. The uric acid content of the blood is increased, but this alone does not precipitate an acute attack. The disease occurs chiefly in middle-aged men.

Acute attacks commence suddenly with pain, swelling, and tenderness in a joint (toes, fingers, or knees). There is an effusion into the joint cavity of fluid containing crystals of sodium biurate. These crystals also become deposited in surrounding soft tissues, where they elicit some foreign body reaction and chronic inflammation. A tophus is a chalky deposit of the crystals in the subcutaneous tissue, in cartilages of the ear, or occasionally in the eyelids (p. 38 and Fig. 2-7).

Tumors. Only rarely do tumors arise from joint structures, but chondromas, lipomas, synoviomas, spindle cell sarcomas, and chondrosarcomas have been described.

Synovial sarcoma. The synovial sarcoma is a malignant tumor arising from the lining cells of the synovial membrane of a joint or bursa. Histologically it shows a distorted picture suggestive of synovia, but the appearance in various examples is far from uniform. A mixed picture of sarcomatous and pseudoepithelial structures is frequently present. There is a groundwork of rounded or spindle cells, with tissue spaces that vary from slitlike clefts to glandlike spaces or pavementlike areas of tissue suggesting low epithelium. Mucinous or serous fluid may be present in glandlike spaces. Papillary villuslike structures or cell tufts are sometimes formed. Recurrence often follows local removal of the tumor, and pulmonary metastasis may occur. Amputation is usually necessary for cure. The less common, well-differentiated synoviomas may be of giant cell type or may be composed of synovial-like spaces lined by cells closely resembling glandular epithelium and may have a better prognosis.

TENDONS

Inflammation. Tenosynovitis is an inflammation of tendon sheaths at the wrist or ankle. It may be traumatic, suppurative, or tuberculous. In the latter, with fibrin in the exudate, there may be formed ovoid melon seed bodies.

Ganglion. Ganglion is a cystlike swelling arising from a tendon sheath or joint capsule. It is most common on the back of the hand or wrist. There is proliferation of fibrous tissue of the sheath, with mucoid degeneration, producing the cystlike swell-

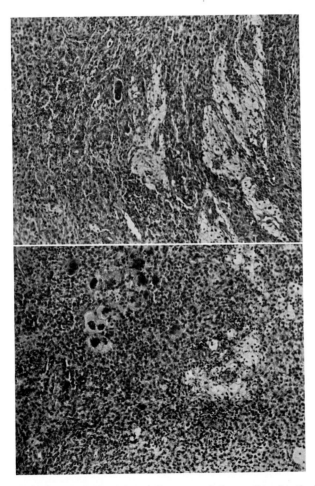

Fig. 24-14. Xanthomatous giant cell tumor of the tendon sheath. Note the xanthoma cells with distended foamy cytoplasm.

ing. There is no true lining, and the ganglion does not communicate with the cavity of the tendon sheath.

Various other types of synovial or bursal cysts occur. The *popliteal cyst (Baker's cyst)* is one of the most frequent. It may be bursal in origin, or it may be a herniation from the knee joint. The cyst lining may be synovial or may be simply fibrous tissue, with or without an inflammatory exudate.

Tendon sheath tumors. Giant cell tumor (xanthoma) of a tendon sheath is a yellow or yellowish brown tumor, which arises near the tendinous insertion, most often in the hand. It has a groundwork of fibrous tissue in which there are scattered giant cells and aggregates of large, lipid-containing foam cells (xanthoma cells). The xanthoma cells are found when there are deposits of iron and cholesterol. Except for this xanthomatous tendency, the tumor is similar to the giant cell epulis and the benign giant cell tumor of bone.

Palmar fibromatosis (**Dupuytren's contracture**). Fibrosis of the palmar fascia, with thickening and shortening, causes flexion of the fingers, with deformity and inability to make normal use of the hand. Although the etiology has been considered inflammatory, it is characterized mainly by a proliferation of fibrocytes, which may produce nodular masses and may be mistaken for fibrosarcoma.

Plantar fibromatosis. Plantar fibromatosis is similar to palmar fibromatosis but does not ordinarily lead to contractures. Nodular masses of well-differentiated proliferating fibrocytes arise within the plantar fascia, more commonly on the medial side. The condition is benign, and fibrosarcoma arising in this region is very rare. It has been suggested that the condition is a reactive fibrous hyperplasia as a result of degeneration of the plantar fascia that may follow trauma. Complete excision of the plantar fascia is necessary to prevent recurrence.

Chapter 25

The nervous system

STRUCTURE AND REACTION TO INJURY

The nervous system and its supporting structures include ten basic cells or tissues, each of which exhibits several common types of response to injury. Some of these reactive changes appear to be specific, e.g., the rounding up of microglia to produce fat-granule cells when myelin is destroyed. Many, however, are nonspecific, and the microscopic changes are interpreted with greater difficulty.

Notochordal tissue. Remnants of this tissue are commonest in the following locations: (1) along the clivus, (2) in the hypophysial fossa, (3) deep to the posterior wall of the pharynx, (4) in the dens, (5) in the nuclei pulposi of the intervertebral discs, and (6) in the sacrum. Pathologically notochordal tissue is encountered as a tumor (p. 874) and in herniation or displacement of intervertebral discs. Posterior protrusion of an intervertebral disc may compress the spinal cord or nerve roots, causing symptoms of root pain. The nucleus pulposus may herniate after trauma and degeneration of disc tissue. This usually occurs in later life and most commonly involves the lumbar region. Notochordal tissue (nucleus pulposus) is identifiable microscopically by its larger vacuolated mucus-containing cells, set in a thin fibrillar stroma of elastic and collagenous tissue.

Ependyma. The ependymal lining cells of the ventricular system of the brain and the central canal of the spinal cord retain an epithelial character. Very often they are flattened and in some regions may appear in folds or tufts, particularly in the third ventricle. During the developmental period the ependymal cells are ciliated, and some ciliated ependymal cells may be found in later life. The more common reactions associated with ependymal tissue include proliferation, subependymal gliosis, and inflammation. *Proliferation,* manifested by reduplication to several layer of cells, may appear as an aging process. This is common in lower levels of the spinal cord, sometimes to such an extent that the central canal appears obliterated. *Subependymal gliosis* seems to be a response to a chronic toxemia or anoxia as in alcoholism, the subependymal layer becoming greatly thickened and densely sclerotic. *Inflammation (ependymitis)* is seen in septic conditions of the ventricles and as a result of irritation of the lining cells by other agents, such as *toxoplasma*. The subependymal layer is swollen and infiltrated with neutrophilic leukocytes, and the lining cells are reduplicated, festooned, and swollen, or they may be eroded.

Neuroglia. The intramedullary supporting glial cells are astrocytes and oligodendroglia. In sections stained by hematoxylin and eosin they must be differentiated by nuclear configuration. The nucleus of the astrocyte is large, oval, pale, and vesicular, with chromatin material deposited in small dustlike particles on a fine linin net. The nuclei of the oligodendroglia are about one-third smaller, more rounded, and stain darkly, with clumped chromatin masses. Special stains show that the astrocytes possess sucker-foot attachments to blood vessels and a great many fibrillar processes. The oligodendroglia have very few processes. Astrocytes appear in greater number in gray than in white matter. Ogilodendroglia are equally numerous in both gray and white matter, forming the "satellite cells" of the neurons and the "interfascicular supporting cells" of the nerve fibers.

Astrocytes may undergo either regressive or reactive changes. Regressive changes are most commonly seen as degenerative processes in tumor cells or in severe toxemia and are manifested by shrinkage and gemistocytosis. *Shrinkage* is identified by pyknosis of the nucleus with fragmentation and extrusion. *Clasmatodendrosis* is a regressive change with cytoplasmic swelling, loss of cytoplasmic processes, and nuclear pyknosis. In *gemistocyte formation* or *swelling* the cells swell and cytoplasm becomes stainable by routine methods. The nuclei are eccentric and may be multiple. These cells are often referred to as "fat astrocytes." Reactive changes in astrocytes are represented by *proliferation,* an increase in the number by amitotic division and by *gliosis,* a production of glial fibrils forming a dense fibrous network and entering into repair phenomena.

Oligodendroglia may present reactive changes. *Acute swelling* and vacuolation is a nonspecific alteration that may occur as an agonal phenomenon. *Satellitosis* is an apparent increase in the number of oligodendroglia neighboring a nerve cell body and is seen in certain toxic states. It has been referred to as incidental to neuronophagia (p. 866).

There are a number of alterations in the nervous system, in

which the parent reacting element is obscure but glial cells may take part. *Glial nodes* are nests of proliferated glial cells that are prominent in rickettsial and other encephalitides and may be seen near infarcts. As they are often aggregated close to vessels and house intracellular organisms, the cells may be derived from perithelial cells of vascular adventitia. *Glial plaques* (Alzheimer) are sclerotic nodules representing focal degeneration. They may contain glial fibers and cells with an admixture of fragmented nerve fibers. *Corpora amylacea* are concentric hyaline bodies of disputed origin. They are common in persons after 40 years of age and often are conspicuous in premature senility. They stain with iodine but contain neither amyloid nor fat. They resemble corpora amylacea of the prostate or the lung.

Choroid plexus. The choroid plexus may be regarded as a pia-ependymal membrane invaginated by subarachnoid vasculature. The ependymal epithelium with a thin fibrous substrate is disposed in a foliated or villous pattern with a highly vascular core composed of loose trabecular tissue resembling arachnoid. Alterations in the choroid plexus are common but usually are unimportant. Most often encountered are *cyst formation,* the thin-walled, translucent cysts appearing most frequently at the confluent part of the lateral ventricles; *concretions* (brain sand), amorphous firm bodies sometimes quite numerous; and *sclerosis,* a fibrosis of the choroid core.

Neurons. The neurons are the functional units of the nervous system and by their interrelationships provide the physical basis for nervous activity. Each consists of a cell body and its processes. Microscopically the best criterion for identification is the nucleus. It is large, round, and vesicular and contains a large nucleolus. The nuclear membrane is distinct. The cytoplasm contains varying amounts and patterns of basophilic material known as Nissl substance. Special stains enable identification of neurofibrils, which traverse the cell body and continue into the processes. The shape of the cell body varies greatly; it may be multipolar or unipolar, and the size ranges from a diameter of a few to over 100μ, depending on location and function. From the cell bodies arise a varying number of processes. The axon is the process over which a nervous impulse is conveyed to an adjacent neuron or to an end organ. Those axons (axis cylinders) attaining a diameter greater than 1.5μ possess a fatty covering, the myelin sheath. In the central nervous system this sheath is limited externally by the network of fibrillar processes of supporting cells (oligodendroglia). In peripheral nerves the myelin is encased in a wrapping supplied by sheath cells (Schwann). Each sheath cell has distinctly marked linear limits, which form a constriction (node of Ranvier) around the axis cylinder, at which point the myelin layer is obliterated. The axis cylinders terminate in buttonlike knobs (boutons), which provide the contact points at the synapse or in special peripheral structures in muscle or gland.

Changes in the body of nerve cells. Changes in the body of nerve cells are difficult to interpret because of the complex nature of the neuron and the distances over which the processes spread. The common reactions of the cell body are shrinkage, swelling, vacuolation, pigment changes, chromatolysis, and neuronophagia. *Shrinkage* is indicated by great irregularity in the shape of the cell, pyknosis of the nucleus, clumping and condensation of Nissl substance, and sclerosis or contortion of processes. Shrunken cells are common in senility and other cerebral atrophies and also may appear in chronic infections. Fixation artifacts may mimic shrinkage or sclerosis of cells. *Swelling* of nerve cells clouds the irregular surface contour. The cytoplasm stains faintly, the processes fragment, and the cell may be evident in outline only. This change, apparently reversible, occurs in acute toxic states and mild infections. It is the most prominent change in tetanus. *Vacuolation* of nerve cells is unusual but occurs in toxic states. It may be seen normally in the hypothalamus, posterior pituitary, and peripheral spinal and autonomic ganglion cells. The appearance of light brown or yellow pigment in a perinuclear position or in cytoplasmic blotches is observed commonly and is referred to as *pigment degeneration*. This degenerative process should not be confused with the normal pigment in cells of certain locations (locus ceruleus and substantia nigra). In *chromatolysis* the Nissl substance becomes fine, dispersed, and peripheralized or loses its staining properties altogether. The nucleus of the involved cell is eccentric in position. Because this change is believed to be a specific retrograde response to axon injury, it has been widely used to identify the nuclear or ganglionic origin of damaged fiber bundles in the central and peripheral nervous systems. *Neuronophagia* involves reaction of macrophages as well as nerve cells. Phagocytosis of nerve cells is common only in inflammatory diseases and is conspicuous only when the death of the cell is brought about by an intracellular agent. It is a characteristic occurrence in poliomyelitis. A mass of macrophages may be seen occupying the position of, or within, a nerve cell body. In satellitosis, on the other hand, the cells are seen around but not within the nerve cell body. The phago-cytic cells may be mononuclear cells from the blood or microglia.

Reactions of the axis cylinder. The reactions of the axis cylinder to injury include changes in the neuraxis, alterations at the synapse or end organs, and neuroma formation. By coating the argyrophilic neurofibrillar structure with reduced silver salts, the morphology of the axis cylinder and its terminal boutons is seen to vary under pathologic influence. The neuraxis may swell in irregular nodules or fragment and become granu-lar. The synaptic change may be a loss of structure, or it may be an accentuation by beading and reduplication of terminal bulbs. Diffuse encephalomyelitis induces the most profound synaptic changes. In peripheral nerves the end organs undergo dissolution after severe damage to the nerve. Neuroma formation occurs as a regrowth reaction to traumatic interruption of nerve fibers. The neuroma is a tangle of regrowing neurofibrils, each spearheaded by a bulbous expansion, the growth cone. Neuro-mas may develop along the trunk of a nerve at a point of trauma or at the extremity of an amputated limb, or stump. The micro-scopic appearance is complicated by growth of fibrous tissue or by sheath cell proliferation. In a *traumatic neuroma* of some duration these supporting elements remain, and the argyrophilic substance of the neuraxes disappears. A different type of neuroma *(plantar digital neuroma)* occurs in Morton's meta-tarsalgia (Morton's toe). This is a tumefacient swelling of a plantar digital nerve, usually the fourth, characterized by de-generation and loss of nerve fibers and fibrosis.

Myelin degeneration. The loss of myelin substance (demye-lination) is a prominent pathologic change in both central and peripheral nervous systems. In considering demyelination as an index of injury it is essential to remember that some fibers nor-mally possess no myelin. This fatty substance, a complex of at least four lipids, is deposited around fibers of both central and peripheral neuraxes. Injury to the cell body or axis cylinder causes a degeneration of the myelin, or its dissolution may occur spontaneously without apparent nerve injury. Demon-stration of the demyelination depends principally upon the use of three staining procedures. The Weigert technique stains normal myelin blue or black. Demyelinated areas do not stain and hence are identifiable by contrast. This procedure is applicable to normal tissue and to old degenerations. Since the Marchi technique stains the altered lipids of degenerating myelin directly, this procedure demonstrates active degeneration. Osmic acid will blacken normal myelin. It is used principally in peripheral nerve study, and the failure to take osmic acid implies loss or absence of myelin.

The demyelinating process and accompanying changes occurring secondary to trauma or interruption of peripheral nerves is called *wallerian degeneration*. This proceeds in both distal and proximal directions from the point of injury. Proximally the observable alterations in the myelin are usually arrested at the next node of Ranvier. The node probably plays no role in this, since the same limitation of retrograde change is seen in the central nervous system. Proliferation of neurofibrils proximal to the injury occurs within a few hours. Distally the axis cylinders become granular and fragment, and the myelin undergoes dissolution and forms fat droplets. The products of degeneration are removed, mainly by macrophages, in a few weeks. Simultaneously, regenerative changes occur. The sheath cells (neurilemma, Schwann) proliferate, enlarge, and migrate from both proximal and distal stumps into the defect, bridging it and providing cytoplasmic channels for the regrowing neurofibrils from the proximal stump. The endoneural connective tissue per-

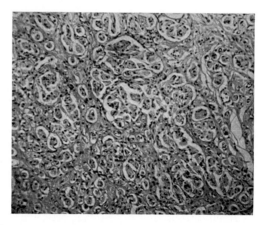

Fig. 25-1. Amputation "neuroma."

sists, reinforcing the neurilemmal cells. Regrowth may be inhibited by scar tissue and by poor apposition of the stumps. Regrowing neurofibrils will progress at the rate of 0.25 mm. per day through the scar and 3 to 4 mm. per day through the peripheral stump. Certain of the regrown fibrils slowly enlarge within the Schwann cells and accumulate a myelin sheath. The original status of an individual myelinated peripheral nerve fiber is reestablished in nine to twelve· months. The complete restitution of all fibers of a peripheral nerve probably does not occur.

In the central nervous system there is a somewhat different process of demyelination. The sheath cells are replaced by oligodendroglia, which lack the remarkable regenerative properties of the former. Central nerve cell processes may be as inherently capable of regrowth as peripheral cells, but only those that possess a neurilemmal sheath can be restored. Consequently, functional repair of interrupted central neuraxes does not occur, although abortive neurofibrillar attempts at regrowth are constantly observed. Hence disruption of nerve tissue with accompanying demyelination in the central nervous system is an irreversible reaction. In the area of injury or softening, where a large amount of myelin is broken down, the degenerative fatty products are removed by macrophages (microglia). The degeneration of myelin progresses distally from the point of injury. The myelin appears in droplet form and acquires staining reactions, which imply chemical alteration. The droplets will, however, remain in position for months, or even years, and mark the degenerating tract. Proximally (toward the cell body) the process may progress for a short distance but ordinarily is insignificant.

A second type of demyelination occurs in the central nervous system without apparent cause. (See demyelinating diseases, p. 890.)

Sheath and capsule cells. A membranous covering for peripheral nerve cell bodies and neuraxes is provided by capsule and sheath cells. Microscopically their nuclei appear as rounded forms satellite to ganglion cells and as elongated structures along peripheral nerves. The sheath cells form a cylindric tube threaded by a neuraxis and separated from it by a concentric sheath of myelin. When myelin is absent, the neuraxis is covered intimately by the thin-walled sheath cell. Applied to the outside of the Schwann sheath are the collagenous elements of the endoneurium. The reactions to which sheath and capsule cells are subject are, principally, hypertrophy and proliferation, and these occur prominently in repair of peripheral nerves.

Meninges. The coverings of the central nervous system include the dura (pachymeninx) and the pia-arachnoid (leptomeninx). The dura is adherent to the cranial periosteum (external layer of dura) but is separated widely from the periosteum of the vertebral canal. The pia follows the surface of the brain closely and is separated from the arachnoid, which is in apposition with the dura, by the subarachnoid space. This space contains cerebrospinal fluid and is bridged by a spongy network of filaments, the arachnoid trabeculae. The principal histologic element of all membranes is collagenous tissue. Elastic fibers appear in the pia-arachnoid and in the innermost layer of the dura. Flattened mesothelial cells (meningothelium) line the subarachnoid and subdural spaces and cover the arachnoid trabeculae. In addition to the lining cells, fibroblasts and fixed histiocytes are identifiable in the membranes. Nests of epithelial-like cells are occasionally encountered buried in the dura. These are arachnoid granulations. The common reactions of the meninges to injury include the production of macrophages and false dura formation. The macrophages are derived from meningothelium or fixed histiocytes, or both, and appear in great number in inflammatory conditions. False dura formation amounts to a rapid repair process in which a coagulum forms, later to be invaded by fibroblastic cells. This occurs when dural continuity is interrupted and in walling off hemorrhage.

Vasculature and related structures. Intimal, medial, and adventitial changes in cerebral vessels are similar to those occurring elsewhere. There are, however, three peculiarities in cerebral vasculature that play prominent roles in reactive phenomena: (1) Vessels less than 70μ in diameter contain little or no muscle in the media after 40 years of age. (2) In passing through the subarachnoid space the vessels acquire a meningothelial sheath and, in penetrating to an intramedullary position, carry a second, outer sheath derived from the pia lining. These concentric wrappings establish a perivascular space (of Virchow-Robin). This space is the morphologic basis for the reaction of perivascular infiltration or cuffing. Drainage from the interstitial spaces of the medullary substance passes through the Virchow-Robin channels and in so doing may load the space with inflammatory cells or products of degeneration. In addition, exudate reaches the perivascular space through the vessel wall. (3) Vascular adventitial elements provide the parent tissue, which reacts to form an abscess wall in response to invasion by certain bacteria.

Microglia (mesoglia). Microglial cells are believed to be mesodermal elements derived from perivascular tissues and are distributed widely throughout the nervous system in postnatal life. Normally they appear to be at rest (fixed), in which form only the nucleus is evident in ordinary sections. Compared to the neuroglia, the microglial nucleus is small, very compact, and may be irregular in shape (round, elongated, or curved). The scanty cytoplasm and thin branching processes require special staining to be demonstrated. These cells respond to the products of myelin degeneration. In this *fat-granule cell* reaction the cell processes are pulled in and the nucleus elongates, becoming bipolar. This *rod cell* migrates to the site of injury, where the nucleus becomes rounded and lighter staining. As fat products are engulfed, the cytoplasm becomes globular and the nucleus eccentric. These fat-laden macrophages (fat-granule cells, compound granular corpuscles) often migrate into the perivascular

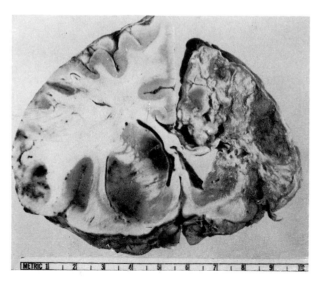

Fig. 25-2. Cerebral infarction.

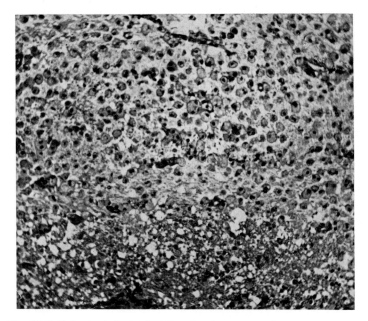

Fig. 25-3. Infarct of the brain. The edge is shown, and many compound granular corpuscles (microglia) are evident.

spaces. They are the characteristic cells in an area of cerebral softening.

Cerebrospinal fluid. The cerebrospinal fluid forms a circulatory system peculiar to nervous tissue, perhaps taking the place of the absent lymphatics. The fluid is formed from blood by the choroid plexus of the cerebral ventricles, probably by a process of dialysis, although there may be an active secretory mechanism as well. Formed mainly in the lateral ventricles, the fluid passes through the interventricular foramina (of Monro) into the third ventricle and through the narrow cerebral aqueduct (of Sylvius) to the fourth ventricle. From the roof and lateral extensions of this ventricle it escapes through the lateral apertures (of Luschka) and the medium aperture (of Magendie) to reach the subarachnoid space. From the large subarachnoid cisterns at the base of the brain it passes downward into the subarachnoid space of the spinal cord and upward through the narrow aperture of the tentorium cerebelli to bathe the surface of the brain. Most of the fluid is resorbed into the venous bloodstream around the region of the vertex by way of the arachnoid villi, which project into the lumina of the venous sinuses. Some diffusion of fluid probably occurs through the perivascular or Virchow-Robin spaces by means of which interstitial fluid of the brain tissue is added to the cerebrospinal fluid.

The cerebrospinal fluid reflects by its changes many important disease processes. Normally the volume is about 125 ml. It is clear and colorless, has a specific gravity of 1.006 to 1.009, and contains fewer than twelve cells (mononuclear) per cubic millimeter in persons after 12 years of age. In disease there may be color changes caused by fresh hemorrhage or xanthochromia, a yellowish tinge derived from hemoglobin and implying stasis after hemorrhage. The cell content may be altered in both number and character, and chemical and serologic changes occur that are valuable aids in diagnosis. The most striking change involving cerebrospinal fluid is the mechanical effect resulting from obstruction to its flow (hydrocephalus).

TUMORS OF THE NERVOUS SYSTEM AND RELATED TISSUES

Intracranial tumors as a group have certain peculiarities as a result of their position and the nature of the cells from which they arise. Occurring within a rigid bony box, their increase of bulk causes damage in increasing intracranial pressure. This is contributed to also by edema of the nervous tissue around the growth and often by obstruction to the pathway of cerebrospinal fluid, with some degree of hydrocephalus. A relatively small tumor may press upon or involve vital areas of the nervous system. Most of the intracranial tumors arise from supporting structures, i.e., neuroglia, sheaths of the brain (meninges) or cranial nerves, and blood vessels. Their greatest incidence is in middle age, but certain types occur mainly in childhood. Most of them do not metastasize, but they may be locally malignant and invasive. Others are quite benign biologically but are serious because of their position. In children the majority of brain tumors are found in the cerebellum, the most frequent being cystic astrocytomas, medulloblastomas, and ependymomas of the fourth ventricle. In elderly persons brain tumors are found mainly in the cerebrum and are predominantly highly malignant astrocytomas (glioblastoma multiforme).

Classification

Chordoma
Primary intramedullary neurogenic tumors
  Gliomas (supporting cell tumors)
    Ependymoma
    Oligodendroglioma
    Astrocytoma
    Glioblastoma multiforme
  Nerve cell tumors
    Medulloblastoma
    Neurocytoma
    Neuroblastoma
    Retinoblastoma
Primary extramedullary neurogenic tumors
  Supporting cell tumors
    Neurofibroma
    Neurilemoma
    Malignant schwannoma
  Nerve cell tumors
    Ganglioneuroma
Tumors of vascular and perivascular structures
  Angioma
  Sarcoma
  Malignant lymphoma
Meningiomas
Mixed tumors
Hypophysial tumors
Pineal tumors
Metastatic tumors

Chordoma. Chordomas are rare, slowly growing tumors derived from notochordal rests and are found most commonly in the sacrum and along the clivus. Grossly the mass is gelatinous or mucinous and tends to compress or invade bone. Microscopically they are composed of large polyhedral cells disposed in lobules or cords surrounded by a myxomatous matrix. Both cytoplasm and nucleus may contain mucus. Because of inaccessibility, complete removal is difficult and recurrence is usual.

Intramedullary tumors. Tumors of nervous tissue proper include the gliomas and nerve cell tumors. Gliomas constitute almost half of all intracranial tumors, whereas tumors of nerve cells are much less common.

Gliomas. Gliomas represent neoplasia of supporting tissues and their stem cells.

Kernohan and associates have suggested a simplified classification and grading of the gliomas. This is based on the concept that the more rapidly growing gliomas represent greater degrees of anaplasia or dedifferentiation rather than undifferentiation. Thus the astrocytoma, astroblastoma, and glioblastoma multiforme are considered to be the same type of neoplasm but of different degrees (or grades) of malignancy. There is a gradual transition between the lowest and highest grades of malignancy. Division into four grades is arbitrary but useful.

EPENDYMOMA. Ependymomas comprise about 6% of the gliomas. They are derived from ventricular lining cells and appear commonly in the fourth ventricle, along the central canal, and in the filum terminale. Although slow growing, they often interfere with cerebrospinal fluid flow, producing an acute increase of intracranial pressure. Grossly they are usually distinctly demarcated from brain tissue. The histology is complex, and they have been classified as (1) papilloma choroideum, a papillary tumor of the choroid plexus, closely simulating the normal structure but with taller epithelium and numerous vacuoles containing mucus; (2) papillary ependymoma, a tumor similar to the foregoing, without mucus in the tumor cells but with abundant myxomatous degeneration in the stroma; (3) epithelial ependymoma, a tumor composed of tubular channels resembling the central canal, having cells free of vacuoles and mucus and often containing blepharoplasts; and (4) cellular ependymoma, a highly cellular tumor containing fragments of tissue conforming to the other patterns and often dotted with pseudorosettes. In these ependymomas mitoses are uncommon. A more undifferentiated form, *ependymoblastoma,* occurs that grows rapidly and is highly malignant. *Colloid cyst* of the third ventricle may represent another form of ependymoma, but it has been suggested also that these may arise from paraphyseal tissue. They are benign

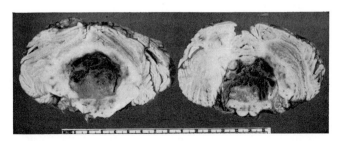

Fig. 25-4. Ependymoma of the fourth ventricle.

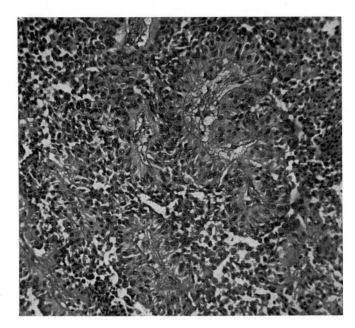

Fig. 25-5. Ependymoma.

and grow slowly but cause symptoms by ventricular blockage. Kernohan and associates have proposed that the ependymomal group of tumors may be graded 1 to 4 according to the degree of anaplasia or dedifferentiation and that such grading of malignancy correlates with the postoperative survival period.

OLIGODENDROGLIOMA. Oligodendrogliomas grow very slowly and appear most commonly in the cerebral hemispheres of adults. The tumors often contain calcium (roentgenographically visible) and tend to become cystic. Histologically they are extremely cellular and exhibit very little stroma. The nuclei are small, dark staining, and surrounded by a halo of clear cytoplasm. *Oligodendroblastomas* are rare, highly malignant, rapidly growing variants of this tumor. Attempts at grading of these tumors have not shown good correlation with survival periods.

ASTROCYTOMA. About one half of the gliomas, or one fourth of all intracranial tumors, are astrocytomas. They occur diffusely throughout the nervous system and are grayish white, fairly firm, and poorly demarcated grossly. They grow slowly and ap-

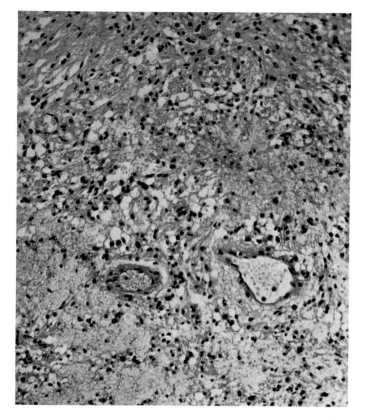

Fig. 25-6. Astrocytoma. Note the uniformity of nuclei and the abundance of fibers.

pear benign histologically. The cells are usually uniform, with nuclear structure comparable to that of a normal astrocyte, but the astrocytes appear increased in number. Giant nuclei and mitoses are absent or rare. More cytoplasm is evident than in normal cells, and stroma is densely fibrillated. Very often gemistocytes are formed, and occasionally they dominate the histologic picture (gemistocytic astrocytoma). *Astroblastomas* are made up of larger cells with short thick vascular processes and are often arranged in a radial pattern around a blood vessel. They exhibit more rapid growth. *Polar spongioblastomas* also may be considered a variety of astrocytoma. They are dom-

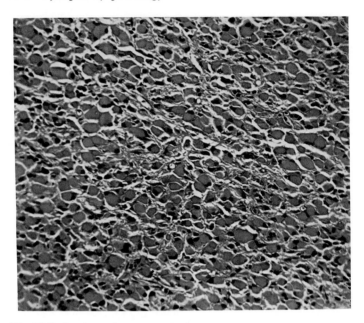

Fig. 25-7. Gemistocytic astrocytoma.

inated microscopically by bipolar or unipolar cells, which are thought to be the immediate stem cells from which astroblasts develop. Microscopically they resemble neurofibromas. The cells and nuclei are regular in size and exhibit no mitoses. They grow slowly. According to Kernohan's classification, well-differentiated astrocytoma would be *astrocytoma, grade 1;* and astroblastoma as well as polar spongioblastoma would be *astrocytoma, grade 2.*

GLIOBLASTOMA MULTIFORME. Glioblastoma multiforme is the second most common of the gliomas. The cellular source of these tumors is obscure. Microscopically representatives of many stem cells can be identified, lending the variability of cellular form characteristic of the tumor. They are exceedingly malignant, rapidly expansive, and invasive. They are often grossly hemorrhagic, and their line of demarcation from cerebral tissue is indistinct. Microscopically there is great variation in size and shape of cells, with giant and multinucleated forms and numerous bizarre mitoses. There is frequently an endothelial hyper-

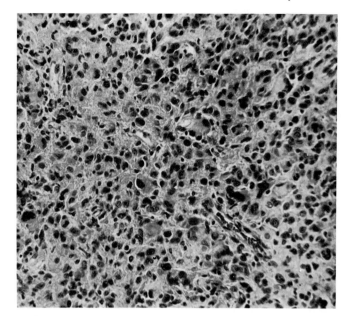

Fig. 25-8. Glioblastoma multiforme.

trophy and reduplication, imparting the appearance of extremely thick-walled vessels. Patches of necrosis surrounded by radiating clumps of small nuclei are very common. Some of the complex vascular formations appear to be caused by thrombosis and organization. Kernohan considers glioblastoma multiforme as *astrocytoma, grades 3 and 4.*

SYRINGOMYELIA. Syringomyelia is a cavitation occurring in the center of the spinal cord. It appears as a slowly progressive gliosis with subsequent cyst formation. The cavity may be focal and round, fusiform and linear, or multiple. The cause is unknown, and although it has been regarded by some as a variety of astrocytoma, its neoplastic character is questionable.

Nerve cell tumors. The second group of primary intramedullary tumors consists of those stemming from the medulloblast in the direction of the nonsupporting element of the nervous system, the neurocyte. They are often mixed (neuroastrocytoma).

MEDULLOBLASTOMA. Medulloblastomas are rapidly growing midline cerebellar tumors of children. They spread by implanting

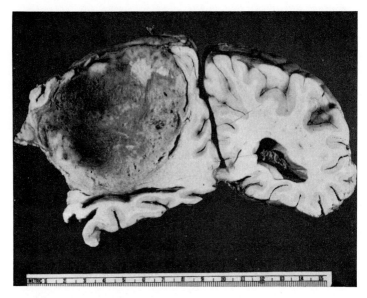

Fig. 25-9. Glioblastoma multiforme.

along the ventricles or in the meninges. Microscopically the cells are small and pear shaped, with a tapered cytoplasmic extremity. They tend to line up in incomplete circles, forming partial pseudorosettes. The tumor cells are radiosensitive, but the response to radiation is temporary.

NEUROCYTOMA (GANGLIONEUROMA). Neurocytomas are rare tumors characterized by the presence of mature nerve cells in which Nissl substance is demonstrable. They grow very slowly.

NEUROBLASTOMA. Closely related to medulloblastomas, neuroblastomas are rare tumors composed of neuroblasts, identifiable by large vesicular nuclei in small rounded cells, with little cytoplasm and no Nissl substance. Neuroblasts can often be identified in medulloblastomas.

RETINOBLASTOMA (NEUROEPITHELIOMA). Occurring in childhood and often familial, retinoblastomas arise from the retinoblast, the representative of the neuroblast in the retina. Closely related to the medulloblastomas, they resemble them in behavior, implanting along meningeal spaces. They tend particularly to invade the optic nerve. Microscopically the cells are small and round, with little cytoplasm, and tend to form rosettes.

Extramedullary neurogenic tumors. Neurogenic tumors developing outside the substance of the brain and spinal cord are tumors of peripheral ganglion cells and nerves and of the stem cells of these structures. In addition, there are a number of neurogenic tumors arising in the adrenal medulla (p. 715) and chromaffin structures (p. 718). Rarely neurogenic tumors microscopically resembling neuroblastoma or medulloblastoma may be found in odd sites, such as bone, skin, muscle, etc., where the stem cell is obscure but is probably related to the migrant cell. The principal extramedullary primary neurogenic tumors are ganglioneuromas, neurofibromas, and neurilemomas.

Ganglioneuroma. Ganglioneuromas are the peripheral counterpart of the central neurocytoma. Grossly they appear as fleshy masses, are often large, and are usually located along the thoracic and lumbar sympathetic trunk, bulging into the mediastinum or retroperitoneal region. They grow slowly and are benign. Microscopically they show mature nerve cells in a profuse stroma of sheath cells, fibrous tissue, and varying amounts of neurofibrils and myelin. (See Fig. 20-30.)

Peripheral nerve tumors. Three sources contribute to the morphology of the peripheral nerve: neuraxes of the nerve cells, sheath cells, and fibroblastic tissue from endoneural and perineural supporting structures. The contribution of neuraxes to the nerve tumors is insignificant. Tangles of neuraxes appear with their growth cones primarily in reparative processes (amputation neuroma). The relative importance of sheath cells or perineurium in the formation of nerve tumors is a much debated and still unsettled question. These tumors occur along cranial or peripheral nerves and at their endings.

Tumors of peripheral nerves (or nerve sheaths) can be classified into three groups. Although there are variations of opinion regarding derivation and terminology, the three types are most commonly called schwannoma (neurilemoma), neurofibroma, and malignant schwannoma.

SCHWANNOMA. Schwannoma (neurilemoma, perineural fibroblastoma) is a solitary encapsulated benign tumor composed of Schwann cells of the nerve sheath. The nerve from which it arises passes to one side or spreads out over the surface of the tumor so that it often can be surgically enucleated with preservation of the parent nerve and without risk of recurrence or malignant change. The larger tumors tend to be cystic. The acoustic nerve is a common site (acoustic neuroma), the tumor occupying the cerebellopontine angle. The elongated component cells are ar-

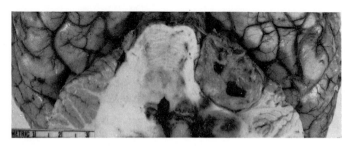

Fig. 25-10. Acoustic neuroma forming a tumor at the cerebellopontine angle. The hemorrhagic cerebellar area is a surgical operative wound.

ranged in irregular or twisted bundles wth palisading of nuclei. (See Fig. 11-8.) Fascicular (Antoni type A) tissue arranged in an organoid formation has been referred to as a Verocay body. Reticular (Antoni type B) tissue forms a loose network of reticulin fibers about minute cystic spaces.

NEUROFIBROMA. Neurofibroma is a diffuse or unencapsulated proliferation of nerve elements, sometimes single but more often multiple (von Recklinghausen's neurofibromatosis). Patches of excessive melanin pigmentation of the skin (café-au-lait spots), pigmented moles, and soft fibromas of the skin (fibromata mollusca) are common stigmas accompanying von Recklinghausen's disease. A neurofibroma cannot be enucleated from the parent nerve, since the nerve fibers run through the center of the tumor instead of around it. Neurofibromas may undergo malignant change. Histologically neurofibromas show an irregular reticular growth of Schwann cells, fibrous tissue, and nerve fibrils (shown by special stains). Proliferation of the tumor may occur within nerve sheaths, causing the involved nerves to become thick and tortuous (plexiform neurofibroma).

MALIGNANT SCHWANNOMA. Malignant schwannoma (neurogenic sarcoma) is composed of cells derived from the nerve sheath and may show some of the whorled interlacing bundles and nuclear palisading seen in neurilemomas. Nuclear hyperchromatism, cellularity, and rapid growth indicate the malignant character. The appearance may simulate fibrosarcoma or leiomyosarcoma. Insidious local infiltration occurs so that the

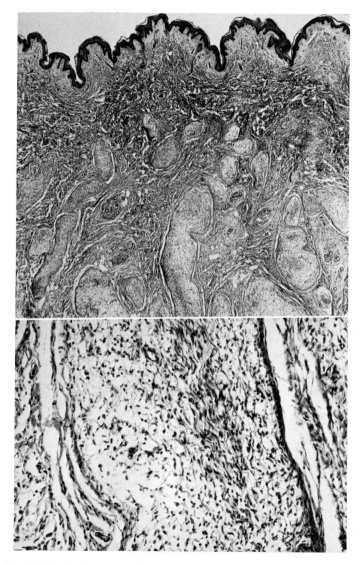

Fig. 25-11. Plexiform neurofibroma.

tumor is likely to recur unless surgical resection is wide. Distant metastasis occurs mainly by the bloodstream.

Tumors of vascular and perivascular structures. Tumors of vascular and perivascular structures include hemangioma, hemangioendothelioma, sarcoma, and malignant lymphoma.

Hemangioma. Hemangioma is a vascular malformation that occurs most commonly over the surface of a cerebral hemisphere as a tangle of tortuous large and small vessels. Microscopically it is similar to angiomas in other locations (p. 315).

Hemangioblastoma. Hemangioblastomas (hemangioendotheliomas) are commonest in the cerebellum of adults. They appear as a small, firm, reddish "mural nodule" in the wall of a large smooth cyst. Histologically they are composed of many immature blood vessels with swollen endothelial lining cells. If they are associated with retinal angiomatosis, the condition is called von Hippel disease. Occasionally there may be hemangioblastoma of the spinal cord and syringomyelia. The tumors are capillary or cavernous hemangiomas, often associated with visceral lesions (Lindau's disease), and they are similar whether in the retina, cerebellum, or spinal cord. The endothelial cells may accumulate lipid, so that the tumor acquires some resemblance to hypernephroma. Visceral lesions, most often polycystic lesions of the pancreas and kidneys, or renal hypernephromas, also may be present, and there may be an associated polycythemia. A familial factor is demonstrable in about 20% of cases. The disease is transmitted as a modified mendelian dominant and is not sex linked.

Sarcoma. Malignant, rapidly growing sarcomatous lesions occur in the brain, growing especially around blood vessels. These have been classified variously as fibrosarcomas, spindle cell sarcomas, and polymorphocellular sarcomas.

Malignant lymphoma. Malignant lymphomas occur infrequently in the epidural space and within the substance of the brain or cord.

Tumors of the meninges. *Meningiomas* comprise about one fifth of all intracranial neoplasms, being second only to gliomas in frequency. They are essentially benign tumors, which grow slowly and compress the brain by expansion. The commonest sites are over the cerebral hemispheres, along the sagittal sinus, over the cribriform plate, and along the lesser wing of the sphenoid. They often erode the bone and sometimes stimulate bone growth into the tumor. They are encapsulated, distinctly

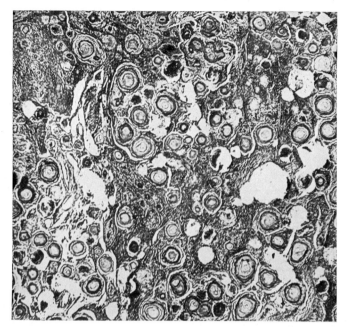

Fig. 25-12. Meningioma. Very numerous rounded psammoma bodies are shown.

demarcated from brain tissue, and are always attached to meninges. The microscopic appearance varies greatly but is often highly cellular and with a pronounced whorled arrangement. The central portion of the whorls undergoes degeneration and calcification, forming psammoma bodies. Meningiomas infiltrating soft tissues of the scalp may simulate carcinomas histologically. Loose edematous meningiomas may be confused with astrocytomas, or the palisading of cells may suggest the appearance of a neurilemoma. The exact origin of the tumor is still debated, but it is commonly believed that they are of arachnoidal origin. In rare instances a meningioma may not be localized but involves the brain surface over a wide area. Malignant fibrosarcomatous forms also occur. Fibrosarcomas of the dura resemble extracranial fibrosarcomas in histology. Pigmented meningiomas and melanomas of the meninges are rare. The latter are highly malignant.

Mixed tumors. Mixed tumors include *epidermoid tumors* (pearly tumors, cholesteatomas), *dermoid tumors,* and *teratomas.* These tumors are thought to arise from congenital cell rests. Morphologically they are similar to their counterparts elsewhere (p. 290).

Hypophysial tumors. Hypophysial tumors include the pituitary adenomas and craniopharyngiomas (pp. 665 and 671).

Pineal tumors. Pineal tumors are described on p. 701.

Metastatic tumors. Metastatic tumors of the brain occur commonly from the lung and somewhat less commonly from a malignant melanoma, the large intestine, testis, breast, stomach, kidney, adrenal, and prostate. Skin tumors involving the orbit sometimes invade the brain. Secondary tumors usually can be identified by their globular shape, sharp demarcation, and frequent multiplicity. Microscopically they resemble the primary growth.

Developmental and congenital disorders

Disorders related to faulty closure of bony structures. Related to faulty closure of the bony structures housing the medullary tube are numerous developmental disorders, which vary primarily in degree of involvement. *Rachischisis* is a failure of formation of the dorsal arch throughout the length of the vertebral column, with exposure of the unclosed neural groove. *Myelocele* is a spina bifida with protrusion of the spinal cord. *Meningocele* is a leptomeningeal protrusion through a local defect in bone and dura with the leptomeninx underlying the skin. This may occur in the vertebral column or skull. *Meningomyelocele* is similar to meningocele, with the inclusion of spinal cord tissue in the protruding part. If the brain is the part involved, the condition is called *encephalocele. Syringomyelocele* is similar to meningomyelocele but with the addition of considerable distention of the central canal. *Spina bifida occulata* is a congenital local dorsal arch defect (usually lumbar or sacral), in which the gap is filled with connective tissue to which the cord membranes are attached.

Malformations primarily involving brain tissue. Malformations may primarily involve brain tissue. *Anencephaly* is the condition wherein the forebrain and calvaria are absent. Often there are significant pathologic changes elsewhere, such as atrophy of adrenal glands. It probably is caused by defective organization in primordial tissues. *Porencephaly* is an abnormal cavitation within the brain substance, the cavities usually communicating with the ventricles. The condition is looked upon as a partial agenesia and is associated with maldevelopment elsewhere. *Heterotopias* are persistent islands of tissue that, although normal for certain developmental stages, are abnormal when found in the mature brain. Malformation of gyri is a common occurrence. Unusually large gyri are called *macrogyri;* unusually small ones, *microgyri*. Disturbances in brain volume are said to exist when brain weight in the adult varies beyond certain extremes. The average weight is around 1,350 grams and it is not uncommon to encounter brains weighing as little as 1,000 or as much as 1,700 grams. *Microcephaly* is the term applied to very small brains, *macrocephaly*, to very large brains. Each condition is often associated with hydrocephalus. *Oxycephaly* is a condition in which a tower-shaped skull is associated with premature synostosis of cranial sutures. Mental deficiency, papilledema, and eventually blindness result from disproportionate growth of the brain in the deformed skull.

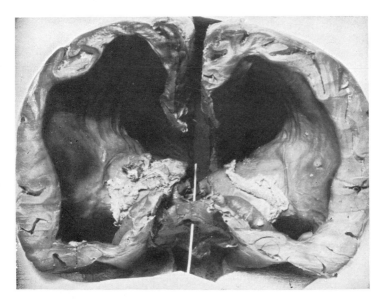

Fig. 25-13. Hydrocephalus. Note the extreme dilatation of the ventricles and the thinness of the cerebral substance.

Congenital hydrocephalus is the condition of an abnormal amount of intracranial cerebrospinal fluid present at, or shortly after, the time of birth. Several descriptive terms are applied to the condition, depending upon gross variations. *External hydrocephalus* describes the condition wherein most of the fluid accumulates over the surface of the atrophic brain. *Internal hydrocephalus* exists when the ventricular system is distended. *Hydranencephaly* exists when the forebrain is represented only by a thin membranous sac filled with water. The head size may be normal and the fontanelles close appropriately. In *hydromacrocephaly* the head is enlarged with the fontanelles and sutures widely open. The ventricular system is dilated, sometimes to a volume of several liters. Often the chambers are confluent. Considerable brain tissue often persists in the outer shell. These cases represent the condition most often referred to as hydrocephalus. *Communicating hydrocephalus* exists when abnormally increased fluid is present, although the connections between the ventricular system and the subarachnoid space are patent.

Theoretically the production of hydrocephalus may be brought about in three ways: (1) by overproduction of fluid, (2) by obstruction to its flow, and (3) by interference with its absorption into the venous system.

The production of cerebrospinal fluid fluctuates with venous pressure. An obstruction to venous return from the choroid plexus might cause excessive production of fluid. However, there is little evidence to incriminate excessive production of fluid as a cause of hydrocephalus. Exuberant growth or cysts of choroid plexus are commonly found associated with infantile hydrocephalus but probably are not causative.

Obstruction to the flow of cerebrospinal fluid is noted commonly in the following locations: (1) interventricular foramina (of Munro), (2) cerebral aqueduct (of Sylvius), (3) apertures of the fourth ventricle (of Magendie and Luschka), and (4) the subarachnoid space at the constricted tentorial aperture. The etiology of the obstruction is often obscure, but there have been noted congenital atresia of the cerebral aqueduct, occluding tumors of the aqueduct in infants, and ependymitis with inflammatory changes producing obstruction, particularly at the interventricular foramina and aqueduct of Sylvius. Recently, toxoplasma has been incriminated as the inciting organism. The infection is thought to be transmitted in utero since the defect produced often can be allocated to early pregnancy by the stage of development of certain structures. This may be an important cause of congenital hydrocephalus (p. 223). Arachnitis from meningeal infection may obstruct cerebrospinal fluid flow by exuberant fibrous proliferations over the foramina of Luschka and Magendie and in the interpeduncular and superior cisterns at the tentorial aperture. This condition has been found in infants but is probably more important in generating adult hydrocephalus.

Interference with absorption of cerebrospinal fluid may occur from destruction of arachnoid granulations by meningitis. This mechanism of the development of hydrocephalus also occurs in expanding central lesions of the brain, which by compressing the brain against the skull, obliterate the subarachnoid space over the vertex (see adult hydrocephalus, p. 909).

Other malformations of cerebral tissues include spastic diplegia, tuberous sclerosis, mongolism, and amaurotic familial idiocy.

Cerebral palsy (spastic diplegia, Little's disease) is characterized clinically by spasticity of the lower extremities, choreiform movements, and sometimes mental deficiency resulting from central neuronal degeneration. Grossly the brain is usually small and shrunken, with patches of microgyri, and there may be gross defects in the cerebellum and pons. Although the cause is usually a defect in development, perinatal trauma and inflammatory disease may also cause cerebral palsy. The syndrome is duplicated in infantile encephalomyelitides and in toxic reactions. Microscopically the atrophied areas show gliosis.

Tuberous sclerosis is a congenital and familial disease manifest a few months to a few years after birth in mental deficiency, epileptiform seizures, cutaneous tumors similar to sebaceous adenomas, and often tumors of other organs. Grossly the brain is small, firm, and dotted by areas of macrogyri, which are pearly white in color and often nodular in form. Similar firm nodules may project into the ventricles. The nodules are composed of dense glial tissue and contain irregular giant cells and atypical glial elements. Hyperplasia of the sebaceous glands of the nose and cheeks (adenoma sebaceum), rhabdomyomas of the heart, and hamartomas of the kidneys are common accompaniments. The clinical syndrome characterized by mental changes and adenoma sebaceum of the skin in association with tuberous sclerosis of the brain is called *epiloia*.

Mongolism (Down's syndrome) is characterized by mongoloid

features in an idiotic child of Caucasian parents. It has been recently discovered that it is caused by the presence of an additional small acrocentric chromosome. The head is usually small, the tongue is prominent, and the musculature is hypotonic. The brain is small, and there may be gross defects in the gyri. There is apparently a diminished number of cortical neurons, and the cortical architecture is distorted. Hypophysial changes have been described (p. 669). The condition appears to cause some predisposition to leukemia.

Amaurotic familial idiocy (Tay-Sachs disease) is a familial condition that occurs in infantile and juvenile forms. The infantile form is found mainly in Jewish people. Progressive muscular weakness develops in the early months of life, and mental development fails. There is a characteristic peculiar cherry-red spot in the retina, and later optic atrophy and blindness develop. The brain is atrophic and firm. The cerebellum may share in the atrophy. The characteristic histologic feature is distention of many of the nerve cells by a granular deposit of lipid (ganglioside) in the cytoplasm. The lipid deposit also involves cell processes. The degeneration of nerve cells and processes is followed by widespread gliosis.

In the juvenile form, which is more common in Gentiles, the cherry-red spot in the macula is absent, and the lipid in nerve cells stains well with the usual fat stains.

DEMYELINATING DISEASES

The process of demyelination has been described as a secondary phenomenon after damage to continuity of nerve tissue (p. 867). A similar process is, however, observed frequently in the absence of any established primary cause. A group of diseases occurs that is characterized by demyelination, which may be patchy or diffuse.

Diffuse leukoencephalopathy. Under the terms *leukodystrophy* and *diffuse leukoencephalopathy* is included a large heterogeneous group of diseases varying in age of appearance from infancy to adolescence, in onset from acute to gradual, and in course from a few months to many years. Familial or hereditary trends in some types are described. All are characterized by diffuse dissolution of white matter, usually bilateral and symmetric, and beginning in the occipital lobes with extension forward. The terminus is often by aspiration pneumonia, which interrupts the process at various stages. Grossly the brain is soft and the white matter gelatinous, or it may be sclerotic. Weigert stains show absence of myelin with sparing of the short associational axons at the cortical margin. Older areas of degeneration show glial proliferation with formation of many bizarre cell forms and various areas of gliosis. Areas of active degeneration show a fat-granule cell reaction, with perivascular cuffing by fat-laden macrophages, and the meningeal spaces may contain large numbers of these cells. There may be diffuse sclerosis or none at all. References to this condition may be found under the terms *diffuse sclerosis, leukoencephalopathy without sclerosis, progressive degenerative subcortical encephalopathy, encephalitis periaxialis diffusa, Schilder's disease, Krabbe's disease,* and *Pelizaeus-Merzbacher disease.*

Disseminated sclerosis. Disseminated sclerosis (multiple sclerosis) is a relatively common disease of undetermined etiology. The three main hypotheses regarding causation, all unproved, are that it is ischemic (resulting from thromboses), that it is infective (bacterial or viral), and that it is allergic (provocative antigen unknown). The onset usually is between the ages of 20 and 40 years. The symptomatology is varied, as would be expected from the irregular distribution of the lesions. Transient paresis, sensory disturbance, nystagmus, and retrobulbar neuritis are common features. A classic triad consists of nystagmus, intention tremor, and slurring speech. The disease clinically may have periods of remission and relapse, sometimes over a period of years. There are widespread scattered irregular lesions, predominantly in the white matter, which appear grossly as yellow-gray areas on the cut surface of the brain or cord. These stand out prominently as pale areas in Weigert preparations. They are most prominent in the long tracts of the cord, and lesions of the stem and cord figure conspicuously in the symptomatology. Microscopically the lesion is a sharply outlined plaque of demyelination, and in degenerated areas of long standing there may be gliosis. The early degeneration appears to spare the axis cylinders, accounting for transient remissions. As in diffuse sclerosis the microscopic picture depends on the duration of the lesion. In the active process fat-granule cells are operative, form perivascular cuffs, and spill into the subarachnoid space. The optic nerve is often involved. If the optic neuritis dominates and is associated with an acute patchy encephalomyelitis, the condition is called *ophthalmoneuromyelitis (Devic's disease).*

Subacute combined degeneration. In subacute combined degeneration there is patchy degeneration affecting the posterior and lateral columns of the spinal cord. It is associated with macrocytic (pernicious) anemia and achlorhydria. The early lesions are focal areas of destruction of axis cylinders and myelin sheaths, with softening and removal of degenerated material by microglial cells. Fusion of the areas and ascending and descending degeneration of cord tracts result in extensive damage of the posterior and lateral columns. Inflammatory reaction is absent, and little glial repair occurs. The damaged areas show only a delicate, spongy network of glial fibers. Since repair does not occur in the central nervous system, therapy will not undo the damage. Peripheral nerve demyelination is also common in pernicious anemia, and improvement in nervous symptoms after therapy is mainly caused by repair of peripheral nerve degenerations.

NEUROMUSCULAR DISORDERS AND MUSCULAR DYSTROPHIES

Disorders of muscle may occur with pathologic involvement of the central nervous system, peripheral nerves, or muscles, and hence are conveniently described as neurogenic atrophy and myopathy (primary muscle disease).

Neuromuscular disorders. In the neurogenic disorders the muscle involvement is secondary to lesions in the spinal cord or nerves, or both.

Amyotonia congenita (Oppenheim's disease). Amyotonia congenita has as its essential feature a paucity of cells in the anterior horn of the spinal cord. As the term is used clinically for a weak hypotonic infant, several distinct conditions may be so designated. In a related condition (Werdnig-Hoffmann type) there is actual degeneration of the ganglion cells and neuronophagia. There is weakness of muscles lacking their proper nerve supply, and microscopically the muscle fibers show great variation in appearance, many being of embryonic type.

Friedreich's ataxia. Friedreich's ataxia is one of a group of hereditary diseases in which ataxia is prominent. Degenerative changes occur in cerebellum and tracts of the spinal cord, so that the cord appears smaller than normal. Myelin sheath degeneration, particularly in the spinocerebellar and posterior columns, is shown by light unstained areas in Weigert preparations. The degeneration apparently begins in the cells of Clark's column. Late in the disease the pyramidal tracts may be involved. Gliosis follows the myelin degeneration.

Amyotrophic lateral sclerosis. Amyotrophic lateral sclerosis appears in later life and runs a fairly rapid course to fatal termination. The pathologic changes are similar to those of progressive muscular atrophy with an added bilateral degeneration of the pyramidal tracts starting at the cerebral cortex. It appears to be a motor neuron disease in which demyelination is secondary to alterations in motor nerve cells.

Traumatic injury. Traumatic injury to a peripheral nerve results in muscular atrophy.

Hypertrophic neuritis. Hypertrophic neuritis is a nodular proliferative condition of sheath cells along a peripheral nerve. There may be an associated degeneration of posterior columns if the disease involves the posterior roots.

Peroneal muscular atrophy. Peroneal muscular atrophy is a degeneration of the peroneal musculature with an associated neuritis. There is atrophy of the calf muscles, with foot drop and clubfoot. The disease is hereditary and occurs in the first decade.

Myopathic muscular atrophies (dystrophies). Some disorders of muscle are of unknown etiology and are without demonstrable primary lesions in the nervous system.

Myasthenia gravis. (See p. 699.)

Myotonia congenita. Myotonia congenita is characterized by sustained contraction on voluntary movement. The muscles often are hypertrophied.

Progressive muscular dystrophy. Progressive muscular dystrophy is a primary disease of muscles characterized by a prolonged course and great muscular weakness. The muscles may show a severe pseudohypertrophy. Microscopically great variation in fiber size is apparent. Terminally the muscle is replaced by connective tissue. Creatine appears in the urine.

DISEASES OF EXTRAPYRAMIDAL MOTOR SYSTEM

In diseases of the extrapyramidal motor system the lesions are localized or predominant in extrapyramidal parts known to affect motor activity. These parts include the thalamus, basal nuclei (caudate, putamen, globus pallidus, claustrum, amygdaloid), and several lower stem nuclei (subthalamic body, nucleus ruber, substantia nigra). Clinically there are disturbances in motor activity manifested by tremor, choreiform movement, torsion spasm, or rigidity without true motor paralysis. The symptomatology varies with the topography of the lesion.

Progressive lenticular degeneration (Wilson's disease). Progressive lenticular degeneration is a genetic defect in copper and ceruloplasmin metabolism, appearing in an adolescent or young adult, its varying course progressing to a fatal ending in a few months to ten years. There is a bilateral symmetric degeneration and cavitation of the putamen and, occasionally, the caudate nucleus. The involved tissue develops a spongy consistency. Microscopically there is a distinct glial proliferation with the production of giant astrocytes. Associated with the disease in the basal nuclei there is a cirrhosis of the liver. An increased copper content has been demonstrated in the liver and the brain and—in the latter—particularly in the putamen, caudate nucleus, and globus pallidus. In addition to the tremor and spasticity of skeletal muscles often there is striking emotional disturbance. A characteristic feature is the appearance of greenish pigmentation along the corneal margin (Kayser-Fleischer ring).

Acute chorea (Sydenham's chorea). Acute chorea usually appears between the ages of 5 and 15 years. It is commonly associated with rheumatic fever. There may be an associated rheumatic myocarditis. The cerebral lesions are difficult to localize, but such striatal involvements as areas of softenings, focal degenerations, toxic changes in striatal cells, and inflammatory foci of mild degree have been described. Clinically the disease is characterized by rapid, involuntary, purposeless movements and considerable incoordination, especially of the upper extremity. Mentally is not affected. Recovery occurs in a few weeks to several years.

Chronic progressive chorea (Huntington's chorea). Chronic progressive chorea is a familial progressive disease appearing in persons after 30 years of age. Sporadic cases are said to occur also. Profound mental changes are associated with the grimacing, gesticulation, and incoordination of the chorea. The corpus striatum is severely shrunken, with dissolution predominant among the smaller cells, and degeneration is found in the supragranular layers of the cerebral cortex. Secondary gliosis is present in lesions of long standing. The hereditary pattern of transmission of the disease is autosomal dominant.

Paralysis agitans (Parkinson's disease, shaking palsy). Paralysis agitans is characterized clinically by coarse tremor (at rest) and muscular rigidity, which is most prominent in the upper extremity. Ordinarily the condition is progressive, with the eventual appearance of the tremor in the lower extremity, jaw, and tongue and a significant alteration in gait. Two distinct forms, essential and secondary, are recognized. Idiopathic paralysis agitans, or Parkinson's disease, begins during or after the involutional period and progresses slowly. The secondary form (postencephalitic parkinsonism) is associated with epidemic encephalitis. A secondary parkinsonism may also follow chronic manganese poisoning or severe carbon monoxide or nitrous oxide intoxication. There are degenerative changes in the basal nuclei, which rarely may be evident grossly as lacunar softenings associated with vascular disease. Often the changes in the basal nuclei are evident only on quantitative study. Loss of nerve cells and nonspecific cellular changes (pigmentation, degeneration, swelling, and shrinkage) predominate. The substantia nigra and locus ceruleus are the principal sites of involvement in idiopathic paralysis agitans. In the postencephalitic form the degeneration is more widespread.

DISEASES OF INTRACRANIAL VESSELS

Meningeal vasculature. The vascular system of the meninges includes three distinctive sets of vessels: the dural sinuses and their tributaries (emissary veins and superficial cerebral veins), the meningeal arteries, and the subarachnoid arteries. The dural sinuses and their tributaries are important in regard to both infections and hemorrhage, and the meningeal and subarachnoid arteries are important principally in relation to hemorrhage.

Sinus thrombosis. Sinus thrombosis is essentially a thrombophlebitis of a dural sinus. Cavernous sinus thrombosis is related to infections of the nose, upper lip, cheek, orbit, and sphenoid and posterior ethmoid paranasal sinuses. Superior sagittal sinus thrombosis occurs as a sequel to frontal sinusitis. Transverse sinus thrombosis is most often related to middle ear and mastoid infections. Superficial infections of the scalp and neck and retropharyngeal abscesses can also give rise to sinus thrombosis by conduction along appropriate emissary veins. There is usually an associated leptomeningitis, and sinus thrombosis is thought to be important in the pathogenesis of some brain abscesses (p. 903).

Epidural hemorrhage. Epidural hemorrhage ordinarily refers to blood in the temporal region from traumatic rupture of the middle meningeal artery or its branches, but rarely it is caused by a tear of an emissary vein as it enters a dural sinus. This may be found in the posterior fossa from rupture of the mastoid emissary as it enters the transverse sinus. The hemorrhage is limited in extravasation to individual bone areas because of the dural attachments at the suture lines. The clot forming between the dura and bone compresses the underlying brain tissue.

Dural or subdural hemorrhage (subdural hematoma, pachymeningitis hemorrhagica interna). Dural or subdural hemorrhage occurs when bleeding from dural vessels extravasates in a subdural or intradural position, forming a hematoma. The hematoma is limited by granulation tissue, probably with fibroblasts of arachnoidal and dural origin. The bleeding point may be difficult to localize, but in recent traumatic cases it can often be traced to the junction of superficial cerebral veins with dural sinuses. Usually there is a small amount of subarachnoid extravasation resulting from arachnoid tears. The hematoma is most frequent over the frontal and parietal areas and is often bilateral. Although generally regarded as traumatic, spontaneous cases have occurred in blood dyscrasias, infections, and toxemias.

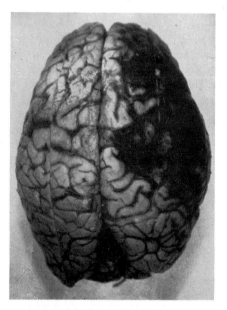

Fig. 25-14. Subarachnoid hemorrhage.

The hematoma organizes at its periphery, usually retaining a fluid center. Its clinical effects result from the fact that it is a space-occupying mass.

Subarachnoid hemorrhage. Subarachnoid hemorrhage is from subarachnoid arteries which lie superficially in the subarachnoid spaces of the base of the brain and deep in the sulci over the other surfaces, or from subarachnoid veins, which occupy a superficial position over the vertex. Bleeding from the latter vessels occurs as a result of trauma, blood dyscrasias, or rupture of a surface angioma. Blood may also appear in the subarachnoid space by rupture from a hemorrhage in brain tissue or by conduction with cerebrospinal fluid from an intraventricular hemorrhage. However, subarachnoid bleeding most commonly is from a ruptured aneurysm. The aneurysms are usually basal in position at points of vessel branching. The most important aneurysms are congenital or mycotic and only rarely can be ascribed to arteriosclerosis and syphilis.

"Congenital" aneurysm. Congenital aneurysms (p. 312) are of fairly frequent occurrence. The angles of bifurcation of the arteries about the base of the brain are common sites. They are

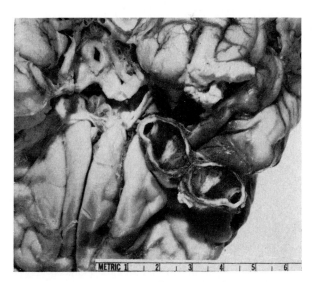

Fig. 25-15. Thrombosed aneurysm of the middle cerebral artery.

caused by congenital weakness of the media at the point where the vessel branches. The aneurysm itself is not always congenital, although the defect in the vascular wall is a congenital or developmental abnormality. It may be associated with other developmental abnormalities such as polycystic kidney. Small leakages may occur through the wall of the sac, giving rise to pigmentation and thickening of meninges in the neighborhood of the aneurysm. Rupture of the aneurysm results in a subarachnoid hemorrhage, which is often rapidly fatal. The subarachnoid space about the region of the aneurysm (hence usually at the base of the brain) is found filled by a recent blood clot. The clot may easily hide the aneurysm unless it is carefully removed. Occasionally the hemorrhage extends into the ventricles. Aneurysms may be associated with cerebral infarction, and sometimes other complications such as intracerebral hematoma and subarachnoid block with hydrocephalus.

Mycotic aneurysm. Mycotic aneurysms are produced by infected emboli lodging in cerebral vessels. Subacute bacterial endocarditis is the commonest source of the embolus, and the middle cerebral artery is the commonest site. Emboli bearing organisms of high virulence usually produce abscess or meningitis rather than mycotic aneurysm.

Birth injury. Birth injury may result from molding of the head during birth, which puts a strain upon the falx of the dura and the tentorium over the cerebellum. A tear may result, sometimes with involvement of the dural sinuses of the great cerebral vein (of Galen), and some subarachnoid hemorrhage may be found also.

INTRAMEDULLARY VASCULAR DISEASES

Arteritis and vascular degeneration, with resulting thrombosis or hemorrhage, occurs as a result of vascular damage from many poisons (carbon monoxide, arsenic), in septic conditions (scarlet fever, pneumonia), blood dyscrasias (purpura, leukemia), polyarteritis nodosa, Buerger's disease, and syphilis. The brain tissue shows multiple small hemorrhages or softenings. Atherosclerosis and hypertension are the two important causes of intramedullary vascular disease.

Arteriosclerosis. Cerebral vessels are similar in structure to vessels elsewhere, although the small arteries contain a disproportionately large amount of connective tissue in their walls. With advance in age muscle decreases, the internal elastic lamina undergoes reduplication, and there is a medial fibrosis. Arteriosclerosis of the larger vessels at the base of the brain is of the atheromatous type. Through weakening of the wall aneurysms may form. Cerebral arteriosclerosis may have no direct correlation with sclerotic changes elsewhere in the vascular system and has no constant relationship to hypertension. However, cerebral hyaline arteriolosclerosis is not uncommon with hypertension. Narrowing of the vascular lumina diminishes the blood supply and exerts a serious effect on brain tissue Multiple perivascular zones of atrophy may be found in the brain as a result of arteriosclerosis, in addition to larger softenings from thrombosis. Particularly susceptible to diminished blood supply are the striatum, hippocampus, dentate nucleus, and cerebral cortex.

Thrombosis. Thrombosis develops in cerebral vessels from the same causes as elsewhere. A sclerotic vessel is usually involved, and arteriosclerosis is the most frequent underlying cause of cerebral infarction.

Embolism. Embolism of cerebral arteries originates from thrombi in the lung or more commonly from the left side of the heart. Paradoxical embolism occurs from emboli breaking off in the right circulatory field and gaining access to the left side of the heart through an open foramen ovale. Air and fat also act as emboli (p. 102). Massive infarction results most commonly from occlusion of branches of the middle cerebral artery, probably because this vessel is a direct continuation of the internal carotid artery. Consequently the middle cerebral artery is in direct line for receiving emboli, as well as being subject to the wear and tear of direct pressure effects from the heart.

Infarction. Occlusion of a cerebral artery results in infarction of the region supplied by the vessel unless adequate collateral circulation is available. Even though abundant anastomoses are present, they may be insufficient to maintain nutrition if an artery is blocked. Cerebral infarcts are characterized by softening. The clinical effects depend upon the area of nervous tissue involved. The appearance of a cerebral infarct depends upon its age. A recent infarct may be indistinguishable in a fresh brain, but after fixation it remains soft in comparison with surrounding tissue. If its age is greater than two or three days, it appears as a soft, semifluid area with a slightly yellowish color and an edematous, sometimes hemorrhagic, edge. Later, when the necrotic and liquefied material has been removed, the region is shrunken and depressed. If the infarcted area is large, it may have a cystlike center containing yellowish fluid *(apoplectic cyst)* encapsulated by glial tissue.

Microscopically a very recent infarct transiently contains neutrophilic leukocytes, but they soon disappear. Nerve cells, axis cylinders, and neuroglial cells degenerate, and lipid of the myelin sheath is broken down and liquefied. The fatty and necrotic material undergoes phagocytosis and is removed by the ameboid microglial cells. These scavengers appear abundantly as rounded cells with a foamy or vascuolated cytoplasm (fat-granule cells, compound granular corpuscles). Healing occurs by proliferation of a granulation tissue composed of astrocytes, capillaries, and a few fibroblasts of the adventitia of adjacent vessels. Eventually a dense neuroglial scar is formed. The damage is permanent, as there is no regeneration of the injured nerve cells and fibers.

Cerebral hemorrhage. Hemorrhages into the brain tissue itself may be either small petechial or perivascular hemorrhages or a massive hematoma. *Acute hemorrhagic leukoencephalitis* is an acute condition localized in the white matter of the cerebrum and characterized by focal perivascular hemorrhage, edema, demyelination, and necrosis. The cut surface of the white matter shows multiple hemorrhagic areas varying from minute points to several millimeters in diameter. The etiology is unknown. Small petechial hemorrhages result from many types of trauma and may be found near gross cerebral lacerations. Petechial hemorrhages also may result from poisons such as carbon monoxide and arsphenamine, from cerebral fat embolism, or from purpuric or leukemic conditions.

Massive intracerebral hemorrhage is caused by vascular disease with or without high blood pressure. It is a frequent end result of hypertensive cardiovascular-renal disease. The vessels most commonly affected are the lenticulostriate branches of the middle cerebral artery, involving the basal ganglia and internal capsule. Less frequently there is hemorrhage into the white matter of the cerebrum or into the pons or cerebellum. The actual mechanism of the hemorrhage is debatable, and it is usually impossible to find the point of vascular rupture. The brain bulges slightly on the side of the hemorrhage, where there is some flattening of the convolutions. Cutting through the brain tissue reveals the area of hemorrhage lacerating the brain substance. Rupture into a ventricle often occurs, and in such cases blood appear in the spinal fluid. Hemorrhage into cerebral tumor tissue may be grossly indistinguishable from the ordinary type of cerebral hemorrhage. Microscopic examination is necessary to confirm or rule out this possibility.

DEGENERATIVE ENCEPHALOPATHIES

Various degenerative lesions of the nervous system are caused by soluble toxins, chemical poisons, anesthesia, uremia, diabetic coma, hypoglycemia, pentylenetrazol (Metrazol) and shock therapy, and deficiency diseases.

The group caused by soluble toxins includes tetanus, botulism, and a heterogeneous group of undetermined etiology referred to as "toxic" encephalopathy. *Tetanus* (p. 122) exerts its effect by its neurotropic toxin.

Chemical poisons, such as arsenic, lead, manganese, carbon monoxide, and alcohol, may give rise to degenerative changes in the nervous system. The mechanism is ascribed to actual toxic necrosis, implicating vascular structures primarily, or to relative or absolute anoxia. Pathologic alterations include edema, congestion, focal softenings, and hemorrhages. Actual inflammatory changes are rare. The changes being nonspecific, demonstration of the toxic substance is essential to diagnosis. *Streptomycin* may cause degeneration and necrosis of neurons of the eighth cranial nerve nuclei, resulting in deafness and some vestibular dysfunction. *Anesthetic agents* such as ether, chloroform, nitrous oxide, cyclopropane, and barbiturates have all been incriminated as occasional causes of death. Relative anoxia usually is described as the mechanism by which neuronal degeneration is induced. The cerebral changes produced by *anoxia* (e.g., as in high altitude flying), circulatory arrest, carbon monoxide poisoning, hypoglycemia, and anesthetic agents are all very much alike, apparently influenced by both vascular and metabolic factors. Similar anoxic changes are found in fatalities after fever therapy. Ether and chloroform, as strong fat solvents, have been known to precipitate demyelination and are generally regarded as dangerous in any patient with a demyelinating disease. Microscopically there may be found satellitosis, glial proliferation with the formation of glial nodes, and nonspecific changes in the nerve cell bodies, such as shrinkage and nuclear pyknosis. *Uremia* may be accompanied by severe edema of the brain, with pressure marks and coning, and by cerebral anemia, believed to be caused by the swelling of the brain. The nerve cells are swollen, and sometimes there is perivascular cuffing. The pathogenesis is obscure. *Diabetic coma* is usually accompanied by little morphologic change. It is usually considered to result from relative anoxia rather than toxemia. *Hypoglycemia* caused by insulin therapy or a tumor of pancreatic islet tissue may exhibit cerebral signs. Changes in the nervous system include chromatolytic, vacuolar, and pyknotic nerve cell alterations (nonspecific), formation of pseudogiant cells, gemistocytosis, degeneration of axis cylinders, and petechial hemorrhages. *Metrazol* and *electroshock therapy* may produce cerebral brain damage similar to that of hypoglycemia. Hemorrhage may be prominent, particularly in electric therapy. *Vitamin deficiency diseases,* particularly pellagra, beriberi, rickets, and scurvy, may have associated nonspecific degenerative changes in the nervous system (p. 249). *Burns,* when extensive and severe, may result in cerebral edema, hyperemia, and small hemorrhages. Ganglion cells may show toxic changes, swelling, chromatolysis, and eccentric nuclei, and there may be small areas of demyelination. Degenerative changes in the brain, as well as in the peripheral nerves (neuropathy), occasionally occur as an unexplained remote effect of visceral cancers, e.g., bronchogenic carcinoma.

ENCEPHALITIS

Inflammatory diseases of the central nervous system may be caused by parasitic and fungous infections, syphilis, bacterial infections, rickettsial diseases, and viral diseases.

Parasitic and fungous infections. Parasitic and mycotic infections of the nervous system include those caused by toxoplasma, trichina, pork tapeworm (cysticercosis), malaria, and actinomycosis (Chapter 9). *Torula (Cryptococcus)* affects both the meninges and brain (p. 210). *Syphilis* frequently involves the central nervous system (p. 190).

Bacterial infection. Bacterial infection of the central nervous system may produce suppurative encephalitis or brain abscess. Staphylococci are the commonest organisms, although streptococci, pneumococci, and others may be causative. Cultures at autopsy often yield mixed agents. The organism may be introduced by direct implantation (trauma, surgery), contiguous extension (e.g., from erosion of bone and dura over an otitis media), or metastatic extension (e.g., from bronchiectasis). A centrally located abscess sometimes has no identifiable primary focus, although it is assumed that all are secondary to some other focus of infection, which is presumed to have disappeared while

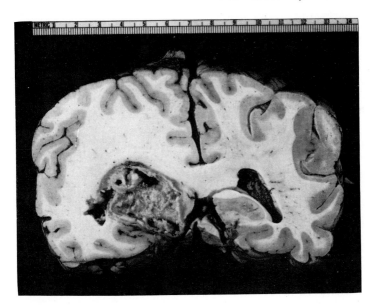

Fig. 25-16. Abscess of the brain.

the brain abscess was developing. Lesions with which brain abscess is commonly associated include otitis media, sinus thrombosis, bronchiectasis, empyema, lung abscess, bacterial endocarditis, and congenital heart disease.

Brain abscesses occur most commonly in the temporal lobe and cerebellar hemispheres. If embolic, they are usually multiple. Grossly the abscess is encapsulated and has a fluid purulent center. The developing abscess goes through the changes of focal necrosis, invasion by leukocytes, liquefaction and formation of pus, fat-granule cell reaction, peripheral fibrinous exudate, surrounding hyperemia and fibroblastic proliferation, and mild marginal gliosis. The fully formed abscess thus has four microscopic layers from within outward: (1) a central necrotic core (cavity of the abscess), (2) a vascular granulomatous border (reactive zone), (3) a zone of hyperemia and fibrosis, and (4) an external zone of gliosis (encephalitic zone). Spontaneous resolution of a cerebral abscess probably does not occur. Rupture of an abscess results in disseminated suppurative encephalitis and purulent meningitis. Usually encapsulation occurs in a variable time of a few days to a few weeks. Abscesses caused by aerobic bacteria tend to form better capsules than those caused by anaerobic bacteria or mixed infections.

Various *viral* and *rickettsial* infections produce encephalitis (Chapter 7).

MENINGITIS

Pachymeningitis. Inflammation of the dura may develop by spread from overlying bone. Hence it may complicate osteomyelitis of the skull, compound fracture, etc. The dura tends to localize the lesion with the production of an *epidural abscess*. The overlying area of the scalp is swollen, congested, and edematous (Pott's puffy tumor). Spinal epidural abscess may cause paraplegia. *Subdural abscess* may occur secondary to neighboring infections. This consists of a broad limited sheet of purulent material or organized exudate. *Peripachymeningitis* is an inflammatory condition associated with Pott's disease (p. 839). *Pachymeningitis cervicalis hypertrophica* is a pronounced thickening of the dura in the cervical region that may be associated with syphilis.

Leptomeningitis. Inflammations of the leptomeninx may be purulent, caused by bacterial or actinomycotic infections, or nonpurulent, caused by tuberculous, syphilitic, lymphocytic, or torula meningitis.

Purulent meningitis. Purulent meningitis may be caused by meningococci, pneumococci, streptococci, staphylococci, gonococci, influenza bacilli, actinomyces, and rarely colon bacilli in infants. The most important of these is the meningococcus, which gives rise to the epidemic form of meningitis as well as to occasional sporadic cases. In meningococcal meningitis the organism may reach the meninges by passage through the nasopharynx, where it leaves no trace, and then along the perineural sheath of the olfactory nerve, and through the cribriform plate of the ethmoid to reach the meninges. However, the probable route of meningeal infection is by the bloodstream. Acute fulminating forms of meningococcal infection are septicemic and systemic with hemorrhagic spots in the skin, hence the term *spotted fever*. The purulent exudate is most abundant over the base of the brain, and extension commonly occurs to the spinal meninges. The infection usually spreads to the choroid plexus and the interior of the ventricles. Some degree of acute internal hydrocephalus results from an increased permeability of the

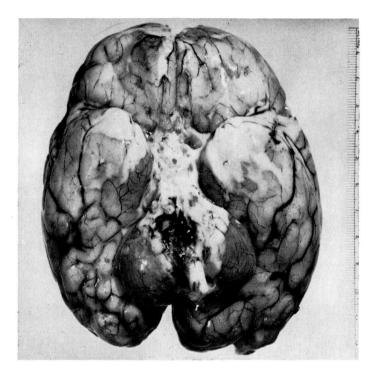

Fig. 25-17. Purulent meningitis.

choroid plexus, an outpouring of exudate into the ventricles, and interference with outflow caused by inflammatory swelling about the narrow ventricular openings. This condition, along with edema, congestion of blood vessels, and subarachnoid exudates, increases the intracranial pressure.

The other purulent meningitides resemble the meningococcal form both grossly and microscopically, necessitating identification of the organism for diagnosis. Streptococcal and pneumococcal exudates appear most abundantly over the vertex, whereas meningococcal exudate tends to aggregate at the base. In meningitis caused by the influenza bacillus, the exudate is most abundant and diffuse.

Nonpurulent meningitis. A variety of infections may cause a meningitis with a nonpurulent type of exudate.

TUBERCULOUS MENINGITIS. Tuberculous meningitis is a non-purulent meningitis, which is secondary to a tuberculous lesion elsewhere and often only a part of a generalized miliary tuberculosis. In other cases it is the most prominent active focus of tuberculosis in the body. It is almost invariably fatal. The brain is swollen, and a gelatinous, translucent, slightly greenish exudate may be evident in the subarachnoid space. If exudate is abundant, it usually involves the base of the brain and spreads through the sylvian cisterns. Tiny opaque yellowish flecks, which represent minute tubercles, are evident along the course of subarachnoid vessels or on the choroid plexus. Microscopically the inflammatory reaction and exudate are in general similar to tuberculosis elsewhere but tend to show more neutrophilic leukocytes. The predominant cells, however, are large mononuclear cells, lymphocytes, plasma cells, and epithelioid cells. Small areas of caseation and definite tubercles may be found. Giant

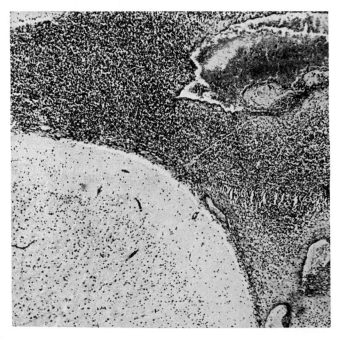

Fig. 25-18. Acute meningitis. Note the involvement of blood vessels.

cells are not numerous. Since the inflammatory process often involves the superficial portions of the cortex, the condition is really a meningoencephalitis. Blood vessels passing through the exudate show adventitial inflammation and intimal thickening (tuberculous arteritis). Fibroblastic proliferation causes a meningeal thickening. Tubercles may be found involving the choroid plexus and ependyma.

The pathogenesis of tuberculous meningitis is a matter of dispute. The three main theories are (1) hematogenous infection of the cerebrospinal fluid, (2) hematogenous spread to choroid plexus, with the development there of a tubercle that later infects leptomeninges, and (3) hematogenous spread to superficial cerebral cortex with the development of a localized tubercle, which later ruptures or spreads infection to meninges.

Tuberculoma of the brain is a large solitary tuberculous lesion. Its symptomatology may cause confusion with a neoplasm. The microscopic structure is similar to that of tuberculous lesions elsewhere.

LYMPHOCYTIC CHORIOMENINGITIS. Lymphocytic choriomeningitis is believed to be caused by a virus and has a transitory, non-

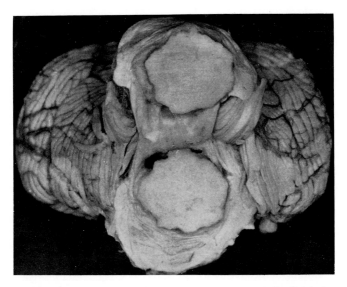

Fig. 25-19. Tuberculoma of the pons. (Courtesy Dr. S. B. Pessin.)

fatal course. There is considerable lymphocytic infiltration of the subarachnoid spaces, with the appearance of large numbers of lymphocytes in the cerebrospinal fluid (p. 165).

TORULA MENINGITIS. Torula meningitis is a chronic meningeal irritation caused by a fungus, *Cryptococcus hominis* (p. 210).

SYPHILITIC MENINGITIS. (See p. 190.)

DISEASES OF PERIPHERAL NERVES

The diseases of peripheral nerves, other than the neoplasms that were discussed previously, fall into the three ill-defined categories of neuralgia, neuritis, and traumatic injury. The changes resulting from peripheral nerve trauma are those of wallerian degeneration and neuroma formation (p. 867).

Neuralgia. Neuralgia refers to pain in the distribution of a nerve supply, the principal ones affected being trigeminal and sciatic. *Protrusion of intervertebral discs* usually involves nerve roots, but particularly in cervical areas, it may result in degenerative lesions in the spinal cord, involving especially the anterior horns, lateral columns, and anterior part of the dorsal columns. These changes may result from a reduction of blood supply in the distal distribution of the anterior spinal artery.

Neuritis. Neuritis is a term used loosely in referring to any condition associated with inflammatory or degenerative changes in peripheral nerves. When many nerves are involved, the condition is described as *polyneuritis;* if one nerve is involved, as *mononeuritis.* Various changes that may be found include hyperemia of the nerve sheath, transudation and swelling, cellular exudate, myelin degeneration, and swelling and fragmentation of axis cylinders. Once continuity of fibers is broken, secondary wallerian degeneration occurs. From an etiologic standpoint, the neuritides may be grouped under the following headings: (1) viral (herpes), (2) bacteriotoxic (scarlet fever), (3) deficiency or metabolic (beriberi), (4) chemical (lead), (5) focal mechanical (tumor pressure), and (6) focal infectious (leprosy). A large number of etiologic agents operate in each category.

The so-called *infectious polyneuritis* or polyradiculitis *(Guillain-Barré syndrome),* is a polyneuritis of sudden onset with widespread flaccid paralysis and increased protein in the spinal fluid without a corresponding increase in the number of cells. The etiology and pathogenesis have not been established, but one concept is that it is an allergic phenomenon, and some cases have been associated with infectious mononucleosis. Recovery is usually rapid and complete. The mechanism may be a sudden swelling of spinal cord roots, resulting in constriction of radicular nerves at their points of penetration of the spinal meninges. Changes in the nervous system are predominantly degenerative and are nonspecific.

INTRACRANIAL TENSION

The relative rigidity of the cranial vault leads to increased intracranial tension from changes in volume of its contents. For this reason space-occupying lesions, conditions limiting the flow of cerebrospinal fluid, and edema of the brain give rise to an elevated intracranial pressure. This brings about certain pathologic changes of great clinical importance.

Changes in extramedullary fluid volume. (See also p. 888.) In the adult, hydrocephalus occurs in a number of chronic diseases as a moderate dilatation of the ventricular system and often along with a slight external hydrocephalus (distended subarachnoid space). This may be seen in syphilis, possibly in chronic alcoholism, and chronic subarachnoid obstructions such as may follow meningitis. Very often the mechanism is obscure. In syphilis, involvement of the arachnoid villi may inhibit absorption of fluid. In addition to thickening after meningitis, chronic arachnitis has been observed after repeated subarachnoid hemorrhage (seeping aneurysm). At autopsy such brains usually exhibit a moderate internal hydrocephalus. In cerebral atrophy associated with senility there is often a severe external hydrocephalus. The absence of ventricular dilatation in such cases indicates that pressure phenomena had little to do with the accumulation of fluid over the atrophied brain. A more acute ventricular distention in the adult occurs in purulent meningitis and with intraventricular block.

Changes in intracranial tissue volume. Changes in tissue volume within the cranium may be brought about by (1) accumulation of intramedullary (interstitial) fluid *(edema)*, (2) increase in vascular volume *(congestion)*, and (3) new tissue growth *(tumor)*. The subarachnoid space often is obliterated, and the surface of the brain is dry. Underlying gyri are compressed and very flattened, and the sulci are obscured. The opposing walls of the ventricles may be in apposition. A distinctive characteristic is the appearance of pressure marks along the base of the brain. The cerebellar tonsils may be shoved over the brim of the foramen magnum, grooving the cerebellum (coning). In addition, the swollen temporal lobes may spread over the free margins of the tentorial aperture with a consequent linear grooving on their medial surfaces. Edema may be related to cardiac decompensation, generalized septic and toxic states, and cachexia. Microscopically the brain tissue is vacuolated, the cells appearing widely separated. Congestion occurs in many inflammatory conditions as well as in cardiac failure and polycythemia. With congestion alone, increase in total tissue volume is usually not excessive, as is shown by the absence of pressure marks.

References

CHAPTER 1—THE CELL AND ITS BEHAVIOR

Ashworth, C. T., et al.: Arch. Path. **75**:212, 1963 (hepatic cell degeneration).

Bourne, G. H., editor: Cytology and cell physiology, ed. 3, New York, 1964, Academic Press, Inc.

De Robertis, E. D. P., Nowinski, W. W., and Saez, F. A.: Cell biology, Philadelphia, 1965, W. B. Saunders Co.

Freeman, J. A.: Cellular fine structure, New York, 1964, McGraw-Hill Book Co.

Irwin, S., and Egozcue, J.: Science **157**:313, 1967 (chromosome abnormalities in LSD-25 users).

King, D. W., editor: Ultrastructure aspects of disease, New York, 1966, Paul B. Hoeber, Inc., Medical Book Division, Harper & Row, Publishers.

Majno, F., et al.: Virchows Arch. Path. Anat. **333**:421, 1960 (necrosis).

Sandberg, A. A., et al.: Cancer Res. **21**:678, 1961 (chromosomes in leukemia).

Thompson, J. S., and Thompson, M. N.: Genetics in medicine, Philadelphia, 1966, W. B. Saunders Co.

Trump, B. F., et al.: Lab. Invest. **14**:343, 1965 (necrosis).

CHAPTER 2—RETROGRADE DISTURBANCES

Biava, C. G., et al.: Amer. J. Path. **44**:349, 1964 (renal hyaline arteriolosclerosis—electron microscope study).

Brown, D. B., and Eguren, L. M.: J. Path. Bact. **83**:107, 1962 (hyaline droplet degeneration).

Cohen, A. S.: The constitution and genesis of amyloid. In Richter, G. W., and Epstein, M. A.: International review of experimental pathology, vol. 4, New York, 1965, Academic Press, Inc., pp. 159-243.

Cohen, A. S.: Lab. Invest. **15**:66, 1966 (amyloid fibrils).

Cooper, J. A., and Moran, T. J.: Arch. Path. **64**:46, 1957 (ochronosis).

Fonnesu, A, and Severi, C.: Brit. J. Exp. Path. **34**:341, 1953 (cloudy swelling).

Heller, H., et al.: J. Path. Bact. **88**:15, 1964 (amyloidosis).

Jeghers, H.: New Eng. J. Med. **231**:88, 122, and 181, 1944 (skin pigmentation).

Kennedy, J. A.: J. Path. Bact. **83**:165, 1962; Lab. Invest. **15**:85, 1966 (amyloidosis).

Lichtenstein, L., et al.: Amer. J. Path. **32**:871, 1956 (gout).

MacDonald, R. A.: Arch. Intern. Med. **107**:606, 1961 (idiopathic hemochromatosis).

McGee, W. G., and Ashworth, C. T.: Amer. J. Path. **43**:273, 1963 (fine structure of hypertensive arteriopathy).

Nyhan, W. L.: Arthritis & Rheum. **8:**659, 1965 (uric acid metabolism and cerebral function).

Olcott, C. T.: Amer. J. Path. **24:**813, 1948 (argyria).

Oliver, R. A. M.: J. Path. Bact. **77:**171, 1959 (transfusional siderosis).

Panabokké, R. G.: J. Path. Bact. **75:**319, 1958 (fat necrosis).

Smith, B. F.: J.A.M.A. **144:**1074, 1950 (tattooing and hepatitis).

Soergel, K. M., and Sommers, S. C.: Amer. J. Med. **32:**499, 1962 (pulmonary hemosiderosis).

Stettin, D., Jr., and Stettin, M. R.: Physiol. Rev. **40:**505, 1960 (glycogen).

Sweetman, L., and Nyhan, W. L.: Nature **215:**859, 1967 (genetic disease of purine metabolism).

Talbott, J. H.: Gout, New York, 1957, Grune & Stratton, Inc.

Teilum, G.: Ann. Rheum. Dis. **11:**119, 1952; Amer. J. Path. **24:**389, 1948; Lab. Invest. **15:**98, 1966 (amyloidosis and paramyloidosis).

Uys, C. J., et al.: S. Afr. J. Lab. Clin. Med. **6:**1, 1960 (siderosis of liver).

Wagner, B. M., and Siew, S.: Significance of the extracellular hyaline substances. In Sommers, S. C.: Pathology annual, vol. 2, New York, 1967, Appleton-Century-Crofts.

CHAPTER 3—INFLAMMATION AND REPAIR

Benditt, E. P.: Gastroenterology **40:**338, 1961 (mechanisms).

Editorial: J.A.M.A. **177:**445, 1961 (basophils).

Editorial: J.A.M.A. **179:**285, 1962 (plasma cells).

Fisher, E. R.: J.A.M.A. **173:**171, 1960 (tissue mast cells).

Gorer, P. A., et al.: Nature **189:**1024, 1961 (transplantations).

Lawrence, J. S.: J.A.M.A. **157:**1212, 1955 (functions of leukocytes).

Marchesi, V. T.: Quart. J. Exp. Physiol. **46:**115, 1961 (emigration of leukocytes).

McCutcheon. M.: Arch. Path. (Chicago) **34:**167, 1942 (chemotaxis).

McGovern, V. J.: J. Path. Bact. **73:**99, 1957 (inflammation).

Movat, H. Z.: Amer. J. Med. Sci. **236:**373, 1958 (fibrinoid).

Paff, George H., et al.: Cancer Res. **7:**798, 1947; Anat. Rec. **121:**579, 1955; **126:**165, 1956 (mast cells).

Rebuck, J. W., editor: The lymphocyte and lymphocytic tissue, New York, 1960, Paul B. Hoeber, Inc., Medical Book Division, Harper & Row, Publishers.

Rich, A. R.: Studies in hypersensitivity, Toronto, 1957, Charles Mickle Lecture, University of Toronto Press.

Spector, W. G.: J. Path. Bact. **72:**367, 1956; **74:**67, 1957 (inflammation).

Thomas, L., Uhr, J. W., and Grant, L., editors: International symposium on injury, inflammation and immunity, Baltimore, 1964, The Williams & Wilkins Co.

Zweifach, B. W., Grant, L., and McCluskey, R. T., editors: The inflammatory process, New York, 1965, Academic Press, Inc.

CHAPTER 4—DISTURBANCES OF BODY WATER, ELECTROLYTES, AND CIRCULATION OF BLOOD

Bland, J. H.: Clinical metabolism of body water and electrolytes, Philadelphia, 1963, W. B. Saunders Co.

Edelman, I. S., and Leibman, J.: Amer. J. Med. **27:**256, 1959 (body water and electrolytes).

Elton, N. W., Elton, W. J., and Nayareno, J. P.: Amer. J. Clin. Path. **39:**252, 1963 (acute salt poisoning in infants).

Mills, L. C., and Moyer, J. H.: Shock and hypotension; pathogenesis and treatment, New York, 1965, Grune & Stratton, Inc.

Thal, A. P., and Sardesai, V. M.: Amer. J. Surg. **110:**308, 1965 (shock and circulating polypeptides).

Weisberg, H. F.: Water, electrolyte, and acid-base balance, ed. 2, Baltimore, 1962, The Williams & Wilkins Co.

CHAPTER 5—BACTERIAL INFECTIONS

Amies, C. R.: J. Path. Bact. **67:**25, 1954 (diphtheria).

Anderson, D. R., et al.: J. Bact. **90:**180 and 1387, 1965; J. Nat. Cancer Inst. **36:**139, 1966 (structure of *Mycoplasma*).

Baker, A. B.: J. Neuropath. Exp. Neurol. **1:**394, 1942 (tetanus).

Chanock, R. M., et al.: Amer. Rev. Resp. Dis. **88** (pt. 2):218, 1963 (*Mycoplasma* in respiratory disease).

Ferguson, J. H., and Chapman, O. D.: Amer. J. Path. **24:**763, 1948 (meningococcal infections).

Francis, E., and Callender, G. R.: Arch. Path. **3:**577, 1937 (tularemia).

Jao, R. L., et al.: Arch. Intern. Med. **117:**520, 1966 (*Mycoplasma* in respiratory infections).

Mufson, M. A., et al.: J.A.M.A. **192:**1146, 1965 (*Mycoplasma* in pharyngitis).

Spink, W. W.: Lancet **2:**161, 1964 (brucellosis).

CHAPTER 6—TUBERCULOSIS

Auerbach, O.: Amer. J. Path. **20:**121, 1944 (miliary tuberculosis); Amer. J. Dis. Child. **75:**555, 1944 (tuberculosis in children).

Auerbach, O., and Green, H.: Amer. Rev. Tuberc. **42:**707, 1940 (healing of tuberculosis cavities).

Brown, R. C.: Int. Path. **6:**86, 1965 (atypical mycobacteria).

Davson, J.: J. Path. Bact. **49:**483, 1939 (pulmonary apical scars).

Doege, T. C.: J.A.M.A. **192:**1045, 1965 (tuberculosis mortality, United States).

Middlebrook, G.: The mycobacteria. In Dubos, R. J., and Hirsch, J. G., editors: Bacterial and mycotic infections of man, ed. 4, Philadelphia, 1965, J. B. Lippincott Co., pp. 490-529.

Myers, J. A.: J.A.M.A. **194:**1086, 1965 (natural history of tuberculosis).

Reported tuberculosis data, Public Health Service Publication No. 638, Washington, D. C., 1965 edition, U. S. Department of Health Education and Welfare.

Rich, A. R.: The pathogenesis of tuberculosis, Springfield, Ill., 1944, Charles C Thomas, Publisher.

Schepers, G. W. H.: Amer. J. Cardiol. **9:**248, 1962 (pericarditis).

CHAPTER 7—RICKETTSIAL AND VIRAL DISEASES

Adams, J. M., et al.: J.A.M.A. **195:**290, 1966 (inclusion bodies in measles encephalitis).

Birdsong, M., et al.: J.A.M.A. **162:**1305, 1956 (cytomegalic inclusion disease).

DeCoursey, E.: Wisconsin Med. J. **53:**325, 1954 (epidemic hemorrhagic fever).

Dudgeon, J. A., et al.: Brit. Med. J. **2:**155, 1964 (rubella).

Elton, N. W., et al.: Amer. J. Clin. Path. **25:**135, 1955 (yellow fever).

Enders, J. F., et al.: New Eng. J. Med. **261:**875, 1959 (measles and giant cell pneumonia).

Horsfall, F. L., Jr., and Tamm, I., editors: Viral and rickettsial infections of man, ed. 4, Philadelphia, 1965, J. B. Lippincott Co.

Lillie, R. W.: Arch. Path. **10:**241, 1930 (pathology of smallpox).

McGavran, M. H., et al.: Amer. J. Path. **40:**653, 1962 (psittacosis).

Pinkerton, H., Smiley, W. L., and Anderson, W. A. D.: Amer. J. Path. **21:**1, 1945 (giant cell pneumonia).

Sigel, M. M., and Beasley, A. R.: Viruses, cells, and hosts, New York, 1965, Holt, Rinehart & Winston, Inc.

Sheridan, M. D.: Brit. Med. J. **2:**536, 1964 (rubella in pregnancy).

Spaulding, W. B., and Hennessy, J. N.: Amer. J. Med. **28:**504, 1960 (cat-scratch disease).

Tamm, I., editor: Amer. J. Med. **38:**649, 1965 (symposium on viruses).

Walsh, J. J., et al.: Arch. Intern. Med. **108:**376, 1961 (influenza).

Wolbach, S. B., Todd, J. T., and Palfrey, F. W.: The etiology and pathology of typhus, Cambridge, Mass., 1922, Harvard University Press.

CHAPTER 8—SPIROCHETAL AND VENEREAL DISEASES

Brown, T. M., and Nunemaker, J. C.: Bull. Hopkins Hosp. **70:**210, 1942 (rat-bite fever).

D'Aunoy, R., and von Haam, E.: Arch. Path. **27:**1032, 1939 (lymphogranuloma venereum).

Ferris, H. W., and Turner, T. B.: Arch. Path. **24:**703, 1937 (yaws).

Getzoff, P. L.: J. Urol. **55:**670, 1946 (balanitis).

Rosahn, P. D., and Black-Schaffer, B.: Arch. Intern. Med. **72:**78, 1943; Amer. J. Syph., Gonor. Ven. Dis. **28:**27 and 142, 1944 (syphilis).

Sheldon, W. H., and Heyman, A.: Amer. J. Path. **22:**415, 1946 (chanchroid).

Sigel, M. M., editor: Lymphogranuloma venereum, Coral Gables, Fla., 1962, University of Miami Press.

von Haam, E.: Amer. J. Trop. Med. **18:**595, 1938 (venereal fusospirochetosis).

CHAPTER 9—MYCOTIC, PROTOZOAN, AND HELMINTHIC INFECTIONS

Anderson, W. A. D., Michelson, I. D., and Dunn, T. M.: Amer. J. Clin. Path. **11:**344, 1941 (histoplasmosis).

Arean, V. M.: Schistosomiasis. In Sommers, S. C., editor: Pathology annual, vol. 1, New York, 1966, Appleton-Century-Crofts, pp. 68-126.

Ash, J. E., and Spitz, S.: Pathology of tropical diseases, Philadelphia, 1945, W. B. Saunders Co.

Baum, G. L., and Schwartz, J.: Amer. J. Med. Sci. **238:**661, 1959 (North American blastomycosis).

Boyd, J.: J. Trop. Med. Hyg. **64:**1, 1961 (amebiasis).

Cox, L. B., and Tolhurst, J. C.: Human torulosis, Melbourne, 1946, Melbourne University Press.

Emmons, C. W., Binford, C. H., and Utz, J. P.: Medical mycology, Philadelphia, 1963, Lea & Febiger.

Furcolow, M. L., et al.: J.A.M.A. **177:**292, 1961 (histoplasmosis).

Georg, L. K., et al.: J. Bact. **88:**477, 1964 (actinomyces).

Hutter, R. V. P.: Cancer **12:**330, 1959 (mucormycosis).

Katz, A. M., and Pan, C.: Amer. J. Med. **25:**759, 1958 (*Echinococcus* disease).

Koppisch, E.: J.A.M.A. **121:**936, 1943; Puerto Rico J. Public Health Trop. Med. **16:**385, 1941 (schistosomiasis).

Littman, M. D., and Zimmerman, L. E.: Cryptococcosis, New York, 1956, Grune & Stratton, Inc.

Morrison, D. B., and Anderson, W. A. D.: Public Health Rep. **57:** 90 and 161, 1942; Arch. Path. **33:**677, 1942 (malaria).

Morse, K. T., editor: Ann. N. Y. Acad. Sci. **64:**152, 1956 (toxoplasmosis).

Mostofi, F. K.: Bilharziasis, New York, 1967, Springer-Verlag, New York, Inc.

Murray, J. F., et al.: Amer. Resp. Dis. **83:**315, 1961 (nocardiosis).

Naji, A. F.: Arch. Path. **68:**282, 1959 (aspergillosis).

Sanger, P. W., et al.: J.A.M.A. **181:**88, 1962 (*Candida* infection).

Stansfeld, A. G.: J. Clin. Path. **14:**565, 1961 (toxoplasmic lymphadenitis).

Straatsma, B. R., et al.: Lab. Invest. **11:**963, 1962 (phycomycosis).

Walshe, J. M.: J. Path. Bact. **67:**371, 1954 (echinococcosis alveolaris). 1945, W. B. Saunders Co.

Wartman, W. B.: Medicine **26:**333, 1947 (filariasis).

CHAPTER 10—CHEMICAL POISONS, RADIATION INJURIES, AND NUTRITIONAL DISTURBANCES

Adelson, L.: Amer. J. Clin. Path. **22:**509, 1952 (common poisons).

Benson, J.: J. Forensic Sci. **1:**119, 1956 (poisonous fish).

Campbell, J. A. H.: Arch. Dis. Child. **31:**310, 1956 (kwashiorkor).

Díaz-Rivera, R. S., Collazo, P. J., Pons, E. R., and Torregrosa, N. B.: Medicine **29:**269, 1950 (phosphorus).

Dutra, F. R.: Amer. J. Path. **24:**1137, 1948; Arch. Derm. Syph. **60:** 1140, 1949 (beryllium).

Editorial: J.A.M.A. **163:**118, 1957 (poisonous fish).

Finck, P. A.: Milit. Med. **131:**1513, 1966 (carbon monoxide).

Follis, R. H., Jr.: The pathology of nutritional disease, ed. 2, Springfield, Ill., 1958, Charles C Thomas, Publisher.

Lowry, T., and Schuman, L. M.: J.A.M.A. **162:**153, 1956 (silo-filler's disease).

Odom, E. T., and Capel, W.: Milit. Surg. **113:**460, 1953 (arachnidism).

Pease, C. N.: J.A.M.A. **182:**980, 1962 (hypervitaminosis A).

Penny, J. R., and Balfour, B. M.: J. Path. Bact. **61:**171, 1949 (vitamin C).

Schepers, G. W. H.: Int. Arch. Gewerbepath. **19:**1, 1962 (berylliosis).

Smith, A. G., and Margelis, G.: Amer. J. Path. **30:**857, 1954 (camphor).
Smith, J. P., et al.: J. Path. Bact. **80:**287, 1960 (cadmium).

CHAPTER 11—DISTURBANCES OF GROWTH

Ackerman, L. V., and del Regato, J. A.: Cancer—diagnosis, treatment, and prognosis, ed. 3, St. Louis, 1962, The C. V. Mosby Co. (general reference).

Batson, O. V.: Amer. J. Roentgen. **78:**195, 1957 (vertebral vein system).

Berenblum, L.: Arch. Path. **38:**233, 1944 (irritation, trauma, and tumor formation).

Boyd, W.: The spontaneous regression of cancer, Springfield, Ill., 1966, Charles C Thomas, Publisher.

Boyland, E., editor: Brit. Med. Bull. **14:**73, 1958 (carcinogenic agents).

Bush, H., Byvoet, P., and Smetana, K.: Cancer Res. **23:**313, 1963 (nucleolus of cancer cell).

Editorial: J.A.M.A. **161:**66, 1956 (keloids).

Evans, R. W.: Histological appearances of tumours, ed. 2, London, 1966, E. & S. Livingstone, Ltd. (general reference).

Everson, T. C., and Cole, W. H.: Spontaneous regression of cancer, Philadelphia, 1966, W. B. Saunders Co.

Foulds, L.: J. Chronic Dis. **8:**2, 1958 (natural history of cancer).

Gellhoren, A.: Seminars Hemat. **3:**99, 1966 (gene control in cancer cells).

Hobbs, C. B., and Miller, A. L.: J. Clin. Path. **19:**119, 1966 (endocrine function in tumors).

Holtz, F.: Cancer **11:**1103, 1958 (liposarcoma).

Huxley, J.: Biological aspects of cancer, London, 1958, George Allen & Unwin, Ltd. (general reference).

Kit, S., and Griffin, A. C.: Cancer Res. **18:**621, 1958 (cellular metabolism).

Lawrence, W., Jr., Jegge, G., and Foote, F. W., Jr.: Cancer **17:**361, 1964 (embryonal rhabdomyosarcoma).

Lieberman, P. H., et al.: J.A.M.A. **198:**1047, 1966 (alveolar soft-part sarcoma).

Musgrove, J. E., and McDonald, J. R.: Arch. Path. **45:**513, 1948 (desmoids).

Nicholson, G. W. de P.: Studies on tumor formation, St. Louis, 1950, The C. V. Mosby Co. (general reference).

Oberling, C.: The riddle of cancer, translated by W. H. Woglom, New Haven, Conn., 1952, Yale University Press.

Papanicolaou, G. N., and Traut, H. F.: Diagnosis of uterine cancer by vaginal smear, New York, 1943, The Commonwealth Fund (cytologic diagnosis of malignancy).

Raven, R. W., editor: Cancer, vol. 1. Research into causation, London, 1957, Butterworth & Co. (Publishers), Ltd. (carcinogenic agents).

Raven, R. W., editor: Cancer, vol. 2. Pathology of malignant tumors, London, 1958, Butterworth & Co. (Publishers), Ltd. (general reference).

Roulet, F. C., editor: The lymphoreticular tumours in Africa, Basel, Switzerland, 1964, S. Karger.

Smith, R. R., and Hilberg, A. W.: J. Nat. Cancer Inst. **16**:645, 1955 (seeding in operative wounds).

Stout, A. P.: Cancer **1**:30, 1948 (fibrosarcoma); Ann. Surg. **127**:278 (mesenchymoma), and 706 (myxoma), 1948.

Stout, A. P.: Atlas of tumor pathology, sect. II, fasc. 6. Tumors of the peripheral nervous system, Washington, D. C., 1949, Armed Forces Institute of Pathology.

Stout, A. P., and Hill, W. T.: Cancer **11**:844, 1958 (leiomyosarcoma).

Wells, H. G.: J.A.M.A. **114**:2177 and 2284, 1940 (lipoma).

Willis, R. A.: Bull. N. Y. Acad. Med. **26**:440, 1950 (teratoma); Atlas of tumor pathology, sect. III, fasc. 9. Teratomas, Washington, D. C., 1951, Armed Forces Institute of Pathology.

Willis, R. A.: Pathology of tumors, ed. 4, New York, 1967, Appleton-Century-Crofts (general reference).

CHAPTER 12—THE CARDIOVASCULAR SYSTEM

Adelson, L., and Hoffman, W.: J.A.M.A. **176**:129, 1961 (sudden death from coronary disease).

Anderson, W. A. D., and Dmytryk, E. T.: Amer. J. Path. **22**:337, 1946 (tumors of heart).

Biava, C. G., et al.: Amer. J. Path. **44**:349, 1964 (renal hyaline arteriolosclerosis—electron microscope study).

Boyd, T. A. B.: Amer. J. Path. **25**:757, 1949 (blood cysts).

Burch, G. E., and Winsor, T.: Amer. Heart J. **24**:740, 1942 (syphilitic coronary stenosis).

Chatgidakis, C. B., and Barlow, J. B.: Med. Proc. **7**:377, 1961 (primary mural endocardial disease).

Crawford, T., and Woolf, N.: J. Path. Bact. **79**:221, 1960 (arteriolosclerosis).

Crosby, R. C., and Wadsworth, R. C.: Arch. Intern. Med. **81**:431, 1948 (temporal arteritis).

Duff, G. L.: Canad. Med. Ass. J. **64**:387, 1951; Amer. J. Med. **11**:92, 1951 (arteriosclerosis).

Duguid, J. B.: Brit. Med. Bull. **2**:36, 1955 (arteriosclerosis).

Enos, W. F., et al.: J.A.M.A. **152**:1090, 1953; **158**:912, 1955 (coronary disease).

Freeman, W. A.: Arch. Path. **65**:646, 1958 (rupture after infarction).

Friedberg, G. K.: Diseases of the heart, ed 3., Philadelphia, 1966, W. B. Saunders Co.

Glagov, S., et al.: Arch. Path **72**:558, 1961 (atherosclerosis).

Gore, I.: Arch. Path. **53**:142, 1952 (dissecting aneurysm).

Gould, S. E.: Pathology of the heart, ed. 2, Springfield, Ill., 1960, Charles C Thomas, Publisher (general reference).

Grant, R. P.: Amer. Heart J. **46**:154 and 405, 1953 (hypertrophy of heart).

Hirst, A. E., Jr., Johns, V. J., Jr., and Kime, S. W., Jr.: Medicine **37**:217, 1958 (dissecting aneurysm).

Holman, R. L., et al.: Amer. J. Path. **34**:209, 1958 (natural history of atherosclerosis).

Hueper, W. C.: Arch. Path. **38**:162, 245, and 350, 1944; **39**:65, 117, and 187, 1945 (arteriosclerosis).

918 *References*

James, T. N., and Keyes, J. W., editors: The etiology of myocardial infarction, Boston, 1963, Little, Brown & Co.

Jones, R. J., editor: Evolution of the atherosclerotic plaque, Chicago, 1963, University of Chicago Press.

Kaplan, M. H., and Svec, K. H.: J. Exp. Med. **119**:651, 1964 (immunologic relation of streptococcal and tissue antigens).

Lev, M.: Autopsy diagnosis of congenitally malformed hearts, Springfield, Ill., 1953, Charles C Thomas, Publisher.

Maher, J. F., Mallory, G. K., and Laurenz, G. A.: New Eng. J. Med. **255**:1, 1956 (rupture after infarction).

Mallory, G. K., White, P. D., and Salcedo-Salgar, J.: Amer. Heart J. **18**:647, 1939 (healing of myocardial infarcts).

Manchester, B., et al.: Arch. Intern. Med. **95**:231, 1955 (rheumatic myocarditis and Aschoff bodies).

McGee, W. G., and Ashworth, C. T.: Amer. J. Path. **43**:273, 1963 (hypertensive arteriopathy—fine structure).

McKusick, V. A., et al.: J.A.M.A. **181**:93, 1962 (Buerger's disease).

More, R. H., and Movat, H. Z.: J. Path. Bact. **75**:127, 1958 (arteritis).

Morgan, A. D.: The pathogenesis of coronary occlusion, Springfield, Ill., 1956, Charles C Thomas, Publisher.

Movat, H. Z., More, R. H., and Haust, D. M.: Amer. J. Path. **34**:1023, 1958 (arteriosclerosis).

Mulligan, R. M.: Arch. Path. **65**: 615, 1958 (myocarditis).

Murphy, G. E.: Medicine **339**:289, 1960 (rheumatic myocarditis).

Page, I. H., et al.: J.A.M.A. **164**:2048, 1957 (arteriosclerosis).

Paterson, J. C.: Arch. Path. **22**:313, 1936; **25**:474, 1938; Amer. Heart J. **18**:451, 1939; J.A.M.A. **112**:895, 1939 (coronary artery disease).

Peery, T. M.: Postgrad. Med. **19**:323, 1956 (brucellosis and heart disease).

Pomerance, A.: J. Path. Bact. **81**:135, 1961 (Lambl's excrescences).

Rich, A. R., and Gregory, J. E.: Bull. Hopkins Hosp. **73**:239, 1943 (rheumatic myocarditis and Aschoff bodies).

Richardson, H. L., et al.: J.A.M.A. **195**:254, 1966 (intramyocardial lesions in sudden death).

Sako, Y.: J.A.M.A. **179**:36, 1962 (experimental atherosclerosis).

Schechter, M. M.: Amer. J. Med. Sci. **227**:46, 1954 (superior vena cava syndrome).

Scotti, T. M., and McKeown, C. E.: Arch. Path. **46**:289, 1948 (sarcoidosis).

Smith, R. R., and Tomlinson, B. E.: J. Path. Bact. **68**:327, 1954 (subendocardial hemorrhage).

Sokoloff, L.: Amer. Heart J. **45**:635, 1953 (rheumatoid arthritis).

Spain, D. M.: Sci. Amer. **215**:48, Aug., 1966 (atherosclerosis).

Spain, D. M., and Handler, B. J.: Arch. Intern. Med. **77**:37, 1946 (cor pulmonale).

Spiro, D., et al.: Amer. J. Path. **47**:19, 1966 (hyperplastic arteriolar sclerosis).

Still, W. J. S., and Hill, K. R.: Arch. Path. **68**:42, 1959 (arteriolar sclerosis).

Stout, A. P.: Cancer **2**:1027, 1949; Lab. Invest. **5**:217, 1956 (hemangiopericytoma).

Strong, J. P., and McGill, H. C.: Amer. J. Path. **40:**37, 1962 (natural history of coronary atherosclerosis).

Thomas, W. A., et al.: New Eng. J. Med. **251:**327, 1954 (endomyocardial fibroelastosis).

CHAPTER 13—THE KIDNEYS, URINARY TRACT, AND MALE GENITALIA

Allen, A. C.: Amer. J. Med. **18:**277, 1955 (nephrosis).

Allen, A. C.: The kidney; medical and surgical diseases, ed. 2, New York, 1962, Grune & Stratton, Inc.

Anderson, W. A. D.: Arch. Path. **27:**753, 1939 (hyperparathyroidism and renal disease).

Davidson, W. M., and Ross, G. I. M.: J. Path. Bact. **68:**459, 1954 (absence of kidney).

Franks, L. M.: J. Path. Bact. **68:**603, 1954; **72:**603, 1956 (prostatic carcinoma).

Franks, L. M.: J. Path. Bact. **68:**617, 1954; Ann. Roy. Coll. Surg. Eng. **74:**92, 1954 (prostatic hyperplasia).

Hartroft, P. M.: Ann. Rev. Med. **17:**113, 1966; Bull. Path. **8:**165, 1967 (juxtaglomerular complex).

Henthorne, J. C.: Amer. J. Clin. Path. **8:**28, 1938 (lymphatic cysts of kidney).

Heptinstall, R. H.: Pathology of the kidney, Boston, 1966, Little, Brown & Co.

Jaenike, J. R.: J. Exp. Med. **123:**523 and 537, 1966 (renal damage from hemoglobinemia).

Johnson, F. R., and Anderson, J. C.: J. Path. Bact. **66:**39, 1953 (developmental remnants in kidney).

Kassirer, J. P., and Schwartz, W. B.: New Eng. J. Med. **265:**686 and 736, 1961 (glomerulonephritis).

Kimmelstiel, P., and Wilson, C.: Amer. J. Path. **12:**83, 1936 (diabetic glomerulosclerosis).

Krickstein, H. I., Gloor, F. J., and Balogh, K., Jr.: Arch. Path. **82:**506, 1966 (hereditary nephritis).

Lucké, B.: Milit. Surg. **99:**37, 1946 (hemoglobinuric nephrosis).

Mallory, T. B.: Amer. J. Clin. Path. **17:**427, 1947 (hemoglobinuric nephrosis).

Mavromatis, F.: J.A.M.A. **193:**191, 1965 (tetracycline nephropathy).

McGee, W. G., and Ashworth, C. T.: Amer. J. Path. **43:**273, 1963 (hypertensive arteriopathy).

Mostofi, F. K., and Smith, D. E., editors: The kidney, Baltimore, 1966, The Williams & Wilkins Co.

Mostofi, F. K., Thomson, R. V., and Dean, A. L., Jr.: Cancer **8:**741, 1955 (mucous adenocarcinoma of bladder).

Myerson, R. M., and Pastor, B. H.: Amer. J. Med. Sci. **228:**378, 1954 (Fanconi syndrome).

Osathanondh, V., and Potter, E. L.: Arch. Path. **77:**459, 466, 474, 485, 502, and 510, 1964 (polycystic kidney).

Quinn, E. L., and Koss, E. H., editors: Biology of pyelonephritis, Boston, 1960, Little, Brown & Co.

Randall, A.: Int. Abstr. Surg. **71:**209, 1940; Ann. Surg. **105:**1009, 1937 (renal calculi).

Reidenberg, M. M., et al.: Amer. J. Med. Sci. **247**:26, 1964 (nephrotoxins).

Relman, A. S., and Schwartz, W. B.: Amer. J. Med. **24**:764, 1958 (kidney in potassium depletion).

Reynolds, T. B., and Edmondson, H. A.: J.A.M.A. **184**:435, 1963 (phenacetin nephritis).

Rich, A. R.: Bull. Hopkins Hosp. **100**:173, 1957 (nephrosis).

Riches, E. W., Griffiths, I. H., and Thackray, A. C.: Brit. J. Urol. **23**: 297, 1951 (urinary tract tumors).

Scowen, E. F., Stansfeld, A. G., and Watts, R. W. E.: J. Path Bact. **77**: 195, 1959 (renal calculi).

Sheehan, H. L., and Moore, H. C.: Renal cortical necrosis and the kidney of concealed accidental hemorrhage, Springfield, Ill., 1954, Charles C Thomas, Publisher.

Sniffen, R. C.: Arch. Path. **50**:259 and 285, 1950 (testicular atrophy).

Sommers, S. C.: Henry Ford Hosp. Med. Bull. **14**:47, 1966 (renal factors in hypertension).

Spence, H. M., Baird, S. B., and Ware, E. W., Jr.: J.A.M.A. **163**:1466, 1957 (cysts of kidney).

Spjut, H. J., and Thorpe, J. D.: Amer. J. Clin. Path. **26**:136, 1956 (granulomatous orchitis).

Strauss, M. B., and Welt, L. G.: Diseases of the kidney, Boston, 1963, Little, Brown & Co.

Teel, P.: Amer. J. Obstet. Gynec. **75**:1347, 1958 (adenomatoid tumors).

CHAPTER 14—THE RESPIRATORY TRACT AND LUNGS

Abell, M. R.: Arch. Path. **61**:360, 1956 (mediastinal tumors and cysts).

Anderson, W. A. D.: Amer. J. Clin. Path. **46**:3, 1966 (lung cancer).

Arias-Stella, J., and Kruger, H.: Arch. Path. **76**:147, 1963 (high altitude pulmonary edema).

Bayley, E. C., Lindberg, D. O. N., and Baggenstoss, A. H.: Arch. Path. **40**:376, 1945 (Löffler's syndrome).

Benoit, H. W., Jr., and Ackerman, L. V.: J. Thorac. Surg. **25**:346, 1953 (pleural tumors).

Carroll, R.: J. Path. Bact. **83**:293, 1962 (lung scars and cancer).

Dickle, H. A., and Rankin, J.: J.A.M.A. **167**:1069, 1958 (farmer's lung).

Divertie, M. B., and Brown, A. L., Jr.: J.A.M.A. **187**:938, 1964 (fine structure of lung).

Esterly, J. A., and Warner, N. E.: Arch. Path. **80**:433, 1965 (pneumocystis pneumonia).

Fienberg, R.: Amer. J. Path. **29**:913, 1953 (cholesterol pneumonitis).

Gore, I., and Tanaka, K.: Amer. J. Med. Sci. **244**:351, 1962 (pulmonary embolization).

Hardy, H. L.: Amer. J. Med. Sci. **250**:381, 1965 (asbestos).

Haugen, R. K.: J.A.M.A. **186**:142, 1963 (laryngeal obstruction—"the café coronary").

Head, R. M., et al.: Amer. Rev. Tuberc. **78**:21, 1958 (Wegener's granulomatosis).

Herman, D. L., Bullock, W. K., and Waken, J. K.: Cancer **19**:1337, 1966 (giant cell adenocarcinoma).

Hewer, T. F.: J. Path. Bact. **81:**323, 1961 (pulmonary metastases resembling alveolar carcinoma).

Hopps, H. C., and Wissler, R. W.: Amer. J. Path. **31:**261, 1955 (pulmonary changes in uremia).

Kent, G., Gilbert, E. S., and Meyer, H. H.: Arch. Path. **60:**556, 1955 (pulmonary microlithiasis).

Kreyberg, L.: Histological typing of lung tumors, Geneva, 1967, World Health Organization.

Liebow, A. A.: Atlas of tumor pathology, sect. V, fasc. 17. Tumors of the lower respiratory tract, Washington, D. C., 1952, Armed Forces Institute of Pathology.

Neubuerger, K. T., Geever, E. F., and Rutledge, E. K.: Arch. Path. **37:**1, 1944 (rheumatic pneumonia).

O'Donnell, W. M., Mann, R. H., and Grosh, J. L.: Cancer **19:**1143, 1966 (asbestos and lung cancer).

Reid, L.: The pathology of emphysema, Chicago, 1967, Year Book Medical Publishers, Inc.

Rifkind, D., Faris, T. D., and Hill, R. B., Jr.: Ann. Int. Med. **65:**943, 1966 (pneumocystis pneumonia).

Rosen, S. H., Castleman, B., and Liebow, A. A.: New Eng. J. Med. **258:**1123, 1958 (pulmonary alveolar proteinosis).

Ross, J. M.: Brit. Med. J. **1:**79, 1941 (blast injury).

Saltzstein, S. L.: Cancer **16:**928, 1963 (lymphomas of lung).

Siebert, F. T., and Fisher, E. R.: Amer. J. Path. **33:**1137, 1957 (bronchiolar emphysema).

Spencer, H.: Pathology of the lung, New York, 1962, The Macmillan Co. (general reference).

Spencer, H., and Raeburn, C.: J. Path. Bact. **71:**145, 1956 (bronchiolar carcinoma).

Sutherland, T. W., et al.: J. Path. Bact. **65:**93, 1953 (hamartoma).

Thomson, J. G., and Graves, W. M., Jr.: Arch. Path. **81:**458, 1966 (asbestos).

Thurlbeck, W. M.: Amer. J. Med. Sci. **246:**332, 1963 (emphysema).

Totten, R. S., Reid, D. H. S., Davis, H. D., and Moran, T. J.: Amer. J. Med. **25:**803, 1958 (farmer's lung).

Walton, E. W.: Brit. Med. J. **2:**265, 1958 (Wegener's granulomatosis).

Whitwell, F.: J. Path. Bact. **70:**429, 1955 (atypical hyperplasia).

CHAPTER 15—THE LIVER, GALLBLADDER, AND PANCREAS

Anderson, M. C.: J.A.M.A. **183:**114, 1963 (pancreatitis).

Baker, H. de C., Paget, G. E., and Davson, J.: J. Path. Bact. **72:**173, 1956 (Kupffer cell sarcoma).

Bearn, A. G.: Amer. J. Med. **22:**747, 1957 (Wilson's disease).

Berg, V. V., and Scotti, T. M.: Science **158:**377, 1967 (peliosis hepatis).

Bigelow, N. H., and Wright, A. W.: Cancer **6:**170, 1953 (hepatic tumors in children).

Billing, B. H., and Lathe, G. H.: Amer. J. Med. **24:**111, 1958 (bilirubin and metabolism).

Brolin, S. E., Hellman, B., and Knutson, H.: The structure and metabolism of the pancreatic islets, New York, 1964, The Macmillan Co.

Brown, C. H., and Crile, G., Jr.: J.A.M.A. **190**:30, 1964 (pancreatic adenoma with diarrhea and hypokalemia).

Cameron, R., and Heu, P. C.: Biliary cirrhosis, Springfield, Ill., 1962, Charles C Thomas, Publisher.

Cunningham, J. A., and Hardenbergh, F. E.: Arch. Intern. Med. **97**: 68, 1956 (incidence of gallstones).

Dubin, I. N.: Amer. J. Med. **24**:268, 1958 (chronic idiopathic jaundice).

Edmondson, H. A., Bullock, W. K., and Mehl, J. W.: Amer. J. Path. **25**:1227, 1949; **26**:37, 1950 (pancreatitis).

Edmondson, H. A.: Atlas of tumor pathology, sect. VII, fasc. 25. Tumors of the liver and intrahepatic bile ducts, Washington, D. C., 1958, Armed Forces Institute of Pathology.

Gall, E. A.: Amer. J. Path. **36**:241, 1960 (cirrhosis of liver).

Gibson, J. B.: J. Path. Bact. **79**:381, 1960 (Chiari's disease).

Greider, M. H., Elliott, D. W., and Zollinger, R. M.: J.A.M.A. **186**: 566, 1963 (islet cell adenomas).

Guckian, J. C., and Perry, J. E.: Ann. Intern. Med. **65**:1081, 1966 (granulomatous hepatitis).

Haverback, B. J.: J.A.M.A. **193**:279, 1965 (exocrine function of pancreas).

Kasai, M., Yakovac, W. C., and Kopp, C. E.: Arch. Path. **74**:152, 1962 (biliary atresia).

Knights, E. M., Jr., et al.: J.A.M.A. **169**:1279, 1959 (fibrocystic disease of pancreas).

Koppisch, E.: Puerto Rico J. Public Health Trop. Med. **16**:395, 1941; J.A.M.A. **121**:936, 1943 (schistosomal cirrhosis of liver).

Lisa, J. R., et al.: Cancer **17**:395, 1964 (carcinoma of pancreas).

MacDonald, R. A., and Mallory, G. K.: Amer. J. Med. **24**:334, 1958 (postnecrotic cirrhosis).

MacMahon, H. E.: Amer. J. Path. **24**:527, 1948; Lab. Invest. **4**:243, 1955 (biliary cirrhosis).

Patton, R. B., and Horn, R. C., Jr.: Cancer **17**:757, 1964 (carcinoma of liver).

Schaffner, F., et al.: J.A.M.A. **183**:343, 1963 (alcoholic hepatitis).

Sprinz, H., and Nelson, R. S.: Ann. Intern. Med. **41**:952, 1954 (chronic idiopathic jaundice).

Stary, H. C.: Amer. J. Med. Sci. **252**:357, 1966 (blood vessels in diabetes).

Walters, M. N. I.: J. Path. Bact. **92**:547, 1966 (adipose atrophy of pancreas).

Warren, S., LeCompte, P. M., and Legg, M. A.: The pathology of diabetes mellitus, ed. 4, Philadelphia, 1966, Lea & Febiger.

Zollinger, R. M., and Grant, G. N.: J.A.M.A. **190**:181, 1964 (ulcerogenic tumor of pancreas).

CHAPTER 16—THE RETICULOENDOTHELIAL SYSTEM, SPLEEN, AND LYMPH NODES

Burkitt, D.: Brit. J. Cancer **16**:379, 1962 (lymphomas of African children).

Craver, L. F., and Miller, D. G.: The malignant lymphoma, New York, 1966, American Cancer Society.

Fisher, E. R., and Reidbord, H.: Amer. J. Path. **41:**679, 1962 (Gaucher's disease).

Jackson, H., Jr., and Parker, F., Jr.: Hodgkin's disease and allied disorders, New York, 1947, Oxford University Press, Inc.

Lukes, R. J.: Cancer Res. **26:**1311, 1966 (histologic types of Hodgkin's disease).

Lukes, R. J., and Butler, J. J.: Cancer Res. **26:**1063, 1966; and Lukes, R. J., Butler, J. J., and Hicks, E. B.: Cancer **19:**317, 1966 (Hodgkin's disease).

Lynch, M. J. G., et al.: Cancer **7:**168, 1954 (Letterer-Siwe disease).

Movat, H. Z., and Fernando, N. V. P.: Exp. Molec. Path. **4:**155, 1965 (fine structure of lymphoid tissue).

Rappaport, H., Winter, W. J., and Hicks, E. B.: Cancer **9:**792, 1956 (follicular lymphoma).

Roulet, F. C., editor: The lymphoreticular tumours in Africa, Basel, Switzerland, 1964, S. Karger.

Wadsworth, R. C., and Keil, P. G.: Amer. J. Path. **28:**1003, 1952 (infectious mononucleosis).

CHAPTER 17—THE BLOOD AND BLOOD-FORMING ORGANS

Diggs, L. W.: Amer. J. Clin. Path. **44:**1, 1965 (sickle cell crises).

Fisher, E. R., and Creed, D. L.: Amer. J. Clin. Path. **25:**620, 1955 (thrombotic thrombocytopenic purpura).

Goldberg, G. M., Rubenstone, A. I., and Saphir, O: Cancer **13:**513 and 520, 1960; **14:**30, 1961 (leukemia).

Koneman, E. W., Miale, J. B., and Mason, A.: Amer. J. Clin. Path. **40:**1, 1963 (sickle cell–thalassemia).

Lieberman, P. H., et al.: Cancer **18:**727, 1965 (myelofibrosis).

Miale, J. B.: Laboratory medicine-hematology, ed. 3, St. Louis, 1967, The C. V. Mosby Co. (general reference).

Nakai, G. S., et al.: Ann. Intern. Med. **57:**419, 1962 (myeloid metaplasia).

Nowell, P. C., and Hungerford, D. A.: Seminars Hemat. **3:**114, 1966 (etiology of leukemia).

Quick, A. J.: Hemorrhagic diseases and thrombosis, ed. 2, Philadelphia, 1966, Lea & Febiger.

Rivers, S. L., et al.: Cancer **16:**249, 1963 (acute leukemia).

Sandberg, A. A.: Cancer **15:**2, 1965 (chromosomes and leukemia).

Wright, Z. S., et al.: J.A.M.A. **180:**733, 1962 (nomenclature of blood clotting factors).

CHAPTER 18—THE MOUTH, THROAT, AND NECK

Albers, G. D.: J.A.M.A. **183:**103, 1963 (branchial anomalies).

Azzopardi, J. G., and Smith, O. D.: J. Path. Bact. **77:**131, 1959 (salivary gland tumors).

Chaudhry, A. P., and Gorlin, R. J.: Amer. J. Surg. **95:**923, 1958 (papillary cystadenoma lymphomatosum).

Collins, N. P., and Edgerton, M. T.: Cancer **12:**235, 1959 (branchiogenic carcinoma).

Costero, I., and Barroso-Moquel, R.: Amer. J. Path. **38:**127, 1961 (carotid body tumor).

Custer, R. P., and Fust, J. A.: Amer. J. Clin. Path. **22**:1044, 1952 (epulis).

Foote, F. W., Jr., and Frazell, E. L.: Atlas of tumor pathology, sect. IV, fasc. 11. Tumors of the major salivary glands, Washington, D. C., 1954, Armed Forces Institute of Pathology.

Goodwin, J. T., Foote, F. W., Jr. and Frazell, E. L.: Amer. J. Path. **30**:465, 1954 (acinic adenocarcinoma).

Gorlin, R. J., Chaudhry, A. P., and Pindborg, J. J.: Cancer **14**:73, 1961 (odontogenic tumors).

Gorlin, R. J., Meskin, L. H., and Broday, R.: Ann. N. Y. Acad. Sci. **108**:722, 1963 (odontogenic tumors).

Hertz, J.: Acta Chir. Scand. **102**:405, 1951 (adamantinoma).

Schermer, K. L., et al.: Cancer **19**:1273, 1966 (glomus jugulare tumors).

Schneider, M.: Amer. J. Med. Sci. **244**:628, 1962 (oral cancer).

Stecker, R. H., Devine, K. D., and Harrison, E. G., Jr.: J.A.M.A. **189**:838, 1964 (snuff dipper's carcinoma).

Suoboda, D., et al.: Exp. Molec. Path. **4**:189, 1965 (nasopharyngeal carcinoma).

CHAPTER 19—THE ALIMENTARY TRACT

Altshular, J. H., and Shaka, J. A.: Cancer **19**:831, 1966 (squamous carcinoma of stomach).

Becker, F. F., et al.: J.A.M.A. **194**:559, 1965 (Whipple's disease).

Berg, J. W.: Cancer **11**:1149, 1958 (gastric polyps and cancer).

Boley, S. J., et al.: J.A.M.A. **192**:763, 1965 and **193**:997, 1965 (potassium and small intestinal ulcers).

Burdick, D., Prior, J. T., and Scanlon, G. T.: Cancer **16**:854, 1963 (Peutz-Jeghers syndrome).

Callaghan, P. J., and Del Beccaro, E. J.: J.A.M.A. **180**:333, 1962 (carcinoma of appendix).

Cassella, R. R., et al.: J.A.M.A. **191**:379, 1965 (spasm of esophagus).

Castleman, B., and Krickstein, H.: Gastroenterology **51**:108, 1966 (polyps and carcinoma).

Dungal, N.: J.A.M.A. **178**:789, 1961 (gastric cancer).

Editorial: J.A.M.A. **187**:57, 1964 (Boerhaave syndrome).

Elliott, G. B., and Elliott, K. A.: Amer. J. Roentgen. **89**:720, 1963 (pneumatosis intestinalis).

Fisher, E. R.: J.A.M.A. **181**:396, 1962 (Whipple's disease).

Foltz, E. L.: J.A.M.A. **187**:413, 1964 (peptic ulcer).

Goldgraber, M. B., et al.: Gastroenterology **34**:809 and 840, 1958 (carcinoma and ulcerative colitis).

Hadfield, G.: Lancet **2**:773, 1939 (regional ileitis).

Helwig, E. B., and Hansen, J.: Surg., Gynec. Obstet. **92**:233, 1951 (lymphoma of rectum).

Kutscher, A. H., et al.: Amer. J. Med. Sci. **238**:180, 1959; Amer. J. Dig. Dis. **1**:455, 1956 (Peutz-Jeghers syndrome).

Lane, N., and Lev, R.: Cancer **16**:751, 1963 (familial polyposis).

McGovern, V. J., and Archer, G. T.: Aust. Ann. Med. **6**:68, 1957 (ulcerative colitis).

Ming, S., and Goldman, H.: Cancer **18**:721, 1965 (gastric polyps).

Pettet, J. E., et al.: Surg., Gynec. Obstet. **98**:546, 1954 (pseudomembranous enterocolitis).

Shiffman, M. A.: J.A.M.A. **179:**514, 1962 (familial multiple polyposis).

Shiner, M.: J.A.M.A. **188:**45, 1964 (sprue).

Spratt, J. S., Jr., and Ackerman, L. V.: J.A.M.A. **179:**337, 1962 (adeno-carcinoma of colon).

Valtonen, E. J.: Gastroenterologia (Basel) **104:**309, 1965 (bezoars).

Warren, S., and Sommers, S. C.: Amer. J. Path. **24:**475, 1948 (regional ileitis).

Zarafonetis, C. J. D., et al.: Amer. J. Med. Sci. **236:**1, 1958 (carcinoid tumors).

CHAPTER 20—THE ENDOCRINE GLANDS

Anderson, J. R., et al.: Lancet **2:**1123, 1957 (Addison's disease and autoantibodies).

Batsakis, J. G., et al.: Amer. J. Clin. Path. **39:**241, 1963 (sporadic goiter).

Bieger, R. C., and McAdams, A. J.: Arch. Path. **82:**535, 1966 (thymic cysts).

Brennan, C. F., Malone, R. G. S., and Weaver, J. A.: Lancet **2:**12, 1956 (Houssay's phenomenon in man).

Brewer, D. B.: J. Path. Bact. **77:**149, 1959 (papillary carcinoma of thyroid).

Browne, F. J.: Lancet **1:**115, 1958 (adrenal gland and eclampsia).

Burnet, M.: Northwest Med. **63:**599, 1964 (thymus and autoimmune disease).

Carpenter, C. C. J., et al.: Medicine (Balt.) **43:**153, 1964 (Schmidt's syndrome).

Carpenter, W. B., and Kernohan, J. W.: Cancer **16:**788, 1963 (retroperitoneal ganglioneuroma).

Chatten, J.: Amer. J. Med. Sci. **248:**127, 1964 (thymus in systemic disease).

Cohen, R. A.: Ann. Intern. Med. **61:**1144, 1964 (pineal gland).

Cohen, R. B.: Cancer **19:**552, 1966 (adrenal cortical nodules).

Conn, J. W.: J.A.M.A. **183:**775 and 870, 1963 (hyperaldosteronism).

Conn, J. W., et al.: J.A.M.A. **195:**21, 1966; **193:**200, 1965 (aldosteronism in hypertensive disease).

Cox, T. R., and Krohn, W.: Amer. J. Clin. Path. **27:**24, 1958 (pituitary changes with steroid therapy).

Currie, A. R., Symington, T., and Grant, J. K., editors: The human adrenal cortex, London, 1962, E. & S. Livingstone Ltd.

Delta, B. G., et al.: J.A.M.A. **194:**507, 1965 (thymus and agammaglobulinemia).

Eylan, E., and Zmucky, R.: Lancet **1:**1062, 1957 (thyroiditis and mumps virus).

Foster, M., and Barr, D.: J. Clin. Endocr. **4:**417, 1944 (myxedema).

Fox, F., Davidson, J., and Thomas, L. B.: Cancer **12:**108, 1959 (maturation of neuroblastoma to ganglioneuroma).

Gaillard, P. J., Talmage, R. V., and Budy, A. M., editors: The parathyroid glands, Chicago, 1965, University of Chicago Press.

Giarman, N. J., et al.: Fed. Proc. **18:**394, 1959 (neurohumoral content of pineal body).

Goudie, R. B., Anderson, J. R., and Gray, K. G.: J. Path Bact. **77:**389, 1959 (antithyroid antibodies).

Hazard, J. B.: Amer. J. Clin. Path. **25**:289 and 399, 1955 (thyroiditis).
Hazard, J. B., Hawk, W. A., and Crik, G., Jr.: J. Clin. Endocr. **19**:152, 1959 (medullary carcinoma of thyroid).
Ibanez, M. L., et al.: Cancer **19**:1039, 1966 (thyroid carcinoma).
Kernohan, J. W., and Sayre, G. P.: Atlas of tumor pathology, sect. X, fasc. 36. Tumors of the pituitary gland and infundibulum, Washington, D. C., 1956, Armed Forces Institute of Pathology.
Kitay, J. I., and Altschule, M. D.: The pineal gland, Cambridge, Mass., 1954, Harvard University Press.
Kleinbeld, G.: Cancer **12**:902, 1959 (functioning tumors of parathyroid).
Klinck, G. H., and Winship, T.: Cancer **8**:701, 1955· (occult sclerosing carcinoma of thyroid).
Laragh, J. H., et al.: Circ. Res. suppl. I, vols. 18 and 19, 1966 (aldosterone in hypertension).
Lathem, J. E., and Hunt, L. D.: J.A.M.A. **197**:558, 1966 (pheochromocytoma of urinary bladder).
Lindsay, S., and Chaikoff, I. L.: Cancer Res. **24**:1099, 1964 (effects of radiation on thyroid).
McGowan, G. K., and Sandlor, M., editors: Symposium on the thyroid gland, J. Clin. Path., suppl., May, 1967.
Meachim, G., and Young, M. H.: J. Clin. Path. **16**:189, 1963 (granulomatous thyroiditis).
Meyer, P. C.: Brit. J. Cancer **16**:16, 1962 (nodular goiter and carcinoma of thyroid).
Moon, H. D., editor: The adrenal cortex, New York, 1961, Paul B. Hoeber, Inc., Medical Book Division, Harper & Row, Publishers.
Nichols, J., and Delp, M.: J.A.M.A. **185**:643, 1963 (craniopharyngeal pituitary gland).
Pearse, A. G. E.: J. Path. Bact. **61**:195, 1949; **64**:811, 1952; **65**:355, 1953 (pituitary histology).
Rose, E., and Royster, H. P.: J.A.M.A. **176**:224, 1961 (Riedel's struma).
Russell, W. O., et al.: Cancer **16**:1425, 1963 (thyroid carcinoma).
Schimke, R. N., and Hartmann, W. H.: Ann. Intern. Med. **63**:1027, 1965 (familial pheochromocytoma).
Schutt, A. J., and Hayles, A. B.: Mayo Clin. Proc. **39**:363, 1964 (intersex).
Sclare, G.: J. Path. Bact. **85**:263, 1963 (thyroid in myxedema).
Sheehan, H. L.: Quart. J. Med. **8**:277, 1939; Amer. J. Obstet. Gynec. **68**:202, 1954 (postpartum necrosis of pituitary).
Sherwin, R. P.: Cancer **12**:861, 1959 (pheochromocytoma).
Stowens, D.: Arch. Path. **63**:451, 1957 (neuroblastoma).
Thomison, J. B., and Shapiro, J. L.: Arch. Path. **63**:527, 1958 (adrenal lesions in meningococcemia).
Walstenhalme, G. E. W., and Porter, R., editors: The thymus; experimental and clinical studies, Boston, 1966, Little, Brown & Co.
Warren, S., and Meissner, W. A.: Atlas of tumor pathology, sect. IV. Tumors of the thyroid gland, Washington, D. C., 1953, Armed Forces Institute of Pathology.
Williams, C. M., and Greer, M.: J.A.M.A. **183**:836, 1963 (neuroblastoma).

Williams, E. D., et al.: J. Clin. Path. **19**:103, 1966 (medullary carcinoma of thyroid).

Wilton, A., et al.: J. Path. Bact. **67**:65, 1954 (Crooke's change).

Winship, T.: Pediatrics **18**:459, 1956 (thyroid cancer in childhood).

Witebsky, E., et al.: J.A.M.A. **164**:1439, 1957 (thyroiditis and autoimmunity).

Whitehead, R.: J. Path. Bact. **86**:55, 1963 (hypothalamus in hypopituitarism).

Wolman, L.: J. Path. Bact. **77**:283, 1959 (infundibuloma); **72**:575, 1956 (pituitary necrosis).

CHAPTER 21—THE FEMALE GENITAL ORGANS

Boivin, Y., and Richart, R. M.: Cancer **18**:231, 1965 (hilus cell tumors of ovary).

Browne, F. J.: Lancet **1**:115, 1958 (eclampsia).

Grady, H. G., and Smith, D. E., editors: The ovary, Baltimore, 1963, The Williams & Wilkins Co.

Hou, P. C., and Pang, S. C.: J. Path. Bact. **72**:95, 1956 (choriocarcinoma).

Johnson, L. D., Easterday, C. L., Gore, H., and Hertig, A. T.: Cancer **17**:213, 1963 (carcinoma in situ of cervix).

Lauchlan, S. C.: Cancer **19**:1628, 1966 (Brenner tumors).

Leventhal, M. L.: Amer. J. Obstet. Gynec. **84**:154, 1962 (Stein-Leventhal syndrome).

Mackles, A., et al.: Cancer **11**:292, 1958 (mesonephric tumors of cervix).

Meeker, J. M., Neubecker, R. D., and Helwig, E. B.: Amer. J. Clin. Path. **37**:182, 1962 (hidradenoma).

McAdams, A. J., Jr., and Kistner, R. W.: Cancer **11**:740, 1958 (vulva).

McKay, D. G.: Clin. Obstet. Gynec. **5**:1181, 1962 (origins of ovarian tumors).

Morris, J. L., and Scully, R. E.: Endocrine pathology of the ovary, St. Louis, 1958, The C. V. Mosby Co.

Neubecker, R. D., and Breen, J. L.: Cancer **15**:546, 1962 (embryonal carcinoma of ovary).

Norris, H. J., and Taylor, H. B.: Cancer **19**:755 and 1459, 1966; Obstet. Gynec. **28**:57, 1966 (mesenchymal tumors of uterus).

Novak, E. R., and Woodruff, J. D.: Novak's gynecologic and obstetric pathology, ed. 6, Philadelphia, 1967, W. B. Saunders Co. (general reference).

Park, W. W., and Collins, D. H.: Modern trends in pathology, New York, 1959, Paul B. Hoeber, Inc., Medical Book Division, Harper & Row, Publishers, ch. 10 (disorders of the trophoblast).

Park, W. W., and Lees, J. C.: Arch. Path. **49**:73, 205, 1950 (choriocarcinoma).

Rywlin, A. M., Recher, L., and Benson, J.: Cancer **17**:100, 1964 (clear cell leiomyoma).

Semmens, J. P.: Obstet. Gynec. **19**:328, 1962 (congenital anomalies).

Scully, R. E.: Cancer **17**:769, 1964 (stromal luteoma of ovary).

Spiro, R. H., and McPeak, C. J.: Cancer **19**:544, 1966 (metastasizing leiomyoma).

Teilum, G.: Cancer **12**:1092, 1959 (mesonephric tumors); **11**:769, 1958 (gonocytoma); Acta Path. Microbiol. Scand. **64:**407, 1965 (embryonal carcinoma of ovary).

Teoh, T. B.: J. Path. Bact. **78:**145, 1959 (Brenner tumors); **67:**433, 1953 (Walthard nests).

Tweeddale, D. N., and Pederson, B. L.: Amer. J. Med. Sci. **249:**701, 1965 (serous neoplasms of ovary).

Wolfe, S. A., and Pedowitz, P.: Obstet. Gynec. **12:**54, 1958 (tumors of uterus).

CHAPTER 22—THE BREAST

Berg, J. W.: Cancer **8:**776, 1955 (lymphatic spread of mammary cancer).

Bloom, H. J. G., et al.: Brit. Med. J. **2:**213, 1962 (breast cancer—natural history).

Davis, H. H., et al.: Cancer **17:**957, 1964 (cystic disease and cancer).

Haagensen, C. D.: Clin Obstet. Gynec. **5:**1093, 1962 (lobular carcinoma).

Handley, R. S., and Thackray, A. C.: Brit. J. Cancer **16:**187, 1962 (adenoma of nipple).

Karsner, H. T.: Amer. J. Path. **22:**235, 1946 (gynecomastia).

Kraus, F. T., and Neubacker, R. D.: Cancer **15:**444, 1962 (papillary carcinoma).

Lester, J., and Stout, A. P.: Cancer **7:**335, 1954 (cystosarcoma phyllodes of breast).

Oberman, H. A.: Cancer **18:**697, 1965 (cystosarcoma phyllodes).

Orr, J. W., and Parish, D. J.: J. Path. Bact. **84:**201, 1962 (Paget's disease).

Sandison, A. T.: An autopsy study of the adult human breast, National Cancer Institute Monograph No. 8, Washington, D. C., 1962, U. S. Department of Health, Education and Welfare.

Wellings, S. R., and Roberts, P.: J. Nat. Cancer Inst. **30:**269, 1963 (electron microscopy—sclerosing adenosis and duct carcinoma).

Wolff, B.: Brit. J. Cancer **20:**36, 1966 (histologic grading of carcinoma of breast).

CHAPTER 23—THE SKIN

Ackerman, L. V., and Murray, J. F., editors: Symposium on Kaposi's sarcoma, New York, 1963, Hafner Publishing Co., Inc.

Allen, A. C.: The skin, ed. 2, New York, 1967, Grune & Stratton, Inc.

Binford, C. H.: Southern Med. J. **51:**200, 1958 (leprosy).

Block, G. E., and Hartwell, S. W., Jr.: Ann. Surg. **154:**74 and 88, 1961 (malignant melanoma).

Caplan, R. M., and Curtis, A. C.: J.A.M.A. **176:**859, 1961 (xanthoma).

Chapman, G. B., et al.: Amer. J. Path. **42:**619, 1963 (wart—fine structure).

Clough, P. W.: Ann. Intern. Med. **51:**174, 1959 (Boeck's sarcoid).

Cox, F. H., and Helwig, E. B.: Cancer **12:**289, 1959 (Kaposi's sarcoma).

Cummings, M. M., and Hudgins, P. C.: Amer. J. Med. Sci. **236:**311, 1958 (sarcoidosis and pine pollen).

Curth, H. O., et al.: Cancer **15:**364, 1962 (acanthosis nigricans).

Montgomery, H.: Dermatopathology, New York, 1967, Harper & Row, Publishers.

Pack, G. T., and Davis, J.: Postgrad. Med. **27**:370, 1960 (pigmented mole).

Platt, L. I., and Kailin, E. W.: J.A.M.A. **187**:182, 1964 (sex chromatin frequency).

Talbott, J. H., and Ferrandis, R. M.: Collagen diseases, New York, 1956, Grune & Stratton, Inc.

Teilum, G., and Poulsen, H. E.: Arch. Path. **64**:414, 1957 (lupus erythematosus).

Zimmerman, L. E.: Arch. Ophthal. (Chicago) **56**:548, 1956 (collagen diseases).

CHAPTER 24—THE BONES, JOINTS, AND TENDONS

Albright, F.: J. Clin. Endocr. **7**:307, 1947 (fibrous dysplasia of bone).

Burkhart, J. M., Burke, E. C., and Kelly, P. J.: Mayo Clin. Proc. **40**:481, 1965 (chondrodystrophies).

Caldwell, R. A.: J. Clin. Path. **15**:421, 1962 (senile osteoporosis).

Collins, D. H.: The pathology of articular and spinal diseases, Baltimore, 1949, The Williams & Wilkins Co.

Coventry, M. B., and Dahlin, D. C.: J. Bone Joint Surg. **39-A**:741, 1957 (osteogenic sarcoma).

Coventry, M. B., Ghormley, R. K., and Kernohan, J. W.: J. Bone Joint Surg. **27**:105, 233, and 460, 1945 (intervertebral discs).

Dahlin, D. C., and Henderson, E. D.: Cancer **15**:410, 1962 (mesenchymal chondrosarcoma).

Dawson, I. M. P.: J. Path. Bact. **67**:587, 1954 (gargoylism).

Fine, G., and Stout, A. P.: Cancer **9**:1027, 1956 (extraskeletal osteogenic sarcoma).

Gilmer, W. S., Jr., and Anderson, L. D.: Southern Med. J. **52**:1432, 1959 (myositis ossificans).

Hicks, J. D.: J. Path. Bact. **67**:151, 1954 (synovioma).

Kunkel, M. G., Dahlin, D. C., and Young, H. H.: J. Bone Joint Surg. **38-A**:817, 1956 (benign chondroblastoma).

Lebowitz, W. B.: Ann. Intern. Med. **58**:102, 1963 (heart in rheumatoid arthritis).

Lichtenstein, L.: Bone tumors, St. Louis, 1959, The C. V. Mosby Co.

MacCallum, P., and Hueston, J. T.: Austr. New Zeal. J. Surg. **31**:241, 1962 (Dupuytren's contracture).

Meyer, P. C.: Brit. J. Cancer **11**:509, 1957 (metastatic tumors of bone).

Patterson, C. D., Harrille, W. E., and Pierce, J. A.: Ann. Intern. Med. **62**:685, 1965 (rheumatoid lung disease).

Pearson, C. M., et al.: Ann. Intern. Med. **65**:1101, 1966 (rheumatoid arthritis).

Sbarbaro, J. L., Jr., and Francis, K. C.: J.A.M.A. **178**:706, 1961 (eosinophilic granuloma of bone).

Snapper, I., and Kahn, A. I.: Seminars Hemat. **1**:87, 1964 (multiple myeloma).

Spencer, H., and Whimster, I. W.: J. Path. Bact. **62**:411, 1950 (tumors of tendon sheaths).

Urist, M. E., and Johnson, R. W., Jr.: J. Bone Joint Surg. **25**:375, 1943 (healing of fractures).

CHAPTER 25—THE NERVOUS SYSTEM

Anderson, M. S.: Cancer **19**:585, 1966 (myxopapillary ependymoma).

Blackwood, W., McMenemey, W. H., Meyer, A., Norman, R. M., and Russell, D. S.: Greenfield's neuropathology, ed. 2, London, 1963, Edward Arnold (Publishers) Ltd.

Burstein, S. D., Kernohan, J. W., and Uihlein, A.: Cancer **16**:289, 1963 (reticulum cell sarcoma of brain).

Christoferson, L. A., et al.: J.A.M.A. **178**:280, 1961 (Lindau's disease).

Crawford, T.: J. Clin. Path. **7**:1, 1954 (acute hemorrhagic leukoencephalitis).

Crozier, R. E., and Ainley, A. B.: New Eng. J. Med. **252**:83, 1955 (Guillain-Barré syndrome).

Crue, B. L.: Medulloblastoma, Springfield, Ill., 1958, Charles C Thomas, Publisher.

Kernohan, J. W., and Sayre, C. P.: Atlas of tumor pathology, sect. **X**., fasc. 35 and 37, Tumors of the central nervous system, Washington, D. C., 1952, Armed Forces Institute of Pathology.

Kepes, J., and Kernohan, J. W.: Cancer **12**:364, 1959 (meningiomas).

Pearce, G. W., and Walton, J. N.: J. Path. Bact. **83**:535, 1962 (progressive muscular dystrophy).

Russell, D. S., and Rubinstein, L. J.: The pathology of tumors of the nervous system, London, 1959, Edward Arnold (Publishers) Ltd.

Scotti, T. M.: Arch. Path. **63**:91, 1957 (plantar digital neuroma—Morton's toe).

Young, J. Z.: Physiol. Rev. **22**:318, 1942 (repair of nervous tissue).

Index

A